HUMAN MEDICAL THERMOGRAPHY

Want to incorporate medical infrared imaging into your practice but can't find a book that explains how to do it? Well, this book is for you! Complete, practical instructions are provided on imager choice and care as well as the physical needs of a thermography service from the imaging room layout to the computer requirements. How to acquire, interpret, and report a thermal examination is covered in detail. Fully illustrated with both normal and abnormal images, *Human Medical Thermography* provides practitioners of all types with the knowledge to design and operate a scientifically based thermography practice.

Key Features

- Shows how to select the best thermal imager for your clinical practice, care for it, and use it correctly.
- Explains how to take medical quality thermal images and scale them for maximum visual effect using the guidelines detailed in this book.
- Details myriad ways that thermography can aid in medical diagnosis and improve surgical outcomes.

AF826951

HUMAN MEDICAL THERMOGRAPHY

James Stewart Campbell, EE, MD
M. Nathaniel Mead, MSc

CRC Press
Taylor & Francis Group
Boca Raton London New York

CRC Press is an imprint of the
Taylor & Francis Group, an **informa** business

First edition published 2023
by CRC Press
6000 Broken Sound Parkway NW, Suite 300, Boca Raton, FL 33487-2742
and by CRC Press

4 Park Square, Milton Park, Abingdon, Oxon, OX14 4RN

CRC Press is an imprint of Taylor & Francis Group, LLC

ISBN: 9781032251417 (hbk)
ISBN: 9781032251400 (pbk)
ISBN: 9781003281764 (ebk)

DOI: 10.1201/9781003281764

Typeset in Warnock Pro
by KnowledgeWorks Global Ltd.

Dedicated to Ms. Joyce B. Cary, President of Integrative Life Solutions, Inc., who facilitated the practice of medical thermography that made this book possible.

CONTENTS

ABOUT THE AUTHORS

James Stewart Campbell, EE, MD. Interested in electronics from a young age, Dr. James Stewart Campbell received his bachelor's degree in Electrical Engineering from Lehigh University in 1966 and then went on to study medicine at the Albany Medical College in Albany, NY, receiving his MD degree in 1970. After completing a straight-surgical internship at the University of Washington, he helped found The Country Doctor Clinic in Seattle and practiced general medicine there until 1975.

In 1976, Dr. Campbell settled in Hayesville, North Carolina, where he founded the non-profit Mountain Peoples' Clinic and had a successful practice of general medicine. He also taught electronics at Tri-County Community College in Murphy, NC.

Dr. Campbell took a leave from clinical medicine in 1986 to work in biomedical engineering, specializing in biological-to-electronic interfacing. His design projects have included air plethysmography, non-invasive blood pressure devices, ultrasound imaging and flowmeters, photo-plethysmography, fluorescence microscopy, bio-impedance, bio-acoustics, intra-cardiac sensor-stimulators, and implantable neural probe systems.

In 2010, realizing that thermal signatures were clinically important to detect certain diseases, Dr. Campbell started a thermography service for Integrative Life Solutions, Inc., in Clemmons, NC. Over the next 7 years, the practice became a successful provider of general and breast thermography. After retiring from medical practice in 2017, he assembled the wealth of objective thermal data from the service into a large spreadsheet derived from over 1000 imaging sessions. These thermal images and numerical data, along with much additional research and writing by his co-author, form the foundation of this book.

Dr. Campbell lives in Pfafftown, North Carolina. He is a Life Senior Member of the Institute of Electrical and Electronics Engineers (IEEE) and a Senior Member of the American Academy of Thermology (AAT).

Mark Nathaniel Mead, MSc, earned his master's degree in Nutritional Epidemiology from the UNC Gillings School of Global Public Health. Through his work as a medical-scientific writer, he has over 40 scientific articles listed on PubMed, including papers published in the *International Journal of Cancer, Journal of the National Cancer Institute, Integrative Cancer Therapies, Environmental Health Perspectives,* and *Cancer Treatment Reviews.* In addition to 9 years as a contributing editor to *Natural Health* magazine, Mead served for 20 years as an editorial board member for *Integrative Cancer Therapies* (Sage Publications) and as a research associate for the Block Center for Integrative Cancer Treatment in Skokie, IL. He underwent clinical training in thermography under his co-author and has lectured at the annual scientific session of the American Academy of Thermology.

INTRODUCTION TO HUMAN MEDICAL THERMOGRAPHY

The human body generates heat – a byproduct of metabolism – and must dissipate it to regulate internal body temperature. The majority of metabolic heat is dispersed into the environment by the skin surface. When viewed through a thermal imager, the human body stands out strongly against cooler backgrounds. Variations, patterns, and differences in skin temperature can be readily visualized. The result is a thermogram, a graphic rendering of the pattern of infrared emissions either in color or shades of gray showing the temperature distribution over the body's surface. Actual surface temperatures may be measured on the image, providing a view of the body's thermal pattern that is both quantitative (numerical) and qualitative (visual).

Quantitative thermography involves the analysis of the actual temperature data of thermograms – the "science of thermography." Qualitative thermography – the "art of thermography" – involves properly adjusting the image thermal span to maximize the information presented to the human visual system. In addition, the art of thermography includes selecting the proper equilibration time, imaging protocol, and patient positioning to display the thermal findings. Though certain procedures such as breast thermography are becoming routine, general thermography examinations may be quite varied.

With the ability to display thermal changes, asymmetries, inflammation, and anomalies, infrared imaging provides valid information to augment medical diagnosis and research. Yet thermography may be the most misunderstood and undervalued of all medical imaging technologies. Just as radiologists at first rejected ultrasound imaging fifty years ago, so too they officially dismiss medical thermography today. This misunderstanding has been largely due to the inferior infrared scanners and substandard methodology of yore; however, much has changed in infrared imaging over the past 25 years. No longer can thermography be regarded as an "alternative" or of questionable medical value. Numerous peer-reviewed studies have demonstrated its efficacy in a diverse range of conditions; practitioners around the world today are using thermography to screen, detect, and monitor diseases.

In 1994, military infrared imager integrated circuits were declassified and released for civilian use. By 2000, temperature-calibrated, microbolometer-based integrated circuits coupled with microprocessors and full-color digital display systems allowed practitioners to visualize a thermographic image in exquisite detail, detecting features and patterns of disease and dysfunction that were previously hidden from view. The older thermal scanner technology quickly became obsolete. Today's infrared imagers can detect minute variations in 10-µm (thermal) radiation and record actual surface temperatures over large areas of the body in one image. This book has been written to demonstrate the capabilities of these new 21st-century thermal imagers.

Human Medical Thermography was written with three primary objectives in mind: (1) to illuminate the physics, anatomy, physiology, pathology, and clinical application of thermal imaging; (2) to advance the use of thermal imaging by guiding practitioners in setting up a scientific thermography service to take, format, and interpret the images; and (3) to promote an evidence-based approach by reviewing some of the thermography's benefits for both clinical medicine and laboratory research.

As a *physiological* imaging method, the clinical use of thermography requires a basic understanding of the mechanisms of temperature distribution on the body surface, as well as how and pattern variations might relate to disease. Small differences in skin temperature can have important medical implications, particularly in the detection of circulatory, inflammatory, neurological, and malignant diseases.

The success of clinical thermography depends on its proper use, requiring a clear understanding of thermal physics, imager operation, patient preparation, and the imaging environment. *Human Medical Thermography* devotes considerable attention to imager choice, care, calibration, proper imaging technique, image scaling, and thermogram interpretation. The book highlights simple ways to choose, check, and operate a modern thermal imager. Using software to best visualize and interpret the images and generate professional reports is also covered.

In recent years, thermographic breast cancer screening has garnered renewed interest due to its superior sensitivity when compared to digital mammography. This superior sensitivity is a direct result of modern imagers and preparation protocols. In the 1970s, breast thermography was declared to be inferior to mammography based on a study that used thermal scanners with poor spatial and thermal resolution. The vastly improved qualitative and quantitative thermal findings in breast cancer patients using modern imagers suggest that a repeat of that study is now warranted.

General Thermography, sometimes known as "full-body" thermography, is useful in the detection and follow-up of numerous disease states. The range of possible topics is so broad that it requires two chapters to cover. Chapter 10 explores the general thermal appearance of common conditions and diseases addressed in a head-to-foot order. Thermal artifacts and scams are also discussed. Chapter 11 covers the use of thermography by various medical and surgical specialties; orthopedics, rheumatology, ophthalmology, neurology, vascular, and surgical specialties are featured in detail.

The terminology of thermography has changed over the years. Given the much improved resolution of modern thermographic devices, this book will use the term *imagers* to denote those systems that employ lenses that focus infrared light onto a monolithic, two-dimensional array of temperature-sensing elements. Older electromechanical devices relying on moving mirrors to direct the infrared rays onto a thermal detector will be referred to as *scanners*. Even though these older scanners with their inferior spatial and temperature display resolution are no longer clinically useful, most thermography research before 2000 was performed with those devices. The term *camera* is reserved here for the visual-band cameras that are often incorporated into a modern thermal imager.

When determining the *absolute* temperature of a remote surface, even a modern digital imaging system has a wide offset error band. Without a known temperature reference in the image, a typical microbolometer imager can be off by ±2.0°C (3.6°F) and still be within the specifications for the device. Unfortunately, many research papers offer no information on temperature calibration of the imagers or scanners used for a particular study, and many accept the absolute surface temperatures reported by a single instrument as accurate. As a consequence, many of the absolute temperature measurements quoted in this book may vary considerably, reflecting the uncalibrated data obtained in the respective studies. *Quantitative* (numerical) temperature

DOI: 10.1201/9781003281764-1

measurements are valid only if the imager's offset and gain are corrected using two or more black-body references.

Besides calibrated thermal imagers, the practice of human thermography depends on the preparation of the patient and the environment of the thermography room. To address these important aspects, *Human Medical Thermography* explains the physiological basis of thermal equilibration and the imaging environment. Without knowledge of patient preparation and imaging environment – set and setting – interpretation of thermal images is fraught with error.

The advent of high-resolution, full-color digital display devices has revolutionized the visual appearance of thermograms. The old scanner FAX and analog displays showed a very limited number of color or greyscale values, obliterating the fine details of the image. Modern color displays have greatly improved the *qualitative* (visual) interpretation of infrared images, allowing the thermographer to view body surface temperatures much as a radiologist views a properly exposed X-ray. The range of surface temperatures encountered is converted to a smooth greyscale or spectral color image that best matches the capabilities of the human eye.

Most of the thermal images presented in this book were acquired in the course of seven years of the first author's general thermography practice, which used validated patient preparation protocols, a temperature-regulated thermography room, industrial-quality thermal imagers, and full-color image displays. All images obtained from that practice include the thermographer's initials "JSCMD" for identification (an artist always signs a completed work). Images from other sources are fully referenced and identified. Observers may note the different and often poorly-scaled visual formatting of those other images. This is due to the infrared-to-visual scaling techniques utilized by the thermographers.

As a non-contact and non-invasive imaging method, thermography lends itself to "N = 1" experiments to directly observe the thermal effects of various maneuvers, protocols, or medications. Several examples of N = 1 experiments appear in this book, some of which confirm findings in the scientific literature and some which do not. Thermographers and students are encouraged to serve as the "normals" and perform suitable N = 1 experiments. In addition, students, technicians, and thermographers alike should personally undergo thermographic exams, including any challenge tests, in order to appreciate and respect the patients' experience. A thermologist who can empathize with the patient is better able to reduce any unnecessary stress associated with a thermographic exam.

Human Medical Thermography lays the groundwork for the use of thermal imaging based on established physics and physiology to visualize diseases not readily detected or monitored by other methods. As thermal imaging is relatively inexpensive, compact, portable, involves no ionizing radiation, and requires little electric power, it seems inevitable that medical practices will adopt thermography for disease detection and screening. Because thermal images are easily transmitted even under low-bandwidth conditions, they may eventually be processed at computer centers using Artificial Intelligence (AI) algorithms that return a probability-rated differential diagnosis list to the front-line practitioner within minutes.

Human Medical Thermography represents the culmination of decades of study and progress in the performance of infrared imaging equipment, standardization of technique, and clinical protocols for thermal imaging. Thanks to all the medical professionals, research scientists, and engineers who have contributed to this effort, the future of clinical thermography appears bright. May the field continue to evolve as an integral part of 21st-century medical practice.

James Stewart Campbell, EE, MD
M. Nathaniel Mead, MSc
December 2021

1

A HISTORY OF THERMOLOGY AND THERMOGRAPHY

The story of thermology – the scientific study of heat and its biomedical effects – is almost as old as medicine itself. Writings on papyrus dating back to 2600 BC suggest that ancient Egyptians were aware of the relationship between body heat, health, and healing.[1] By 400 BC, they had recognized the diagnostic value of variations in temperature over different body parts and compared the temperatures of different organs as indicators of underlying disorder; "In whatever part of the body excess of heat or cold is felt, the disease is there to be discovered."[2] Fever was deemed to be a manifestation of not just heat alone, but excesses of various qualities or "humors." "Pains are also the result of cold or heat, either in excess or reversely."[3]

Hippocrates devised a simple yet effective method for assessing thermal changes: covering the body with a thin coating of wet mud and observing the patterns rendered by different rates of mud drying over the surface of the body. If the mud on one area of skin dried rapidly while all other areas remained moist, an underlying "tumor" was suspected. The observed asymmetries and incongruities in temperature distribution were then used to inform the diagnosis and prognosis of disease, as discussed in Hippocrates's *Book of Prognostics.* Hippocrates is also credited with describing an early two-dimensional image of skin temperature by using a moist linen cloth, covering an area of skin to produce an impression of surface temperatures via the changes in cloth color.[4] These appear to be among the earliest explorations of what would later become the science of medical thermology.

Six hundred years later, renowned Greek philosopher-physician Aelius Galen proposed that bodily heat is generated internally by the heart and circulatory system. Innate heat, also called vital or natural heat, was a term that Galen and other physicians of his day used when referring to heat produced within the body. In his treatise titled *On the Usefulness of the Parts of the Body,* Galen wrote, "The heart is, as it were, the hearthstone and source of the innate heat by which the animal is governed."[5] Galen also spoke of the interplay or feedback between the sensory and motor nerves, now known to be central to the mechanism of thermoregulation.[6]

The association between fever (elevated body temperature) and disease was recognized by physicians throughout antiquity. In the first century A.D., the Roman encyclopaedist Aulus Cornelius Celsus (not to be confused with Anders Celsius, 1701–1744, developer of the Celsius temperature scale) laid out detailed descriptions of the symptoms and different varieties of fever, and eventually designated four classical signs of inflammation: *calor* (heat), *dolor* (pain), *rubor* (redness), and *tumor* (swelling). These cardinal signs continue to be part of today's medical vernacular. Without thermometers, the method of sensing bodily heat in those early explorations of thermology was quite basic. Most often, temperature changes were detected by the ability of the physician or healer to sense those changes using his or her hands.

Up to this point, *temperature* had been considered as a general expression of hot or cold, not in terms of objective measurements. The earliest recorded investigations into thermometry have been credited to Hero of Alexandria (10–70 AD). Hero's musings on the subject of pneumatics (the branch of physics concerned with the mechanical properties of gases) introduced the concept that a gas (or liquid) expands when warmed and contracts when cooled. His writings helped usher in a wave of experimentation that led to the invention of the first crude "air thermometer," possibly by Galileo Galilei in 1592. Galileo referred to the device as a *thermoscope.* The instrument consisted of an upright tube with a closed bulb at one end, partially filled with air, and resting in a container of water at the open end of the tube. Using temperature changes to expand or contract the entrapped air in the bulb, the column of water moved down or up the tube. Since both temperature and atmospheric pressure affected the expansion and contraction of the air inside the bulb, the device could have been named a *barothermoscope*; however, the slow and relatively minor influence of barometric pressure was not recognized until the invention of the barometer in 1643.[7]

The first thermoscopes were probably little more than playthings or objects of curiosity. This perception would change abruptly when the toy thermoscopes were fashioned with numerical scales, reflecting the 17th-century trend toward quantification of natural phenomena. In 1611, Galileo's physician-engineer friend, Santorio Santorio, placed the first such scale on a thermoscope, thus creating a very crude clinical thermometer.[8] The accuracy of the instrument must have been rather poor, due to in part to the variability of measurements arising from changing barometric pressures as well as a lack of any standardized scales for quantification. Although the bulb portion of the instrument could have been inserted into a patient's mouth for taking a temperature, it is not likely that the reading would have meant anything of clinical significance.

By the 1650s, enclosed liquid-in-a-glass thermometers were being fashioned by glassblowers in Italy. Ferdinand II, the Grand Duke of Tuscany, is credited with inventing the first hermetically sealed thermometer in 1654, using alcohol as the liquid. Having a sealed tube improved the precision of temperature measurement by eliminating the influence of barometric pressure on the thermometric readings. The thermometers could be inserted into the mouth without concern for fluid leaking out. These early clinical thermometers were highly inaccurate, however, due to a lack of standard calibration.

In 1665, Robert Boyle and Christian Huygens proposed independently that thermometers could be calibrated effectively from a single fixed point.[9] Their work laid the foundation for the development of the mercury thermometer with a standardized scale, invented by Daniel Gabriel Fahrenheit in 1714. This was followed in 1742 by the Celsius scale, conceived by Anders Celsius. The use of these scales enabled the recording of temperature in an accurate and consistent fashion. As the international standard, the Celsius scale presents 100 degrees between the freezing point (0°C, 32°F) and boiling point (100°C, 212°F) of pure water at sea level air pressure.

Public health crises in 19th century Europe provided a strong impetus for further developments in clinical thermometry. The most prevalent diseases of the day were smallpox, typhus, enteric fever, and tuberculosis, with cholera making its debut in the early 1800s. The deadliest of these maladies was smallpox, killing an estimated 400,000 Europeans each year and afflicting commoners and royalty alike.[10] All of these diseases included fever as a primary symptom, hence the umbrella term "fever diseases." In 1802, the London Fever Hospital was established to help accommodate Londoners who were inflicted by infectious disease. A second, larger fever hospital

DOI: 10.1201/9781003281764-2

was established in 1848. These hospitals served as the main facilities for patients with smallpox and other infections.[11]

Amidst all the fear and suffering engendered by these deadly epidemics, German medical professor Carl Wunderlich made the first comprehensive effort to document diagnostic findings with regard to fever. In 1871, Wunderlich began a systematic investigation of clinical thermometry by recording the progression of temperature changes in sick people diagnosed with rheumatic fever and other fever diseases. His thermometers were 12 inches (30.5 cm) long; Axillary temperature measurements took 20 minutes due to a large amount of mercury that had to be heated to body temperature. By charting the daily progress of all of his patients twice a day, he was able to construct a series of temperature graphs for each patient (Figure 1.1). He collected well over a million axillary temperatures. In his treatise, *On the Temperature in Diseases,* he advocates the routine measurement of body temperature and placing temperature charts in hospitals, thus providing a graphic record for tracking each patient.[12] Unfortunately, Wunderlich's published reports offered nothing more than snapshot glimpses of his raw data and neglected to describe his methods of data analysis.[13]

Wunderlich concluded that the mean healthy human body temperature was 37°C (98.6°F) and that 38°C (100.4°F) was the upper limit of normal, i.e., the threshold for a fever. (In principle, a fever is any elevation in body temperature above the normal temperature; in Wunderlich's time, however, the patient was not considered to have a clinically significant fever until the temperature exceeded 38°C.) Better controlled, statistically based research published in 1992 established that average human temperature is actually 36.8°C (98.2°F). A study of human body temperatures over the past 157 years has shown a steady decrease of 0.03°C (0.054°F) per decade, additionally finding that body temperature decreases 0.27°C (0.49°F) from age 40 to age 75.[15] It is now known that the normal body temperature fluctuates by about 1°C (1.8°F) in the same person at different times of the day and varies from person to person.[16] To address this diurnal temperature variation, the 38°C (100.4°F) fever mark has been replaced with fever thresholds based on the time of day.[17]

Wunderlich's study of body temperature may be viewed as a landmark contribution to medical progress because it helped establish several key precepts of clinical thermometry. First, fever is only a sign of disease, not the disease process itself. Second, healthy individuals have an almost identical temperature, regardless of age, race, physical condition, place, and circumstance; and this provides a baseline for determining what constitutes a normal body temperature. Third, deviations from the normal temperature can and should be measured in sick persons, and there may be considerable variation of temperature depending on the severity of the disease. With the introduction of clinical thermometers, allopathic physicians in Europe and America began to measure body temperature as a matter of clinical routine; it later became a *vital sign* along with heart rate, respiration rate, body weight, and blood pressure.

Thermometers were obviously a practical milestone in this regard, but only in terms of measuring internal body temperature. Thermometers were neither useful nor practical for depicting temperature variations of the body surface or over any particular region of the body. The key to accomplishing that feat would have to come from capturing the body's infrared emissions and then converting them into temperature readings.

The emergence of infrared imaging

Radiative heat dissipation was among the many areas of interest for Sir Isaac Newton in the late 1600s. Newton's law of cooling (1701) states that the rate of heat loss of a body is proportional to the difference in temperatures between the body and its surroundings. Two qualifying conditions were later tagged on to this cooling law. First, in the case of heat transfer via thermal radiation, the law holds only for small temperature differences. Second, the nature of heat transfer must remain the same, i.e., the heat transfer coefficient mediating heat losses and temperature differences must remain constant, a condition best met by conductive heat transfer. Newton's law of cooling is applied in engineering to describe how the temperature of an object or material changes as a function of time.[18] In the forensic sciences, the law has been used to help estimate the time since death occurred.[19]

Newton's law of cooling does not apply to live warm-blooded organisms, however, due to the dynamics of internally generated heat dissipation. Instead, a mammal's mechanisms of temperature regulation are best modeled by the hypothetical construct that has been called the "Newtonian animal."[20] Newton's law of

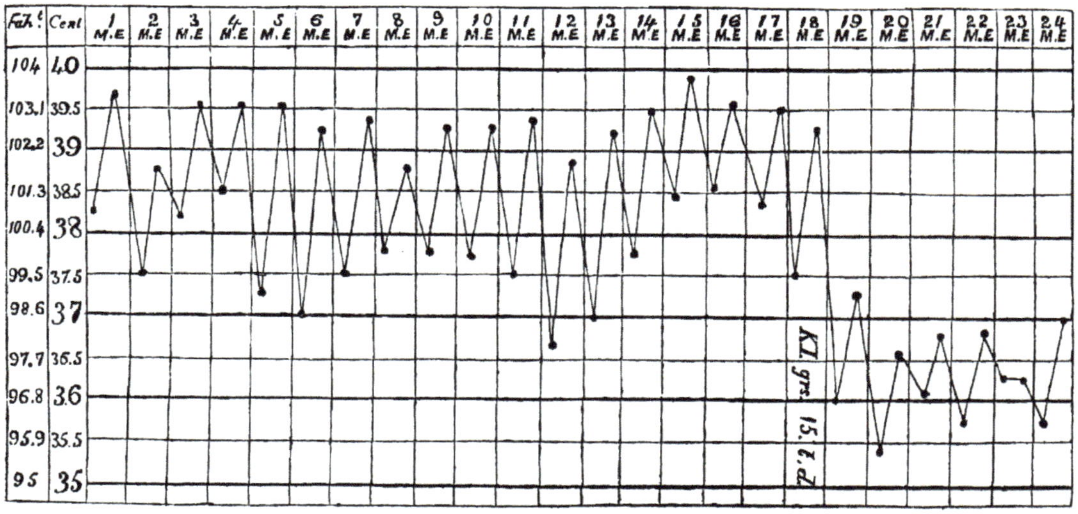

FIGURE 1.1 A graph of temperatures from a patient with syphilitic fever by Dr. Wunderlich. Administration of potassium iodide, a common remedy at that time, reduced the fever.[14]

cooling only applies to a warm body *without* internal heating and surrounded by a cooler environment.[21] This is not consistent with the dynamic reality of homeothermic organisms, which are subject to physiologic, metabolic, and circadian variations in heat output due to variations in blood circulation from the warm core to the body surface.

The phenomenon known as infrared radiation was first identified by Sir William Herschel. In the year 1800, Herschel presented his research findings on infrared with an elegant experiment: splitting sunlight by passing it through a glass prism, then measuring the amount of heat associated with each color of the spectrum using thermometers with blackened bulbs to better absorb the rays (Figure 1.2). Moving from the violet to the red part of the spectrum, Herschel noted a steady increase in temperature. Surprisingly, the highest temperature was just beyond the visible red. This region of the electromagnetic spectrum is now called the *infrared*, which means "below the red." What Hershel actually detected was what we now call near-infrared (NIR) radiation, as the longer wavelength mid-infrared (MIR) detected in human thermography would not have passed through his glass prisms. Hershel's discovery of infrared radiation remains a remarkable achievement. Hershel's experiments also indicated that, under the right conditions, the rays were reflected, refracted, absorbed, and transmitted just like visible light.[23]

In the first three decades following Herschel's discovery, it was confirmed that heat radiation obeyed the basic laws of optics. There was no effective way to visualize this radiation, however, and experimenters were handicapped by the ordinary bulb thermometer. The body's surface temperature could not be reliably measured by any device placed in direct contact with the skin. This was because the skin has a relatively low heat capacity and poor lateral heat conductance, thus its temperature is likely to be altered by contact with a cooler or warmer object. Such contact also alters the temperature of the skin by affecting the local thermosensors and eliciting a series of reflexes in the local or systemic autonomic nervous system, causing dilation or constriction of skin vasculature. Due to these limitations of contact thermometry, it can be said: "The only way the surface temperature of skin can be measured without contact is by remotely sensing the infrared blackbody radiation emitted by it."[24]

Development of sensitive and accurate contact-free detectors of the infrared radiation emitted by the body was needed. The first breakthrough came from the discovery of the thermoelectric effect by Thomas Johann Seebeck in 1821. Seebeck showed that a small electric *current* will flow between different conductive materials (i.e., a closed circuit of two dissimilar metallic conductors) if the two junctions are kept at different temperatures. This discovery helped bring about the discovery of the *thermocouple* in 1829 by the Italian physicist Leopoldo Nobili. The thermocouple is a temperature sensor formed by the electrical junction of two dissimilar metals, which generates a temperature-dependent *voltage*. Any change in this voltage is directly proportional to the

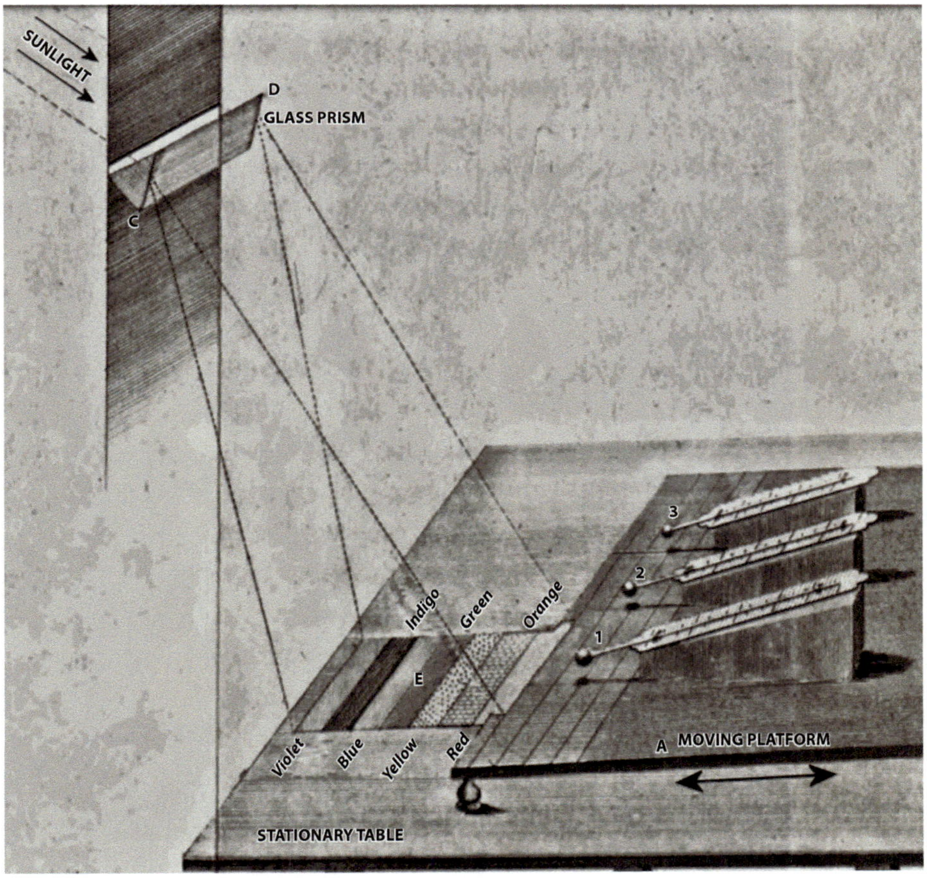

FIGURE 1.2 William Herschel's experimental setup that detected invisible infrared rays. The platform (a) was moved, so the bulb of thermometer #1 measured the heat of various colors from sunlight. The other two thermometers acted as controls.[22]

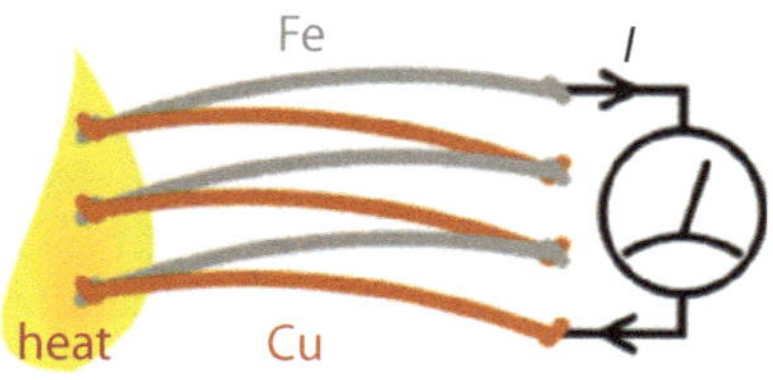

FIGURE 1.3 The Seebeck current (i) in a thermopile made from iron and copper wires. Wires made of other dissimilar metals will also produce a Seebeck current. If this current is interrupted, it will develop a voltage proportional to the temperature difference between the hot and cold junctions.[25]

temperature of the junction as long as the reference end of the two conductors is held at a fixed reference temperature.

The thermocouple was an improved electrical thermometer, essentially a way to measure the temperature difference between the sensing and reference junctions. It would evolve further when Macedonia Melloni made the first *thermopile* by linking several bismuth-copper thermocouples in a series, thus generating a higher measurable output voltage (Figure 1.3). The output voltage of such a structure increases linearly with the number of thermocouples connected in series and with the temperature difference between the junctions. This relationship is quite stable. Common non-contact thermometers available today utilize this same thermopile technology, albeit in integrated circuit form (Figure 1.4). The instruments focus incoming radiation onto the sensing junctions, heating or cooling them relative to the laterally placed reference junctions which are shaded from the incoming rays.

After Sir William Herschel's death in 1840, his son, Sir John Frederick William Herschel, helped bring about the birth of thermography, generating the first-ever infrared image. He accomplished this feat by *evaporography,* a complicated and exacting process that focused a scene through a salt-crystal lens onto an oily suspension in alcohol for 10 seconds. This resulted in a crude yet visible thermal image (Figure 1.5).[27] Sir John named this image a *fixed thermograph* and later called it a *thermogram.* Thus, the earliest mid-infrared thermograms pre-dated electronic infrared imaging devices and capitalized on thermally sensitive rates of evaporation of oil versus water.

The first real breakthrough in electronic detection of thermal radiation came with the invention of the *bolometer* by Samuel Pierpont Langley in 1878. This detector measured electromagnetic radiation by thermally induced changes in resistance of an electrical conductor and was sensitive to differences in temperature of 0.00001°C at the detector. Over the next 20 years, Langley continued to make modifications in his bolometer to improve its performance. He reported that his final iteration of the device was also at least 400 times more sensitive than his first prototype.[29]

Other novel infrared systems were developed during World War I (1914–1918). Infrared detectors have been indispensable for night warfare since then, to help detect enemy movements and to locate wounded personnel under cover of darkness. Infrared methods could distinguish between unconscious and dead casualties by examining the surface temperature of the body from a distance. Other important WWI developments included remote temperature sensing and infrared "flying torpedo" guidance using multiple thermosensors.

Between 1900 and 1920, multiple patents were issued for infrared inventions with applications for detecting artillery, aircraft,

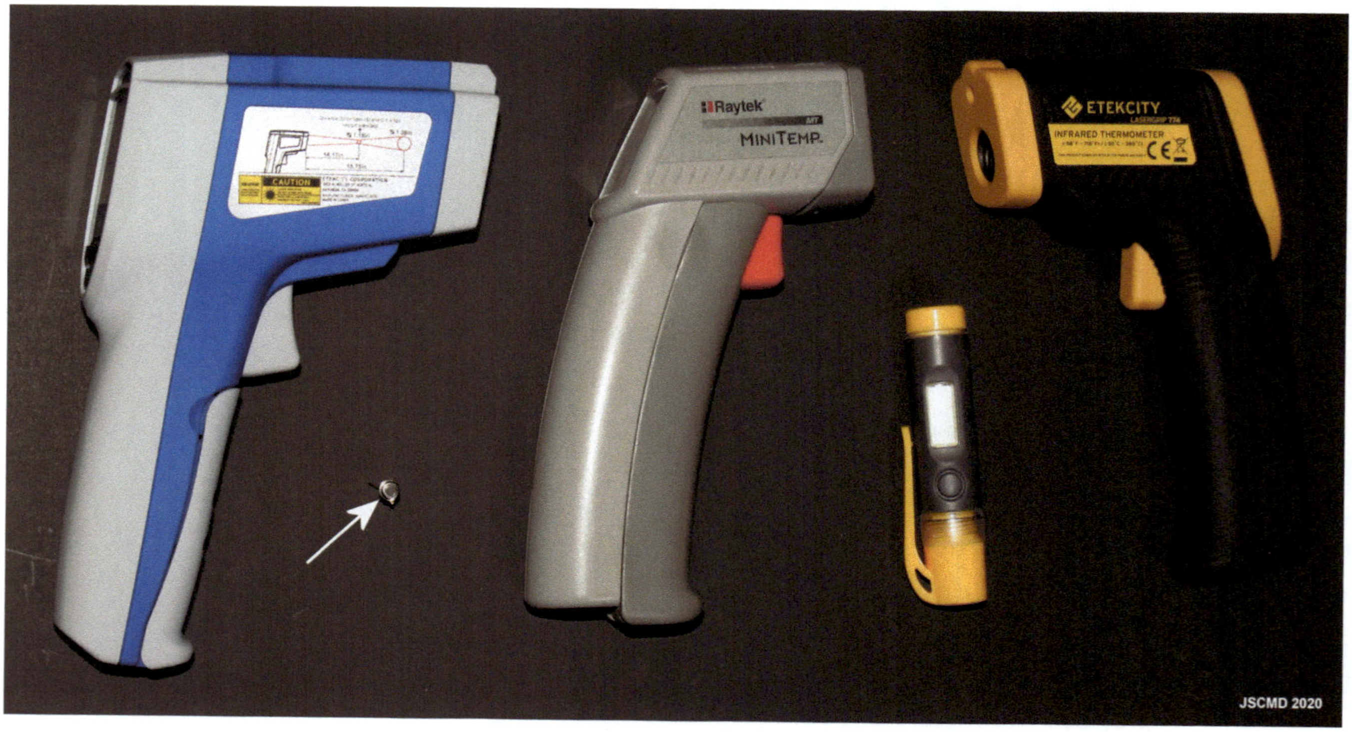

FIGURE 1.4 Modern infrared non-contact thermometers like these four devices use thermopile sensors such as the hermetically sealed integrated circuit thermopile in its windowed metal case (arrow). The tiny window is not glass but a filter that only admits mid-infrared rays longer than 5 µm.[26] Infrared lenses or parabolic mirrors inside the thermometers focus the rays onto the thermopile chip.

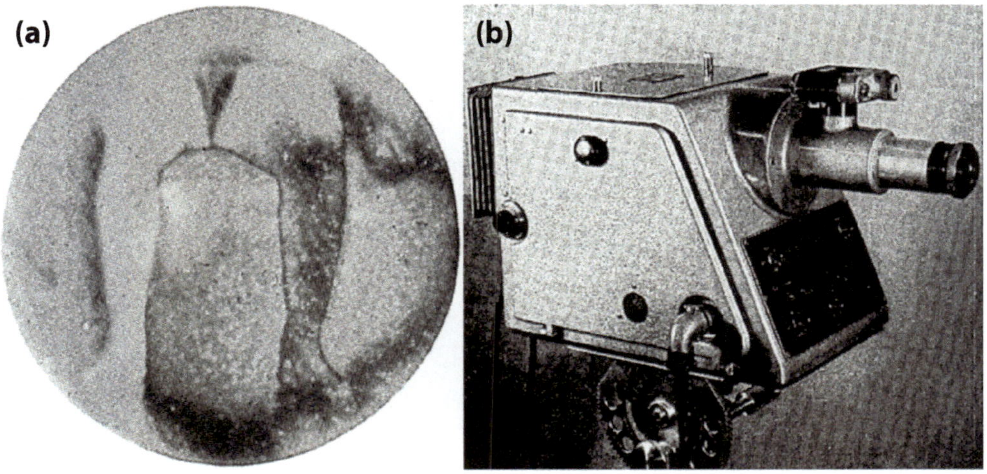

FIGURE 1.5 (a) Evaporogram of a sitting man with left leg phlebitis. (b) A model KR-1 evaporograph instrument circa 1962.[28]

ships, and even icebergs.[30] Shortly after the 1912 tragedy of the Titanic, a device was patented called the "Infrared Eye" which could detect the presence of icebergs and ships by using a curved mirror to focus mid-infrared rays onto a Nobili thermopile/Langley bolometer.[31] In 1928 the field of Human Thermography began when Professor Marius Czerny documented the first infrared image of a human subject.[32] These were the first advanced applications of infrared technology for civilian purposes.

The next important innovation was a photoconducting infrared detector invented by Theodore Case in 1917. The detector utilized thallium sulfide (Tl_2S), which results in a faster response than the other thermal detectors available at that time. The signal generated by Tl_2S comes from direct interaction with photons instead of being sensitive to the increase in temperature caused by the incident radiation. These devices exhibit a linear decrease in electrical resistance when illuminated with infrared radiation from 1.0 to 4.8 μm; for operation, however, they require cooling to liquid nitrogen temperatures.[33] Although photoconducting detectors have undergone extensive improvements since the 1940s, microbolometers are favored in today's high-resolution infrared imagers for medicine because they are generally sensitive to the 10 μm infrared wavelength emitted at body temperatures and can also operate at room temperature.

The medical use of infrared thermography did not begin until 1952 when German physician Ernst Schwamm and physicist Jobst Reeh patented an infrared bolometer for serial thermal measurements of defined regions of the skin for diagnostic purposes.[34] In 1954, Schwamm and Reeh founded the first medical society for thermography, still active today as ThermoMed – International Society of Thermography and Thermology – established 1954, thereby making it the oldest organization with a focus on medical thermography.[35]

The first electronic sensor for infrared imaging, developed in the early 1940s, was made from indium antimonide (InSb) and mounted at the base of a small Dewar vessel to allow cooling with liquid nitrogen. InSb is a photovoltaic substance that generates an electric current when illuminated by infrared radiation. Thermal scans using this sensor were initially taken at the Royal National Hospital for Rheumatic Diseases in Bath, England (now the United Kingdom) in 1959. The prototype scanner, known as the Pyroscan, could assess the heat from arthritic joints (Figure 1.6). By today's standards, these thermal scanners were rather crude and difficult to interpret due to low spatial resolution and the ability to display only a few values of grey.

Although the single thermal detector in the Pyroscan Mark II was accurate to 0.1°C (0.18°F), the Cathode Ray Tube or FAX display devices in these older machines severely limited the thermal

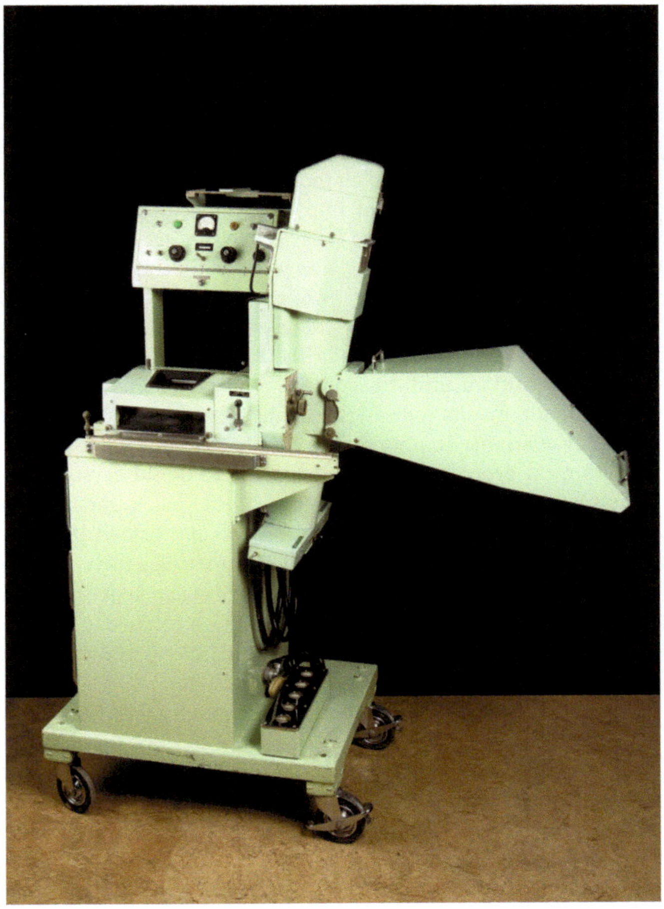

FIGURE 1.6 The mark II-D "Pyroscan" medical thermographic scanner by Smiths Industries Ltd, London, England 1960. The apparatus on the right holds a mirror for scanning horizontal areas. The mirror unit could be removed to scan upright subjects.[36]

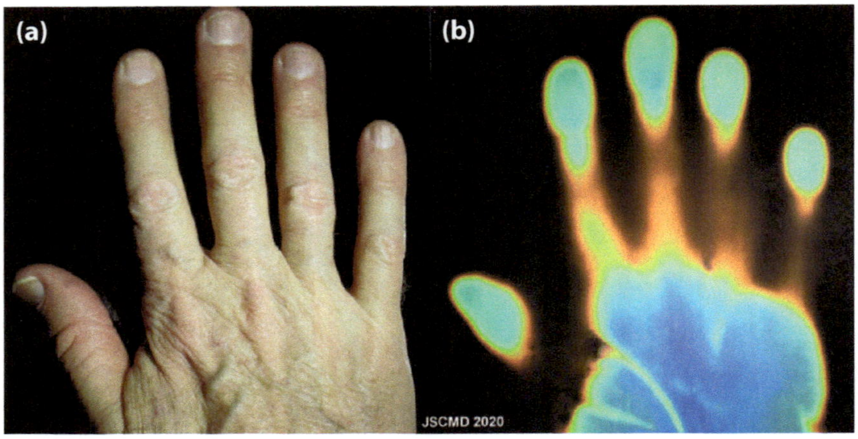

FIGURE 1.7 A demonstration of liquid-crystal thermal display technology. (a) The right hand is pressed against a black, temperature-sensitive liquid-crystal sheet on an insulated mat. (b) The thermal impression as captured by the cholesteric sheet. Blue indicates warm, and orange is cooler. Uniform physical contact with the sheet is difficult to control, leading to major artifacts on surfaces such as the breasts, face, hands, and feet.

resolution visible to the human eye to between 7 and 22 shades of grey. Over a typical 10°C temperature span, this is equivalent to a visible step size ranging from 0.45 to 1.4°C (0.8–2.5°F). These large steps obliterated any fine thermal details in the image. In addition, significant loss of spatial resolution was caused by wobble or timing inaccuracy in the mechanical scanning system, plus the inevitable patient movement during the scan, which could take several minutes to complete.[37] This is why older infrared scanners, such as the Pyroscan (UK), Agema (Sweden), and Bales (USA) devices, could not display or record the fine details seen by today's microbolometer-array imaging technology.

Infrared imaging entered into U.S. medical practice in the late 1950s. Early studies used fairly crude *contact thermography*; liquid-crystal temperature sensors were pressed against the skin to indicate the local surface temperature pattern (Figure 1.7). Though these sheets of liquid cholesteric crystals were reusable and inexpensive, their thermal sensitivity declined steadily over time. In addition, uniform contact with curved body surfaces was difficult; results were highly subjective and not amenable to serial evaluations. To obtain better body contact for breast thermograms, a protocol was developed where liquid crystal paint was sprayed onto the patient after an initial black undercoat of paint was applied. The interpretation was performed by direct observation after a time period to allow the surface to dry and the temperature to stabilize. Permanent records were kept on 35 mm color slides.[38] Besides being of low resolution relative to modern infrared imagers, this method was difficult, messy, and time-consuming for both the patient and thermographer.

During the 1970s, liquid crystal thermography was supplanted by improved electronic infrared scanning devices that brought better-quality non-contact thermal imaging into clinical use. The images generated by thermographers of that era suggested applications in areas as diverse as the detection of breast cancer and neurological disorders. The introduction of mini-computers in the mid-70s paved the way for color displays and basic image analysis, as well as the first iterations of digital image and data storage systems. By the late 1970s, guidelines for clinical thermography were being proposed, and new training centers were graduating medical professionals who would strive to make thermography useful and available to the general public.

By the 1980s, qualitative (false-color) thermography was being combined with quantitative thermography as a matter of clinical routine. A new generation of smaller thermal scanning systems had been introduced in Europe and North America. Nevertheless, the infrared scanners that predominated up until the mid-1990s were grossly lacking in thermal display resolution and spatial accuracy. Even the best scanners of the 1980s were incapable of displaying the subtle changes in skin temperature needed to accurately identify and monitor changes in disease and disability.

The Agema AGA 782 Scanner was developed circa 1985 (Figure 1.8). This was a miniaturized, liquid nitrogen cooled, infrared thermal scanning system made by AGA (Sweden). Two small rotating prisms at right angles scanned the image vertically and horizontally. The original 782 scanner could display eight values of greyscale. Images were stored by photographing the monochrome cathode-ray display screen. Later models used a computer to produce eight artificial colors representing the corresponding gray shades in the original image. These were some of the earliest thermal images that could be stored as a digital file. Despite its limitations, the small size of the AGA scanner family helped usher in the era of portable thermal scanning for medical purposes.

Further progress in medical infrared imaging was hampered for many years during the "Cold War" (1947–1991). Modern microbolometer thermographic imaging chips were considered a military secret. These monolithic silicon image sensors were rugged, small, and capable of operating without liquid nitrogen cooling. They provided soldiers a convenient hand-held capability of detecting the enemy at night or through smoke, even in battlefield conditions. Thus, their development and use were classified until 1992, after which solid-state microbolometer imaging devices were released for civilian use, greatly elevating the visual and spatial resolution of medical infrared images to the level that is standard today.[40]

The emergence of breast thermography

Research showing that temperature irregularities on the body's surface are associated with various disease states spawned interest in recording infrared emissions in medical practice. Earlier

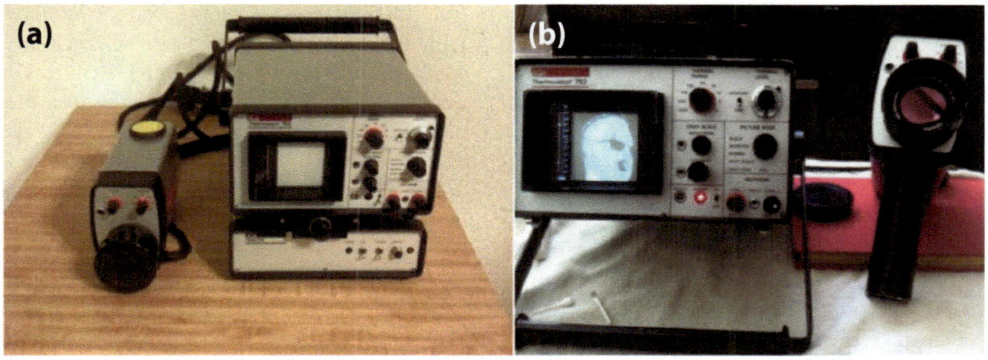

FIGURE 1.8 Two views of an Agema AGA Thermovision 782 infrared scanner with its portable greyscale cathode ray display. The yellow cap on the scanner covers the Dewar flask for the liquid nitrogen to cool the thermal sensor.[39]

work by American physiologist James Hardy had shown that the human skin, regardless of skin color or ethnicity, is a highly efficient radiator of infrared with an emissivity of 0.98, making it an almost perfect black body.[41] This point made thermography an attractive option for diagnosing, assessing, and monitoring a wide range of diseases; most of the initial focus was on arthritis and breast cancer.

The use of infrared imaging to assess breast disease began with the pioneering work of Canadian surgeon Ray Lawson. In 1955, using an Evaporograph imager, Lawson measured skin temperatures overlying a malignant breast tumor and observed that the readings were elevated when compared to those of a symmetrically identical area in the opposite breast (Figure 1.9).[42] He went on to note that benign tumors showed either smaller elevations or sagittal symmetry. Lawson referred to areas of markedly increased temperature as "hot spots," a term that has remained in vogue ever since.[43] In a 1956 paper, Lawson states: "It is fascinating to speculate on the diagnostic possibilities of a heat-sensitive imaging device capable of surveying breasts in much the same manner as mass screening by chest radiography is carried out for the early detection of tuberculosis."[44]

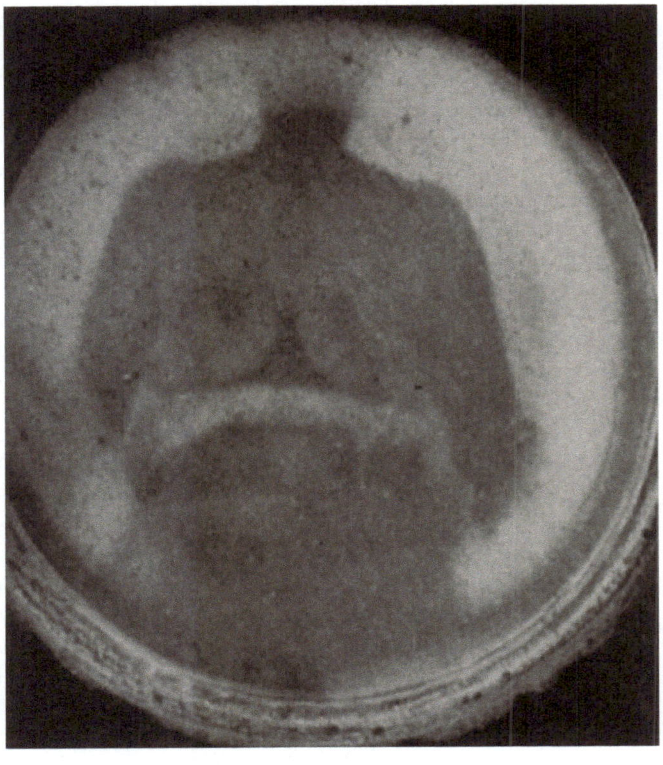

FIGURE 1.9 Infrared evaporograph of a woman with cancer of the right breast by Dr. Ray Lawson.[45]

Lawson also highlighted a rationale for infrared imaging of breast tumors: their increased growth rate when compared to that of the surrounding host tissue. "The malignant propensities ... can be readily detected by estimating temperature changes in the tumor or its immediate environment." Lawson later postulated that the increased infrared emissions may be due to an increased blood supply to the tumor.[46] For Lawson, a heat increase of 0.8–1.4°C (1.5–2.5°F) referred to either a metabolically active benign tumor or to an early-stage malignant tumor; infections and inflammatory conditions of the breast (e.g., mastitis) seemed to average 1.1°C (2°F) or lower.[47] However, as the Evaporograph can only detect thermal differences of about 1°C (1.8°F), these temperature delineations must be viewed as approximations.[48] Also, Dr. Lawson's hypothesis that the main cause of surface warmth associated with breast cancer is due to increased tumor metabolism has been shown to be erroneous. As a pioneer in the field, he was unaware of the importance of tumor-generated nitric oxide (NO) in arteriolar vasodilation, which was not discovered until after 1980.[49]

British surgeon Kenneth Lloyd Williams conducted a comparative study of the thermal contours of the skin between right and left breasts, charting a series of individual measurements. Remarkably, 54 out of 57 breast carcinomas showed a temperature elevation of 1–2°C (1.8–3.6°F). Equally impressive was the finding that 23 out of 24 cysts and benign adenomas were associated with a thermal difference of less than 1°C (1.8°F). These findings confirmed Lawson's hypothesis that temperatures were elevated on the skin surface corresponding to an underlying malignant tumor, in comparison to the contralateral, noncancerous breast area.[50]

The discovery that skin over a breast cancer is warmer than in the surrounding skin helped catalyze a host of investigations into medical thermography.[51] Most clinical studies during the 1960s reported an increase in temperature and abnormal thermographic patterns associated with malignant lesions despite the low-resolution techniques available at the time.[52] Connell and associates proposed that breast thermography could serve as the "first line of attack on cancer of the breast." They went on to say "this approach may provide us with our first major scanning technique among the asymptomatic population."[53] A logical coupling between thermography and mammography had begun to emerge, with thermography focusing on the breast's thermal appearance while mammography addressed the radiological appearance.

It was also becoming increasingly clear that breast thermography should be seriously considered as the primary tool for breast cancer screening.[54] This premise was bolstered by a 1975 review of 10,000 breast exams in which thermography was able to identify many tumors that were not found by mammography.[55] Subsequent studies demonstrated that these "mammographically occult" breast tumors were either too small – generally between 0.5 and 0.9 cm (0.2–0.35 in.) in diameter – or too enmeshed in dense breast tissue to be detected by screening mammography.

Also in the 1970s, information began to emerge about breast thermography's prognostic potential. It was reported that the survival of patients was indirectly related to the temperature over the cancerous breast; in 167 cases, none of the patients with differential temperatures exceeding 2.5°C (4.5°F) over the tumor site survived past 2.5 years.[56] Breast tumor doubling time as measured by mammography and correlated with thermographic evaluation of the affected breast was studied. Doubling times of 400–500 days showed no thermal aberrations compared with doubling times of 40–50 days, where the temperature differences were greater than 3°C (5.4°F) in more than 88% of cases.[57] These findings suggested that thermography could be useful in assessing the growth rate of tumors and provided insight into its prognostic potential as well.

In 1972, the U.S. Department of Health, Education and Welfare announced that thermography was "beyond experimental" for evaluations of the female breast. It was widely believed that infrared imaging could help reduce the proportion of women requiring mammography.[58] Breast thermography was a relatively low-cost and innocuous technique that could help identify those individuals requiring further investigation via X-ray mammography.[59] But would a negative infrared image be sufficient to preclude the use of clinical examination and mammography in the detection of breast cancer?

To answer this question, the U.S. National Cancer Institute (NCI) launched a large multicenter study called the Breast Cancer Detection and Demonstration Project (BCDDP).[60] Beginning in 1973, over 280,000 women at 29 sites were screened annually using clinical examination, thermography and mammography.[61] Unfortunately, the thermographers in the study thought of breast thermography as a simple procedure requiring little if any expertise or patient preparation. They were also hampered by the thermal scanners of the period, which had poor spatial resolution and inadequate visual display systems. In addition, the BCDDP's coordinators evinced a strong bias toward mammography, with only a superficial interest in thermography. For the preceding 16 years, the American College of Radiology had supported and coordinated week-long conferences and workshops aimed at optimizing mammography. All mammograms in the BCDDP were conducted by trained technicians and read by qualified radiologists. While proven expertise in mammography was a prerequisite for becoming a BCDDP screening center, no such requirement applied to infrared imaging. Indeed, no experience with thermography whatsoever was required when the 27 screening centers opened their doors. Thus, most of the physicians and technicians participating in the BCDDP had only a rudimentary understanding of the acquisition and interpretation of infrared images. In some centers, no effort was made to cool the patient prior to the thermal imaging exam, completely undermining the reliability of the imaging process. Other centers lacked any standard procedures. Physicians in most centers evinced a simplistic, unsophisticated attitude toward the interpretation of the thermograms. Infrared imaging was narrowly reported as either normal or abnormal, with no attention given to any grading system or any specific aspects of the thermal signatures.[62]

When this flawed data was examined, the BCDDP Working Group concluded that thermography showed very low sensitivity and was not a viable screening tool compared to mammography.[63] The results gave thermography a ranking of third best after physical examination and mammography. The Working Group also stated that thermography was less effective than mammography overall in detecting small to intermediate-sized tumors; omitting the fact that thermography actually detected the smallest tumors. It was on the basis of these biased conclusions that the medical establishment rejected breast thermography as a valid screening tool, a view that has persisted to the present day. Indeed, the BCDDP's findings are the most frequently cited reason for the decreased use of infrared imaging in medical practice after the 1980s.

Given the BCDDP's lack of thermography expertise and the poor quality of the infrared results used in the analysis, it is not surprising that the thermography arm was discontinued in 1977. Also discontinued was mammographic screening for women under age 50. This latter decision was ascribed to mammography's failure as a screening tool in these younger women, a point that was usually glossed over in the media's reporting of the BCDDP findings. In women under age 50, mammography alone detected only 44% of breast cancers – hardly grounds for claiming success in screening that age group.[64]

The data analysis generated by the massive BCDDP project would leave a dent in the reputation of breast thermography, yet research on the subject continued. Following the poor outcome of the BCDDP, researchers at the Ville Marie Comprehensive Breast Center in Montreal enrolled 100 successive patients with stage I or II breast cancer in two separate series (200 patients total).[65] All 100 patients in each series underwent preoperative clinical examination, mammography, and infrared imaging using a Bales infrared scanner. The two studies found that the sensitivity of suspicious mammograms was 83% and 85%, respectively; the combination of suspicious mammograms and abnormal thermograms increased the sensitivity to 93% and 95%, respectively. In each study, the mean size of tumors detected by thermography was significantly smaller than those detected on mammogram. These findings suggested that infrared thermal imaging could provide additional helpful information when performed in conjunction with mammography.

When evaluating studies of thermography, the century of publication matters. Almost all of the large-scale studies conducted before 2000 relied on relatively low-resolution thermal scanning technology. Modern infrared imaging systems introduced since 2000 have used focal plane detector arrays of uncooled microbolometers, a *major* breakthrough offering clear color images with superb spatial and thermal resolution. It is fair to say that improvements in the image quality of thermograms represent a quantum leap in quality compared to the low-resolution thermal images of the 1990s and earlier (Figure 1.10). Modern infrared imagers are compact, fast, rugged, and easy to use, all in sharp contrast with cumbersome, slow, single-detector thermal scanners, which not only require cryogenic cooling but also a great deal of mechanical alignment and calibration.

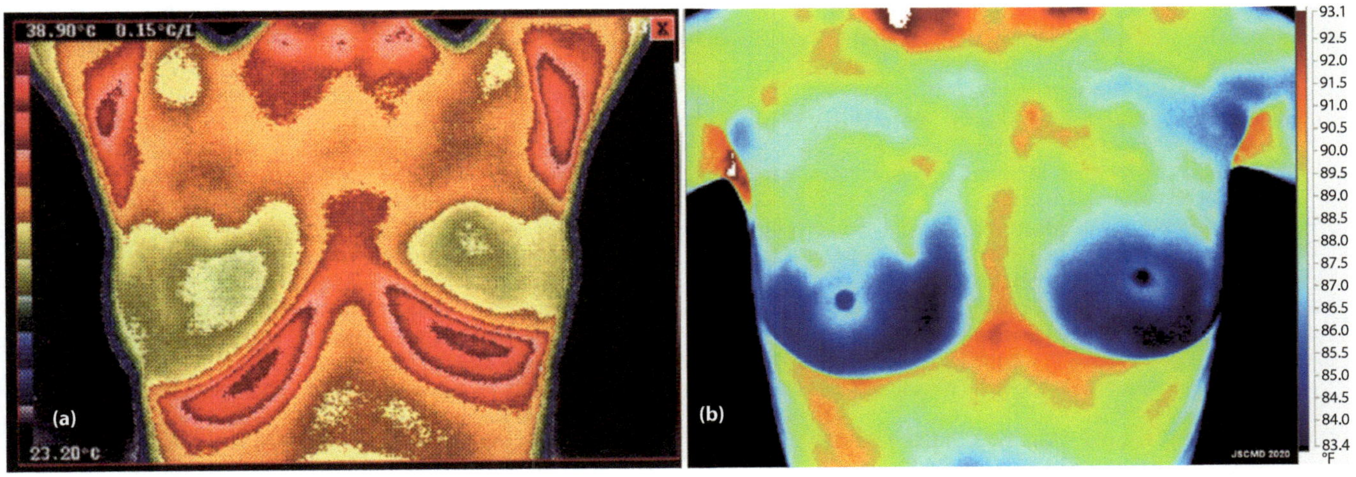

FIGURE 1.10 (a) An infrared breast image taken for the Ville Marie breast study with a Bales infrared scanner circa 1999.[66] (b) A typical infrared breast image taken with a 320 × 240-pixel uncooled microbolometer imager in 2012 showing the vast improvement in spatial and thermal resolution.

Following these major advances in infrared imaging hardware and software, most of the recent breast thermography studies have shown substantially higher sensitivity for thermography relative to mammography when compared to the findings from earlier studies (see Chapter 9). Superior sensitivity means that a normal thermogram has a smaller chance of missing cancer when compared to a normal mammogram. From a pragmatic, epidemiologic standpoint, sensitivity is the key factor in the success of any screening program, because it refers to the effectiveness of a test in detecting a cancer in those who actually have the disease.

Today's thermography systems provide high-speed, high-resolution imaging coupled with computerized digital technology and 24-bit color displays (as compared with the 4 to 5-bit resolution of the older displays), all in a convenient and compact form. This results in clear, detailed color images that can be captured by certified technicians and interpreted by qualified practitioners. Infrared imaging is now widely recognized as a sophisticated science with standardized applications in not only breast health but also neurology, rheumatology, orthopedics, ophthalmology, burn management, and other specialty areas.

Notes

1. Piemonte V, et al. (eds). In: Biomedical Engineering Challenges: A Chemical Engineering Insight 1st Ed, John Wiley and Sons Ltd., 2018; ISBN: 978-1119296041.
2. Hodge, S. In: Thermography & Personal Injury Litigation. Wiley Law Publications. 1987; ISBN: 9780471844693.
3. Hippocrates. In: The Writings of Hippocrates and Galen. Lindsay and Blakiston, Pub. Philadelphia, 1846; http://resource.nlm.nih.gov/56811050R
4. Otsuka K, Togawa T. Physiol Meas. 1997. PMID: 9290139.
5. Galen. Clin Orthop Relat Res. 2003. PMID: 12782854. See also: Galen. Clin Orthop Relat Res. 1997. PMID: 9137171.
6. Romanovsky AA. Handb Clin Neurol. 2018. PMID: 30454596.
7. Roller D. The Early Development of the Concepts of Temperature and Heat: The Rise and Decline of the Caloric Theory. Cambridge, MA: Harvard U. Press, 1950; OCLC Number: 45845692.
8. Kelly, K. Santorio and the Body as a Machine. The Scientific Revolution and Medicine. Infobase Publishing, 2010; ISBN 9781438126364.
9. Berger RL, et al. Methods Biochem Anal. 1984. PMID: 6377012.
10. Barquet N, et al., Ann Intern Med. 1997. PMID: 9341063.
11. Niven J, et al., Edinb Med J. 1883. PMCID: PMC5301626.
12. Wunderlich CA & Woodman WB. On the Temperature in Diseases: A Manual of Medical Thermometry, 2nd Ed, New Sydenham Society. London, 1871; ISBN-13: 978-5518554320.
13. Mackowiak PA, et al., Clin Infect Dis. 1994. PMID: 8011836.
14. Chart by Dr. Carl Wunderlich, *in* On the Temperature in Diseases: A Manual of Medical Thermometry, 2nd Ed, New Sydenham Society, London, 1871, Figure 39, in the Public Domain.
15. Protsiv M, et al. eLife Sciences 2020; https://elifesciences.org/articles/49555
16. Whybrew K, et al., BMJ. 1998. PMCID: PMC28626.
17. Mackowiak PA, et al., JAMA. 1992. PMID: 1302471.
18. Yener Y, et al., Heat Conduction, 4th Ed, CRC Press, 2008; Doi: 10.1201/9780203752166. See also: Özişik MN, Heat Conduction, John Wiley & Sons, New York, NY, 1980; Doi: 10.1002/aic.690260528
19. Rodrigo MR, J Forensic Sci. 2016. PMID: 26213145. See also: Lévesque L. Biomed Opt Express. 2014. PMID: 24688807.
20. Kleiber M. Science. 1972. PMID: 4640063.
21. Strunk TH. J Theor Biol. 1971; 33(1):35–61. PMID: 5130671.
22. From: Herschel FW, Experiments on the refrangibility of the invisible rays of the Sun. Phil Trans Roy Soc. London 1800; 90:284–292. Image in the public domain annotated by JSCMD.
23. Herschel W, Phil Trans Roy Soc London, 1800; 90:293–326.
24. Anbar M. Quantitative Dynamic Telethermometry in Medical Diagnosis and Management, 1st Ed, CRC Press, London, 1994; ISBN-13: 978-0849344091.
25. Graphic: Wikimedia Commons, File: Thermoelectric effect.svg, Author: CMG Lee, Created: 12 December 2018, CC BY-SA 4.0, Annotation by jscmd.
26. Source: Specification Sheet for the ZTP-135SR Integrated Circuit Thermopile. See: https://www.amphenol-sensors.com/en/component/edocman/132-thermometrics-infrared-ir-sensor-ztp-135sr-datasheet/download?Itemid=8465%20%27
27. Sintsov VN. Appl Opt. 1967. PMID: 20062316.
28. Images from: McDaniel GW et al., Appl Opt. 1962; Doi: 10.1364/AO.1.000311 reprinted with permission.
29. Rogalski A. Infrared Phys Technol. 2002; Doi: 10.1016/S1350-4495(02)00140-8
30. Corsi C. Adv Opt Technol. 2012; Doi: 10.1155/2012/838752
31. Bellingham L, US patent 1,158,967, 1913. See also: Parker RD, US patent 1,099,199, 1914.

32. Carpes FP. Adv Physiol Educ. 2018. PMID: 30113221.
33. Thorlabs Inc., Newton, New Jersey, USA, 2019; https://www.thorlabs.com/catalogpages/obsolete/2019/PDA30G-EC.pdf
34. Schwamm E, et al. Hippokrates 1953. PMID: 13142555.
35. Hildebrandt C, et al. Sensors (Basel) 2010. PMCID: PMC3292141 Also see: http://www.thermomed.org/
36. Image Source: © Science Museum Group, London UK. Object: 1988-435, Used with permission.
37. Dummer GWA et al., eds. Medical Electronic Laboratory Equipment 1967–1968. Pergamon Press, 1967; ASIN: B01DSRU326.
38. Davison TW, et al. Cancer, 1972. PMID: 4553757.
39. Images courtesy of: The AGA Museum, Emmen, NL; http://www.aga-museum.nl/, used with permission.
40. Rogalski A. Opto-Electron Rev. 2012; Doi: 10.2478/s11772-012-0037-7. See also: Wood RA, et al., Laser Focus World, 1993. Semantic Scholar Corpus ID: 107420492.
41. Hendler E, et al. J Appl Physiol. 1958. PMID: 13525257.
42. Lawson RN. Can Serv Med J. 1957. PMID: 13460932.
43. Lawson RN. Ann N Y Acad Sci. 1964. PMID: 14237523 Also see: Lawson RN, et al., Ann N Y Acad Sci. 1964. PMID: 14237530.
44. Lawson R. Can Med Assoc J. 1956. PMCID: PMC1824571.
45. Image credit: Lawson R. 1956. PMCID: PMC1824571. Used with permission from Can Med Assoc J.
46. Lawson RN, et al., Ann N Y Acad Sci. 1964. PMID: 14237530.
47. Connell JF Jr, et al. Cancer 1966. PMID: 5901410. See also: Swearingen AG. Radiology. 1965. PMID: 5844518.
48. McDaniel GW et al., Appl Opt. 1962; Doi: 10.1364/AO.1.000311
49. Moncada S, Higgs EA. Br J Pharmacol. 2006; PMCID: PMC1760731.
50. Williams KL, Ann N Y Acad Sci. 1964. PMID: 14237519.
51. Barnes RB, et al., J Albert Einstein Med Cent (Phila). 1963. PMID: 13969372.
52. Harris DL, et al., Br J Cancer. 1966. PMCID: PMC2008153.
53. Connell JF Jr, et al. Cancer 1966. PMID: 5901410.
54. Jakobsson S, Acta Radiologica. 1975; Doi: 10.3109/02841867509132683
55. Amalric R, et al. Bibliotheca Radiologica 1975. PMID: 1180863.
56. Williams KL, Bibl Radiol. 1969. PMID: 5762034. See also: Hobbins WB. JAMA 1979. PMID: 501880.
57. Fournier DV, et al. Cancer 1980; 10.1002/1097-0142(19800415)45:8<2198::AID-CNCR2820450832>3.0.CO;2-7.
58. Institute of Medicine (US) and National Research Council Committee on Technologies for the Early Detection of Breast Cancer; Nass SJ, et al., eds. National Academies Press 2001; URL: https://www.ncbi.nlm.nih.gov/books/NBK222338/
59. Dempsey PJ, J Ultrasound Med. 2004. PMID: 15292555. Note: Breast ultrasound was in its infancy in the 1970s and was not included in the BCDDP.
60. Threatt B, et al., Ann N Y Acad Sci. 1980. PMID: 6931543.
61. Cunningham MP. CA Cancer J Clin. 1997. PMID: 9152170.
62. Head JF, et al., IEEE Eng Med Biol Mag. 2002. PMID: 12613215.
63. Keyserlingk JR, et al. IEEE Eng Med Biol Mag. 2000. PMID: 10834114. See also: Threatt B, et al. Ann N Y Acad Sci. 1980. PMID: 6931543.
64. Hollingsworth AB, Am J Surg. 2019. PMCID: PMC6640096.
65. Keyserlingk JR, et al. IEEE Eng Med Biol Mag. 2000. PMID: 10834114. See also: Keyserlingk JR, et al. Breast J. 1998. PMID: 21223443.
66. Image from: Diakides NA and Bronzino JD, eds., Medical Infrared Imaging. CRC Press, 2008. Used with permission conveyed through The Copyright Clearance Center.

2

THE PHYSICS OF HUMAN THERMOGRAPHY

As depicted in Figure 2.1, humans "glow" with infrared radiation at a 10-micron (μm) wavelength invisible to the human eye. The wavelengths of visible light cover a relatively narrow range of 380–780 nanometers (nm), or about one octave (one octave represents a doubling of frequency or a halving of wavelength). By contrast, the infrared spectrum contains a very wide range of wavelengths, starting just beyond 780 nm and extending up to 1 millimeter (mm), a span of over 10 octaves. Within this spectrum, there are three ranges: near-infrared (NIR, 780 nm–3 μm; ~2 octaves), mid-infrared (MIR, 3–30 μm; ~3.5 octaves), and far-infrared (FIR, 30 μm–1 mm; ~5.5 octaves). These three bands each have unique physical and optical properties requiring specialized emitters, detectors, lenses, and imagers that operate in only a portion of the total infrared band.

There is some disagreement concerning the nomenclature of the infrared bands. The far-infrared is sometimes referred to as "sub-millimeter waves" or the "terahertz band." A major manufacturer of infrared imagers refers to devices that detect 3–5 μm waves as "MWIR" and detectors of 8–14 μm radiation as "LWIR."[2] To avoid confusion, it is better to speak of the wavelength under consideration, not the band. Human thermography utilizes only a small portion of the mid-infrared band (MIR) extending from 5 to 20 μm as shown in Figure 2.2.

Objects emit *peak* radiation at one wavelength depending on their surface temperature. As the surface temperature increases, the peak wavelength emitted *decreases*. Two examples within the physiologic temperature range are: (1) A surface having a temperature of 37°C (98.6°F) – "body temperature" – emits a peak wavelength of 9.34 μm, and (2) a room temperature of 20°C (68°F) has a peak wavelength of 9.89 μm.

The human eye detects visible light emitted by, transmitted through, or reflected off an object's surface. When the skin surface is viewed with an 8–12 μm infrared imager, it detects both self-emitted and reflected infrared radiation. As the human body does not transmit infrared energy to any extent, it may be excluded from this discussion. In human thermography, it is the self-emitted radiation that is medically important. Thus the thermographer must reduce the infrared radiation being reflected from the body surface. Dry human skin is about 98% emissive and 2% reflective to 10 μm radiation.[4] To reduce any thermal reflections, strong infrared sources such as sunlight, flames, smoldering incense, or incandescent light bulbs must be excluded from a thermography room. The skin's reflection of infrared radiation from these hot sources may create significant artifacts in a human thermal image. As the skin also reflects the diffused radiation from the objects in and walls of the thermography room, reflection of the background temperature must be corrected by the thermal imager (Figure 2.3).

The basics of heat transfer and radiative thermometry

Humans cannot directly see infrared radiation. They can, however, feel or sense it in the form of thermal radiation, which produces warming of the surface of the skin. The skin of the human cheek below the eye can normally sense the increased thermal radiation of a warm palm held at a distance of 2 inches (5 cm) at a room temperature of 70°F (21°C).[5]

In physics, the word "heat" can be either a noun or a verb: a warm body will *heat* (verb) a cooler body, increasing the *heat* (noun) of the cooler body. As a noun, heat refers to the total amount of random kinetic energy the molecules of a substance have at any given moment, measured in units of joules (J). Heat as a verb refers to energy transfer from a warm to a cold body. The cooler body increases its internal energy, while the warmer body decreases its internal energy until the *temperatures* of the two bodies become equal. This heat transfer does not stop when the two bodies are at the same temperature. The bodies continue to radiate heat toward one another, but the radiation balances out, so the net energy transfer is zero.

Objects at high temperatures are capable of emitting radiation with shorter wavelengths than infrared, including visible and ultraviolet light. Steel at 1500°C (2732°F, 1773°K) has a peak emitted wavelength of 1.64 μm in the near-infrared band, yet it appears white hot to the human eye due to emitting some radiation in the visible range (see the radiation curves in Figure 2.5). For bodies having physiologic surface temperatures, however, the radiated energy peaks within the 7–14 μm octave of the electromagnetic spectrum and even the shorter wavelengths emitted are invisible to the eye. The human body emits its peak radiation in the 9–10 μm part of the spectrum, thus imagers with detectors sensitive to this radiation are preferred in medical thermography. Imagers capable of viewing other infrared wavelengths are of more practical use in industrial and scientific research settings.

The term "emissivity" in thermal imaging refers to the ability of a surface to emit or absorb radiation within 9–10-μm infrared range. The range of emissivity runs from 1.0 (the ideal emitter/absorber) to 0.0 (the ideal reflector). In physics, a *blackbody* is an object that has an emissivity of 1.0. None of the incident radiation is reflected from or passes through a perfect blackbody. Thus, a blackbody completely absorbs all radiant energy reaching it, and simultaneously emits radiant energy. If not otherwise heated or cooled, it eventually attains a temperature equal to its environment and then maintains that energy balance.

The physical opposite of an infrared blackbody is a surface that is extremely shiny and reflective to infrared. Mathematically, emissivity (ε) plus reflectance (R) add up to unity: ($\varepsilon + R = 1$). Polished aluminum or brass surfaces have an infrared emissivity of 3% ($\varepsilon = 0.03$), meaning that they reflect 97% of incoming rays. A silver-coated glass mirror has a similar high infrared reflectance. Liquid water, though it may appear to have visible reflectivity, has an infrared emissivity of 0.95–0.96 (perpendicular to the water surface), almost as emissive as human skin.[6]

There are four fundamental mechanisms by which the heat generated by the human body is transferred to its surroundings, as discussed in the following text.

Radiation

Radiative heat transfer occurs via infrared waves traveling between two separate objects, which may be at different temperatures. This transfer can occur even through a vacuum. Bodies receive radiated electromagnetic energy emitted by the surroundings, some of which is reflected and the remainder absorbed. Whereas

DOI: 10.1201/9781003281764-3

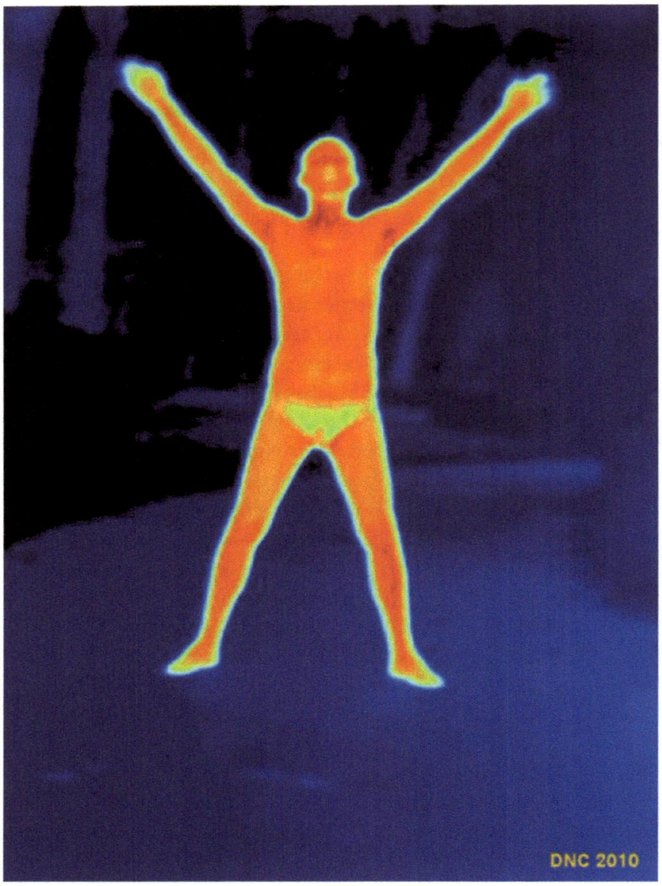

FIGURE 2.1 Infrared image of a warm, fully vasodilated man standing outside at a temperature of 45°F (7.2°C).[1]

emissions of radiant energy entail a decrease in internal energy, absorption results in an increase. Radiance is a directional (vector) quantity. Therefore, if a body maintains a constant temperature it is in *thermal equilibrium*; the energy emitted is counterbalanced by the energy absorbed plus any heat energy produced internally. If a body is at either a higher or lower temperature than its surroundings, the net radiative heat transfer is the difference between emitted and absorbed radiation. In infrared imaging, this radiative heat transfer occurs simultaneously between the human subject and the local environment, of which the thermal imager itself is an integral part. The sum of the infrared radiation emitted and reflected from a surface is what a radiometric thermal imager detects and quantifies as surface temperature. About 60% of the heat lost by the human body is lost through radiation.

Conduction

This describes the transfer of heat by direct physical contact between two bodies or masses having different temperatures. About 3% of human body heat is lost through conduction. Fourier's law of heat conduction states that the rate of heat transfer through a material is proportional to the gradient in the temperature and to the area, at right angles to that gradient, through which the heat flows. Heat conduction is also inversely proportional to the distance through any material separating the two masses; the greater the distance, the less the rate of conductive heat transfer. Conduction of heat within the human body occurs between adjacent structures or regions of the body. Thermal conduction also occurs between the human body and items that touch it, such as furniture. Conductive heat transfer takes place through body tissues even with no blood flow. In the arms and legs, this transference depends on the temperature gradient between the skin surface and underlying muscle as well as the distance from the muscle to the skin. Heat transfer by conduction is facilitated when the temperature gradient between muscle and skin is increased. A subcutaneous muscle warmed by exercise will warm the overlying skin by heat conduction which can be detected by thermal imaging. Heat conduction may work both ways, as when a subject places his or her cold hand on a warm part of their body, thus temporarily decreasing the skin temperature of that part while simultaneously raising the temperature of the hand. Conductive heat transfer may be also be used in thermography by changing the skin surface temperature rapidly and reliably. As an example, the thermal recovery time after removing a cool pack from the skin may differentiate malignant from benign growths.

Convection

Convection refers to heat transfer occurring from the contact of a solid body with a moving liquid or gaseous medium. Within the human body, heat convection occurs via blood flow; blood flowing through the body core is heated and consequently heats the skin layers it passes through. Likewise, blood flowing through cooler skin will be carried back to cool the core. Outside of the body, heat from the body's surfaces is transferred into the surrounding room through airflow governed by fluid dynamics. Air (or water, from swimming, for example) moving over the skin surface facilitates convective heat exchange with the environment. About 15% of the heat from a human body is lost through convection. In the case of an unclothed human standing still, heat convection occurs as the skin surface warms the nearby air, which expands and rises, creating a baseline convective airflow – this is referred to as *natural convection*. Convective heat transport can work both ways; hot air or water can increase skin temperature. Clothing decreases convective heat loss (or gain) by reducing the airflow near the skin. In the practice of human thermography, the convection principle explains why it is necessary to minimize *forced convection* (e.g., from air conditioning vents, HVAC (Heating, Ventilating, Air Conditioning) ducts, or fans) during an imaging

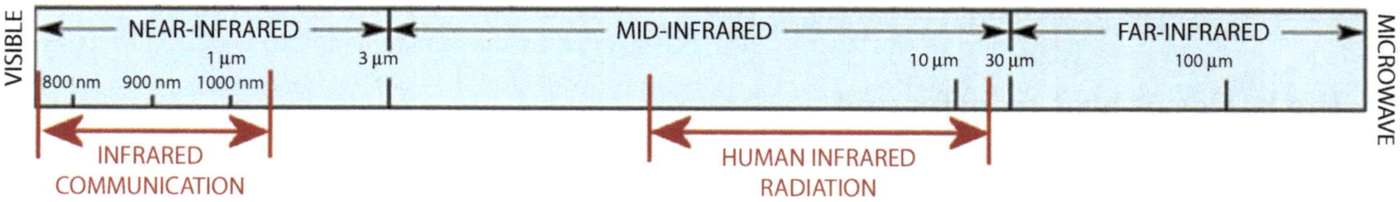

FIGURE 2.2 The infrared bands showing the useable range of human IR emissions located in the mid-infrared band. Infrared communication devices such as IR remote control units utilize the near-infrared band and do not interfere with human thermography.[3]

(a) $T_{corr} = [(T_d - T_{bk})(1 - \varepsilon)] + T_d$

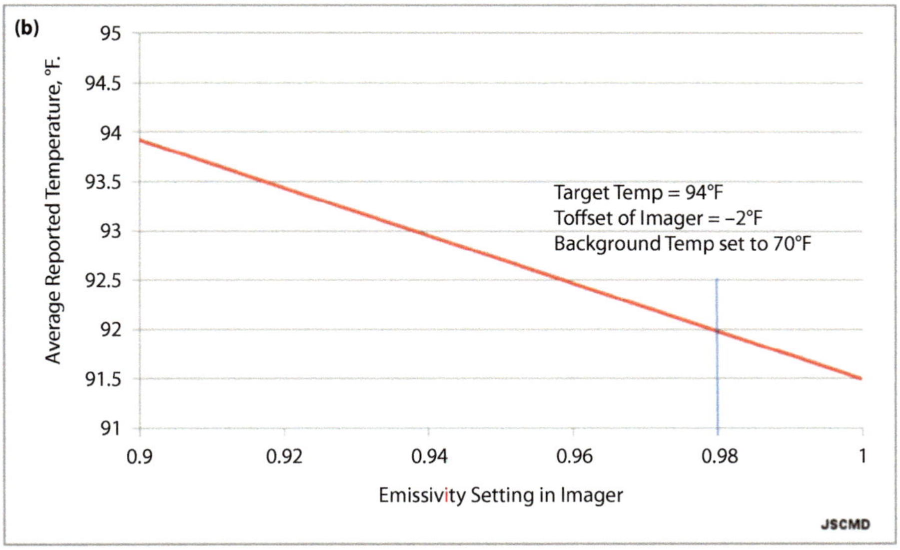

FIGURE 2.3 (a) The formula for correcting the reflected background temperature. Td is the corrected temperature detected by the pixel. Tbk is the background temperature setting entered into the imager. ε is the emissivity value entered into the imager, and Tcorr is the background-corrected temperature reported by the imager. Thermal imaging software may perform these calculations automatically based on operator-entered emissivity and room temperature values. (b) Changing the emissivity correction value of a thermal imager from 0.90 to 1.00 reduced the detected temperature reading of a 94°F target by 2.4°F. This is in agreement with the background correction formula. The linear trendline derived from data is shown.[20]

session. Increased skin cooling from forced convection may occur on the upwind side of a subject, while less cooling takes place downwind and near skin folds, possibly creating temperature artifacts in the images. Very cold-forced convection may also overwhelm the heating effect of blood flow to the skin, an effect known as *dynamic cooling.* Dynamic cooling is used in certain thermographic protocols to increase the thermal contrast between normal and abnormal areas.

Evaporative cooling

Unlike the other three methods of heat transfer, evaporation works only to cool the body. The evaporation of sweat on the skin is the primary mechanism for heat dissipation in hot environments and during intensive physical activity, allowing the body to reduce its core temperature by decreasing the skin surface temperature. Even in cool temperatures and without exercise, water constantly evaporates from the skin surface as *insensible water loss.* About 20% of the heat lost by the body occurs through this basal evaporation, though that amount may be much greater when actively sweating. Evaporation of water, whether insensible or as sweat droplets, requires the input of heat energy. To evaporate 1 cubic centimeter (1 ml) of water requires 2444 J of heat at 25°C, equal to 584 calories (0.584 Calories).[7] This heat must come from the immediate surroundings, cooling the skin by conduction.[8] Note that this evaporative skin cooling only occurs if the sweat stays in contact with the body surface. Cooled sweat droplets reduce the skin surface temperature by conduction, which in turn cools the blood flowing through the dermal veins. This cooled blood then reduces the body core temperature by pumped flow convection. High relative humidity reduces water evaporation, reducing the effect of evaporative cooling considerably. Conversely, airflow and low relative humidity facilitate cooling by increasing sweat evaporation. This is why the relative humidity of a thermography room should be about 40%–70% and why the subject should be sufficiently dry prior to imaging. It should be noted that sweat itself does not significantly alter the thermal emissivity of the skin, as water has an emissivity value close to that of the skin. If liquid sweat droplets form, however, they will generally appear cooler than the surrounding skin due to the evaporative heat loss from the surface of each droplet.

The importance of evaporative skin cooling for human life cannot be overlooked. Humans cannot survive long in very warm and humid conditions because evaporative cooling is severely reduced. Prolonged exposure to "wet-bulb" temperatures exceeding 35°C (95°F) may cause fatal hyperthermia even in unclothed, non-obese humans – despite rest, shade and cooling fans – because the body's metabolic heat production cannot be adequately dissipated by radiation, convection, conduction, and evaporation under such conditions.[9]

The physical laws of thermology

Within a room designed for human thermography, there should be no significant external or additional sources of infrared energy to illuminate or reflect off the subject other than the room background temperature itself.[10] Under these conditions, the major source of 10-μm IR radiation arises from the surface temperature of the body being imaged. The thermal energy naturally emitted by every object does so in accordance with Planck's radiation law, a mathematical relationship that describes the non-linear energy distribution of radiation emitted by a blackbody. Given that human skin's emissivity is only slightly less than 1, it follows that the infrared radiation emitted from human skin can be described fairly accurately using Planck's law.

Planck's law is the mathematical principle behind non-contact radiometry and thermography. The law mathematically expresses the thermal energy radiated by a blackbody at temperature (T) as detected over one wavelength (λ) of radiation. This energy is called Spectral Radiance (B_λ) which can be calculated by Planck's complicated formula (Equation 2.1).

$$B_\lambda(\lambda, T) = \frac{2hc^2}{\lambda^5} \frac{1}{e^{\frac{hc}{\lambda k_B T}} - 1}$$

EQUATION 2.1 Planck's law[11]

where:

h (Planck's constant) = 6.6256×10^{-34}
k_B (Boltzmann's constant) = 1.38054×10^{-23} WsK^{-1}
c (velocity of light in vacuum) = 3×10^8 ms^{-1}
λ (Lambda) = wavelength in µm (microns)
T = absolute temperature (degrees Kelvin)

The SI Units for B_λ in the IR band are $W{\cdot}sr^{-1}{\cdot}m^{-2}{\cdot}\mu m^{-1}$ (watts per steradian per square meter per micron).

To simplify the relationship between temperature and spectral radiance, a graphic representation of Planck's law shows the wavelength at which radiation emitted by a black body of a certain temperature has a maximum (see Figure 2.5). This maximum radiance point shifts linearly with changing temperature following Wien's displacement law: The black-body radiation curve for different temperatures will peak at different wavelengths that are inversely proportional to the absolute (Kelvin) temperature (Equation 2.2). The wavelength of the emitted radiation peak is inversely proportional to its energy.[12] Thus the peak wavelength of radiated energy decreases with rising temperature.

$$\lambda_{\text{peak}} = \frac{b}{T}$$

EQUATION 2.2 Wien's displacement law[13]

where:

T is the absolute temperature in degree Kelvin
b is Wien's displacement constant (b ≈ 2898 µm·K)
λ (Lambda) is the peak radiated wavelength in µm (microns)

Conversely, the lower the temperature of the object, the further its radiation maximum shifts toward longer wavelengths. When a blackbody object is close to a room temperature of 20°C (68°F, 293.15°K), the maximum wavelength radiated is at about 9.89 µm. For a typical human body surface temperature of 32.2°C (90°F, 305.37°K), Wien's Law predicts the peak of the emitted energy at 9.49 µm. Observing the human radiation spectrum curve in Figure 2.5, it can be seen that most of this radiation falls within the mid-infrared band. Heat radiating from human skin has a peak power wavelength at about 10 µm, with a broad −3 dB (half-power) bandwidth extending from 5 to 20 µm.[14] Modern thermal imagers for medical purposes are designed to work best at around 10 µm to take advantage of the maximum thermal emissions from human skin.

Biothermal radiation dynamics

All living things produce heat as a byproduct of metabolism. This heat is considerable, about 75 watts or approximately one-tenth of horsepower for a *resting* human, which comes out to a daily basal heat energy output of 1.8 kilowatt-hours or about 1500 Calories.[15] To experience a heat output of about 75 watts, put your dry hand on the glass bulb of a cool 75-watt incandescent light bulb and turn it on. In about 10 seconds, the bulb will become too hot to touch. This amount of heat must be dissipated constantly into the surroundings to maintain a normal body temperature. An unclothed non-obese resting human is in temperature balance when the surrounding air is between 27°C and 28°C (80.6°F and 82.4°F) at a relative humidity of about 70%, assuming no drafts or breezes. This is about 10°C (18°F) below the human core temperature, creating a thermal gradient that allows controlled shedding of metabolic heat.[16] Warmer ambient temperatures may feel too hot, while cooler temperatures feel too cool.

The infrared emissivity of human skin is just under 1.0 (actually 0.98), making it a near-perfect emitter/absorber of 10-µm infrared radiation at room temperature.[17] Skin emissivity is practically constant in the infrared range from 7 to 14 µm, measuring 0.977 ± 0.007 in a definitive study.[18] The very low standard deviation (±0.007) shows that individual skin variability is minimal. Skin color, whether white, brown, black, red, yellow, or even burnt, has no effect on human infrared emissivity.[19] It is because of this extremely high and uniform emissivity that measurements of infrared radiation emanating from the human body's surface can be converted into accurate skin temperature values.

Setting an infrared imager to emissivity values other than 0.98 may affect the accuracy of the absolute and differential temperature readings by changing the thermal gain of the imager as referenced to the background temperature setting. As shown in the formula (Figure 2.3(a)), background temperature correction can have the following effects: cooler body parts with surface temperatures close to the background temperature setting will show little error in reported surface temperature readings, even with emissivity settings as low as 0.8. Temperatures over warm skin surfaces, however, will be reported considerably warmer than actual due to the increased gain if the emissivity is set lower than 0.96. Conversely, reported temperatures of warm surfaces will be *lower* than actual if the emissivity is set to 0.99 or 1.0. Thermographers are advised to check and adjust both the imager's emissivity and background temperature settings to obtain the most accurate absolute and differential thermal measurements. Incorrect emissivity and background temperature settings may also cause errors when checking the calibration of an imager.

Detected temperatures are significantly affected by the imaging distance; objects warmer than the background appear cooler, and cooler objects than background appear warmer with increasing imaging distance.[21] This is due to the lens and internal structures of an imager scattering an *average* of the incoming radiation onto the sensor leaflets; more background area radiation is scattered onto the image at increasing target distances.[22] Distance effects may be important in studies involving absolute temperature measurements such as fever detection. Differential temperature measurements on the body should not be significantly affected by this distance effect because the two measurements will be altered by about the same amount.

Other sources of thermographic measurement error are clinically less important. The recommended Relative Humidity (RH%) level in the thermography room (40%–70%) does not significantly affect thermal readings unless it is so high that water vapor condenses in the air or on the infrared lens.[23] In addition, infrared attenuation caused by the reflection coefficient at the infrared imaging lens may affect readings, though this is reduced to about 1% with proper optical coatings and is accounted for during factory calibration of the imager/lens combination.[24]

Infrared imaging is not based on direct contact measurement of surface temperatures but rather on receiving the sum of the infrared radiation emitted and reflected from a distant surface. The sensed radiation is diminished as it passes through the atmosphere toward the imager; atmospheric attenuation of 10-μm radiation is negligible within the thermography room, however.[25]

Because infrared radiance from the skin is a directional quantity maximally emitted perpendicular (i.e., at 90°) to the skin surface, the angle of incidence between the skin and thermal imaging axis must also be taken into account when sensing surface temperatures. As the imaging angle increases away from perpendicular, the detected radiance decreases as a cosine function, with the detected temperature value also decreasing. At an angle of 30° (cos 30° = 0.866), small temperature errors are noted. An incident angle of 60° (cos 60° = 0.50) creates significant temperature errors. From a thermographic perspective, an imaging angle of 45 degrees from perpendicular (cos 45° = 0.707) is the recommended maximum for clinical temperature evaluation. At larger angles, the detected temperature will be significantly reduced, as shown in Figure 2.4.[26]

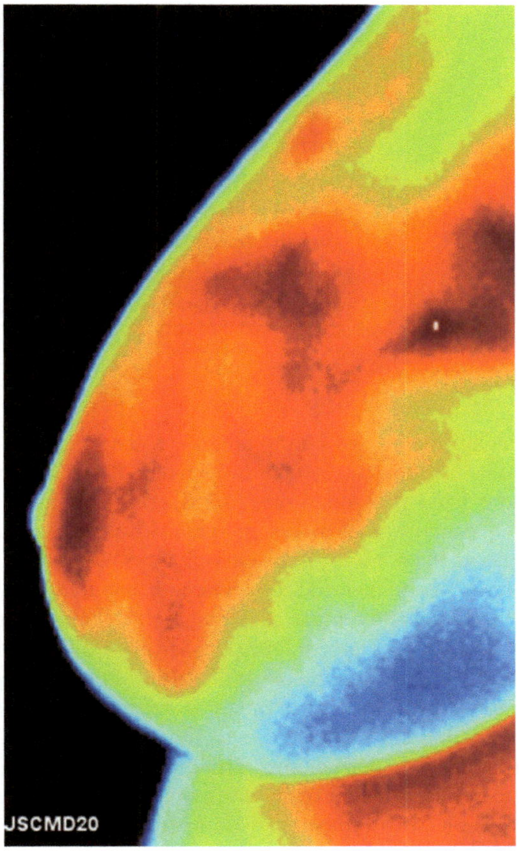

FIGURE 2.4 The yellow-green-blue "fringing" seen at the edge of this breast image is an artifact due to the reduced infrared emissivity from the skin as the imaging angle of incidence approaches 90 degrees. This fringing effect is also seen in Figure 2.1.

Summing up the physical principles of human thermography

The electromagnetic radiance detected by a modern infrared microbolometer chip behind a standard coated germanium crystal lens is shown as a red column in Figure 2.5. The steep sides

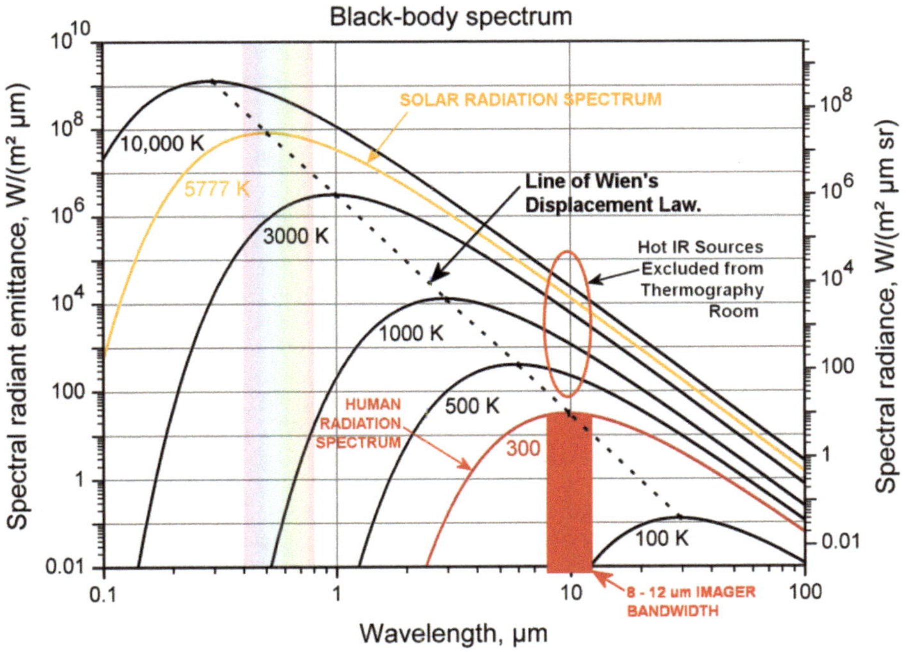

FIGURE 2.5 Nested curves derived from Planck's law showing the thermal radiance detected by an 8–12 μm infrared imager under controlled thermographic conditions (*red column*). The maximum detected radiance varies linearly with Wien's displacement law. Strong infrared sources that might reflect off human skin are kept out of the thermography room by physical design.[27]

TABLE 2.1 Key Temperature and Peak Wavelength Values Encountered in Human Infrared Imaging. λpk = Peak Wavelength at That Temperature Calculated from Wien's Law. NETD = Noise Equivalent Temperature Difference (the Electronic Noise of the Imager). RMS = Root Mean Square

Average body temperature:	98.6°F = 37°C = 310.15°K (λpk = 9.34 μm)
Lowest skin temperature during imaging:	65°F = 18.3°C = 291.48°K (λpk = 9.94 μm)
Highest expected skin temperature Maximum:	105°F = 40.55°C = 313.7°K (λpk = 9.24 μm)
Human infrared signal range:	22.2K° = 7.2% change in thermal radiation
Thermal radiation change from 1°C (1.8°F):	0.32% change
Thermal radiation change at NETD (0.05°C):	0.016% change = typical RMS noise level

of the column are fixed by the optical passband of the lens and the physical properties of the bolometers. The bottom of the column is fixed at absolute zero (0.0°K). It is the slightly curved top of this column that moves up and down with changing temperatures as the summit of the curve follows Wien's Law. As the maximum change in infrared wavelength is only about 0.7 μm over the physiologic temperature range, this change in the area of the column varies almost linearly when electronically detected by the array of microbolometer leaflets. In addition, the signal-to-noise ratio is optimal because the imager detects the signal at the peak of the human radiance curve. Thus the height and area of the detected "radiance column" are directly proportional to the absolute detected Kelvin temperature of the target. Ratios of the signal change with temperature compared to the total area of this radiance column are given in Table 2.1. For reference, a 1°C (1.8°F) temperature change causes a 0.32% change in the detected signal. To prevent this small signal from being overwhelmed by more powerful infrared sources, thermographic protocol excludes any hot radiation sources from the room while images are being obtained. Imaging software can then correct the "raw" thermal signal for surface emissivity, background temperature, target distance, lens attenuation, and the offset and gain of each pixel before assigning the corrected temperature values in the final image.

Notes

1. Image credit: Image taken by Dianne N. Campbell (2010) using a Fluke Model TI55 Thermal Imager.
2. See various imager specifications at https://www.flir.com/
3. Infrared scale from The Photonics Spectrum Reference Chart 2012, Laurin Publishing, Pittsfield, MA. Used with permission. Annotations added by jscmd.
4. Anbar M, et al. Dentomaxillofac Radiol. 1998; PMID: 9656868.
5. This thermosensitive site corresponds to the Quanliao (S.I. 18) point in acupuncture notation.
6. Table of Emissivity of Various Surfaces: https://www.engineeringtoolbox.com/emissivity-coefficients-d_447.html
7. CRC Handbook of Chemistry and Physics – 83rd Ed, Lide DR, ed., CRC Press, Boca Raton, FL, 2002, p.6-3.
8. Evaporative cooling also occurs in the lungs and respiratory tract during normal breathing, mainly cooling the blood flowing through the lungs.
9. "Wet-Bulb" temperatures may be measured by wrapping a temperature sensor (such as a standard thermometer bulb) with a cloth wet with distilled water, then allowing time to reach thermal equilibrium. This will sense the air temperature minus the heat of evaporation.
10. To reduce any other thermal reflections, the thermographer and other aides in the room should wear long-sleeved loose clothing such as a lab coat to cover their warm skin as much as possible. Warm electronics and hot or cold water containers can be covered with a towel or placed behind a screen until needed. Scanning the room with the thermal imager can reveal other hot or cold objects that might affect the clinical picture.
11. Formula from Wikipedia, Entry for Planck's Law, edited 18 December 2019.
12. Richards JA, et al. Modern University Physics. Addison-Wesley Publishing, Reading, MA, 1960.
13. Formula from Wikipedia, entry for Wien's Displacement Law, edited 17 February 2020.
14. The −3 dB bandwidth lies between the frequencies (or wavelengths) where the signal *power* becomes half of its peak value. See Floyd TL, Principles of Electric Circuits, 2nd Ed, Charles E. Merrill, Pub, Columbus, OH, 1985, Section 18-5.
15. In this book, the quantity of heat energy will be referred to as follows: 1 Calorie (capital "C") = 1000 calories (lowercase "c") = 1 kilocalorie = 4186.8 Joules.
16. Diakides NA, Bronzino JD, eds., Medical Infrared Imaging, Section 6.3. CRC Press, Boca Raton, FL, 2008.
17. Jones BF, et al. IEEE Eng Med Biol Mag. 2002; PMID: 12613210. See also Togawa T, et al., Physiol Meas. 1994; PMID: 7994207. See also Togawa T, Clin Phys Physiol Meas. 1989; 10(1):39–48; PMID: 2714059.
18. Sanchez-Marin FJ, et al. J Biomed Opt. 2009; PMID 19405736.
19. Steketee J. Phys Med Biol. 1973; PMID: 4758213.
20. Graph of emissivity correction by Fluke Corp. TiX-500 imager internal firmware. Target: flat black painted ¼ inch thick aluminum plate in a 94°F temperature-controlled chamber. The linear trendline is derived from 12 imager measurements.
21. Experimental data collected by JSCMD at a room temperature of 21.7°C (71°F) and relative humidity of 70%.
22. For a more scientific explanation, see: Bieszczad G, et al. Metrol. Meas. Syst 2011; Doi: 10.2478/v10178-011-0064-6
23. Minkina W, et al. J Sens Sens Syst. 2016; Doi: 10.5194/jsss-5-17-2016
24. Ibid. 16, Section 5.6.2.
25. Ibid. 23.
26. Ibid. 16, Section 22.3.2.3.
27. Original graphic from Wikimedia Commons. https://commons.wikimedia.org/wiki/File:BlackbodySpectrum_loglog_en.svg. Artist: Prog. Created 10 July 2017. CC BY-SA 4.0. Annotations added by jscmd 2019.

3

THERMAL IMAGER FUNDAMENTALS

Dramatic improvements in medical thermal imagers have taken place since the late 1990s, mostly due to ongoing refinements in mid-infrared detector chips, fast electronic digitization, image manipulation software, and improved display systems. These technological advances have transformed the landscape of medical thermography to the extent that the latest infrared imaging systems can be easily integrated into modern medical practice.

Thermal imagers are now capable of generating an image similar to that of a regular camera. But whereas the image produced by a visual camera shows the reflected light from the scene's illumination, the thermographic imager senses the scene's infrared emissions and does not require visible or infrared illumination. Indeed, any strong sources of mid-infrared energy must be kept out of a human thermography room to prevent infrared reflection artifacts. Upon acquiring the infrared emissions, thermal microsensors within the imager transform the radiation into electronic signals. These sensors are capable of detecting electromagnetic radiation of wavelengths around 10 μm. In most systems, a germanium lens blocks the reception of visible light, enabling the imager to detect only thermal infrared emissions.

Once the thermal imaging system converts the infrared emissions into electronic signals, those signals can then be displayed in either colors or gray shades representing various temperature values. The system's software converts each infrared energy level into a corrected temperature reading while simultaneously assigning each temperature a color or shade. The result is a visible false-color image called a thermogram, a dynamic, two-dimensional, graphic representation of the amount of heat emitted from the body's surface by infrared radiation.

The warmer the surface, the higher the energy of the infrared emissions. Using the standard red-blue spectral color palette (also called a rainbow palette), increased heat coming off the body shows up as shades of red, orange, or yellow, while cooler temperatures are displayed in shades of green or blue. A linear greyscale conversion palette is sometimes used to represent the heat signal, with black indicating cool, and white representing warm temperatures. (Note: Some imagers, such as those used for night surveillance, display a *non-linear* grayscale where human temperatures appear almost white against a dark background. These non-linear thermal displays are not suitable for medial thermography.)

The appeal of using infrared imaging in medical practice has grown due to the following advantages:

- As a non-invasive, non-contact technology, thermography allows a comfortable distance between the imager and the subject being imaged.
- When properly performed, the non-contact imaging procedure will not alter the result of the measurement, and the measurments are repeatable.
- As a painless, easily tolerated procedure similar to taking a photograph, thermography lends itself to favorable acceptance as a method that provides useful pathophysiologic information.
- Because modern thermographic imaging takes place in real time, it may be used for the acquisition of rapidly changing thermal patterns. Spatial blurring due to subject movement over time is virtually eliminated. Videothermography at 30 frames-per-second is possible.
- Thermography provides two-dimensional, temperature-calibrated infrared images, thus enabling differential thermal comparisons between areas of the body, even across separate images or imaging sessions.
- Thermography is suitable for repeated use on subjects of all ages because it produces no ionizing radiation or X-rays.
- Unlike ultrasound imaging, thermography emits no mechanical waves or other energy that might damage cells or tissues. Thermography may be used to monitor infants over long periods.

A number of disadvantages must also be understood and properly addressed in order to optimize thermographic applications.

- Human thermography must be performed in a controlled environment because the results are highly dependent on the preparation of the subject as well as the surrounding temperature, airflow, and humidity during imaging. This requires a specially equipped room, staff instruction, and patient education.
- Because infrared images can be difficult to format and interpret, specific thermographic training is required both on the technician and physician levels.
- As the scientific basis for human thermography is widely underappreciated and largely misunderstood by the established medical community, it is not yet accepted as a standard practice. Third-party reimbursement may not be available from all insurance companies due to the abrupt, unexplained removal of CPT billing codes for thermographic procedures in 2009.[1]
- Unlike digital X-ray images, which are stored and displayed in a standard DICOM format, thermal image display is dependent on the device manufacturer's proprietary software, which may be incompatible with other thermal image file formats.[2]
- Finally, despite the recent development of fast and affordable hardware, an infrared imager is still an expensive device. Although the more affordable models (around US$5,000) offer ample spatial resolution (320 × 240 pixels) with a thermal noise level that is sufficient for most medical applications, these devices have recently been supplanted by higher resolution imagers (640 × 480 pixels). Prices for these newest imagers may range from US$10,000 to US$30,000 depending on the NETD noise factor.[3]

Sensors used in modern infrared thermography

The process of converting the infrared radiation to a digital format for computer display begins with a sensor that transforms infrared thermal radiation into an analog signal. The older infrared scanners used thermal detectors that needed to be cooled to cryogenic temperatures (–200°C/–328°F or lower), a requirement that is expensive, bulky, inefficient, and difficult

DOI: 10.1201/9781003281764-4

to maintain. Some modern ferroelectric FPA-based imagers still incorporate cryogenic cooling, but they have equivalent noise specifications that do not meet the requirements for human thermography.[4] Development of infrared imagers that do not require cooling facilitated the use of thermography in clinical settings.

As uncooled infrared detectors, microbolometer sensors provide a resistance proportional to the received thermal radiance. The focal plane array (FPA) chip in a thermal imager consists of tiny bolometer sensors that measure the energy of incoming mid-infrared rays. The FPA-integrated circuit contains 307,200 active pixels for a 640 × 480 array. Each pixel is a microbolometer leaflet measuring as small as 10 µm × 10 µm × 0.5 µm thick, or a little bigger than a human red blood cell. As leaflets become smaller, they become less effective antennas for thermal radiation, resulting in a relative increase in electronic noise (NETD). This cutoff limits the minimum pixel dimensions.

The microbolometer FPA's sensitivity and rapid thermal response are accomplished by the leaflet surfaces having a very low thermal capacity, optimal insulation, and high surface emissivity in an evacuated environment (a vacuum). The silicon base under the leaflet has low emissivity to reduce heat radiation from the leaflet. The pixels can respond to infrared changes with a typical five millisecond time constant (25 ms for a 95% response), which is fast enough to facilitate thermographic video at 30 frames per second (fps). Microbolometer arrays are very specialized and expensive chips, typically priced around $500 apiece as of 2020.

Microbolometer FPA-based infrared imagers have become the mainstay of medical thermography for several reasons. These systems can produce a highly detailed infrared image of the scene or object, with each microsensor (pixel) conferring infrared information from one point on the target. FPA detectors can generate high-resolution infrared images without a cumbersome mechanical scan mechanism or the need for cryogenic cooling. The FPAs offer advantages in terms of data acquisition time, expense, convenience, and ease of use. The rapid development of these lower-cost FPA-based uncooled imagers has driven most of the growth of the thermography market in the 21st century.

Figure 3.1 shows a single leaflet microbolometer "pixel" of vanadium oxide (V_2O_5) suspended on cantilevered legs above a silicon chip. V_2O_5 is chosen for the sensor because of its large resistance change with temperature, approximately 2%–3% per degree Kelvin around room temperature.[7] Minor differences in the multistage photolithographically-controlled micromachining of the pixel leaflets make each one unique, with its own thermal offset and gain that must be determined by blackbody calibration and then corrected digitally.

These microscopic VOx leaflets are extremely fragile and may be damaged by the shock of a 1 meter drop onto concrete. Such damage is depicted on the surface of a microbolometer detector (Figure 3.1). Most microbolometer FPA chips are protected in a

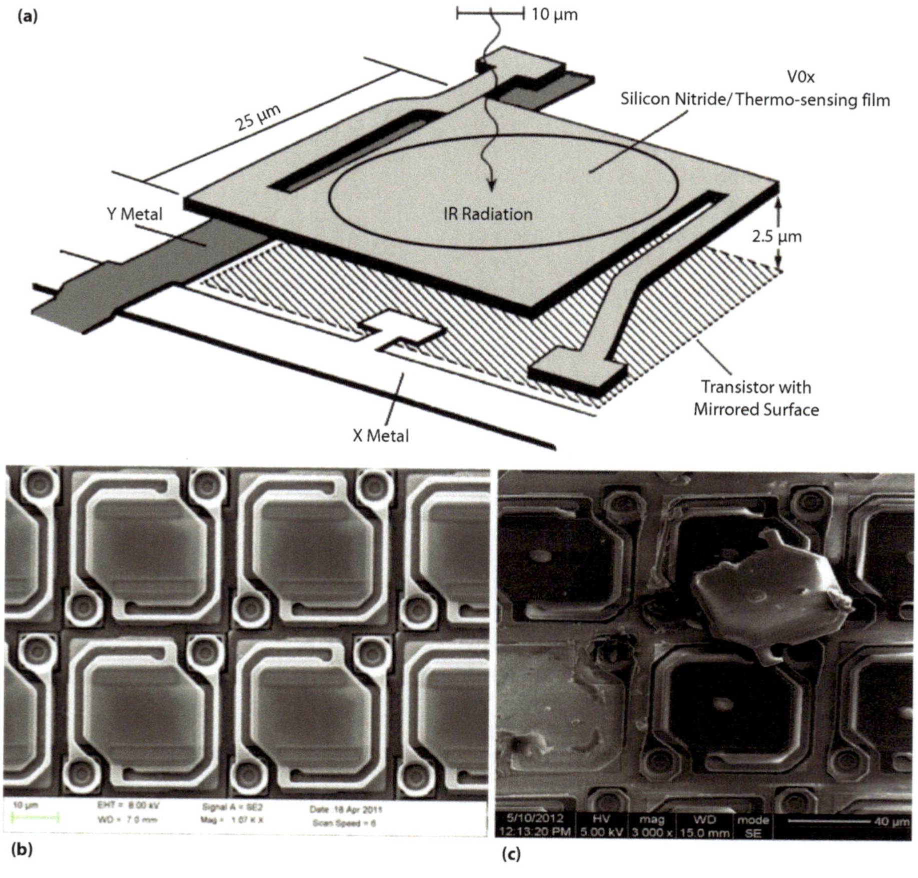

FIGURE 3.1 (a) A single microbolometer leaflet "pixel" consists of a suspended layer of vanadium oxide (V_2O_5) above a silicon chip containing amplifiers and other circuitry.[5] (b) An undamaged microbolometer surface with pixels measuring 37 × 37 µm. (c) The microbolometer detector leaflets damaged by a 1000 g mechanical shock.[6]

sturdy, hermetically sealed vacuum case to reduce any possible damage to the leaflets.

Each pixel's resistance changes in response to the VOx leaflet's temperature, and that change generates an electrical voltage or current signal detected by analog techniques. The resistance of each pixel varies in a linear manner at human body temperatures. Fast 14- or 16-bit Analog-to-Digital (A/D) converters digitize the amplified analog signals. A Digital Signal Processor (DSP) rapidly calculates a radiometric temperature value for each pixel, and generates the greyscale or false-color image. Thermal imagers require an extensive calibration process in which gain and offset values are allocated to each pixel at different black body temperatures and stored in a digital Pixel Correction Memory. To increase the measuring accuracy of the microbolometers, the FPA is often stabilized at a defined chip temperature.

The DSP is essentially the thermal imager's Central Processing Unit or CPU. This processor corrects the signal coming from each vanadium oxide (VOx) pixel separately. As the entire chip package, lens, and imager are glowing in the infrared, this background temperature must be detected and subtracted out by the DSP. When the shutter is closed to calibrate the microbolometer, the pixels sense only the background heat within the imager; these background temperature values for each pixel are stored in memory. Once the shutter opens, thermal infrared emissions from the subject alter the resistance of the VOx leaflets. These open-shutter resistance values minus the closed-shutter values represent the radiance from the target and are stored in *corrected* radiometric memory for display or downloading.

Imager calibration is a complicated process that must be performed by the device manufacturer or a certified laboratory. To calibrate each pixel of a microbolometer, the entire system is checked at several known temperatures. These temperature-calibrated values for each pixel are then stored in the Pixel Correction Memory. The final corrected image is radiometric, meaning each pixel value represents an actual surface temperature value. The corrected radiometric pixel matrix is then converted into a visible image for display.

Up to 1% of pixels may be non-functional on a microbolometer chip. They are usually "corrected" by assigning them the average value of the eight adjacent pixels, thus excluding wildly erroneous pixel values from the final image matrix. Although these flawed pixels are hard to detect, they usually are not clinically significant. Without the merging of analog pixels with digital memory and correction, infrared imaging quality would be quite poor, as illustrated in Figure 3.2.

The components comprising a thermal imaging system are selected with considerable care. Within the 8- to 12-µm portion of the infrared spectrum, thermal radiation can only be focused with optics made of Germanium crystal, potassium bromide, sodium chloride, zinc salts, or surface mirrors.[9] These specially coated infrared lenses represent a significant cost factor in infrared imagers. Germanium crystal is the most frequently used lens material due to its hardness, chemical resistance, good polish qualities, and high refractive index, which enables the use of thinner lenses.[10] Each lens assembly must be calibrated for infrared transmission to facilitate correct thermal measurements. This is especially critical for thermal imagers with interchangeable lenses.

Description of an Imager Block Diagram, Figure 3.3: A warm human subject emits infrared rays in the 10-µm wavelength band. A coated Germanium crystal lens passes over 90% of 7- to 12-µm infrared rays while blocking visible, ultraviolet, and near-infrared light.[11] The lens focuses the infrared emissions from the subject's body onto the microbolometer leaflet array. The normally open shutter closes on command, blocking any external infrared entering through the lens to allow "zeroing" the thermal offset caused by the imager's internal temperature. When the shutter opens, the microbolometer chip inside its hermetically sealed vacuum case senses the heat image radiating from the subject, as shown in Figure 3.4. The amplified electronic output is a timed serial string of pixel-specific uncalibrated analog voltages that are digitized in an A-D converter, digitally corrected to represent calibrated temperature values, and then displayed or transmitted as a radiometric or non-radiometric image.

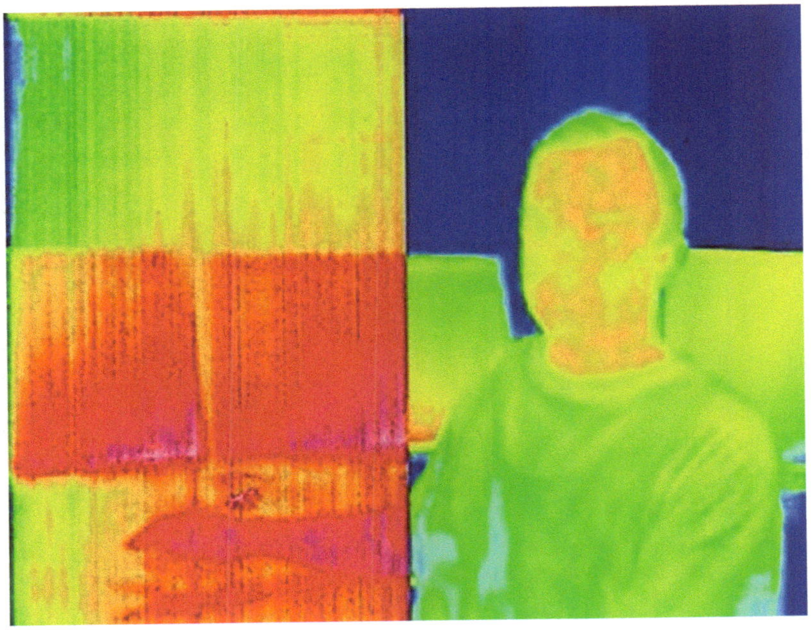

FIGURE 3.2 A thermal image showing uncorrected (*left*) versus corrected (*right*) microbolometer pixels values.[8]

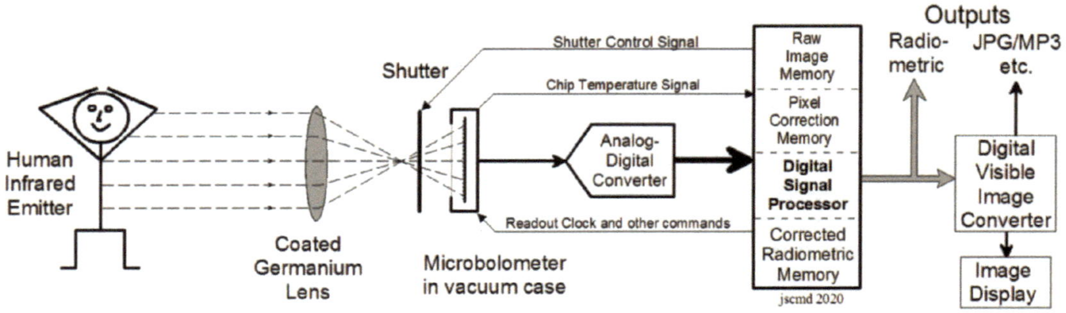

FIGURE 3.3 Flow diagram of an uncooled microbolometer-based digital infrared thermal imager.

Imager sensitivity and thermoelectric noise

When choosing a thermal imager, the sensitivity of the infrared detector is of paramount importance. Sensitivity is inversely related to the amount of noise generated by the system's electronics. All electronic devices develop quantum noise that is experienced audibly as the well-known background radio "hiss." This noise is an unavoidable byproduct of the microbolometer's electronics, which are measuring the amount of infrared heat falling on the bolometer leaflets as a tiny change in resistance. To measure a resistor's value requires passing electric current through it. As electrons flow through the VOx resistor leaflet and into the amplifier, they jump from molecule to molecule, creating a background hiss of white noise. Temperature changes causing signal changes smaller than this electronic noise cannot be measured – they are literally "down in the noise." *Thermoelectric noise* refers to the temperature difference that would cause the same signal change as the intrinsic electronic noise.

One of the key metrics for assessing an imager's sensitivity is the Noise Equivalent Temperature Difference (NETD). This is a measure of how well the detector is able to distinguish between very small differences in infrared radiation represented within the image. More specifically, NETD is the difference between two temperatures needed to generate a variation of the thermal imager signal equal to its quantum noise level. It can be understood as the imager's thermal resolution and is typically expressed in milli-Kelvins (mK) or degrees centigrade (°C), with 100 mK equaling 0.1°C NETD.

A low NETD results in better thermal sensitivity and resolution in the final image, with 50 mK (0.05°C) being the maximum NETD recommended for human thermography. This thermoelectric noise is the main source of measurement and display limitation in modern imagers. The older "Flying Spot" (single-detector) thermal scanners had acceptable sensor NETD values of around 100 mK (0.1°C), but they were incapable of visually displaying temperature differences smaller than 0.5–1.0°C over a 10°C span. Thus the good sensitivity of the thermal sensor was lost due to the poor display technology of that time.

A typical modern microbolometer has a thermal sensitivity of about 50 mK (0.05°C) at 30°C. This NETD level allows accurate infrared difference measurements down to 0.05°C or approximately 0.1°F. Assuming a clinically significant temperature difference of 0.5°C (~1°F), the thermal signal-to-noise ratio will be about a factor of ten. Clinically significant thermographic temperature differences are thus well above the typical noise level of a good microbolometer. When used with a blackbody temperature

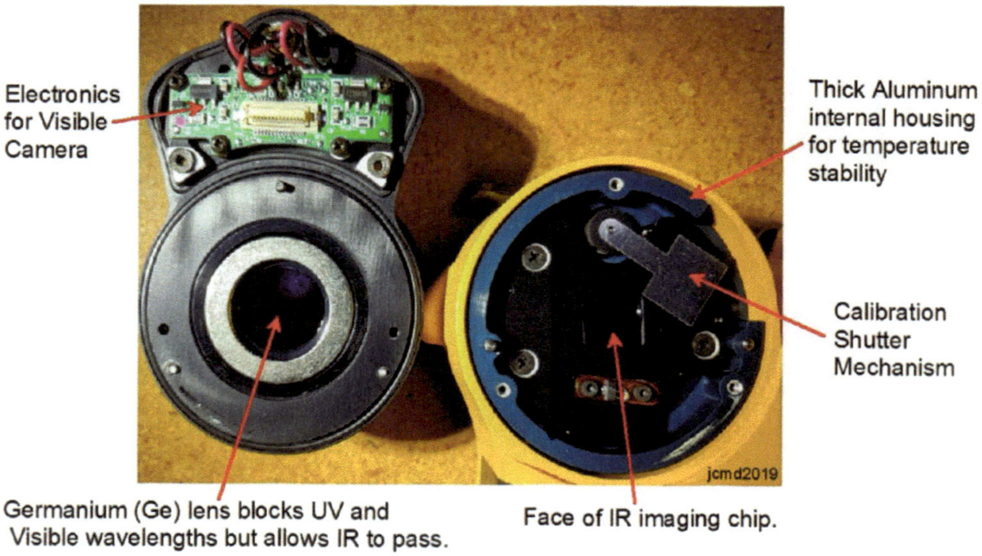

FIGURE 3.4 The interior of an infrared imager showing the optical components, shutter mechanism, and housing. Note that there is no radiation-reducing iris in a thermal imager.[12]

standard in the image, microbolometers have been found to be accurate enough for non-contact fever screening.[13]

Spatial resolution of infrared imagers

Spatial resolution is of vital importance for medical infrared imaging. To maintain sufficient spatial resolution and thereby enable accurate interpretation, the region of interest (ROI) should be positioned close enough to the thermal imager to fill most of the viewable image frame without causing undue spherical or "fisheye" distortion.[14] This is to increase visualization of smaller thermographic findings such as lymphatic inflammation, skin neoplasms, and vascular detail. If multiple views are required for bilaterally equivalent areas of the body, all equipment settings must remain essentially unchanged for these views.

With the recent advent of 640 × 480-pixel microbolometer imagers, spatial resolution recommendations for full-body imaging must be reexamined. In the "portrait" orientation, a typical 640 × 480 imager provides a vertical field of view (FOV) of 34°, and a horizontal FOV of 24°.[15] A 1.83 meter-tall (72 inch/6 foot) subject will subtend an FOV of 34° (640 pixels) at a focal distance of 2.7 meters (107 inches/8.9 feet). At this distance, the target's spot size per pixel is 2.9 mm (0.11 inch) on a side, assuming the pixels are square. This is much larger (i.e., worse) than the maximum spot size of one square millimeter recommended for breast exams.[16] Though this resolution is adequate to detect larger thermal findings such as muscle warmth, large-joint inflammation, and varicose veins, it is inadequate for reliably detecting smaller findings such as lymphatic patterns or fine vascular markings. To detect these smaller details with a 640 × 480-pixel imager, either the camera-to-subject distance must be shortened to less than 0.94 meters (37 inches/3.1 feet), or an infrared telephoto lens must be used.

Focusing the imager: Manual vs. automatic

When it comes to viewing and focusing, thermal imagers function very much like normal digital cameras. Each imager has a sighting area called the FOV, which typically varies between 6° for a telescopic lens and 48° for a wide-angle lens. Standard imager optics have a typical 24° by 34° FOV. Wide-angle lenses may create an undesirable "fisheye" distortion of human subjects. Although telescopic lenses are useful for fever screenings, the FOV they provide is too small for a typical thermography room, and atmospheric IR losses may become significant.

For optimal thermal resolution, there is consensus among breast thermographers that the ROI should fill approximately 75% of the image.[17] When an object is located farther away and thus appears small in the image, it "illuminates" fewer pixels, providing less spatial resolution. Thus, finer details will be harder to distinguish qualitatively. A minimum practical distance from subject to imager will provide the best image resolution.

Manual focus

It can be challenging to manually focus infrared images. Human thermal images are intrinsically blurry because the lateral heat gradient of normal skin is only about 0.1°C per mm (~0.5°F per 1/10th inch).[18] One trick for manually enhancing the sharpness of an image is to focus on a hair, nipple edge, skin fold, or blemish, as shown in Figure 3.5. Focusing on other anatomical edges or

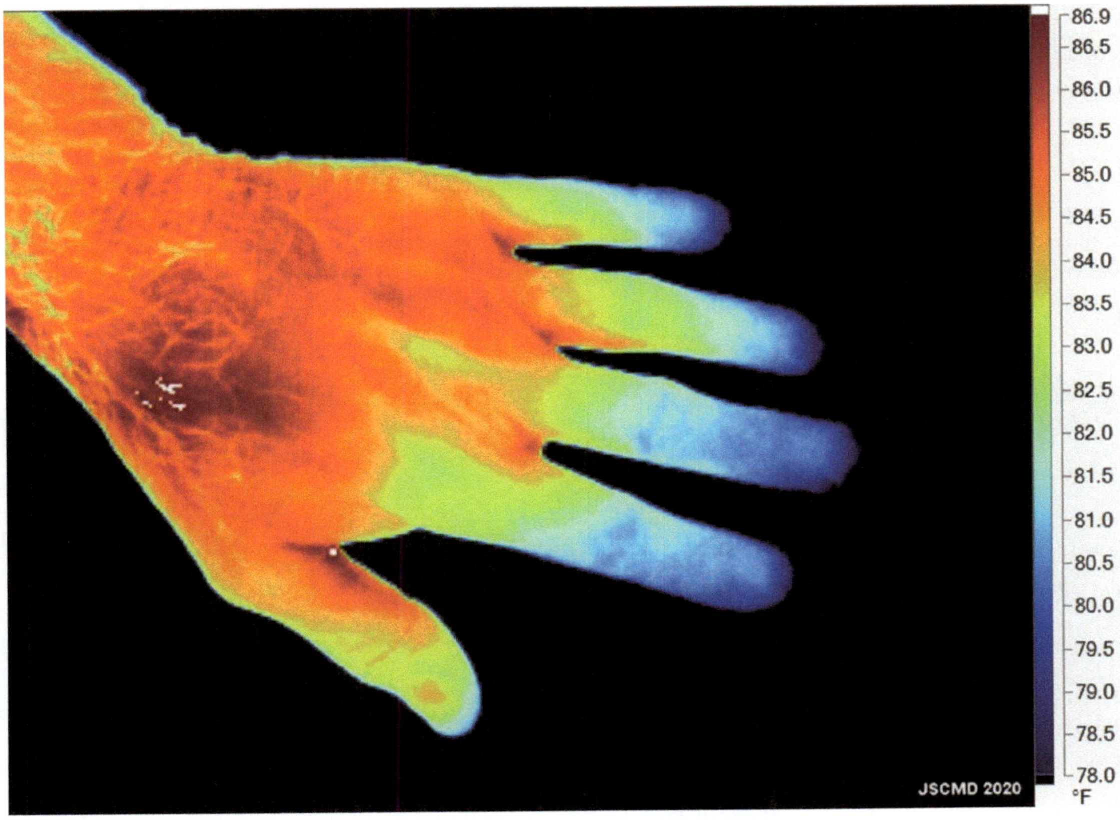

FIGURE 3.5 Appearance of hair in a focused infrared image. Manual focusing can be facilitated by making hairs in the image appear sharp.

contours can be similarly helpful. Small metallic fiducial markers placed on the ROI can also aid manual focusing. Greyscale images may be easier to focus manually than color images. Out-of-focus images impair the detection of smaller thermographic findings and may give significant radiometric temperature errors, with lower temperatures detected in an out-of-focus image.[19]

Automatic laser focus

Automatic focus is highly recommended for producing sharp, clear, and calibrated thermal images. When using a laser focusing mechanism, care should be exercised to avoid directing the light beam into the subject's eyes. Direct the laser toward the forehead or chin when imaging the face. When using laser focus, carefully observe the laser beam on the ROI to be sure the correct area is being measured, not the wall behind. A laser focusing beam is not visible in the thermal image, but it can be seen on the visible-band camera in the imager, if so equipped, or by directly observing the subject. The autofocus feature is useful for documenting the focus distance in a report. The autofocus distance is often stated in the image metadata. Documented distance measurements are useful to assure consistent repeat images of a subject.

Physical considerations in choosing a thermal imager

The major physical formats of professional thermal imagers are as follows:

- Handheld imagers
- Fixed position single imagers
- Multiple fixed-position imager arrays

Some imager types work better than others, depending on the thermography needs of an individual clinic.

Handheld imagers

Handheld imaging techniques allow close-up and custom views as well as standard views in both breast and general thermography exams. Several different types of handheld imagers are shown in Figure 3.6. As the height and body habit of different subjects can vary greatly, this flexibility to direct the image axis and distance is very useful. The thermographer can hold the imager at the proper height, angle, and distance from the ROI in order to produce the best thermal image possible. Nevertheless, with handheld imaging, it may be difficult to closely reproduce the same image angle and distance in future imaging sessions. This makes session-to-session image comparison more challenging for the image interpreter.

High-quality handheld thermal imagers are available in a "pistol-grip" format. These are usually less expensive than swiveling-head imagers because the physical packaging and electronics inside the unit are easier to manufacture. Such imagers are well suited for standard breast and upper body imaging sites; however, areas such as the top of the scalp may require special positioning of the subject. In some cases, the thermographer may need to kneel or crouch down on the floor for a proper imaging angle of the lower legs or underside of the breasts.

For ease in full-body imaging, handheld imagers are available with viewing screens that rotate in relation to the imager lens. These are called "Swiveling-head" imagers. An imager head that can swivel in relation to the viewing screen makes it much easier to image subjects from below or above, allowing images of the scalp, underside of the breasts, shins, or Achilles tendons without the thermographer having to kneel, stoop, or stand on tiptoes. Swiveling handheld thermal imagers are available from several manufacturers with specifications well suited for human thermography.

Fixed-position imagers

Fixed tripod-mounted thermal imagers allow for standardized views such as those used in breast imaging. These imagers may not have a built-in viewing screen. Instead, the thermal image appears on a remote computer screen that may be in a separate control room. The obvious advantage of these imagers is their ability to maintain a consistent viewing height, angle, and distance to the subject from one imaging session to the next.

Even with the tripod technique, however, direct image comparison between sessions is difficult.[22] The subject's position must be directed by the thermographer in order to obtain the frontal, oblique, and lateral breast views, this is likely to introduce positioning errors. Imaging the underside of pendulous

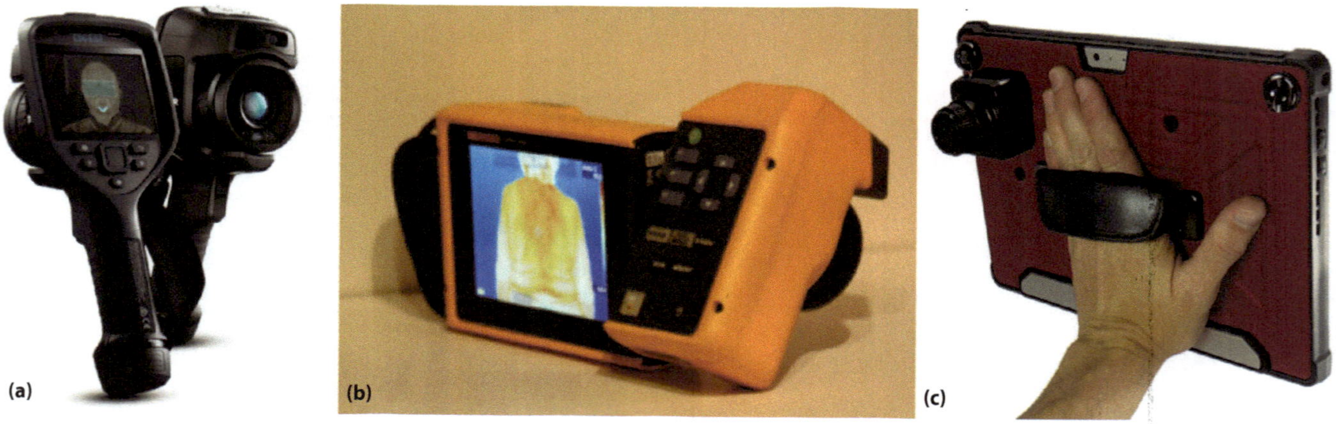

FIGURE 3.6 Handheld imagers: (a) A "pistol-grip" thermal imager optimized for physiologic temperatures.[20] (b) An infrared imager with a swiveling head which facilitates imaging at steep angles. (c) A small infrared imager attached to a tablet computer which displays the image.[21]

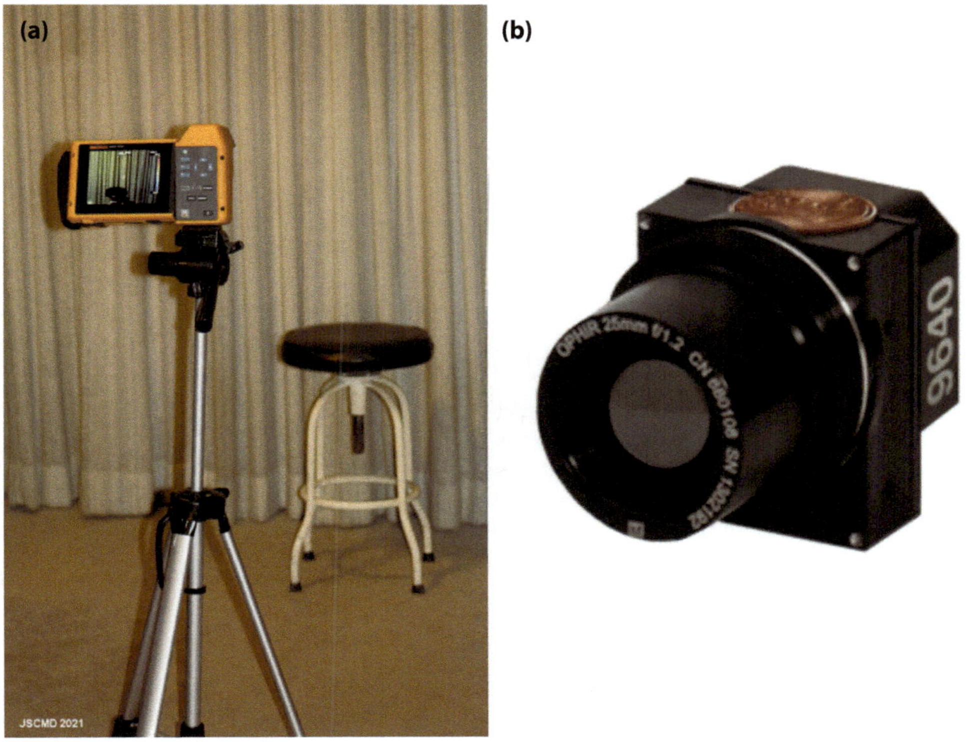

FIGURE 3.7 Fixed position imagers: (a) A fixed, tripod-mounted imager for breast thermography. (b) Small radiometric thermal imagers like this model can be mounted in arrays to facilitate routine examinations.[23]

breasts is a problem with the single fixed-imager technique, and some clinics will omit this very important view because of the positioning difficulty. In general thermography, fixed-position imagers are not recommended for high-resolution full-body thermal imaging.

For a high-volume thermography clinic such as one dedicated to breast imaging, multiple precision thermal imagers may be placed in an array at the proper positions and angles to obtain the four or more views of the exam simultaneously (see the chapter on Breast Thermography for details on these views). Very small radiometric thermal imagers are available for this purpose (Figure 3.7). Three such imagers can be mounted on an apparatus that can be adjusted for the subject's breast height level to obtain the frontal and oblique views. A fourth imager may be mounted near the floor and directed upward to obtain the underside image of the breasts. These small imagers typically do not have a monitoring screen; instead their imaging axis and focus are monitored on a computer in the imaging control room. Focusing all the imagers in the system to accommodate different size subjects may be a problem. For this reason, autofocusing imagers are recommended. Generating thermography reports for multi-imager systems may require specialized software to facilitate the process.

Software considerations in choosing a thermal imager

Perhaps more important than the physical aspects of an imager is the imaging interpretation and report writing software that is usually supplied with an imager. Without this interpretation software, the imager and its radiometric image files are useless for thermographic viewing, measuring, editing, and reporting. Unfortunately, there is no accepted universal radiometric file format at this time. Almost all imager manufacturers have their own proprietary radiometric file format that can only be read by their software. A thermographer who has image files in a certain format is compelled to rely on that manufacturer's imagers and software. If a manufacturer decides to no longer support a certain radiometric file format, or if the company should close, all files in that format may become obsolete and useless to interpretation.[24] To use the Latin phrase, *caveat emptor* – let the buyer beware – the thermographer uses the software at his or her own risk in the absence of any universal file format system.

Radiometric files and images

Every valid pixel value in an infrared radiometric file *is* the detected and corrected surface temperature of that spot on the target surface. Radiometric files are the most accurate for analysis of actual surface temperatures, and the visual color or greyscale images are derived from them. These files can be opened by the imager manufacturer's proprietary software as thermal images, which can then be scaled to maximize the qualitative information provided by the data. These radiometric thermal images can be visually adjusted, annotated, and analyzed with point, line, and area temperature measurements. Being a proprietary format, however, radiometric files are usually not readable by other imaging or thermographic software. The imager manufacturer may provide numeric output of the radiometric data in matrix spreadsheet format, but specialized programming and software are required to analyze, image, or interpret this numeric data.

Radiometric files may also contain a wealth of metadata. This metadata is useful because it records the date and time of the image, the emissivity setting, lens and imager type, the imaging

File Location	C:\Thermography Files\[illegible]3\IR_00915.IS2
Image Time	[illegible]/2017 4:18:14 PM
Emissivity	0.98
Background Temp	70.0 °F
Transmission	100%
Image Range	68.3 °F to 94.1 °F
Average Temp	79.2 °F
Severity	
Camera model	TiX500
IR Sensor Size	320 x 240
Camera Manufacturer	Fluke Thermography
Calibration Range	-4.0 °F to 176.0 °F
Camera serial number	TiX500-1[illegible]
Lens description	FLK-LENS/TELE2
SOC Version	4.2.2

FIGURE 3.8 Typical proprietary metadata within a radiometric image file. Emissivity, background temperature, IR transmission, and "severity" notations are manually entered into the imager. An internal clock provides the image time to the second. The other data is known or detected by the imager.[25]

distance, and other important information, as shown in Figure 3.8. This metadata may not be available except via the imager manufacturer's proprietary interpretation software.

Non-radiometric thermal images

At present, the best way to share or compare edited and annotated images taken with different manufacturers' imagers is to convert them to a universal digital image format such as JPG, PNG, or TIF once they are fully measured and labeled on the radiometric image. PNG and TIF formats are preferred as they are "lossless" non-compressed formats as opposed to the standard JPG format, which can distort an image. Image conversion from radiometric to a non-radiometric format may require the use of a screen "snipping tool" to capture and save an image at high resolution from the interpretation software display screen, as shown in Figure 3.9. The copied image can be easily stored in a file or "pasted" into a report. Images exported via a command in the manufacturer's software may have poor resolution.

A qualitative image (JPG, TIFF, PNG, etc.) requires an accompanying temperature scale for quantitative temperature estimations. Even with a scale or digital color-comparison analysis, these images are not accurate for precise absolute or differential temperature measurements unless radiometric temperatures over the points or areas of interest are displayed on the image.

Thermal image transfer

In the process of selecting a thermal imager, learn how the device transfers the image files for later interpretation and report generation. Ideally, the system enables not only a secure image transfer but also a high degree of convenience. Such a tradeoff occurs when transferring removable physical media (i.e., flash drive, Secure Digital card, or microSD card), which requires removing the media from the imager and then reading it on the office computer, before eventually returning it to

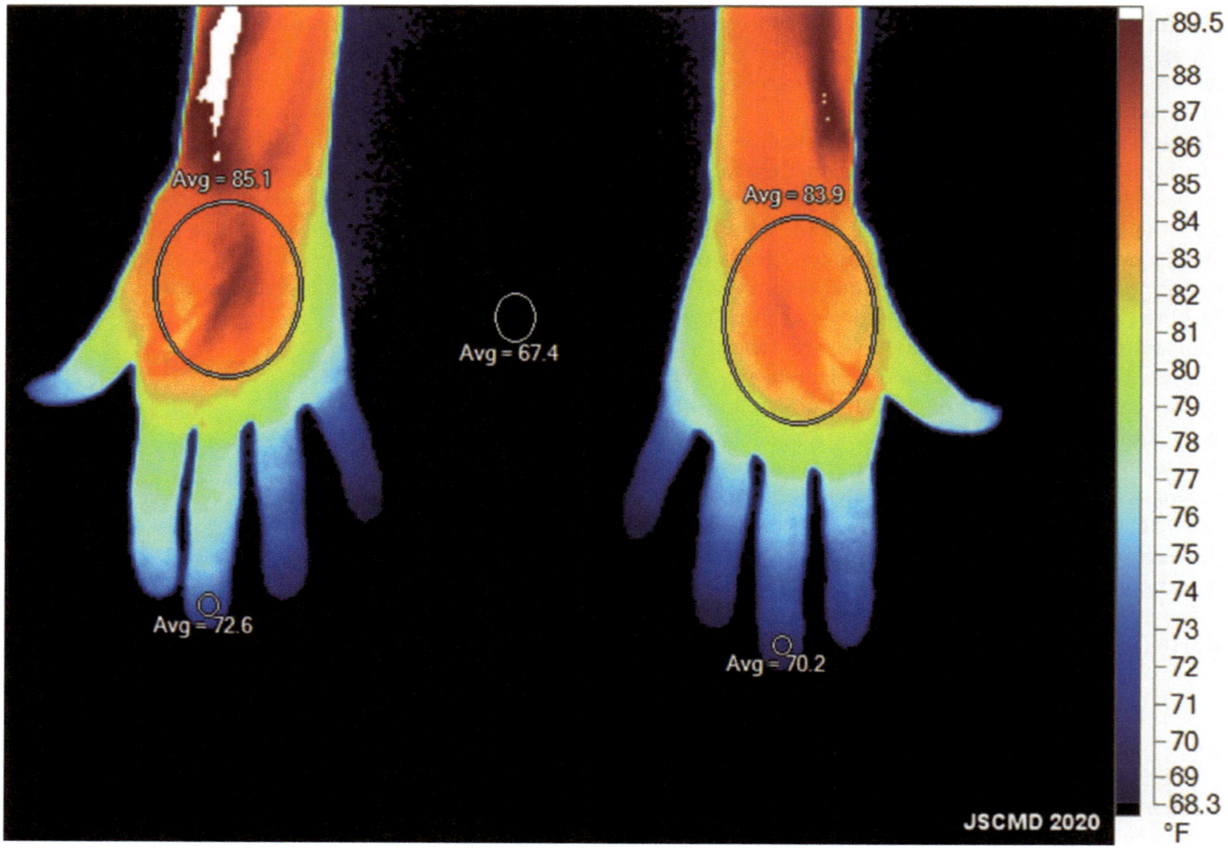

FIGURE 3.9 A non-radiometric (PNG) "Screengrab" with the color palette span and area temperature data added while the image was in the radiometric format. Further temperature measurements or color span adjustments are no longer possible in this format.

the imager. This method is secured from hacking, but not from damage, loss, or theft.

Universal Serial Bus (USB) or Ethernet wire transfer requires plugging a cable from the imager directly into the computer (not through a router or hub), then directing the software to transfer the images. This connection is secure as it is a dedicated point-to-point line. Images on the imager may also be deleted through the wired interface, however. Such an accidental deletion is one way to completely lose image files.

Wireless (Wi-Fi) transfer is convenient as long as the connection works properly. There may be a problem initiating or maintaining a connection, especially in the event of imager software updates, Wi-Fi router problems, or computer system changes. The possibility of medical files being hacked or copied is ever-present in any wireless communication. As with a USB connection, the original files on the imager may be deleted by a command sent over the Wi-Fi connection; caution is advised to prevent the deletion of non-replaceable files.

If file transfer by Wi-Fi is activated on the imager, the USB connection may not work, or vice versa. Other problems may arise from both hardware and software. It is advisable to set the imager to store the image files on a removable physical memory, such as an SD card or USB memory stick. This removable memory can then be used to perform a manual image transfer in case other connections fail.

For transfer of the thermography clinic's patient files for off-site backup and interpretation, automatically encrypting USB hard-disk drives can hold patient files safely. Even if stolen, these drives are unreadable without the passcode. Encrypted email may also be used to transfer patient files for off-site interpretation. File storage and sharing through an internet server ("the cloud") should only be used if all files are encrypted before uploading. Thermographers should always maintain safe backup copies of all patient files because there is always the possibility that an employee may delete or alter files either accidentally or deliberately.

Standard imager care tips

- Protect the imager from marked heat or cold. Recommended imager storage temperatures are typically −4°F to +122°F (−20 to +50°C). Because these temperatures may be exceeded in a vehicle during winter or summer conditions, bring the imager indoors whenever confronted with extreme temperatures.
- Use the thermal imager only after it has been equilibrated to room temperature to avoid errors from temperature offset drift.
- Protect the imager from mechanical shock or drops. Keep the imager in a safe area or protective case when not in use, especially during transportation.
- Never expose the imager lens to sunlight or powerful laser light; common laser pointer beams will not damage the imager. When not in use, attach a lens cap to protect the valuable lens.
- The shutter is normally OPEN, thus the delicate microbolometer is always exposed to focused incoming thermal radiation which may damage the VOx leaflets.
- Industrial-grade imagers can usually withstand direct sunlight into the lens, though temporary image "ghosting" may occur. Damage to the imaging chip is possible.
- Remove or change the imager lens only in dry, dust-free, and low-infrared conditions. When the lens is removed, the infrared-transparent window of the microbolometer chip is fully exposed.
- Carefully clean the infrared lens, viewing screen, and visible camera lens occasionally as advised in the imager instructions.

SIDEBAR 3.1 INFRARED IMAGING AND FDA APPROVAL

Just as the US Food and Drug Administration (FDA) does not dictate to an individual medical practitioner which digital camera and display program may be used for evaluating, documenting, or following the *visual* appearance of a medical problem, FDA should not require listing of a properly calibrated 10-µm thermal imager and its standard display software for the evaluation, documentation, or follow-up of the *infrared* appearance of a medical problem. Actually, the FDA has been concerned less with thermal imagers than with practitioners promoting thermography as a stand-alone diagnostic method. The agency considers any thermal imaging system intended for stand-alone use in diagnostic screening a Class III (highly regulated) device, requiring a massive amount of clinical data and studies for approval. To date, no infrared imaging system has met this regulatory requirement.[26] The FDA approved breast thermography devices in 1982 only for use on an adjunctive basis with mammography and other diagnostic modalities, not as a stand-alone test.

Under the US law, thermal imagers are considered medical devices when they are *marketed* for use in the diagnosis of disease or other conditions or in the cure, mitigation, treatment, or prevention of disease. As long as a thermal imager or system is not marketed for medical purposes, it should not fall under the scope of the law. The FDA acknowledges it is not authorized to regulate the practice of medicine. A private practitioner may use any drug or device to help their patient without interference from FDA, though state law may limit medical practice and devices in that state.

Some infrared imaging systems designed and marketed specifically for medical purposes *are* FDA listed via 510(k) certification, meaning that they are "grandfathered in" because the technology existed before federal control of medical devices became law. These infrared imagers are currently classified as Class I devices, which are the *least* regulated. They are referred to as "Telethermographic Systems," which must be functionally equivalent to the long outmoded "predicate" thermal scanners of 1976. Being granted 510(k) certification only indicates that the device is "listed" with the FDA; it does not imply any *approval* per se. No clinical studies, actual thermal images, spatial resolution specifications, or temperature calibration data are required in the application for 510(k) listing.[27]

FDA-listed thermography systems may not be as well-calibrated, convenient, versatile, or well-supported as a commercial "off-the-shelf" thermal imager and software product, and they will likely cost far more. Regardless of FDA status, thermographers are advised to be sure their imagers are fully calibrated and used clinically under the controlled thermographic conditions delineated in this book. Practitioners are also cautioned not to claim capabilities for human thermography that are beyond the scope of the field and not supported by valid clinical studies.[28]

Notes

1. The CPT (Current Procedural Terminology) reimbursement codes are maintained and copyrighted by the American Medical Association.
2. DICOM: Digital Imaging and Communications in Medicine. The international standard to transmit, store, retrieve, print, process, and display medical imaging. See more at https://www.dicomstandard.org/
3. *See* Fluke Corporation Ti401 PRO, Ti480 PRO, TiX501, and TiX580 Infrared Camera Specification Sheet 2019 *and* FLIR Model T860-24 Specification Sheet 2019.
4. See various thermal imager NEDT noise specifications at the SPI Corporation website: https://www.x20.org/shop
5. Illustration from Moreno M, et al., Ch 2 of Bolometers, Prof. Unil Perera (Ed.), InTechOpen 2012; ISBN: 978-953-51-0235-9, CC-BY-3.0.
6. Images B and C from: Chen Chao, et al., J Vibroengineering 2015; 17(5). © 2015 JVE International Ltd. CC-BY-4.0.
7. Forsberg F, et al. IEEE J Sel Top Quantum Electron. Jul/Aug 2015; 21(4). Doi: 10.1109/JSTQE.2014.2358198
8. Image from: Budzier H & Gerlach G, J Sens Sens Syst. 2015. Doi: 10.5162/irs2015/1.1 (CC-BY-4.0)
9. Source: Diakides NA, Bronzino JD, eds., Medical Infrared Imaging, Section 5.6. CRC Press, Boca Raton, FL, 2008.
10. Dakin JP & Brown RGW, eds., Handbook of Optoelectronics, Vol I, 2nd Ed, Section 18.2.7. CRC Press, 2017. ISBN 9781482241785.
11. *See* Thorlabs, Newton NJ USA: Germanium Window Specification Sheet, accessed March 2022: https://www.thorlabs.com/thorproduct.cfm?partnumber=WG91050-G
12. The interior of a Fluke Ti55 thermal imager is shown.
13. Ghassemi P, et al. PLoS One. 2018. Doi: 10.1371/journal.pone.0203302
14. https://aathermology.org/organization-2/guidelines/guidelines-for-breast-thermology/, Section 3.1.
15. *From*: Specifications for the TiX501 Infrared Camera, 640 × 480, 60 Hz, Fluke Corporation, Everett, WA 2019.
16. https://aathermology.org/organization-2/guidelines/guidelines-for-breast-thermology/, Section 3.2.
17. Breast Thermography Guideline 3.1, 2018, Am. Acad. Thermology, Greenville, SC. https://aathermology.org/
18. Anbar M, Quantitative Dynamic Telethermometry in Medical Diagnosis and Management, 1st Ed, CRC Press, London, 1994, p. 112.
19. *See:* Fluke Corp Thermal Imaging Blog. https://www.fluke.com/en-us/learn/blog/thermal-imaging/thermal-camera-accuracy
20. Image courtesy of FLIR Systems Inc., Wilsonville, OR. Used with permission.
21. Image courtesy of ICI – Infrared Cameras Inc., Beaumont, TX. Used with permission.
22. Ring F, et al., eds. Infrared Imaging, A Casebook in Clinical Medicine, IOP Publishing LTD, Bristol, UK, 2015, Chapter 2 by Karl Ammer, p. 2-1.
23. Photo courtesy of ICI – Infrared Cameras Inc., Beaumont, TX. Used with permission.
24. Goodman M. Understanding Proprietary Infrared Image Files. IRINFO.ORG, Burlington, NJ. https://irinfo.org/04-01-2006-colbert/
25. Data metafile information as shown by Fluke SmartView version 4.3.122.0. Identification information redacted.
26. See: U.S. Code of Federal Regulations 21CFR Sec. 884.2980 Telethermographic system, 1 Apr 2019.
27. For example, see: FDA 510(k) Application K171928, approved 8 Dec 2017.
28. See: Aicher RH, Is the FDA Regulating the Practice of Medicine? Aesthet Surg J. 2013; PMID: 23515389.

4

VERIFYING THERMAL IMAGER CALIBRATION

Why should a thermographer be so concerned with the physical principles, operation, and care of a thermal imager? Because with any complicated combination of microscopic analog devices, mechanical mechanisms, and compensatory digital software, a great deal can go wrong. Sometimes the problem is readily discerned. The imager may freeze up or reboot frequently. The device may fail to turn on in the first place, or the image may become streaked or speckled with noise. At other times, however, significant problems are far more subtle and may even go unnoticed because the imager seems fully operational, generating clear and complete images. The primary focus of this chapter is on those subtle yet critical errors that can be overlooked unless they are checked at regular intervals.

Thermal imagers measure microbolometer leaflet resistance, not temperature. Thus, they must be calibrated at the factory using a series of known blackbody temperatures and sensing the resultant resistance values, as shown in Figure 4.1. During calibration, a reference table is produced containing the digitized temperature/resistance measurements entered into the calibration software. Every microbolometer pixel within the imager's FPA chip has a slightly different temperature offset and gain. To produce an accurate thermogram, these different gains and offsets must be corrected to a normalized value. The manufacturer's calibration software accomplishes this via non-uniformity correction (NUC), which uses multi-point correction of both thermal gain and offset of each pixel. The pixel calibration is stored in the imager's memory as a numeric table that relates resistance values to blackbody temperatures. Later, when the imaging system takes a measurement, it utilizes the calibration data to calculate the sensed surface temperature.

Up to 1% of the pixels in a microbolometer array may produce outputs far outside of a correctable range. Ideally, the NUC process identifies these faulty pixels and replaces them using a nearest-neighbor averaging algorithm. Faulty pixels are difficult to detect during routine imager operation due to the NUC process. Fortunately, these faulty pixels are not clinically significant as long as the bad pixels are scattered throughout the detector matrix and not adjacent to one another.

As pixel offset and gain may change with time, the imager needs to be recalibrated periodically, typically every two years. This chapter is concerned with checking the imager's calibration to assure these offset and gain values remain within specified limits over all regions of the image.

The following three measurements are necessary when manually verifying the calibration of a thermal imager:

1. **Thermal Gain.** An actual 1.0°C (1.8°F) temperature difference between two locations on a target should be detected and displayed as a 1.0°C (1.8°F) temperature difference by a properly calibrated thermal imager; i.e., the Thermal Gain should be 1.0. This 1:1 relationship should remain constant whether the measurement is near room temperature (Troom, ~20°C/68°F), body temperature (Tbody, ~37°C/98.6°F), or at any temperature in between. If the thermal gain is in error, a 1.0°C (1.8°F) temperature difference on a target may be displayed by the imager as only 0.2°C (0.36°F) or some other wrong value, making the quantitative measurements erroneous, yet the qualitative image may still appear completely normal by adjusting the color span.[2] As the quantitative interpretation of human thermograms relies heavily on differential temperature measurements, assuring a Thermal Gain between 0.95 and 1.05 (preferably 1.0) across the physiologic temperature range is of paramount importance.
2. **Temperature Offset.** This refers to the temperature difference between the target surface temperature detected by the infrared imager and the actual temperature of that surface. Temperature offset and thermal gain are related: if the imager's offset value is stable across the physiologic temperature range, the thermal gain will be 1.0 over those temperatures. Stable offset values up to ±2°C (3.6°F) are typical for professional microbolometer imagers.
3. **Temperature Flatness.** "Flatness" measures the consistency of a constant temperature object as sensed at different regions of the image, usually measured at the center and four corners of the image at Troom. The imager should be fully warmed up before this test so that the imaging chip has reached a stable temperature. The flatness of the image at Tbody can also be measured by using a Blackbody Calibrator.

Procedures for verifying thermal calibration of an imager

What follows is a description of simple ways the thermal GAIN, OFFSET, and FLATNESS of an imager can be checked without sending it off to the calibration laboratory. If any of these tests indicate that the imager is out of specification, then professional recalibration is essential. There is no way the imager can be adjusted by the user. Contact the imager manufacturer for the best way to accomplish calibration. Private companies can also recalibrate an imager, but they may not be able to perform repairs if necessary, creating more delay in returning a functioning and calibrated unit.

The contact and non-contact thermometers (NCTs) described here are invaluable for quick-and-easy calibration verification of infrared imagers, and they are always useful for checking the temperatures of the thermography room, spot points on the thermography subject, and any water baths used in the imaging procedures. A serious thermography center should include both contact and non-contact thermometers and keep them calibrated to NIST standards. The electronic displays of the thermometers should have a minimum resolution of 0.05°C (~0.1°F).

Measuring the imager thermal GAIN

This test should be performed in a proper thermographic environment without infrared heat sources such as sunlight or incandescent lighting. Additionally, there should be minimal airflow and a room temperature of about 21°C (70°F). This is the simplest, quickest, and least expensive way to validate the GAIN of a thermal imager at physiologic temperatures via a two-point calibration.

Equipment Needed:

- A calibrated non-contact thermometer (NCT), thermopile type; the unit should be at room temperature.

DOI: 10.1201/9781003281764-5

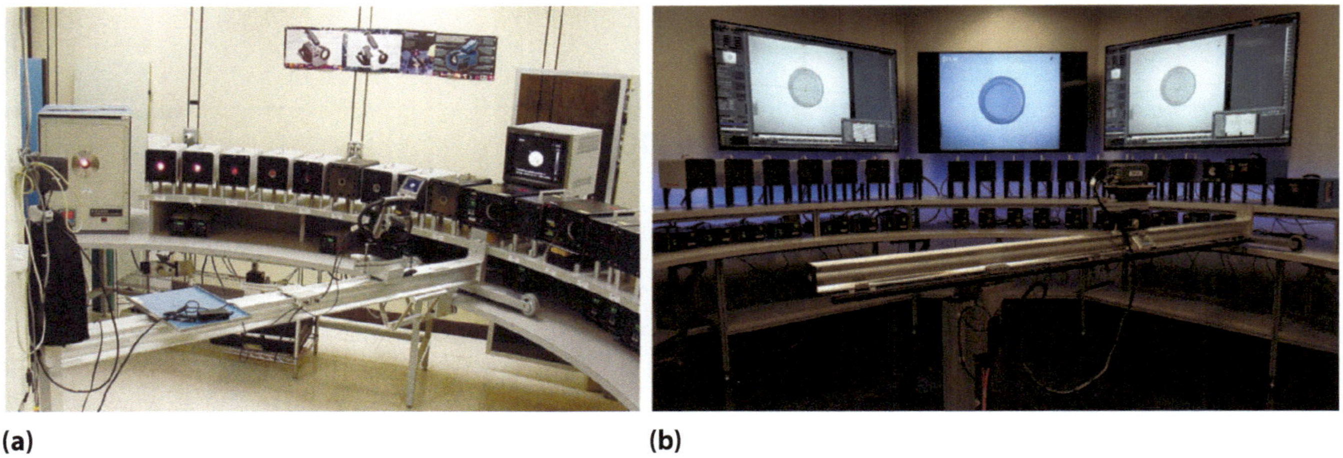

FIGURE 4.1 (a) An early thermal imager calibration laboratory. Note that some of the blackbody temperature standards on the left side are glowing red. (b) A modern calibration laboratory also arranged in a semicircle of temperature standards.[1]

- The imager being tested (IMGR), turned on, and fully warmed up.
  - The Emissivity setting of the imager should match the emissivity value of the NCT.[3]
  - The Background Temperature setting of the imager should match the actual room temperature.
- A room-temperature matte target such as foam-core art-board (Troom).
- A stable blackbody temperature reference between 32°C and 38°C (90°F and 100°F) (Tbody)
  - Tbody may be a simulated by a human forehead or a blackbody calibrator.

Procedure:
In quick succession, to minimize any temperature drift:

A. With the NCT, measure Troom off the matte surface and record the value as "Troom(NCT)"; ignore any Temperature offset (Figure 4.2a).
B. With the same instrument, measure a surface with a temperature representing Tbody, and record the value as "Tbody(NCT)." Tbody may be generated by a normal human forehead as shown in Figure 4.2b or by a Blackbody Calibrator (see Figure 4.9, page 34). Using an observation mirror increases the accuracy of this operation.

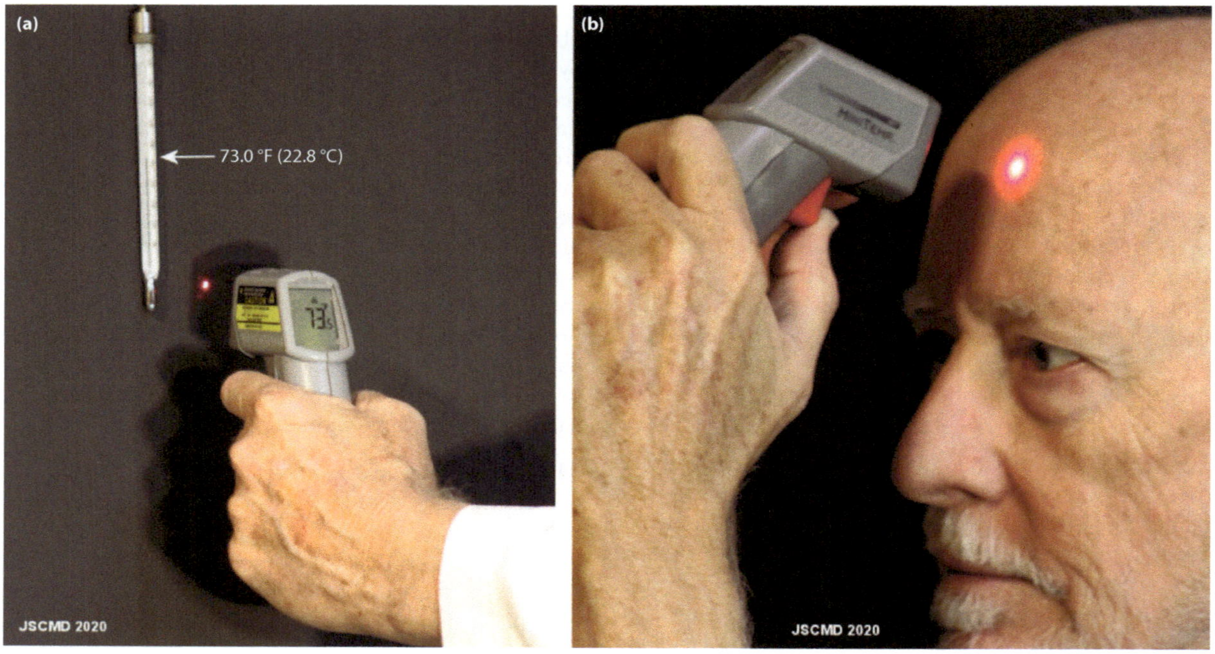

FIGURE 4.2 (a) Measuring Troom with a thermopile non-contact thermometer (NCT). (b) Measuring Tbody at the forehead with the same non-contact thermometer.

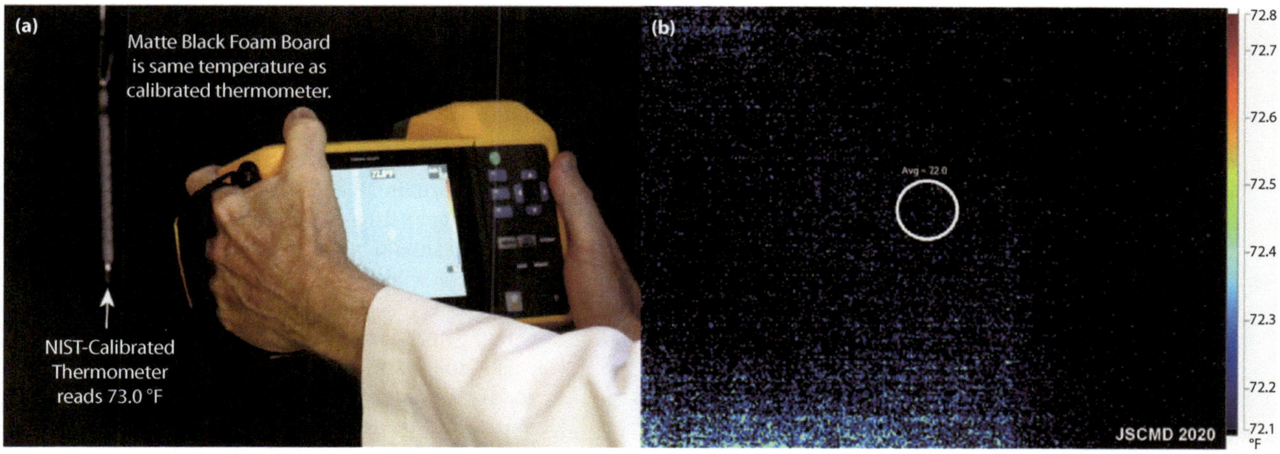

FIGURE 4.3 Measuring Troom with the imager. (a) A focused thermal image is taken of a matte board of known temperature. (b) An area at the center of the image is selected to determine Troom(IMGR).

C. Now with the imager, measure Troom by taking a *focused* image of the matte board as shown in Figure 4.3a and record the value as "Troom(IMGR)." For best accuracy, Troom is an average area measurement taken near the center of the image (Figure 4.3b).

D. Continuing with the imager, measure Tbody at the same site measured by the NCT (see Figure 4.4). Record the value as "Tbody(IMGR)." Using a mirror to observe the monitor and focusing laser may simplify this operation. For best accuracy, Tbody is an average area measurement as shown. Tbody may be taken from a forehead or from a Blackbody Calibrator.

E. Now calculate the following *difference values*. Note that any IMGR or NCT temperature offsets will be subtracted out at this step if their emissivity values have been set to the same value:

$$\textbf{For the Thermometer (NCT): Tbody} - \textbf{Troom} = \Delta\textbf{Tnct}$$

and

$$\textbf{For the Imager (IMGR): Tbody} - \textbf{Troom} = \Delta\textbf{Timgr}$$

F. Subtract these two difference values to quantify any GAIN error:

$$\Delta\textbf{Tnct} - \Delta\textbf{Timgr} = \textbf{Temperature Detection Difference (TDD)}$$

G. TDD should be within ±0.55°C (±1°F) for imager GAIN validation.

H. If TDD remains out of range after correcting any settings errors explained in the notes, the imager will need to be sent out for calibration.

Notes on Checking Thermal GAIN:

1. After obtaining a suitable forehead image to determine Tbody, delineate an area approximately the same place as the NCT reading was taken. The image may reveal abnormal warm spots over the forehead, such as a pimple, insect bite, or other lesion. If such abnormalities are present, use another subject's more isothermal forehead or a stable 35°C (95°F) Blackbody Calibrator to simulate Tbody.

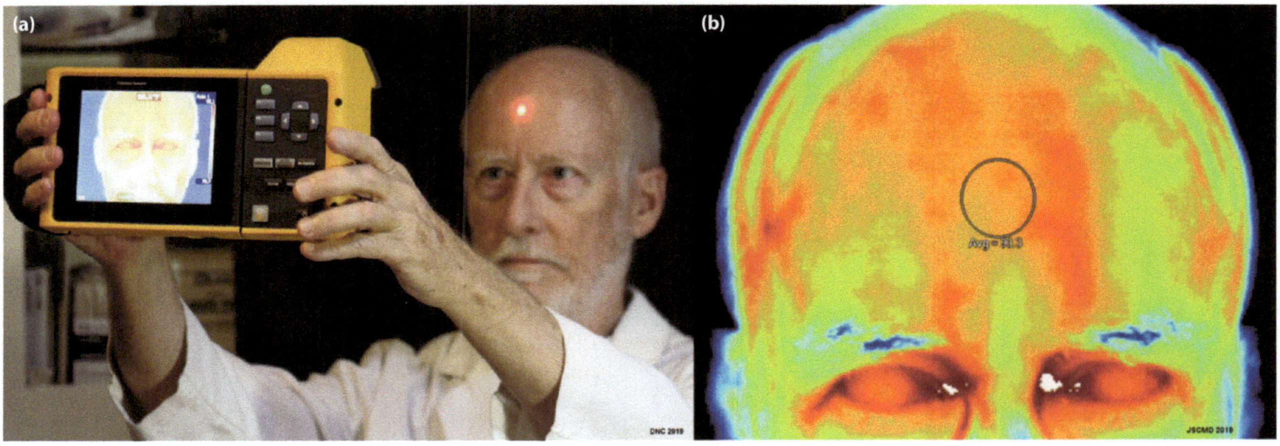

FIGURE 4.4 Measuring Tbody with the imager. (a) Focusing the imager using the laser focus. (b) The thermogram taken by the imager showing the area of temperature measurement.

2. As the minimum temperature change from Troom to Tbody is about 11°C (20°F), a maximum Temperature Detection Difference (TDD) over this range of 0.55°C (1°F) represents a 5% GAIN error and is generally acceptable for clinical measurements. A 5% gain error in a clinically significant difference measurement of 1°C (1.8°F) would cause an acceptable error of ±0.05°C (0.09°F), about the same as a typical NETD of an uncooled microbolometer.
3. If the Thermal GAIN of the Imager Under Test (IUT) is out of specification, be sure the imager's emissivity is set to match that of the NCT, and the Background Temperature value entered into the imager matches the actual room temperature. High-end thermopile NCTs may have adjustable emissivity settings, in which case both units should be set for 0.98 if using a forehead as Tbody. Non-adjustable thermopile NCTs usually have a default emissivity of 0.95, in which case setting the imager (IMGR) to match the emissivity value of the NCT will give the best test accuracy. Check the NCT device manual to find its emissivity setting. Be sure to reset the imager's emissivity to 0.98 after any adjustments.
4. Some imagers allow adjusting the "transmission value," which corrects for any infrared attenuation when imaging through a protective thermal window. This value should be set at 100% as these windows are not used in human thermography. Lower transmission values will cause all temperature readings to be too high, and the GAIN will also be high. Infrared transmission may also be slightly attenuated by increased relative humidity (RH).[4] If an atmospheric correction algorithm is present in the imaging software, setting the RH to about 50% and the imaging distance to 3 meters (10 feet) is generally appropriate.

Measuring temperature offset and image flatness at room temperature

After validating the imager GAIN, the next procedure is to check the imager Temperature OFFSET at a stable room temperature. Using the procedures described here, FLATNESS can also be determined.

Equipment Needed:

1. A stable-temperature room around 21°C (70°F) without drafts, infrared sources, or windows (i.e., a standard cool thermography room).
2. A piece of foam-core artboard with a dull, matte finish (ε will be approximately 0.95). The board color is not important as long as it has no shine or reflectivity to its surface. The board should be touched only at the edges.
3. A NIST-traceable bulb or digital thermometer calibrated in the 18–35°C (65–95°F) range monitoring the temperature of the Foam Board.[5] Note: Although common NCTs may be used to measure the foam board's surface temperature, they are not as accurate as a contact-type thermometer in temperature equilibrium with the board, and may add or subtract an additional offset error to the result.
4. The IUT, turned on and fully warmed up, with the emissivity setting adjusted to match that of the board or target.

Procedure:

Allow at least 30 minutes for the foam board and thermometer to equilibrate to room temperature. Then take a *focused* image close-up so that the foam board fills the entire image (Figure 4.5). The center axis of the image should be perpendicular to the board surface.

For best accuracy, Timgr is an average area measurement taken near the center of the image and adjacent to the calibrated thermometer.

To calculate the imager OFFSET at room temperature, use this formula:

$$\textbf{Toffset} = \textbf{Timgr} - \textbf{Tstd}\ @\textbf{Troom}$$

where

- **Timgr** is the temperature of the board as detected by the imager.
- **Tstd** is the temperature reading on the NIST-calibrated thermometer.
- **Toffset** is the imager temperature difference compared to the standard.
- **@Troom** means the image target is at a nominal room temperature.

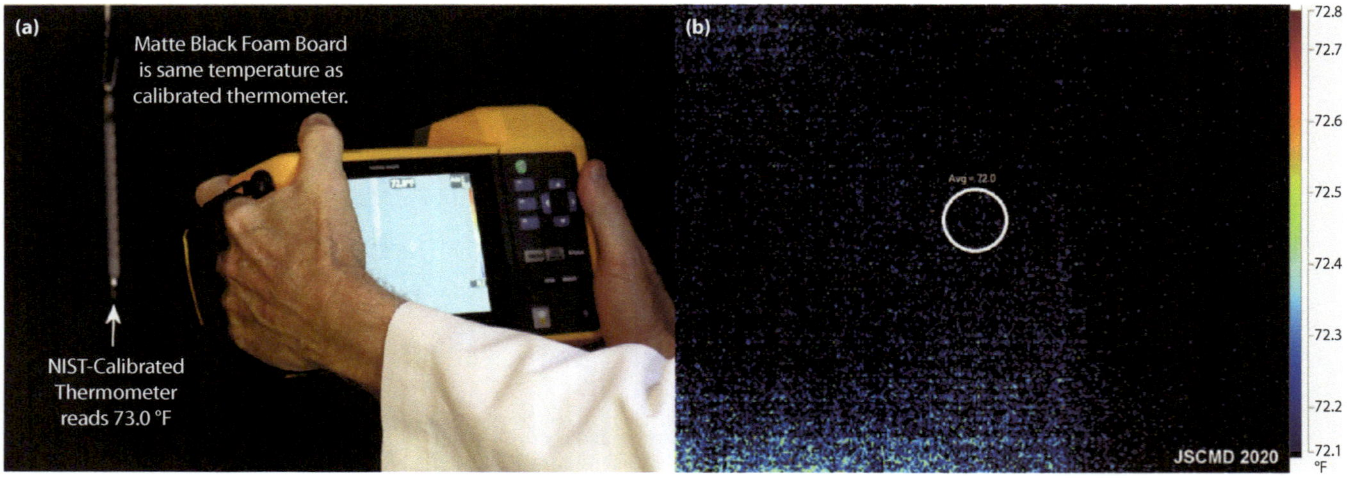

FIGURE 4.5 (a) Taking a focused close-up image of a matte surface at room temperature to measure the offset at room temperature. (b) The resulting image and center area measurement (Timgr) is shown.

The OFFSET for a calibrated microbolometer is typically ±2°C (3.6°F) across its full temperature detection range, and usually ±1°C (1.8°F) at physiologic temperatures.

If the imager's OFFSET is greater than the specified maximum error, off to professional recalibration it goes! Be sure to tell the technicians to calibrate it carefully at the 18–40°C (~65–105°F) physiologic range and be less concerned about other temperatures.

Image flatness at room temperature

Although checking image FLATNESS is becoming less important with the newer low-power imagers that develop less internal heat, it should be checked when the unit is first put into service and at least annually. This test can be performed using the same image taken for the OFFSET measurement (Figure 4.5b).

Equipment Needed:

- Same as that required for the OFFSET measurement described above.
- The NIST-traceable bulb or digital thermometer is not required here.
- A stable room-temperature blackbody device may be used (optional).

Procedure:

Using the image already taken for the OFFSET measurement, make four additional area measurements, one in each corner of the image. The absolute FLATNESS for the image is the lowest of the five measurements subtracted from the highest measurement. Some image interpretation software applications can automatically find and measure the highest and lowest temperatures detected across an image, making this measurement simple and more universal.

$$\textbf{Tflatness} = \textbf{Tmax} - \textbf{Tmin}\ \textbf{@Troom}$$

where

- **Tflatness** is the maximum temperature difference over the image.
- **Tmax** is the maximum temperature reading among the measurements.
- **Tmin** is the minimum temperature reading among the measurements.
- **@Troom** means the image is taken at a nominal room temperature.

In this example (Figure 4.6a), Tflatness = 72.2–71.9 = 0.3°F (0.17°C) @Troom. A FLATNESS value of 0.17°C (0.3°F) with this simple test is acceptable. There will often be a slight temperature gradient across the foam board due to air convection. This same imager gave a FLATNESS value of 0.0°C (0.0°F) using a Blackbody Calibrator as shown in the five-image sequence (Figure 4.6b).

Bucket calibration

Another calibration verification method suitable for a human thermography clinic is referred to as "Bucket Calibration."[6] A variation of Bucket Calibration is explained here. This method is inexpensive, semi-automated, and requires little equipment. Bucket Calibration tests both the imager GAIN and OFFSET, but not image FLATNESS.

A common thin-walled metal bucket with the outside painted flat black is filled with hot tap water at about 43°C (~110°F). The water temperature is monitored by a NIST-calibrated remote-reading, long-stem thermometer. The infrared imager under test is aimed to measure an area temperature on the black portion of the bucket, while the visual camera in the unit records the remote readout of the immersed thermometer (Figure 4.7).

Imager Emissivity should be set to 0.95 (approximately equal to the blackened bucket surface, see **reference 9**) and the Background Temperature set to the room temperature. The environment should be at nominal room temperature with little air movement and no radiant infrared sources or sunlight.

The thermometer temperature and the bucket temperature as detected by the imager are recorded over time. The imager is set to automatically record both visual and infrared images at 30-minute intervals. It will take 7–8 hours for the water in

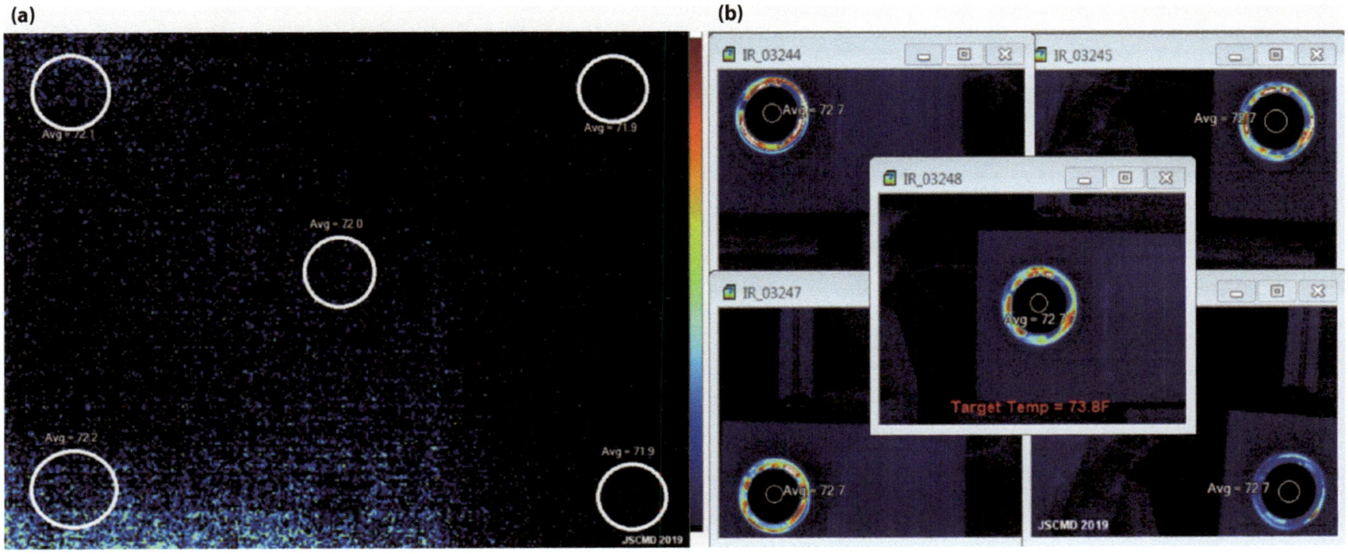

FIGURE 4.6 (a) An infrared image of a room-temperature matte-surfaced board to check image flatness. (b) Five sequential infrared images of a stable-temperature blackbody will also check the imager for thermal flatness.

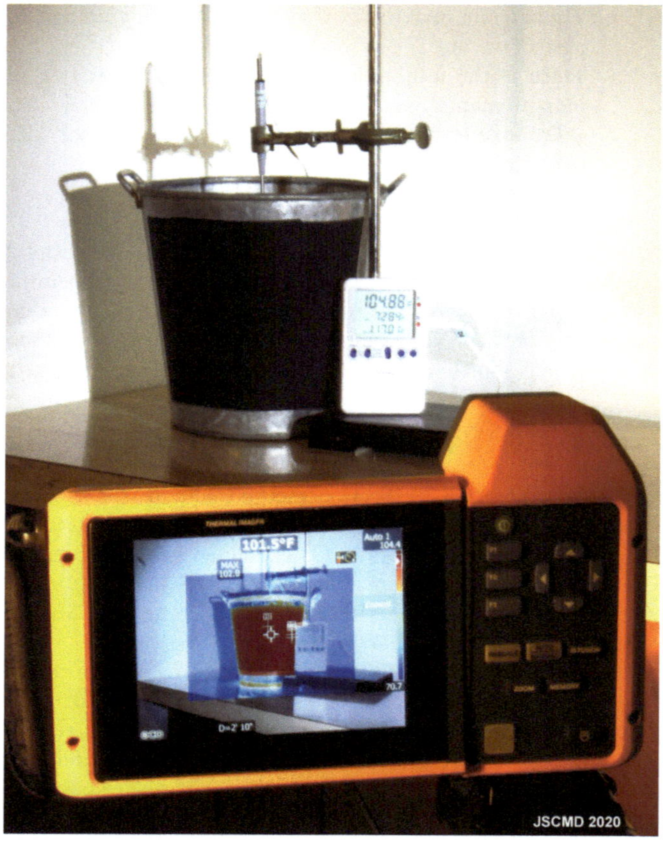

FIGURE 4.7 A setup for performing "bucket calibration" with the imager mounted on a stable tripod and focused on the bucket. A remote-reading contact thermometer is suspended in the water with its readout display placed to be visible in the imager's camera.

the bucket to settle near room temperature, providing serial temperature readings spread across the physiologic range. It may be convenient to begin this calibration at the end of the day and let it run overnight at a stable room temperature. Thus, the imager may be returned to service the next day, pending calibration results. When the bucket has cooled, the pictures from the imager are analyzed. The infrared image gives the bucket surface temperature recorded by the imager (Timgr), while the visual camera picture provides the simultaneous thermometer reading (Tstd). These two readings are entered into a spreadsheet and graphed over time to observe any change in imager offset with temperature (see Figure 4.8). Temperature OFFSET *variation* should be less than ±1°C (1.8°F) from 24°C to 37.8°C (75–100°F). Maximum temperature OFFSET should be within the manufacturer's specification for that particular imager. These parameters may be displayed in more detail by graphing Timgr minus Tstd over time (not shown).

Using a laboratory blackbody calibrator

In order to fully check the thermal calibration of an infrared imager, it is necessary to generate a stable, calibrated infrared source about 15°C (27°F) above room temperature (Figure 4.9). That is the purpose of a Blackbody Calibrator, which essentially acts as a "surrogate forehead" to provide Tbody temperatures.

A small, countertop blackbody calibrator costs about the price of one professional calibration; a calibrator is a worthwhile purchase for a professional thermography center. The calibrator can be used to check 5-point FLATNESS and OFFSET at Tbody temperatures of 32.2–37.8°C (90–100°F), where it can be a more reliable temperature reference than a human forehead. When used with a blackbody at room temperature (Troom), Imager GAIN can be verified as described above.

If purchasing a Blackbody Calibrator, be sure it can generate the temperatures necessary for human thermography, with a minimum temperature setting of 90–100°F (32.2–37.8°C). Calibrators should emulate the physiologic human surface temperature (Tbody), allowing the imager OFFSET at Tbody to be measured. Imager OFFSET at Troom is then checked by the method shown in Figure 4.5. The calibrator's blackbody target may also be used to emulate Troom if the device is unplugged and equilibrated to room temperature.

Blackbody calibrators may introduce significant temperature errors. The actual temperature of the blackbody surface may vary ±1.4°C (2.5°F) from the front-panel set point, and the stability of the blackbody surface may cycle ±0.3°C (0.5°F) over time. Use a calibrated NCT to check the actual blackbody target temperature

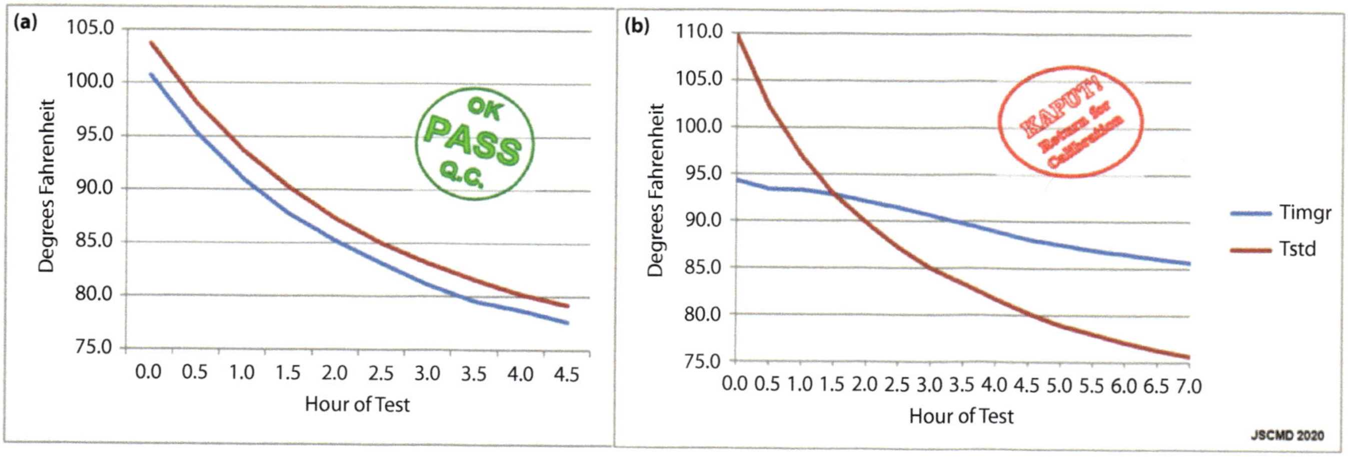

FIGURE 4.8 (a) This imager displays an approximate −1.4°C (−2.5°F) stable offset with temperature and passes the bucket test. (b) This imager does not pass! Its offset varies widely with changes in observed temperature. Timgr = temperature reading from imager; Tstd = temperature sensed by the immersed contact thermometer.

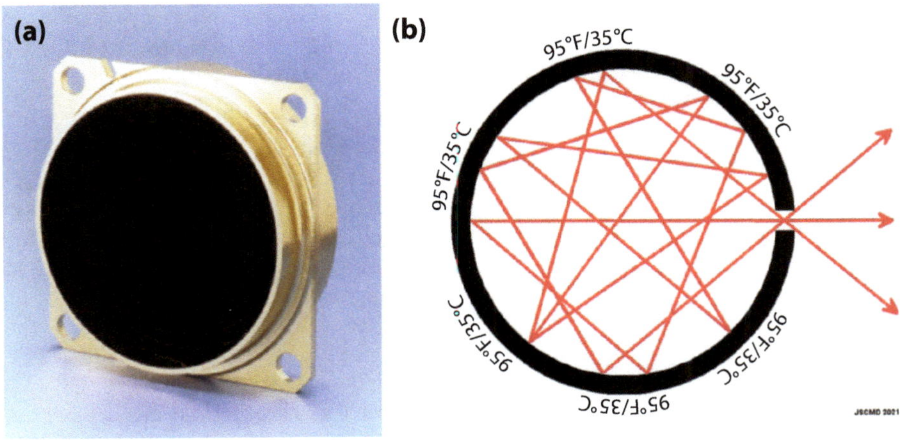

FIGURE 4.9 Blackbody calibrators. (a) A "plate-type" blackbody module. The machined metal block has internal heating elements and temperature monitoring thermistors. The black "target" has a typical emissivity of 0.95.[7] (b) Schematic cross-section of a cavity-type blackbody. The cavity wall is diffusely heated to the desired temperature. This type of blackbody has a typical emissivity of 0.98.

to be sure the calibrator is correct. The emissivity of the blackbody target is usually fixed at 0.95, close but not equal to the 0.98 emissivity of human skin. This may cause small errors in absolute temperature measurements, but GAIN calculations should not be affected as long as the IMGR and NCT device emissivities are set the same.

SIDEBAR 4.1 MAKING A SIMPLE, ACCURATE, AMBIENT TEMPERATURE BLACKBODY

Blackbodies for ambient temperature reference (Troom) are relatively easy to make because they require no heating or cooling mechanisms, power, or precise electronic controls. All that is required is a large metallic mass with a matte surface, a suitable NIST-calibrated thermometer, and a protective case.

In this example (Figure 4.10), a 5/8-inch (1.59 cm) thick aluminum block is suspended on a piece of fiberglass material to insulate it from the plastic case. The tip of a long-stem electronic thermometer fits snugly in a hole drilled into the center of the block and is thermally coupled to it with a small amount of heat sink grease. The front surface of the block is coated with carbon black by using a candle flame to build up layers of soot until no visual reflection of strong light can be seen. This coating approximates an infrared emissivity of 0.95.[8]

A protective aperture coated internally with flat-black paint blocks most external infrared energy. The aperture in this device is the cone from an old X-ray unit, but a 3-inch (7.6 cm) length of 2-inch (5 cm) plastic plumbing pipe fastened to the front of the case will suffice. A protective aperture cover (not shown) is recommended to prevent damage to the delicate carbon-black surface when the reference is not in use. To preserve the high emissivity of the coating, never allow anything to touch the blackbody surface.

To use the ambient temperature blackbody, place it in a room at a temperature about 20°C (68°F) for at least one hour until the temperature of the metal block stabilizes. Then aim an imager directly into the aperture and focus on the blackbody

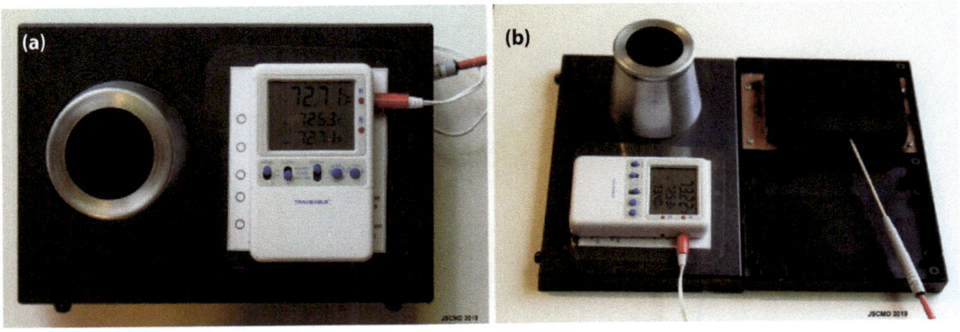

FIGURE 4.10 (a) The front of the ambient temperature blackbody device. Inside the aperture on the left is the blackbody surface. The monitoring thermometer readout is seen on the right. (b) The interior of the ambient temperature blackbody device is shown. The front cover is seen on the left. The blackened aluminum block and monitoring thermometer probe are mounted on the back cover (right).

surface. An area measurement of the carbon-black surface compared to the reading of the thermometer will give the temperature OFFSET at Troom for the imager. The OFFSET of an NCT device can similarly be determined by aiming the device directly into the aperture at close range. The blackbody also makes a convenient way to check the FLATNESS of an infrared image (see Figure 4.6).

Calibrating the calibration thermometers

Standard industrial non-contact thermopile infrared thermometers are inexpensive. How can the thermographer be sure that these devices – or any of the temperature-measuring devices, for that matter – are accurate?

Here we turn to the stable freezing temperature of water by using **"Tin-Cup Calibration."** The freezing point of pure water is virtually the same around the world and is not affected by altitude, RH, or other factors. Thus, it makes a perfect check to see if a bulb-type thermometer or non-contact IR thermometer is accurate at 0.0°C (32°F).

Equipment Needed:

- A thin-walled metal vessel painted with flat black paint (the Tin Cup).[9]
- Pure ice – frozen distilled water is best, but common ice is acceptable.
- Pure water – distilled is best, but filtered tap water will also work.
- A wooden or plastic stirring rod.
- The thermometer(s) being tested. Non-contact units should be at room temperature.
- An infrared-free area if testing NCTs, i.e., no sunlight or incandescent lights.

Procedure:

These tests are best performed at a nominal room temperature in still air. Fill the Tin Cup with a mixture of ice and water, and stir occasionally for 5–10 minutes. The ice-water mixture will reach an equilibrium temperature of 0.0°C (32°F). If testing a non-contact IR thermometer (NCT), continue stirring while measuring the painted surface of the cup with the device (Figure 4.11a).

Water condensation may occur on the outside of the cup but will not affect the reading. Allow time for the NCT reading to settle. It should read close to 0.0°C (32°F) with little, if any, OFFSET. Generally, these devices will show a maximum OFFSET of ±0.25°C (~0.5°F). Record this OFFSET value.

If testing a contact-type thermometer, gently stir the ice-water mixture with the sensing portion of the thermometer while observing its reading (Figure 4.11b). Generally, these devices will also show a maximum OFFSET of ±0.25°C (~0.5°F) at equilibrium with the freezing point. Record this OFFSET value.

Once the thermometer has been tested at the freezing point, it is tested at room temperature as shown in Figure 4.12 to complete two-point verification. If the thermometer has OFFSET readings at both freezing and room temperature that are within 1°C (1.8°F), it has passed two-point verification.

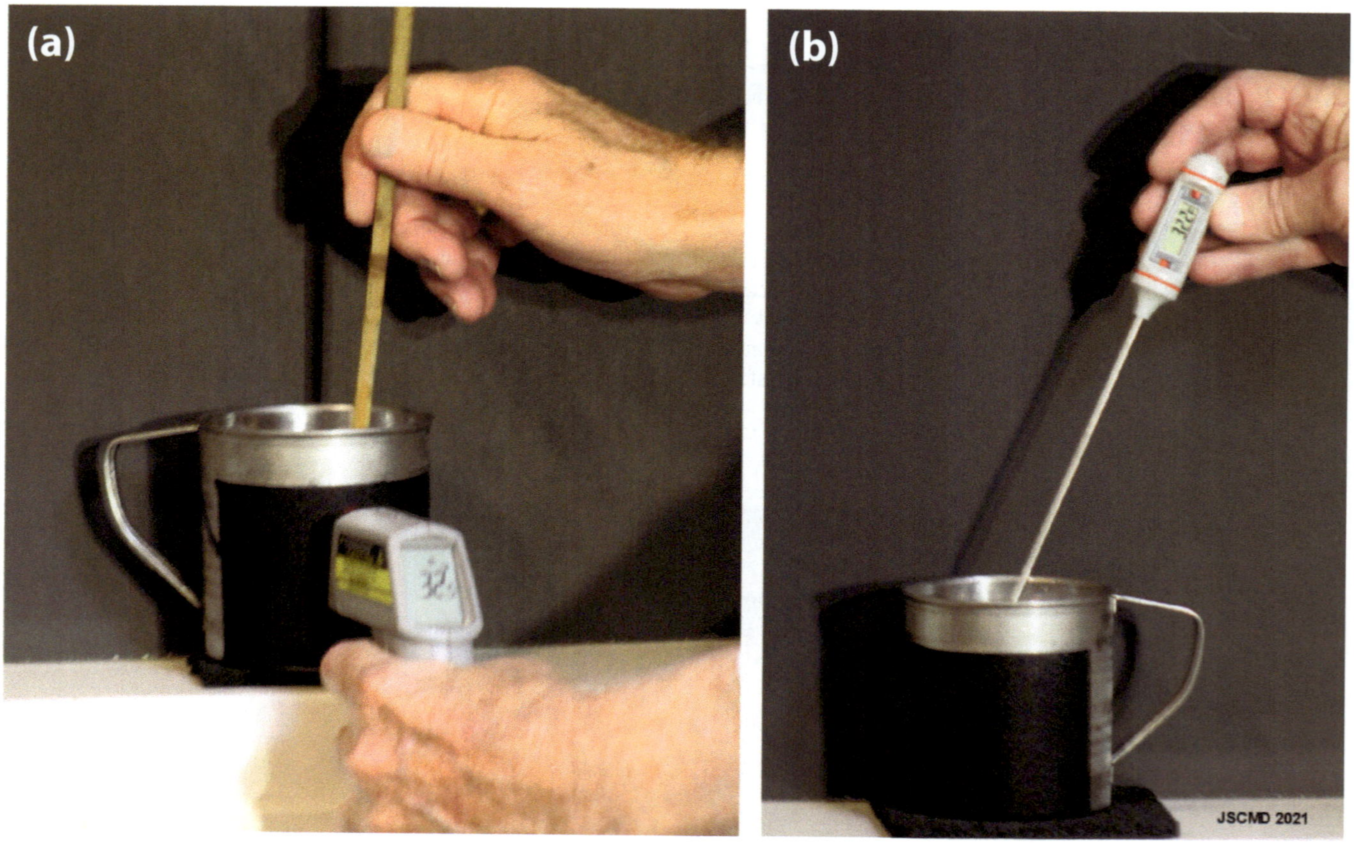

FIGURE 4.11 Calibrating thermometers at the freezing point, 0.0°C (32°F). The cup is filled with a stirred ice and water mixture. The cup is sitting on an insulating pad. (a) Testing a non-contact thermometer by aiming at the flat-black surface. (b) Testing a contact thermometer by immersing it in the ice water.

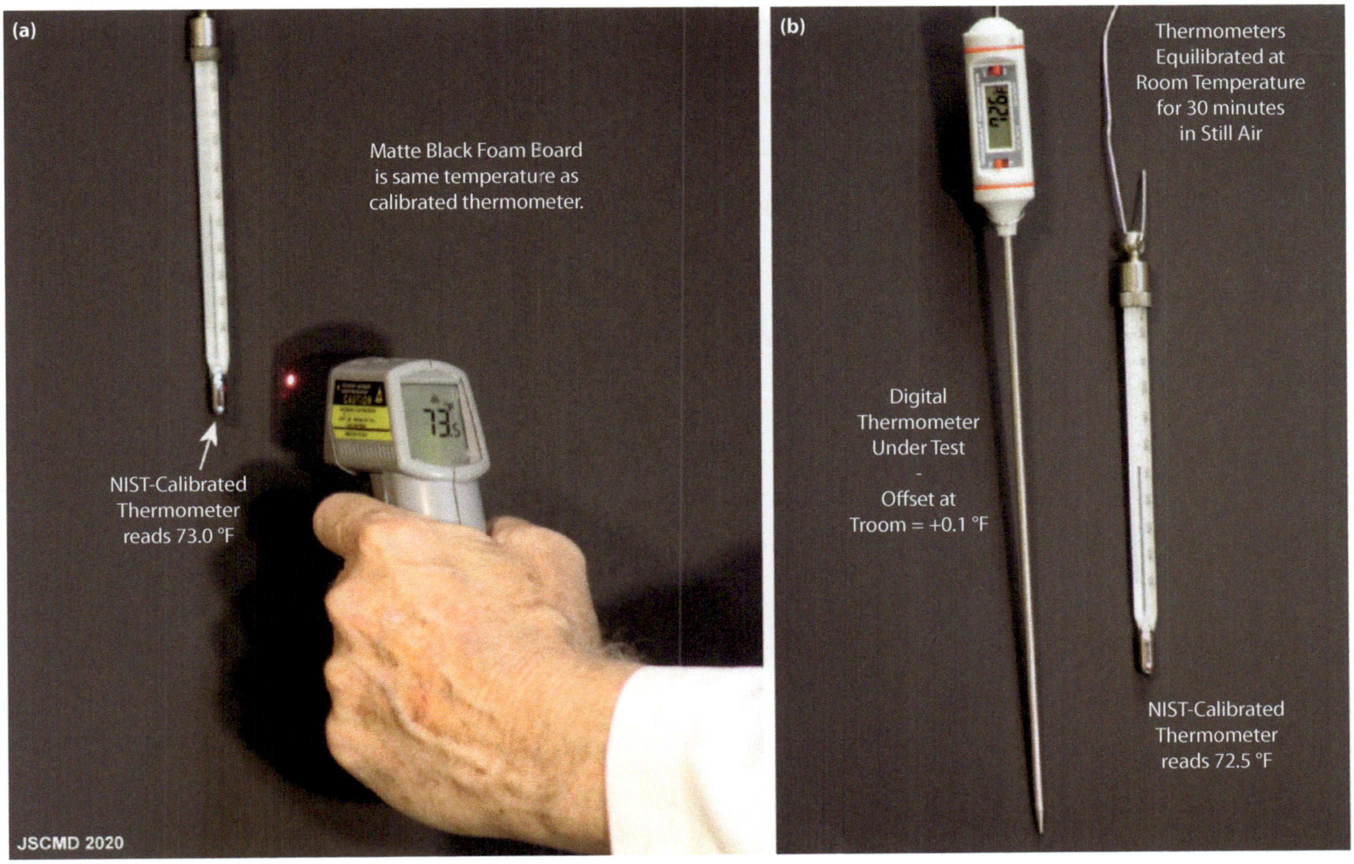

FIGURE 4.12 Two-point calibration of a thermometer requires checking it at room temperature (Troom) as well as freezing. Contact thermometers are usually more accurate than non-contact types. (a) Non-contact calibration; (b) Contact thermometer calibration.

A typical non-contact infrared thermometer incorporating a thermopile sensor has a specified accuracy of ±2°C (3.6°F), which is a rather wide range. Usually, NCTs are far more accurate than that at physiologic temperatures. As for differential measurements, for a two-point calibration with the points 20°C (36°F) apart (room temperature minus freezing temperature), a 5% error would occur if the two temperature offsets vary by 1°C (1.8°F). A 5% offset error in a clinically significant difference measurement of 1°C (1.8°F) would cause an acceptable error of ±0.05°C (0.09°F), about the same as caused by the intrinsic thermo-electronic noise (NETD) of an uncooled thermal imager. This error is clinically acceptable.

SIDEBAR 4.2 WHEN SHOULD YOU SEND YOUR IMAGER OFF FOR LABORATORY RECALIBRATION?

For the high-quality infrared imagers used in clinical practice, full calibration adjustments must be performed by the manufacturer in a calibration laboratory. This is done to detect and correct any problems with the temperature OFFSET and GAIN for each pixel in the entire image field. Any problems with the shutter mechanism, internal temperature detector, readout electronics, autofocus, and infrared lens are also examined. Using specialized software during an intensive calibration process, the manufacturer employs a multi-point approach in which black bodies at precise points across the desired temperature range provide known infrared radiance levels to the imager. Each pixel is checked and automatically corrected for minimum offset to the blackbody temperatures.

Checking the unit across its full specified temperature range to make any needed calibration corrections is the best way to check imager calibration. This approach is expensive, however, costing a minimum of $1000 US and often much more if any mechanical or electronic repairs are required. In addition, damage or loss may occur in shipping, and the imager may be out of service for up to a month before it is returned. Thus, it is often best to send an imager out for professional calibration only when needed, not necessarily on a set schedule. By regularly checking and documenting the imager GAIN, OFFSET, and FLATNESS in the clinic, the thermographer can rely on the qualitative and quantitative results of the images. If any parameters drift out of specification, send the imager for full calibration. Just remember the old adage: "If it isn't broken, don't fix it ..."

Notes

1. Images courtesy of FLIR Systems, Inc., Wilsonville, OR. Used with permission.
2. Personal experience of jscmd. See the Bucket Calibration section for a response graph of a defective camera with poor thermal gain.

3. Common Non-Contact Thermometers usually have a fixed emissivity value of 0.95. Higher-end units may be adjustable, in which case both CAM and NCT devices should be set to match the emissivity of the target surface for the most accurate absolute and differential temperature measurements.
4. Chen CC, Attenuation of Electromagnetic Radiation by Haze, Fogs, Clouds, and Rain. A Report prepared for the US Air Force Project Rand, R-1694-PR, April 1975. URL: https://www.rand.org/content/dam/rand/pubs/reports/2006/R1694.pdf
5. NIST = US National Institute of Science and Technology, Gaithersburg, MD.
6. As proposed by Jose Quesada and Ricardo Vardasca in Ch. 12, p. 300 of Application of Infrared Thermography in Sports Science, Springer, 2017. ISBN: 978-3-319-47410-6.
7. Photo courtesy of NASA, The National Aeronautics and Space Administration, USA 2006.
8. Infrared Services Inc., Littleton, CO. Emissivity Values for Common Materials. Table URL: https://www.infrared-thermography.com/material-1.htm.
9. The infrared emissivity of the paint surface depends on which type of flat (matte) paint is used. Example emissivities at 10 μ are: Krylon, flat black – 0.956; Oil Paint, various colors – 0.94; Krylon, flat white #1502 – 0.989; SOURCE: Infrared Services Inc., Emissivity Values for Common Materials.

5

THERMAL PHYSIOLOGY AND THERMOREGULATION

Humans are *endothermic homeotherms*, meaning that they produce body heat and regulate internal temperature, with an average core temperature of 36.5°C (97.7°F), plus or minus 0.5°C (0.9°F).[1] This relatively high core temperature is achieved through heat production as a result of internal metabolism and neuromuscular activity. The term *core*, in this context, refers to the internal portions of the head, thorax, and abdomen, including organs such as the heart, brain, and liver. The resting core temperature normally shows small fluctuations occurring in a range of 36.7–37.5°C (98.1–99.5°F) for men and 36.8–37.1°C (98.3–98.8°F) for women.[2]

More than just an indicator of health, keeping body temperature within narrow limits is also a matter of survival. The human body is always adjusting to maintain a core temperature that is neither too hot nor too cold. Temperature changes outside the normal range can critically disrupt the biochemical processes necessary for normal functioning. Significant swings in the core temperature are a definite indication of dysfunction and can eventually prove fatal.

With prolonged immersion in cold water, the human body loses heat faster than it can produce it, with about 90% of the heat loss occurring through the skin. Continued exposure will drop the body temperature to about 35°C (95°F), causing mild hypothermia, which slows brain activity, breathing, and heart rate resulting in fatigue, lethargy, and confusion.[3] In severe hypothermia, body temperature drops below 27°C (82°F), where neuromuscular, respiratory, cardiovascular, and hematological changes can prove fatal.[4] The survival time of individuals immersed in cold water without having proper thermal insulation is about 2 hours at a water temperature of 5°C (41°F).[5]

Increased core temperature or *heatstroke*, is common among those who work in hot, humid environments. Exposure to "wet-bulb" temperatures exceeding 35°C (95°F) for prolonged periods may be fatal even in the shade and with forced-air convection. A wet-bulb thermometer measures the ambient temperature minus the heat loss from water evaporation. Hyperthermia results when the body's core temperature rises above 40°C (104°F). If this temperature continues to rise and exceeds 42°C (107.6°F), cellular damage occurs.[6] This manifests as progressive organ and neuronal dysfunction, eventually causing multi-organ failure.[7] Active cooling is paramount for averting death in this situation.

In physical terms, healthy thermoregulation means that the body's heat generation equals its heat losses while retaining a core temperature around 36.5°C (97.7°F). The direction of heat transfer always occurs down a thermal gradient, i.e., from hot to cold.[8] As the human body is often the warmest object in a given space, it will normally lose heat to its immediate surroundings through some combination of radiation, conduction, convection, and water evaporation. When the core temperature drops in a cold environment, dermal vasoconstriction, piloerection, and muscular shivering will be stimulated. Prolonged cooling lasting over 30 minutes may create skin temperature instability.[9] Under moderate cooling conditions – the thermoneutral zone – core temperature remains stable, adrenergic sympathetic vasoconstriction controls skin surface temperatures, and the heat patterns detected by thermal imaging show autonomic dysfunction more clearly. Under warming conditions, a cholinergic sympathetic increase in skin blood flow alters the thermal patterns as heat loss via sweat evaporation becomes the primary means of heat dissipation.

Blood circulation and thermal dynamics

As cooled venous blood returns from the extremities, adjacent arteries warm it by conduction. The slightly warmed blood enters the thorax to be carried toward the right atrium of the heart by the great veins. These veins are located adjacent to deposits of Brown Adipose Tissue (BAT). This heat-producing fat is stimulated by cold conditions to help re-warm the returning blood to maintain body temperature. Metabolic heat production in all the active body organs, especially the liver, also heats the returning blood.

The venous blood enters the right ventricle, which adds about 10 Calories of heat per day as it pumps the blood through the lungs. There the blood is exposed to the inspired air, which may cool or warm the blood depending on the environmental air temperature. In the usual case of the air being cooler than the blood, exhaled air removes heat from the body in two ways. First, heat is conducted out of the blood, equilibrating with the cooler air filling the alveoli. Exhalation then expels the heat by forced convection. Second, water is evaporated from the alveolar lining to be expelled in the breath as "insensible" fluid loss. This removes about 220 Calories per day of evaporative heat, which is supplied by the nearby capillary blood, cooling it.

After passing through the lungs, the blood is pumped through the left chambers of the heart. The left ventricle muscle contraction work adds at least 50 Calories of heat per day to the flow.[10] The blood then passes through the aorta and great arteries of the thorax, where it is again warmed if needed by the adjacent BAT before flowing out of the chest and abdomen, carrying warm, oxygenated core blood back to the head and extremities, heating the returning venous blood on the way.

Physiology of whole-body temperature regulation

It is useful to think of body temperature regulation in terms of two physiological domains, the central core and the peripheral "shell" or skin. Core temperature generally remains quite stable. Skin temperature can vary from ambient to core temperature mainly via autonomic control. Peripheral blood flow increases with a sufficiently high core temperature, augmenting heat transfer from the extremities.[11]

Skin temperature is normally a reliable indicator of the heat exchange activity of the body. The average temperature of the skin is about 32.5°C (90.5°F) or 4°C (7.2°F) lower than the body's core temperature under thermoneutral conditions.[12] At a room temperature of 25°C (77°F), local skin temperatures may vary within a range of 4–5°C (7.2–9°F) depending on physiologic, anatomic, and pathologic factors.[13] In a warmer environment, the temperature of the skin increases toward core temperature as blood flow through the skin increases. The human body is

DOI: 10.1201/9781003281764-6

generally warmer than the ambient temperature, allowing a flow of heat from the core to the environment. Even with clothing for insulation, heat is steadily lost from the body. During cold stress, blood flow through exposed skin is reduced, leading to a decrease in skin temperature and conservation of core body heat. Skin temperature in the periphery may approach the ambient temperature during cooling, with the nose, ear, finger, and toe temperatures becoming about 17°C (30.6°F) lower than normal core temperature when the body is equilibrated to an air temperature of 20°C (68°F).

Physiologically, internal temperature control is coordinated by the hypothalamus.[14] Thermoreceptors located in both the periphery and central core provide constant neural input to the hypothalamus. These thermoreceptors occur in two basic subtypes, those responding to warm and those responding to cold (Figure 5.1). In central (core) areas such as the brainstem, spinal cord, viscera, and great veins, warm thermoreceptors are more abundant than cool thermoreceptors. The opposite is true in the periphery, where cool thermoreceptors outnumber their warm counterparts.

The hypothalamus integrates inputs from thermoreceptors in both the skin and core organs. Activation of warm thermoreceptors may cause inhibition of cold receptors.[16] Specialized neuronal thermoreceptors in the hypothalamus constantly compare arterial blood temperature to an internal set point. This temperature setting may vary with individuals and with circadian rhythms; core temperature typically fluctuates between average values of 36.4°C (97.5°F) in the morning and 36.9°C (98.4°F) in the evening.[17] Various pathological processes can induce either systemic or local thermal anomalies; for example, core temperature may increase due to infection, inflammation, trauma, and malignancy, while limb temperature may decrease due to ischemia or increase due to inflammation.

Other physiological mechanisms that modulate the thermoregulatory response include muscle activity, dermal blood flow, shivering, sweating, and stimulation of brown fat. With regard to muscle activity, running at 16 km/h (10 mph) increases basal body heat production by twenty-fold, generating about 1500 watts (2 HP) of heat.[18] This heat is conducted through tissues to the skin and is also transported throughout the body by the circulation of blood (circulatory convection). The hypothalamus detects the increase in blood temperature and transmits nerve signals to activate various heat loss processes, including peripheral vasodilation, perspiration, exhalation, and a drop in the metabolic rate. Vasodilation occurs in active muscles, increasing circulatory thermal transport. *Vasoconstriction* occurs in the inactive

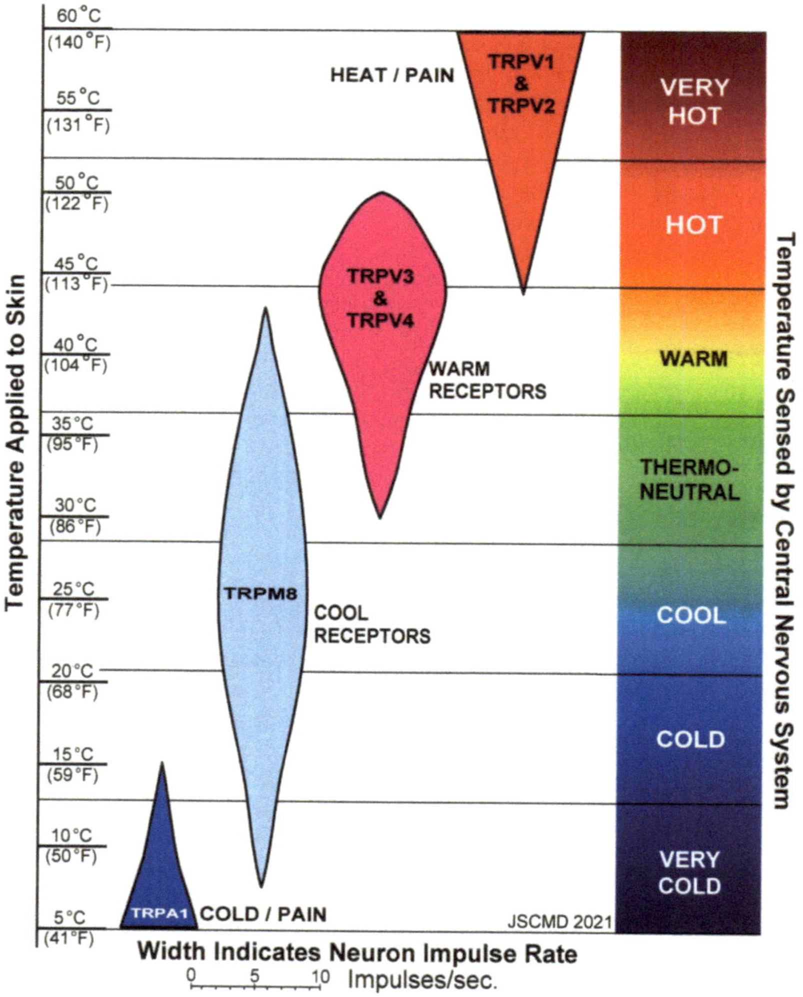

FIGURE 5.1 Types of neural thermal receptor responses over temperature. The TRP channels which sense the various temperatures are shown. The four receptor active zones overlap, providing uninterrupted temperature information to the hypothalamus.[15]

muscles. Regulation of blood flow is thus a key physiological feature of exercise, with adjustments in blood flow to the skin and muscle areas being achieved mainly through the interaction of central and peripheral mechanisms.[19]

Shivering generates muscular heat as part of the body's natural response to cold. The shivering reflex manifests as rapid rhythmic contractions of the skeletal muscles and is triggered whenever the core temperature drops below a certain set point. The increased muscular activity warms the body by increasing metabolic heat generation. Maximum shivering can increase basal body heat production by four or five times, producing about 375 watts (0.5 HP) of heat.[20] The hypothalamus serves as the primary driver for shivering.[21] Shivering can also be a response when developing a fever: the hypothalamic set point for core temperature is raised, causing the body temperature to rise by creating the sensation of feeling cold and ramping up physiologic heat production and conservation until the new core temperature set point is reached.

The most important thermoregulatory response to hyperthermia is the production of eccrine sweat. Sweat glands in the dermis can greatly increase evaporative heat loss when stimulated by cholinergic sympathetic neurons.[22] The core temperature threshold for sweating is typically 0.2°C (0.36°F) higher than the threshold for vasoconstriction. Nevertheless, sweating begins within seconds of the onset of exercise, even before any changes in internal temperature.[23] During exercise, sweating can remove 1000 Calories of heat per hour, assuming all the sweat evaporates in contact with the epidermis and does not run off.[24] Sweat evaporation during repetitive limb movement can be efficient enough to keep the distal skin surfaces cool, thus extracting heat from the core more rapidly by providing an increased thermal gradient. After exercise, the skin temperature rises in a glomus AVA pattern, increasing heat loss via convection and radiation.[25]

Evaporation of sweat leads to a reduction in skin temperature as long as the maximum evaporative power of the environment is not exceeded.[26] Evaporative cooling is the sole means of heat loss when ambient temperatures exceed the core temperature.[27] When the ambient temperature is 35°C (95°F) and the relative humidity is above 90%, the typical human cannot lose enough heat by sweating, even at rest with forced air circulation, and will eventually die from hyperthermia unless cooled by artificial means (Figure 5.2).[28]

In summary, thermoregulation is the process by which the body maintains a constant core temperature mainly by adjusting peripheral heat exchange with the environment. Continuous heat production from internal body processes must be balanced by continuous heat loss. When heat production minus heat loss is zero, the core temperature is stable and the body is in thermal balance. This dynamic balancing act between heat gain and heat loss maintains a physiologic core temperature.

Skin blood flow and thermoregulation

The skin is the largest organ of the human body and serves as the primary barrier between the body's internal milieu and the outside world. With its multi-layered structure, the skin shields the body from the local environment and regulates core temperature. Normally, only a small amount of blood flow is needed to deliver nutrition to skin cells, hair follicles, and glands (Figure 5.3a). Skin blood flow may increase greatly, however, to reduce regional and whole-body temperature.

Temperature of the skin's surface largely reflects blood flow through the dermal microvasculature, though larger superficial veins may also warm the skin surface enough to be detected by thermal imagers (Figure 5.3b). Approximately 4% of cardiac output flows through the skin under thermoneutral conditions. This perfusion can increase by more than tenfold via maximal cutaneous vasodilation in response to heat stress, or quickly drop to near zero under severe cold stress.[30] Cutaneous blood flow depends mainly on blood circulation in the smallest blood vessels (between 10 and 100 μm in diameter), primarily the arterioles, capillaries, and venules. Whereas the capillary network supplies nutrients and oxygen to the dermal structures, the arterioles are essential for blood flow regulation.[31] The regulatory mechanisms include flow-induced vasodilation from wall shear stress,

NWS Heat Index

Temperature (°F)

Relative Humidity (%)	80	82	84	86	88	90	92	94	96	98	100	102	104	106	108	110
40	80	81	83	85	88	91	94	97	101	105	109	114	119	124	130	136
45	80	82	84	87	89	93	96	100	104	109	114	119	124	130	137	
50	81	83	85	88	91	95	99	103	108	113	118	124	131	137		
55	81	84	86	89	93	97	101	106	112	117	124	130	137			
60	82	84	88	91	95	100	105	110	116	123	129	137				
65	82	85	89	93	98	103	108	114	121	128	136					
70	83	86	90	95	100	105	112	119	126	134						
75	84	88	92	97	103	109	116	124	132							
80	84	89	94	100	106	113	121	129								
85	85	90	96	102	110	117	126	135								
90	86	91	98	105	113	122	131									
95	86	93	100	108	117	127										
100	87	95	103	112	121	132										

Likelihood of Heat Disorders with Prolonged Exposure or Strenuous Activity

Caution | Extreme Caution | Danger | Extreme Danger

FIGURE 5.2 The likelihood of human hyperthermia is affected by both temperature and relative humidity.[29]

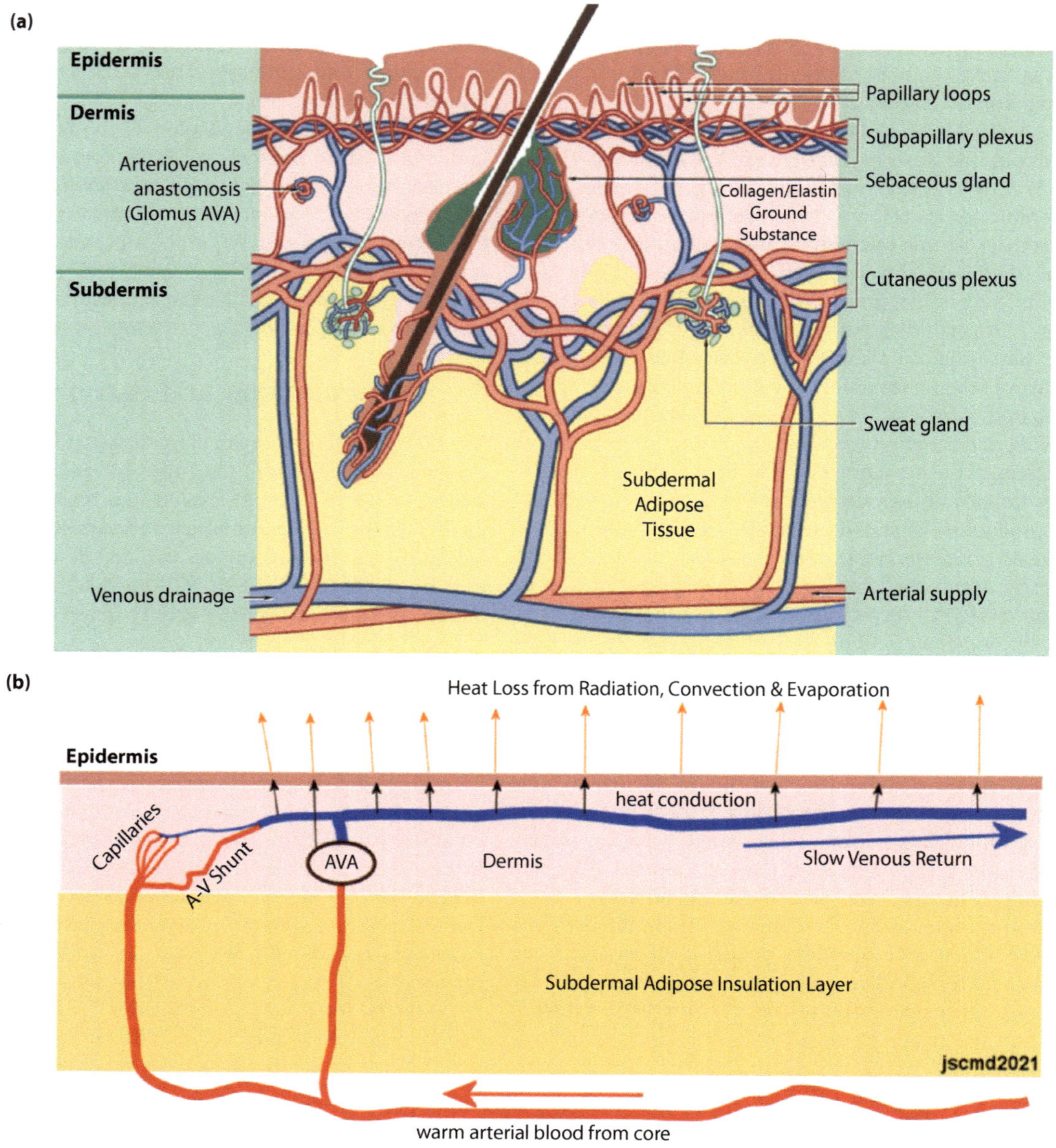

FIGURE 5.3 (a) Diagram showing the anatomical location of the arteries, veins, capillary networks, and glomus bodies (AVAs) within the dermis.[38] (b) Simplified schematic showing the blood flow paths through the skin. Skin capillaries provide nutrients to the dermis, but are relatively flow-limited. Small, thick-walled A-V shunts create a high-volume pathway that dilates from cholinergic sympathetic stimulation. The glomus bodies (AVAs) allow a regulated flow of blood inhibited by adrenergic sympathetic stimulation. The warm arterial blood flows into superficial dermal veins where the heat is dissipated by conduction to the nearby skin surface.

arteriolar myogenic response, and metabolic and autonomic nervous control.[32]

Both human skin and skeletal muscle display an extraordinary capacity to boost their blood flow 50- to 100-fold, an increase due to local vasodilation.[33] Depending on temperature exposure, blood flow to the skin may vary from nearly zero in extreme cold to about 7 liters per minute when core temperature increases. Maximal skin blood flow can reach 300–400 milliliters per minute per 100 grams of skin when the cutaneous vascular smooth muscles are completely relaxed.[34]

While blood flow to the skin may be affected by local metabolites as well as local warming and cooling; autonomic regulation plays the major role. Significant increase in local skin circulation is produced by chemical or surgical disruption of the lumbar sympathetic trunks.[35] As an indicator of skin blood flow, thermographic assessment of skin temperature is useful for obtaining quantitative data regarding the functioning of the autonomic nervous system.[36]

Skin can be divided into two basic types: glabrous and nonglabrous skin. In some disciplines, glabrous skin is referred to as acral (distal), while nonglabrous skin is labeled non-acral. Glabrous skin is smooth and hairless; the type found on the palms, soles, penis, eyelids, and lips. Glabrous skin is innervated mainly by adrenergic sympathetic vasoconstrictor nerves, which increase their tone in response to cold, causing vasoconstriction. Warm conditions increase cutaneous blood flow through passive vasodilation when adrenergic sympathetic activity decreases.[37] Nonglabrous (hair-bearing) skin covering most of the body's surface is innervated by both cholinergic vasodilator and adrenergic vasoconstrictor nerves.

The role of dermal arteriovenous shunts

Glabrous skin of the palms and soles contains a large number of glomus bodies, also known as arteriovenous anastomoses or AVAs.[39] Although only about 0.5 mm (0.02 in.) in diameter, glomus AVAs can produce substantial changes in blood flow to the skin. The highest concentration of AVAs is found in the nail beds of the fingers and toes (600 AVAs/cm^2) and in the skin of the palms and soles (100 AVAs/cm^2).[40] Glomus bodies are also found scattered over many areas of the non-glabrous skin surface. Glomus AVAs are within a firm capsule. An afferent arteriole enters the glomus body, becoming tortuous with a small lumen and a thick, muscular wall. Richly endowed with sympathetic nerves, this intra-glomus vessel links up with a thin-walled vein that eventually drains into larger superficial skin veins. When the core temperature rises, adrenergic sympathetic tone decreases, opening the intra-glomus vessels. Warm blood then flows directly from artery to vein, bypassing the capillary beds. In this way, the glomus bodies modulate heat exchange and work in parallel with the capillaries and A-V Shunts of the skin.

The anastomosing vessels that pass through the glomus bodies are controlled by adrenergic sympathetic neurons, which excrete norepinephrine. When the core temperature drops, a centrally controlled increase in sympathetic tone elicits rapid vasoconstriction of the AVAs within two to four heartbeats. Maximal sympathetic stimulation can completely close the lumen of an AVA, dramatically limiting blood flow to the skin.

On the other hand, the withdrawal of sympathetic tone leads to glomus vasodilation that is exclusively passive and can take up to 10 or more heartbeats to complete. The increasing blood flow into the dermal venous plexus results in increased heat loss from the skin's surface (Figure 5.4). The veins also dilate when warm, increasing skin heat loss from the greater exposed vein area. When cool, the superficial skin veins contract, reducing skin heat loss by shunting venous blood into the deeper veins.

Between the cool (fully vasoconstricted) and warm (fully vasodilated) states lies the "thermoneutral zone," an environmental temperature range in which the blood flow through the AVAs is modulated by the hypothalamus. Rather than being steady or constant, this neural signaling occurs in bursts of adrenergic sympathetic activity every 15–30 seconds, and is most active in the middle of the thermoneutral zone (~31°C, 88°F). Each rapid adrenergic vasoconstriction is followed by a slower, passive vasodilation. Vasoconstrictive sympathetic bursts may occur from sensory stimulation of another area of the body and even from mental stimulation. Norepinephrine antagonists such as clonidine and adrenergic receptor blocking drugs may reduce AVA constriction. Without sympathetic stimulation such as in the case of local anesthetic nerve blockade, the AVAs remain open.

The rhythmic AVA fluctuations normally occur almost simultaneously in all four limbs, thus differential quantitative thermal measurements taken from the same image should not be affected in a normal subject. These fluctuations in flow are similar to the 15–60 second volume fluctuations detected in the distal fingers via plethysmographic techniques, and both phenomena may be due to the same neural mechanism. Local peripheral nerve block or sympathectomy obliterates both types of fluctuation.[41] These centrally controlled AVA fluctuations are not affected by local warming to 43°C (109.4°F), though skin blood flow through arteriolar A-V Shunts increases. Below a local skin temperature of 21.5°C (70.7°F), the AVAs remain closed. When cooled to several degrees above freezing, however, the AVAs will remain tightly constricted for 5–10 minutes, at which point the AVAs open abruptly for 10–20 minutes before constricting again.[42]

In hot environments, the dermal heat loss from the relaxation of AVA dilation may not be sufficient to cool the core. If the total body heat loss is insufficient after removal of active vasoconstriction, then a further increase in skin blood flow can occur via active arteriolar A-V Shunt dilation controlled by acetylcholine from sympathetic cholinergic nerves (Figure 5.5). This initiates an increase in total cutaneous blood flow from 300 milliliters per minute up to or exceeding eight liters per minute.[46] Other chemicals that may play a role in active vasodilation include nitric oxide, vasoactive intestinal peptide, substance P, histamine, prostaglandins, and transient receptor potential V1 receptor activation. Of these, the most important with regard to thermography is nitric oxide.

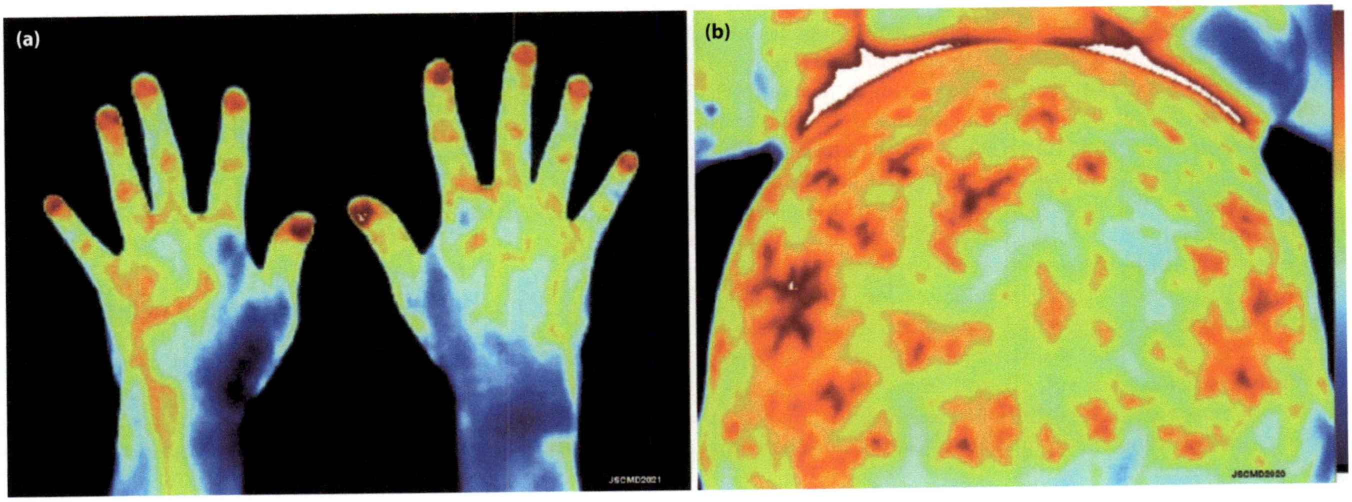

FIGURE 5.4 (a) Thermographic appearance of glomus AVA dilation in the hands. Note the warm fingernails and veins – 34 yoF. (b) A non-acral glomus dilation pattern may accompany the hand pattern. This is the abdomen of a rested, cooled 64-year-old female. The venules draining the AVAs are visible as "starburst" patterns.

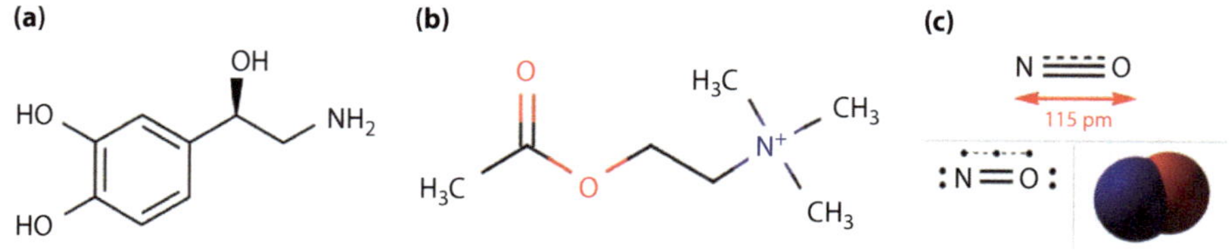

FIGURE 5.5 The three major vasoactive substances: (a) Norepinephrine – sympathetic AVA vasoconstricting neurotransmitter.[43] (b) Acetylcholine – promotes sweating and A-V shunt vasodilation.[44] (c) Nitric oxide – a potent vasodilating diffusible gas. Note the small molecular size.[45]

Nitric oxide and skin circulation

Nitric oxide (NO) is a toxic, colorless, free-radical gas and one of the principal oxides of nitrogen. Inhaling a 100 ppm (120 mg/m^3) concentration of nitric oxide can be dangerous to life and health.[47] Within the human body, however, NO is a highly diffusible intercellular signaling molecule involved in a wide range of biological effects. It is one of the smallest molecules involved in intercellular signaling. The gas is highly reactive and short-lived, with a half-life of only a few seconds, yet it diffuses freely across biological membranes.[48] These attributes make NO an ideal transient signaling molecule for events such as vasorelaxation and neurotransmission. Once converted to nitrites or nitrates by reaction with oxygen and water, the signaling activity of NO ceases.

NO's role in skin temperature regulation centers on its effects on the smaller arteries. It signals the vascular smooth muscle in the tunica media to relax, resulting in vasodilation and increased blood flow. This potent vasodilator plays a major role in establishing both whole-body and regional "vascular tone." So prominent are its vasodilating effects that NO is also known as endothelium-derived relaxing factor (EDRF). It is synthesized endogenously in essentially all tissues by nitric oxide synthase (NOS). Synthesis of NO requires the amino acid L-arginine, oxygen, and various cofactors, notably NADPH.

The most extensively studied NOS isozymes are cytokine-inducible NOS (iNOS) and endothelial NOS (eNOS), both of which generate free NO when upregulated. The expression of iNOS is often induced by inflammatory and immune stimuli, notably microbial endotoxins and the proinflammatory cytokines associated with cancer, autoimmune processes, and other diseases. In human skin, iNOS is associated with cutaneous immune responses.[49] Once induced, the iNOS isozyme is active for relatively long periods of time, thereby generating large quantities of NO. Shorter pulses of NO production are mainly associated with maintaining vascular tone. Thus, while transient increases in NO are a part of normal physiological functioning, larger amounts of NO, produced for extended periods of time are often associated with disease states.[50] This NO overproduction can be detected thermographically if it occurs near the skin surface.

Direct warming of the skin produces a local increase in the activity of NOS and cutaneous NO concentration.[51] Local heating to 42°C (107.6°F) causes maximal vasodilation. Some NOS isoforms are involved in vasodilation from local skin warming, while others appear to be involved in the vasodilation response to whole-body heating.[52] NO-mediated vasodilation is attenuated by NOS inhibition.[53]

NO is also an intermediate chemical messenger between the nervous system and vascular smooth muscle. The initial vasodilation from NO is transient, and is modestly reduced and shortened by NOS inhibition.[54] This reaction is followed by a slow reversal of the vasodilation due to adrenergic sympathetic vasoconstrictor activity. The vasoconstriction with local skin cooling is brought about, in part, by NOS inhibition and postsynaptic upregulation of adrenergic receptors. Local cooling also elicits an early vasodilator response that is commensurate with the rate of cooling. The mechanism for this transient vasodilation is inhibited by intact sympathetic vasoconstrictor and sensory nerve functioning.[55]

Another small toxic gaseous molecule, hydrogen sulfide (H_2S), works in synergy with NO to produce vascular dilation by relaxing the muscular layers of the blood vessels. H_2S increases the local concentration of NO by upregulating a nitric oxide synthase enzyme (eNOS) present in the vascular wall.[56] Though profound thermal effects of H_2S have been seen in experimental animals, research into the thermographic effects of varying H_2S concentrations in humans is lacking at this time.[57]

SIDEBAR 5.1 THE VASODILATION EFFECT OF AMYL NITRITE, AN NO DONOR MOLECULE

Amyl nitrite (AmNO), a volatile organic liquid, is a potent vasodilator that is readily absorbed by inhaling the vaporized liquid. It is used medically as a fast-acting substitute for nitroglycerine, another therapeutic NO donor. Systemic symptoms of headache, lightheadedness, and tachycardia may occur within 30 seconds of inhaling AmNO, and last about 5 minutes before "wearing off." Oddly enough, vasodilation of the fingers as monitored by thermal imaging does not occur until *after* the systemic effects begin to fade (Figure 5.6). This may be due to the time required for the enzymes xanthine oxidoreductase and/or mitochondrial aldehyde dehydrogenase 2 to release active NO from the amyl nitrite.[58] The side effects of AmNO may be due to the chemical itself, with the therapeutic vasodilatory effect occurring later as the drug is metabolized, releasing active NO.

Nitric oxide and human pathology

Excessive NO concentrations in tissues appear to be associated with multiple disease states and with profound changes in circulatory and immune system functioning; the nature of these changes is generally dependent on the magnitude and duration of NO synthesis. This may explain the thermal imaging differences between normal and malignant states. These differences may be caused by the ability of some tumor cells to produce NO, causing dilation of nearby vessels.[59] Tumor tissue releasing NO relatively close to the surface of the breast or other body region produces elevations in

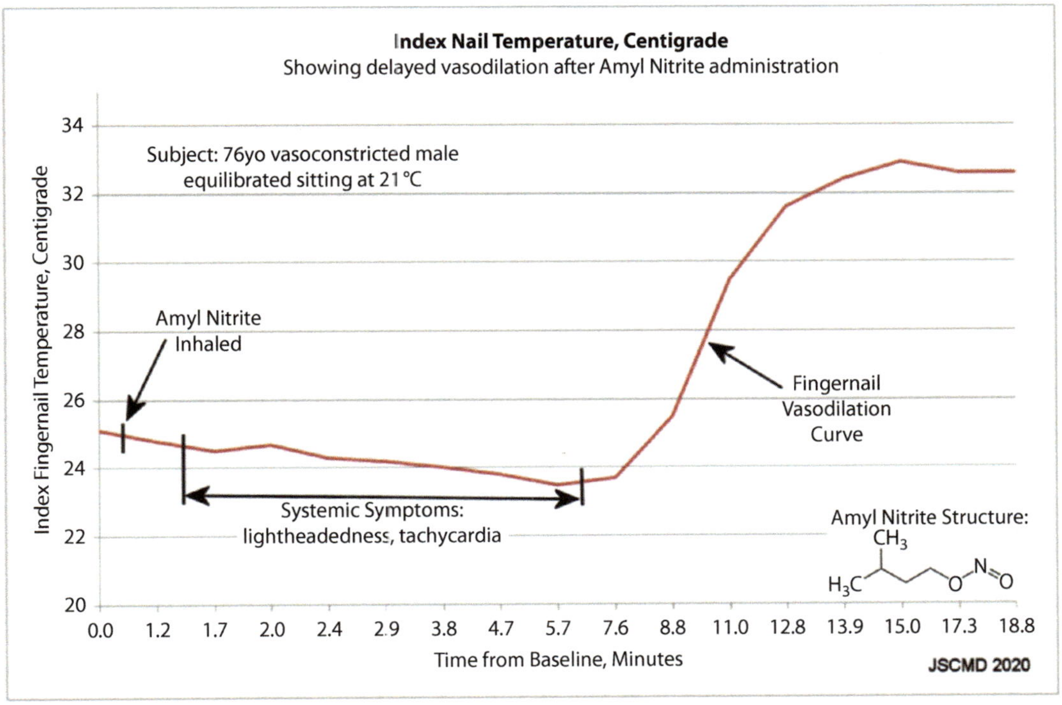

FIGURE 5.6 Vasodilation after inhaling amyl nitrite vapor is delayed by about 5 minutes in the fingers.

local skin temperature. Tumors that generate ample amounts of NO will increase their own vasodilation and nutrient delivery to the mass of cancer cells.[60] NO diffuses widely into surrounding tissue, increasing vasodilation and making the nearby skin hyperthermic (the "nitric oxide blush," as depicted in Figure 5.7). This would explain how a small volume of NO-generating malignant tissue situated 10 mm deep can be detected thermographically by virtue of its effects on skin thermoregulation.[61]

Medical thermography utilizes effects from the NOS system to assess inflammatory disorders. The inflammatory immune response is generally associated with enhanced activity of macrophages that are known to generate NO, which then diffuses freely beyond the confines of its point of origin. Therefore, if NO is overproduced in a certain part of the body, it will diffuse throughout the surrounding tissues (with the exception of bone), resulting in local hyperperfusion. If the affected region is in relatively close proximity to the skin, such hyperperfusion will manifest as a localized increase in heat on the body's surface. This mechanism explains the association between skin surface hyperthermia and a number of inflammatory disorders.[62] Indeed, significant correlations have been found between skin temperature and the severity of arthritic knee pain, suggesting that infrared imaging is a reliable method for assessing inflammation in arthritis.[63]

Heat generation by brown adipose tissue

BAT is a thermogenic fat located primarily in the supraclavicular area of the neck as well as along the sides of the thoracic vertebral bodies.[64] BAT is brown because of the high concentration of mitochondria in the adipocytes. Brown fat, when activated, can

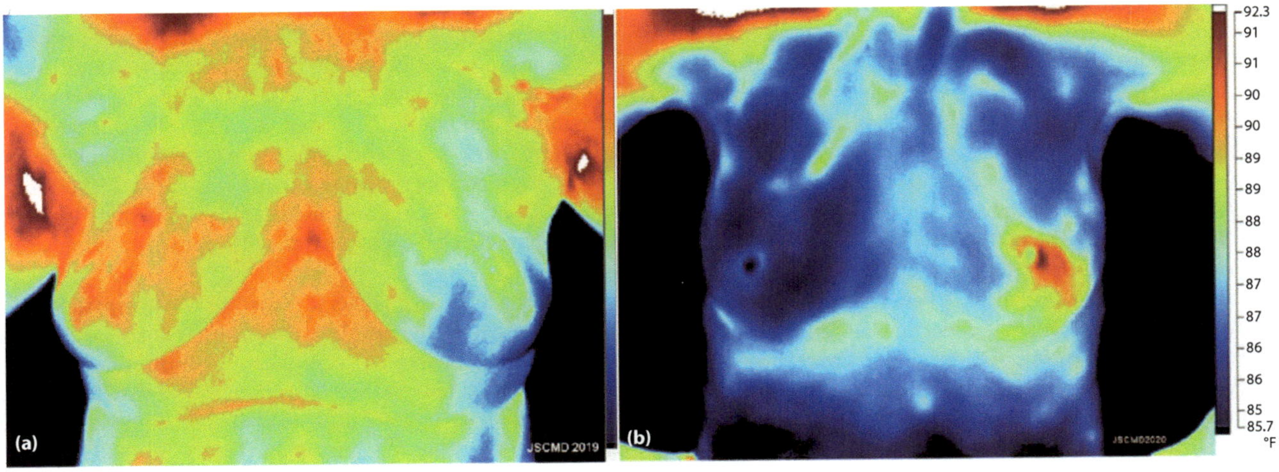

FIGURE 5.7 (a) Diffuse nitric oxide blush over a palpable mass in the mid-right breast – 56 yoF. (b) A more intense NO blush affecting the left breast, areolar, and nipple skin surfaces. Pathology unknown – 47 yoF.

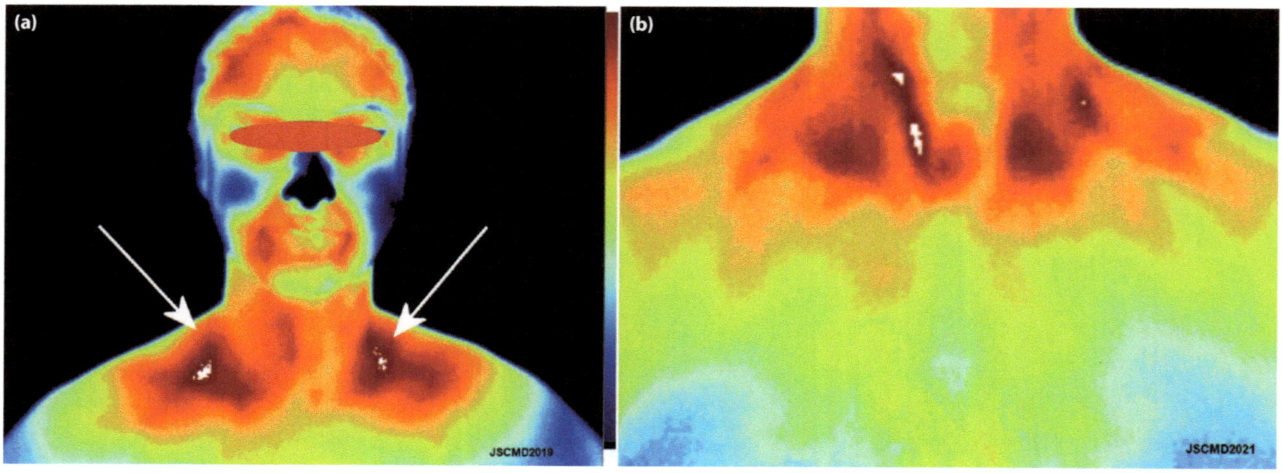

FIGURE 5.8 (a) Brown adipose tissue (BAT) thermal pattern (arrows) in a cooled 63-year-old female subject. (b) BAT pattern in a cooled 54-year-old male. The right anterior jugular vein is also visible.

generate about 300 watts of heat per kg of tissue.[65] This heat can be detected with infrared imaging of the supraclavicular fossa – the area of the neck just above the medial clavicle (Figure 5.8). The heat is transferred from the BAT tissues to the overlying skin by thermal conduction. BAT activity is greater in females, young individuals, and those with a low body-mass index (BMI). When BAT is activated, whole-body energy expenditures increase.[66] A 1.5°C (2.7°F) rise in BAT temperature may be brought on by hydrocortisone or isoproterenol as well as by eating a standard meal.[67]

Interest in BAT focuses on its potential use in the treatment of metabolic disorders, notably obesity and diabetes.[68] BAT activity is inversely correlated with fasting glucose levels, and there is less BAT activity in humans with Type 2 diabetes.[69] In addition, 10 days of cold exposure increases insulin sensitivity in adults with Type 2 diabetes, suggesting that BAT modulation may be a key treatment for obesity and diabetes.[70] Nonetheless, the majority of studies report that BAT activation does not influence body weight and metabolic control in humans.[71]

Although PET-CT is considered the gold standard for assessing BAT, thermography has emerged as a noninvasive and safe way to indirectly assess the activity of BAT in humans.[72] The supraclavicular thermogenic response that occurs upon exposure to cold is mainly generated by BAT activity. Supraclavicular skin temperature responses are rapid, occurring within 10 minutes of the cold exposure.[73] MRI investigations have confirmed the rapid response phenomenon.[74] The BAT thermal response peaks at 25 minutes, then decreases with ongoing cold exposure; the response gradually diminishes until finally stopping altogether.[75]

In most studies in which participants are first cooled, an increase in thermographically-measured supraclavicular skin temperature is noted. The increase in supraclavicular skin temperature in response to cold temperatures indicates increased BAT metabolic activity in adults.[76] Few studies have taken into account the thickness of the subdermal fat layer when taking BAT measurements, however. Obese subjects may show less BAT activity on thermography for two reasons: their core is better insulated from a cold environment, and their thicker subdermal fat layer in the neck insulates the heat generated by BAT from reaching the skin. Nevertheless, because of its safety and non-invasiveness, thermography can be a useful tool for metabolic determinations.[77]

Sympathetic anatomy and skin temperature

The two sympathetic trunks, which are located paraspinally from the second cervical vertebra to the coccyx, control the vasomotor, piloerector, and sudomotor activity of the entire skin surface (Figure 5.9).[78] Thus a difference of the "tone" along or between the sympathetic trunks is often visible to thermography. Central nervous system control of sympathetic vasoconstrictive tone appears to be primarily inhibitory, thus increased sympathetic constriction of the skin vasculature occurs with spinal cord disruption or hemispheric stroke. There is cranial-caudal distribution of neural signaling in each sympathetic trunk, but apparently no direct signaling between the right and left trunks except at the caudal end, where they fuse together near the coccyx. Thus, a difference in the sympathetic tone between the trunks produces qualitative and quantitative thermographic differences from one side of the body to the other, with the *cooler* side having *greater* adrenergic sympathetic tone due to increased vasoconstriction (Figure 5.10a). If generalized along one entire sympathetic trunk, the entire ipsilateral hemi-body from head to foot will be affected. This produces *sympathetic imbalance* or *sympathetic dominance*, an important phenomenon to recognize, especially in breast thermography, where it can adversely affect the accuracy of the exam interpretation.

Interruption of one or both sympathetic trunks produces a profound and predictable thermographic appearance, depending on where the sympathetic disruption occurs. If the cervical portion of one trunk is isolated from the thoracic section, the ipsilateral neck, head, and face can be expected to be warmer. If the lumbosacral portion of one trunk is isolated (L3 vertebra and below), the ipsilateral groin and leg will be warmer. Transection of the thoracic portion of a trunk will appear as a warm arm and cool leg.

With the advent of bilateral transthoracic sympathectomy for the treatment of hyperhidrosis, Corposcindosis, or "split body syndrome," may occur as a complication. This produces a distinct thermographic appearance in which the sympathetic nervous system has been divided into two distinct body regions above and below the level of transection (Figure 5.10b). Compared to the indistinct thermal division caused by spinal cord transection, local transection of a sympathetic trunk creates a well-demarcated thermal appearance. The upper body appears warm due

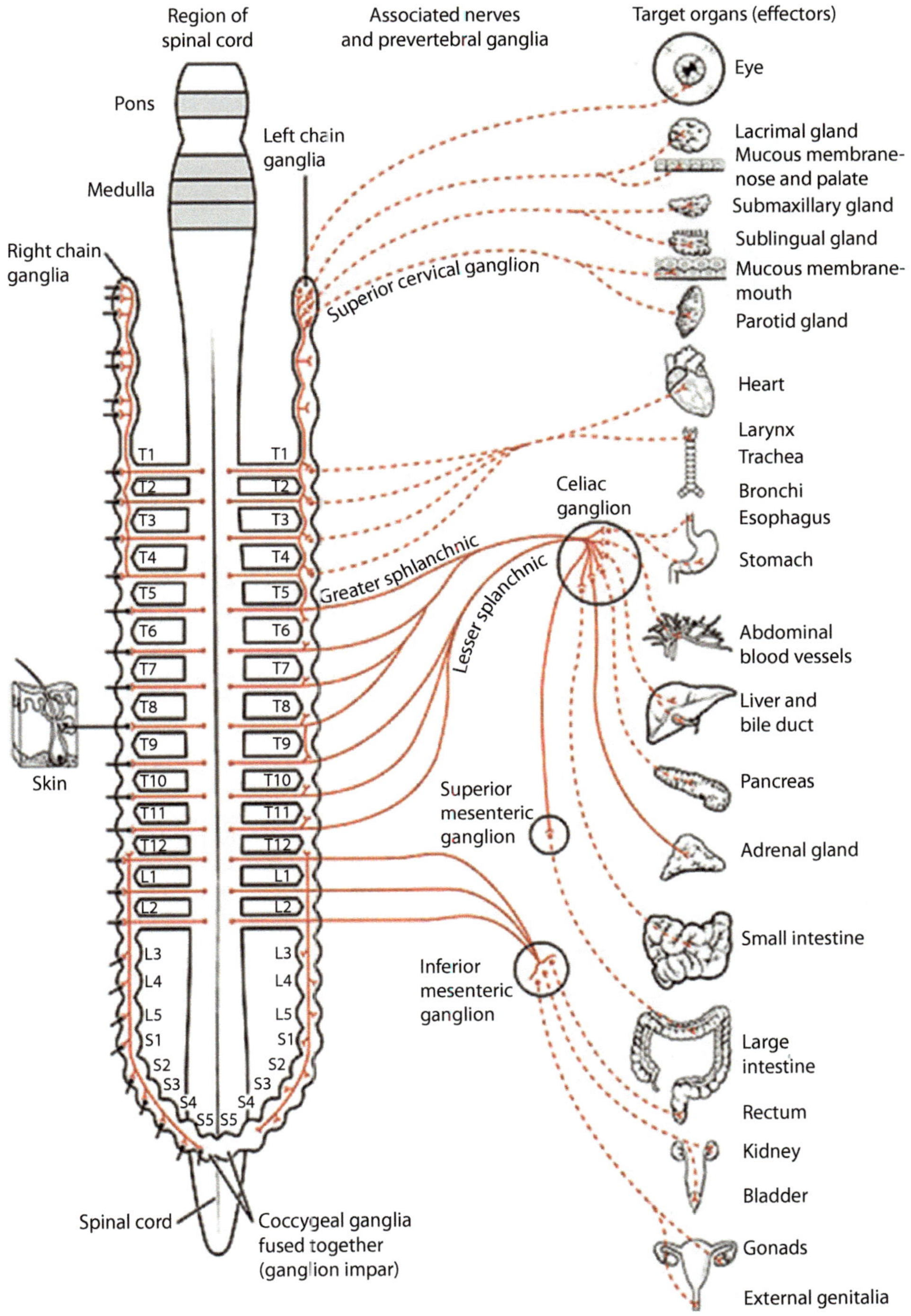

FIGURE 5.9 A schematic diagram of sympathetic nerve connections. The upper third of the trunks have intersegmental connecting fibers from T1 through T5. T6 through T11 have little interconnection between segments, and the lower third connects with the spinal cord via T12, L1, and L2. Although this schematic shows the right sympathetic trunk enervating the skin and the left innervating only the organs, the neural connections are actually anatomically bilateral.[79]

to overactive CNS inhibition of sympathetic vasoconstriction. Below the sympathetic transection, the body appears cool due to compensatory hyperactivity of the sympathetic trunks.

The sensitivity of thermal imaging to changes in sympathetic stimulation provides a useful and non-invasive method for evaluating the effectiveness of local blocks of the sympathetic ganglia or peripheral nerves. Thermographic monitoring of the affected region and its contralateral site, both before and during nerve block, can detect a successful blockade within minutes if conducted under cooling conditions. With a successful block, skin temperatures in the affected area should increase, with differential temperatures rising from 1.5 to 7.5°C (2.7 to 13.5°F) above the contralateral site.[81] The temperature differences should persist as long as the block is effective.

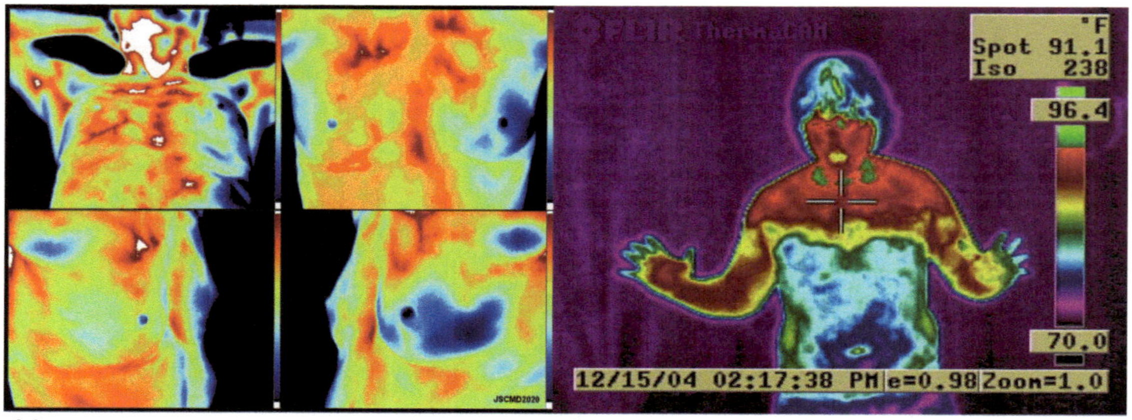

(a) (b)

FIGURE 5.10 (a) Sympathetic dominance on the left, imaged during a routine breast examination in a 67-year-old female. The left abdomen, thorax, arm, neck, and face are all visibly cooler than the contralateral areas. (b) Male subject imaged 2 years after bilateral endoscopic thoracic sympathectomy, showing corposcindosis, or split-body syndrome.[80]

Thermal appearance of the vascular system

Structurally speaking, the human vascular system can be described in terms of arteries, veins, capillaries, and lymphatics. In this section, the thermal effects of the blood-carrying vessels will be examined, as they control thermal convection within the body as well as from the body core to the skin surface. Though the lymph system has much less thermal effect than the blood-carrying vessels, lymphatics may become visible thermographically when inflamed or blocked.

Arteries carry core body heat to the skin surface, where it is dissipated or conserved to maintain the body core temperature within tight limits.[82] Although arterial blood is warm, arteries are rarely visible thermographically outside of certain anatomical sites where they run close to the skin surface (Figure 5.11). These sites include the antecubital fossa at the elbow, the inguinal fold, the popliteal fossa behind the knee, the radial and ulnar arteries at the wrist, and the posterior tibial and dorsalis pedis arteries in the foot. Increased arterial warmth may be due to arteritis or aneurism. Anatomically, arteries are almost always accompanied by one or more veins, making it difficult to determine arterial from venous warmth. Arteries over the scalp, though located close to the skin surface, are rarely visible because the usually warm cranium tends to mask their appearance. When scalp arteries show up thermographically, arterial inflammation should be considered.

At other anatomical sites in the neck, chest, abdomen, and limbs, the major arteries run in deep locations where they are insulated from the skin surface by muscles, fat, or veins. Thus, they cannot be visualized thermographically. When vascular patterns are visualized over most body areas, they are almost always venous, not arterial.

The arteries carrying the warm core blood to the dermis enter through the subdermal fat layer, which can vary widely in thickness from less than 0.5 to 5 centimeters or more. This layer acts as a thermal insulator, passively keeping the heat of underlying muscles,

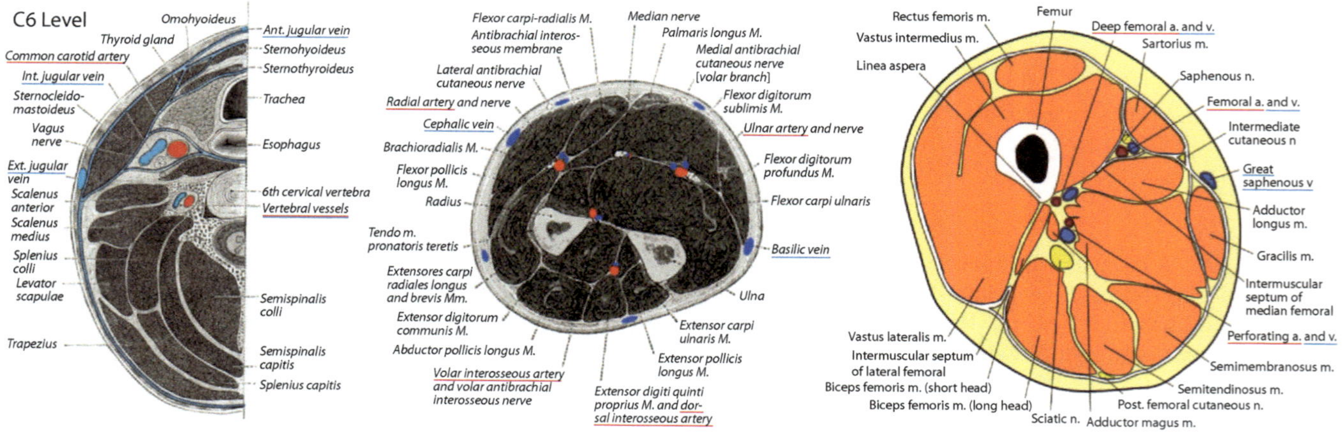

(a) (b) (c)

FIGURE 5.11 Anatomical cross-sections showing the major arteries in red and veins in blue. (a) Neck (left side) at C6 level. The external and anterior jugular veins are located in the subdermal adipose layer, where they may be visible to thermographic imaging. The arteries are too deep to be detected.[83] (b) Mid forearm. Note the deep location of the arteries embedded between muscle groups. The largest forearm veins are located in the subdermal adipose layer.[84] (c) Mid upper leg. The arteries and most veins are located deep, surrounded by muscle tissue. Only the greater saphenous vein is normally visible thermographically.[85]

nerves, and other tissues from being conducted to the dermis. Multiple small arteries perforate the subdermal fat layer, bringing a copious supply of blood to the dermis, more than is needed for its nutrient supply. When arterial blood flow to the dermis is increased, the arteries "short circuit" the insulation of the adipose layer by carrying warm core blood directly through to the dermal layer.

The dermis consists of a 2 mm (0.080 inch) thick layer of tough collagenous ground substance. Within the dermis is a rich matrix of arteries and veins arranged in two planes: a superficial plane in close contact with the epidermis, and a deep plane situated next to the subdermal fat. Blood gets from the dermal arteries to the veins via three distinct paths: (1) the nutrient capillaries, (2) the anastomosing arterioles (A-V Shunts), and (3) the glomus AVAs (see Figure 5.3b).

Blood flow through the nutrient capillaries is limited due to small vessel size. In contrast, the A-V Shunts and AVAs allow large flows when dilated. They open under sympathetic command to shunt warm arterial blood into the plexus of slower-flowing dermal veins. Heat from these warm veins is then conducted through the epidermis to be dispersed into the surrounding atmosphere by radiation, convection, or evaporative cooling.

The epidermis is the tough outer layer of skin about 0.5 mm (0.020 inch) thick. It is a good conductor of heat and, being thin, can conduct heat from the underlying dermis to the ambient surroundings easily. There are no blood vessels in the epidermis, but there are arteriolar loops in close contact with the underside of the layer (Figure 5.3a). The epidermis receives nutrients by diffusion from the dermis, and water evaporates constantly through the epidermal layer into the atmosphere as an "insensible" fluid loss.[86] This water evaporation amounts to approximately 500 milliliters per day in an adult and continuously cools the surface of the skin as the heat required for the evaporation is taken from the epidermis itself. This baseline evaporative heat loss amounts to about 270 Calories per day.

The three-layer organization of the skin implements control of the heat lost to the surroundings. When heat needs to be conserved to increase the body core temperature, noradrenergic sympathetic nerves constrict the AVAs of the dermis. This vasoconstriction may also be triggered by local skin cooling. The distal (acral) regions of the skin – that is, the hands, feet, nose, cheeks, and ears – respond strongly to this stimulation, reducing local heat loss from blood flow to almost zero in those locations. Additionally, in the hairy regions of the trunk and limbs, adrenergic sympathetic nerves stimulate vasoconstriction and piloerection ("goosebumps"), slightly reducing heat loss from those areas.

With hyperthermia, *cholinergic* sympathetic tone increases, stimulating the sweat glands and dilating the A-V Shunt arterioles, allowing up to 10 times the blood flow provided by AVA dilation.[87] Severe hyperthermia may increase skin blood flow up to 60% of cardiac output and produce up to 2 liters of sweat loss per hour.[88] Transection of peripheral sympathetic nerves causes the dermis to lose the capabilities to sweat and to fully vasoconstrict.[89] The affected skin thus appears warmer than the surrounding skin due to increased AVA blood flow and lack of evaporative cooling.

After passing through the dilated glomus or arteriolar shunts in the skin, the warm blood is carried by superficial veins where it can dissipate heat to the external surroundings. In the upper extremity, the majority of the warmed blood flows in multiple subdermal veins up to the elbow, where these superficial veins coalesce into the basilic vein. This large vein dives to meet the deeper brachial veins, which continue between the biceps and triceps muscles up to the shoulder, too deep to be detected thermographically. The cephalic vein, however, may sometimes be visualized, coursing up the lateral upper arm and across the anterior shoulder.

In the feet, non-exercise glomus dilation appears less often and less intense than in the hands (Figure 5.12a). The foot veins, while initially located in the subdermal fat over the metatarsals and tarsals, dive deep at the ankle to accompany the anterior tibial artery. This deep venous system is invisible to infrared imaging until

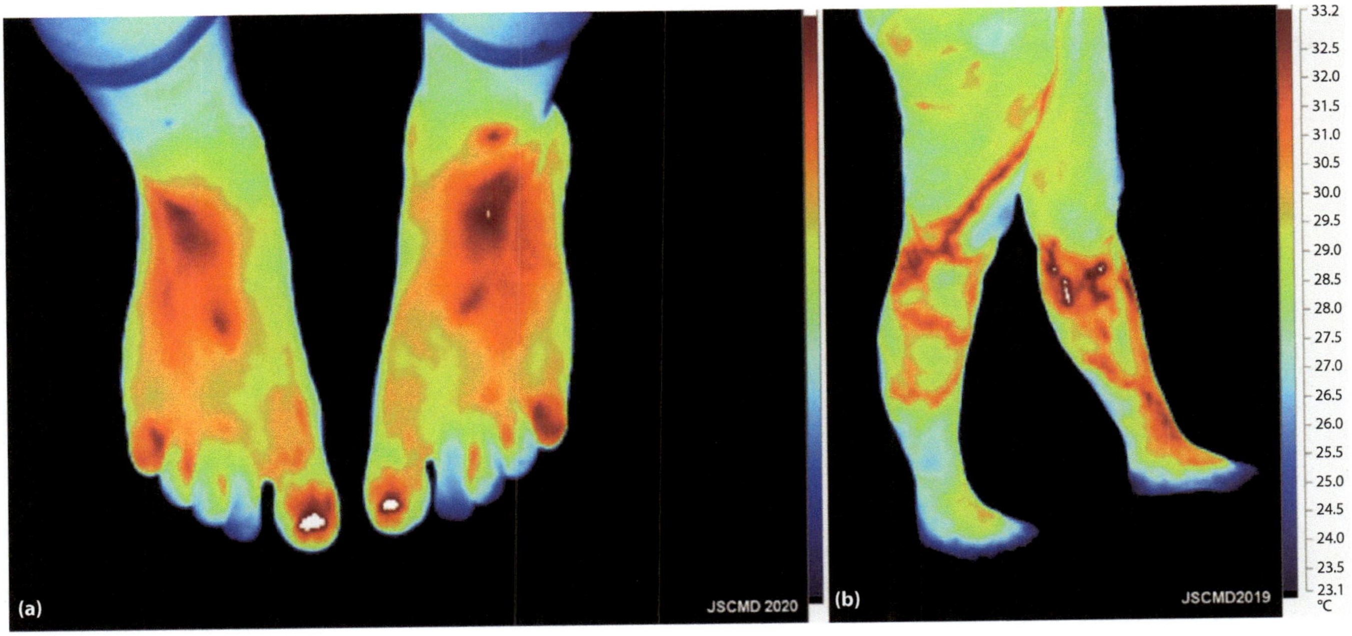

FIGURE 5.12 (a) Glomus dilation pattern in the feet. Digits ii–iv are not involved in this example – 36 yoF. (b) Bilateral lower limb varicosities of the saphenous veins – 67 yoF.

reaching the groin. The subdermal great saphenous vein progresses up the medial leg from just in front of the medial malleolus of the ankle to the groin, where it meets the larger femoral vein. The small saphenous vein starts behind the lateral malleolus of the ankle and runs subdermally up the back of the leg to the knee. Both saphenous veins may be seen by infrared occasionally, and these veins frequently generate varicosities that are thermally visible, smaller superficial leg veins may also become varicose (Figure 5.12b).

SIDEBAR 5.2 ACUTE ARTERIAL OCCLUSION CREATES ADJACENT THERMAL EFFECTS

When thermographically observing a warm, vasodilated, healthy subject, occluding all blood flow into a finger causes an expected drop in temperature of that digit as there are no muscles in the distal finger to create heat, and all warm arterial blood is excluded. For this test, a small one-inch (2.5 cm) wide occluding cuff over the proximal phalanx of digit III is inflated to 200 mmHg, which is not painful to the subject. As expected, the occluded finger will begin to lose heat to the surrounding ambient temperature (22.9°C/73.2°F) per Newton's law of cooling (Figure 5.13). A surprise finding, however, is that *all* the other digits of the hand simultaneously decrease in temperature by 0.5–1°C (0.9–1.8°F), and then gain 1–2°C (1.8–3.6°F) when the cuff is released. This occurs even in digit V, which is supplied by the ulnar nerve (digit III is supplied by the median nerve). This indicates that the reaction of the non-occluded digits is due to mechanisms in either the sympathetic trunk, central nervous system, or both. More research into this phenomenon may provide clinically useful information.

The thermal appearance of muscles and tendons

Exercising muscles (generating pulling force via their tendons) are much more metabolically active than muscles at rest; muscles cannot push, they can only pull.[90] This activity generates heat, thereby raising the temperature in the muscles involved. The heat is dissipated by blood convection into the thermographically invisible deep veins draining the muscle, and by conduction through the adjacent tissues. If the active muscle is located just under the subdermal fat layer, this metabolic heat warms the skin by conduction. Deeper muscles have a much smaller impact on skin temperatures as their heat conduction to the skin is attenuated by overlying musculature. Sedentary, non-contracting muscles should appear cool, especially if flaccid paresis is present.

Body tissues that have a low metabolic rate such as fascia, tendons, tendon sheaths, ligaments, cartilage, bone, and bursae generate little heat and require only little blood flow unless inflamed, infected, or injured. Thus, they appear relatively cool in thermographic images when normal. Inflammation, infection, or injury of any of these structures will increase local blood flow, bringing core heat which is then conducted toward the skin surface. Most inflammatory events also increase the production of NO, which causes local dermal vasodilation visible to thermography.

The thermographic pattern of muscle warmth depends on muscle activity during temperature acclimatization. The internal temperature of an exercising muscle increases 0.5–1°C (0.9–1.8°F) above the arterial blood temperature.[91] If the subject is cooled in a walking/standing position, the leg muscles involved with postural balance will be warm (Figure 5.14b). If acclimatization is done in a sitting or supine position, these muscles should appear cool. The upper leg muscles, including the quadriceps, generally appear cool in subjects acclimatized standing still, though the quadriceps and the hamstring muscles may appear warmer after walking.[92] It is important to consider the subject's position and activity during acclimatization when interpreting a thermographic study.

When a subject is cooled in a standing or sitting position, the muscles over the posterior neck and upper back are under constant tension. The atlas bone (first cervical vertebra) supports the entire weight of the cranium, face, and jaw on a pivot posterior to the balance point of the head. The inferior portions of the anterior skull also support the pharynx, larynx, and upper trachea. When the body is upright, the weight of these structures anterior to the atlas pivot would rotate the head forward if not for the pull of the posterior cervical muscles, mainly the trapezius. Any tension in the anterior neck muscles requires the posterior muscles to contract more, as does leaning the head forward.

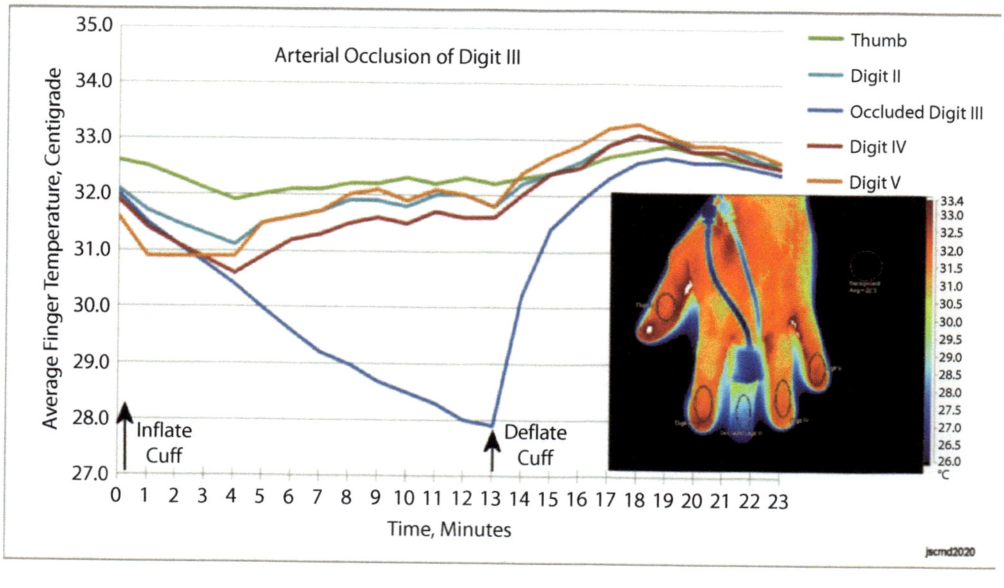

FIGURE 5.13 Occluding the blood flow to the middle finger causes significant temperature fluctuations in all the ipsilateral fingers.

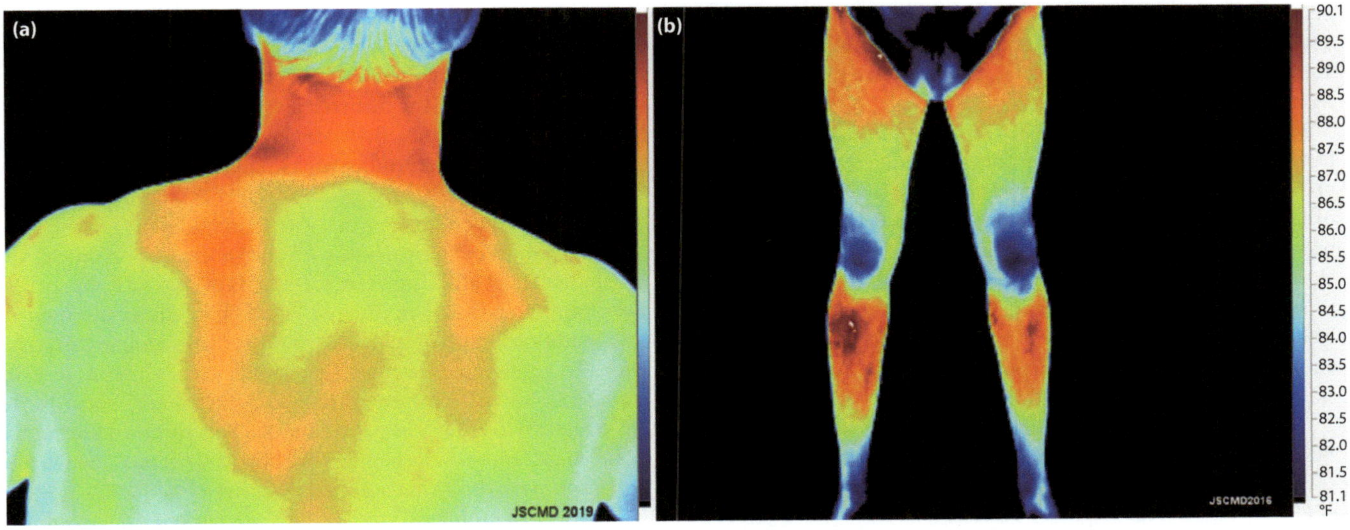

FIGURE 5.14 (a) The gravitational and muscular forces on the anterior skull create a forward rotation when the spine is upright that must be countered by the posterior neck muscles. This gives the appearance of trapezius muscle tension – 56 yoF. (b) legs, anterior view: 33-year-old right-footed male cooled with a walking-standing protocol. The muscles of walking and balance appear warm. The tendinous areas around the knee and ankle appear cool.

Subjects cooled in a standing or sitting position may often show warmth over the trapezius muscles, especially the cervical portions (Figure 5.14a). Warmth of the scapular portions of the trapezius may also be seen due to the tension in the upper shoulders and arm girdle required to support the weight of the arms. To thermographically examine the upper back and neck without these gravitational effects, the subject should be cooled prone with the neck in a neutral position and the arms relaxed. This may require special positioning and imaging on a massage table equipped with face and arm cradles (Figure 6.4, page 63).

Factors that affect thermographic appearance

Age

Children normally have a higher skin temperature than adults.[93] Maximal skin blood flow diminishes with advancing age, and there are functional declines at submaximal levels with age; virtually no one has a "normal" full-body thermographic pattern after age 50.[94] Older individuals show reduced cutaneous vasodilation from local warming, apparently reflecting impaired NO signaling.[95] Mean absolute temperatures of the outer canthus and anterior segment (cornea) of the eye, as measured by infrared thermometry, significantly decrease with age.[96] Altered physiological responses to cold stress can be related to aging, including attenuated peripheral vasoconstriction and reduced cold-induced metabolic heat production.[97] It is also known that older men and women sweat less during passive heat exposure than young gender-matched subjects.[98] In the practical context of infrared imaging, the age-related changes in skin blood flow are most relevant when comparing current thermograms to much earlier thermograms as opposed to comparing annual thermograms. Fortunately, sagittal thermal symmetry is not affected by age.[99]

Body composition

As with all major imaging techniques (ultrasound, X-ray, CT, and MRI), thermographic image quality is adversely affected by obesity. The thickness of subdermal fat has a decisive influence on the heat emitted from the skin surface. Because body fat has the lowest thermal conductivity of any tissue, it is the best insulator (see Table 5.1). Lower skin temperatures are consistently detected by infrared imaging in overweight individuals.[100] Impaired skin microcirculation in regions with high fat content also reduces the heat emission.[101] Overweight individuals release their metabolically generated core heat more slowly than those of normal weight, which means it takes longer for the heat to reach the skin by conduction or blood convection, attenuating temperature changes measurable through infrared imaging.[102]

Heat conduction depends on the existing temperature gradient as well as on the thermal conductivity of various body layers, all of which are in direct contact.[103] The water content of these tissue layers has a major positive impact on thermal conductivity. Because of the low water content of fat, heat flow is significantly hindered by the subcutaneous fat layer. The thicker the fat layer (which can be quite thick in obese individuals), the more it will

TABLE 5.1 Average Thermal Conductivity of Some Body Tissues[104]

Substance	Thermal Conductivity (W/m/°C)
Air	0.03
Blood	0.52
Bone	0.32
Brain	0.51
Breast fat	0.21
Breast gland	0.33
Connective tissue	0.39
Eye (aq. humor)	0.58
Subdermal fat	0.21
Muscle	0.49
Tendon/ligament	0.47
Testis	0.52
Water	0.60

insulate the skin from the heat of underlying muscles, viscera, and other structures. The major arteries and veins are deeply situated in or below the insulating fat, thus they are rarely visualized by infrared imaging.

Measurements of surface temperatures tend to be most reduced in the abdomen and thighs, as these areas of the body have the greatest accumulations of body fat.[105] The surface temperature of these body parts is inversely proportional to the subcutaneous fat thickness, as well as being strongly proportional to the share of visceral fat. Increased glomus activity in the hands leads to enhanced blood flow and may compensate for the reduced heat loss in the torso. This explains why increased body fat percentage tends to increase palm skin surface temperature even as torso skin temperatures are reduced.[106]

Gender

A woman's skin is cooler, on average, than a man's skin; this appears to be related to a higher subdermal fat thickness in women.[107] After adjusting for body composition, a male's higher basal metabolic rate could also be a factor, as this would require higher heat dissipation by the skin.[108] According to Anbar: "Because of the different distribution of body fat in males and females, one expects to see significant gender-related differences not only in the average skin temperature but in the relative temperatures of the skin of different organs, as well as in the skin temperature distribution over specific organs. The difference in skin temperature between men and women is accentuated in a cold environment where women have a lower core to skin conductance than men."[109]

Diabetes and hyperglycemia

Many vascular abnormalities occur in people with diabetes mellitus, especially in the hands and feet. Infrared imaging can assess the peripheral circulation in diabetic individuals by applying a mild cold stress followed by imaging the thermal recovery.[110] Individuals with poorly managed diabetes may show declines in microvascular functioning, which can lead to dangerous foot ulcers. Diabetic neuropathy reduces adrenergic sympathetic vasoconstriction as well as cholinergic sympathetic vasodilation and sweating. Thermography has obvious advantages for monitoring these individuals by following the thermographic appearance of the plantar foot after cold challenge.[111]

Hypertension

Hypertension damages the blood vessels; it can also exacerbate atherosclerosis. Maximal skin blood flow is reduced in hypertension, and may be detected by infrared imaging.[112] Research on peripheral vascular reactivity using thermography to monitor the hand images before and after cold challenge yields significant results; vascular hyperactivity becomes manifest before an abnormal increase in blood pressure is recognized.[113] Medications used to treat hypertension, especially clonidine and Ace-Receptor Blockers (ARBs) may affect glomus AVA functioning, thus altering the thermographic picture. Whether thermographic image interpretation can detect poor or inadequate management of hypertension is an area in need of study.

Female reproductive hormones

Estrogens and other female reproductive hormones exert key influences on autonomic regulation of body temperature. Estradiol and progesterone influence thermoregulation both centrally and peripherally. Whereas estradiol tends to promote heat dissipation, progesterone tends to promote heat conservation and higher body temperatures.[114] Changes in thermoregulation over the course of the menstrual cycle are mediated by hormonal influences on neural control of skin blood flow and sweating.

Different phases of the menstrual cycle are linked with fluctuations in body temperature. Body temperature may be approximately 0.4°C (0.7°F) higher in the luteal phase (after ovulation) than in the earlier follicular phase of the cycle.[115] When exercising in the mid-luteal phase, women with normal menstruation show less effective heat dissipation in comparison with thermoregulation during the mid-follicular phase. Gross measurements of skin heat dissipation were found to be lower in the mid-luteal phase under thermoneutral conditions; moreover, the set point of core temperature also seems to be elevated during that phase.[116] According to an early study, warm breasts compared to a cool sternal area occur in the pre-ovulatory period, while the situation was reversed during the luteal phase. These cyclic changes did not occur in post-menopause subjects or women taking oral contraceptives.[117]

"Estrogen dominance," means having elevated estrogen levels with insufficient progesterone to balance the estrogenic effects. Although it is claimed by certain thermography centers that estrogen/progesterone dominance can be detected by certain breast heat patterns, studies addressing this subject are lacking in the scientific literature. Until such studies are performed, such claims must be evaluated with skepticism.

Exogenous estrogens can have profound effects on breast vasculature and skin temperature if given in high doses (see Figure 5.15). These effects may take over 6 months or more to resolve after stopping the hormone. Estrogenic overstimulation can be followed thermographically, and the effect can be strong enough to change the breast TH classification. On the other hand, progesterone applied transdermally in doses of 20 mg per day appears to have little, if any, effect on the thermographic breast image. Newer transdermal hormone preparations also contain 0.75 mg of estriol, applied once daily. Whether this dose of estriol, a mild estrogen with poor skin absorption, will have discernable thermographic effects remains to be seen. Of greater concern is the advent of non-prescription estriol vaginal suppositories, which contain a therapeutic dose (2 mg) given via a highly-absorbent route. Subjects undergoing thermographic imaging should be questioned about all hormones they may be taking, both prescription and non-prescription "supplements."

Psychological stress

Thermoregulation of the skin is controlled by the autonomic nervous system, which can be profoundly influenced by psychological stress. Transient reductions in skin blood flow occur when people are "under stress."[118] Mental or emotional distress has been shown to elicit an increase in core body temperature, a phenomenon known as "psychogenic fever."[119] When the stress is acute, the impact is transient: sympathetic activation results in peripheral vasoconstriction, which shunts blood into the core, thereby raising core body temperature while lowering skin surface temperature. Outwardly, the thermoregulatory response to mental stress manifests as a short-lived skin cooling (vasoconstriction) followed by skin vasodilation and then recovery.[120]

Even supposedly non-stressful but closely personal social interactions can produce significant increases in facial and upper chest skin temperatures. This reaction is increased if the examiner is of the opposite sex, and if the interaction is more personal in nature.[121] For this, as well as ethical reasons, any interaction with subjects undergoing thermography should be kept strictly professional, avoiding any personal touching or "off-color" humor

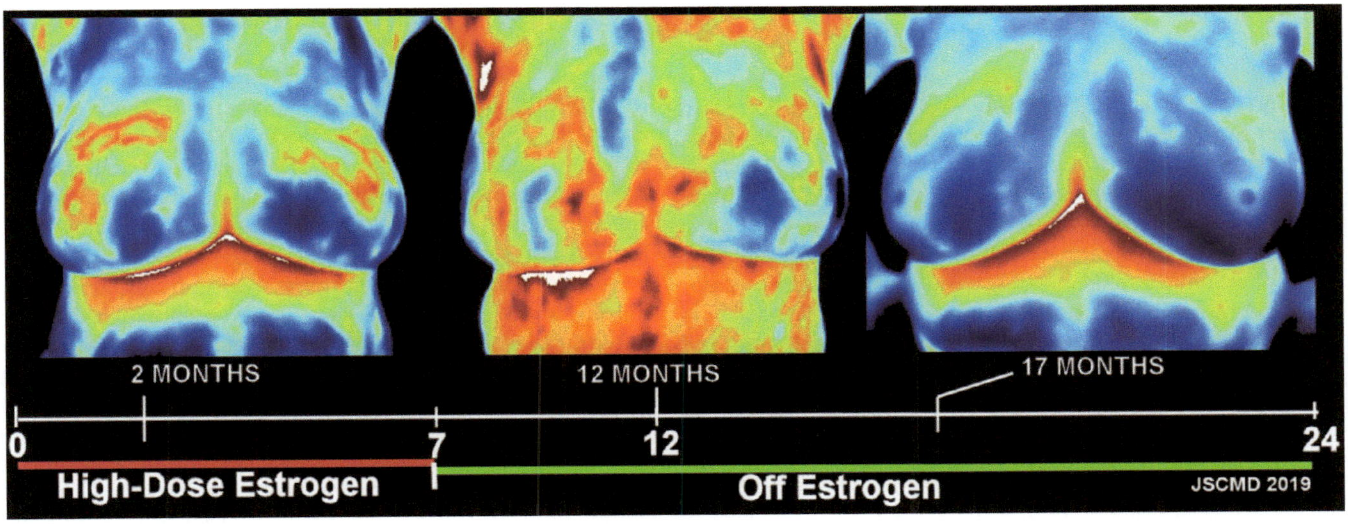

FIGURE 5.15 Thermographic effect of high-dose transdermal cyclical estradiol/progesterone therapy for 7 months: A pattern of increased vasculature over the breasts was visible by 2 months and was still prominent 5 months after stopping the therapy, but had resolved by 10 months. Vessels of the chest wall, axillae, and abdomen were also stimulated.

of an embarrassing nature. Disruptions of patient privacy during thermography, especially if they are unclothed, should be avoided.

Thermal effects of alcohol and drugs

Niacin

Niacin is a B-vitamin that can be obtained from dietary sources. Dietary niacin supplying 50 to 100 mg per day does not appear to have significant thermographic effects. At pharmacologic doses of 1000 to 3000 mg, however, niacin has definite effects on skin blood flow (Figure 5.16). Flushing of the face is one of the most common side-effects associated with ingestion of niacin as well as nitrate medicines (nitroglycerine, isosorbide dinitrate, etc.) and PDE5 inhibitor drugs (sildenafil, etc.). Pharmacologic heat dissipation may be triggered by these vasodilating drugs. All forms of niacin should be avoided for about 8–12 hours before a thermographic exam.

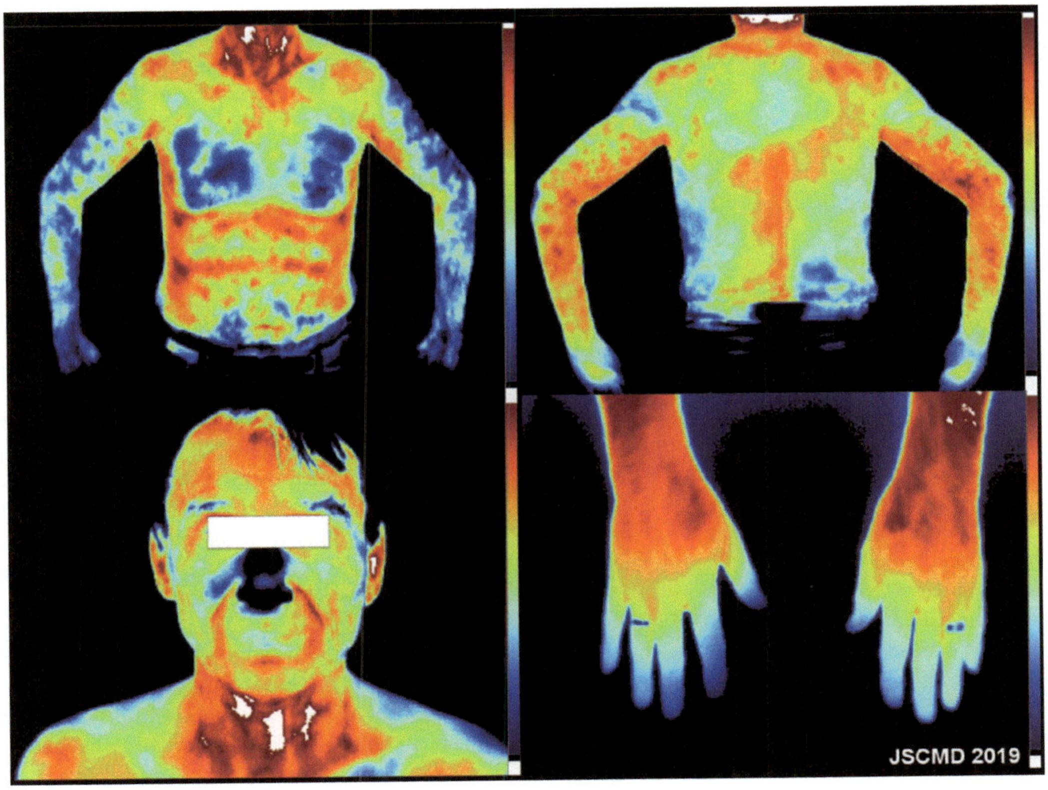

FIGURE 5.16 Niacin flush reaction in a 76-year-old vasoconstricted man. Note that the glomus AVAs under the nails are not dilated, nor is the nose. The ears, however, are vasodilated.

Epinephrine

(Adrenaline) is known to have a strong vasoconstrictive effect. This medication is found in some non-prescription asthma inhalers. Intravenous epinephrine infusions in bovines decreased corneal temperatures significantly, suggesting that autonomic-mediated conjunctival vasoconstriction occurred.[122] Albuterol (salbutamol), a prescription Beta-2 agonist asthma medication available as an inhaler or for oral use, causes an increase in the blood flow to the forearm of up to 45%.[123] Whether albuterol results in thermographic warming of the hand or dilation of glomus AVAs remains to be studied. Thermographic subjects should be asked whether they use asthma medications, what type, and when it was last used.

Alcohol

Moderate alcohol ingestion does not appear to markedly alter the thermoregulatory response to hypothermia.[124] Moderate alcohol intake is defined as ingesting 70 milliliters of pure ethanol per day for males, 53 ml/day for females. Animal studies suggest that high, frequent doses of alcohol may impair both autonomic and behavioral thermoregulation and may lower the set point for the control of body temperature.[125] Hand temperatures are definitely warmer after consuming 10 g of pure ethanol (equivalent to 25 cc of 40% [80 proof] whiskey). This effect is stronger in non-drinkers.[126] Recent alcohol ingestion or the presence of a "hangover" increases breast temperature significantly with a more diffuse pattern than normally seen.[127] Although moderate alcohol intake is unlikely to have any significant thermographic impact, it should be avoided at least 6 hours before a thermographic exam.

Nicotine and stimulant drugs

Nicotine via any delivery method (smoking, vaporizing, chewing tobacco, snuff, gum, transdermal, etc.) has a vasoconstrictive effect. Smoking may have a profound effect on the thermographic appearance of non-smokers, and may cause a drop of up to 3°C in breast surface temperature.[128] A subject undergoing thermography should not smoke or "vape" within 3 hours of the exam; and users of other longer-acting nicotine forms may need to discontinue their use the day before the exam. Other stimulants such as cocaine, caffeine, and certain pungent spices may elicit thermogenic responses to the extent that hypothermia can be delayed upon cold exposure.[129] Due to their thermal artifact potential, subjects should avoid use of these substances prior to an infrared imaging session.

Physiology of the cold stress challenge

Immersion of one or more limbs in cold water, commonly known as the cold stress challenge or cold stress test, is the most common way of providing a thermal challenge to evoke an autonomic response. Immersion of the hands in cold water can absorb about 100 to 200 watts of heat from a warm vasodilated subject; less if the subject is vasoconstricted.[130] The cold stress test typically involves the use of cold water at 12–16°C (55–60°F) applied to the hands or feet.[131] Either one or both hands or feet are immersed in a cold-water bath, which may be unpleasant for an already cooled subject, but is not painful. Any subsequent skin temperature changes are documented by repeat imaging of the bodily regions of interest. Cold stress produces a generalized adrenergic sympathetic vasoconstriction by cooling the blood returning from the immersed limb(s). This reaction may be blocked by restricting venous return with a tourniquet proximal to the immersed limb segment.[132] In addition, the vasoconstriction is temporary, lasting only about 5 minutes.[133] This recovery is most likely due to autonomic stimulation of BAT.

For more severe cold stress testing, ice-water immersion (0°C/32°F) produces a temporary systemic sympathetic response due to the intense cold stimulating the TRPA1 receptors in the skin, causing pain (see Figure 5.1). This can be detected as a transient increase in blood pressure and heart rate, which fades as the cold-sensing nerve fibers slow and cease firing, becoming numb to the stimulus.[134] The different thermographic responses to cold versus ice-water challenge have not been fully explored using modern imagers, and whether one is more useful than the other in the diagnosis of various conditions remains to be studied.

Until the 1990s, the cold stress challenge test was commonly believed to improve the sensitivity and specificity of breast thermography. Sometimes cold stress was applied directly to the breast using chilled air or evaporative sprays. To date, however, no cold stress procedure has shown any advantage over standard thermograms of the breast in vasoconstricted subjects. An observational study of cold challenge responses in 500 patients with normal or persistent abnormal thermograms concluded that it does not enhance the detection of occult cancers in those thermograms.[135]

It should be pointed out, however, that the cold stress challenge has good utility as a test for Raynaud's disease, Complex Regional Pain Syndrome (CRPS), peripheral neuropathy, and other conditions. Clinical research suggests that cold stress testing coupled with thermography may be an effective way to evaluate patients suffering from these diseases.[136]

Dietary influences on skin temperature

Dietary factors can influence skin temperatures by altering vascular dynamics. Omega-3 polyunsaturated fatty acids regulate vasomotor tone by competing with omega-6 fatty acids for metabolic enzymes.[137] Omega-3 fatty acids have been extensively studied in terms of both vasodilatory and anti-inflammatory effects.[138] Whereas fish oil has vasodilatory effects, borage oil may promote vasoconstriction.[139]

Polyphenol-rich foods and food products such as grape products (e.g., grape juice and wine), black and red berries, green and black teas, and cocoa can trigger activating pathways in endothelial cells, increasing formation of NO, and relaxing vascular tone.[140] The juices extracted from polyphenol-rich berries such as blueberry, pomegranate, raspberry, cranberry, and black currant, all support sustained NO formation.[141] Allicin (from garlic) and capsaicin (from chili pepper) induce endothelium-dependent NO-mediated relaxations of arteries.[142] The cocoa in chocolate contains polyphenols, which increase endothelial vasodilation.[143]

Diet-induced thermogenesis refers to the energy dissipated as heat after a meal.[144] The majority of this diet-induced heat is produced as a byproduct of the energy required to convert and store the ingested ingredients. Another thermogenic response elicited by food ingestion occurs in the BAT, which" burns" glucose and fatty acids, producing heat in response to dietary stimuli.[145] A high-fat, high-protein meal is more likely to produce this effect.[146] When dietary protein intake in a single meal exceeds 30 grams, protein oxidation becomes an important driver of BAT thermogenesis.[147] Omega-3 fatty acids from fish oil may activate thermogenic BAT in humans.[148] A number of dietary phytochemicals and botanicals have been shown to stimulate BAT thermogenesis in laboratory animals.[149]

Strong dietary spices such as capsicum, ginger, and other irritants to mucous membranes can cause changes to the thermographic appearance of the face and possibly other body sites. These substances are known to stimulate parasympathetic vasodilatory nerves supplying the central parts of the face around the eyes, nose and mouth.[150] This effect may be detected via facial thermography in a cooled subject (see Figure 10.27). Whether other dietary influences listed in this section have thermographically detectable signatures will require further study.

SIDEBAR 5.3 THERMOGRAPHY REFLECTS ANATOMY

The changes in skin surface temperature detected by thermography are based on human physiology. Once these physiological principles are in play, however, it is the gross and microscopic anatomy beneath the epidermal surface that produces and shapes the thermal findings. The warmth produced by an underlying inflammation will be most intense in the overlying skin. Skin warmth caused by glomus AVA dilation will have a distinct distribution and thermal appearance. Thus, the location and shape of the visualized warm pattern provide information linked to the anatomical structure underneath that is producing the thermal findings. Whether the detected surface warmth is caused by thermal conduction from a superficial muscle, nitric oxide vasodilation from an area of inflammation or neoplasm, a subdermal varicose vein, or changes in vasoconstrictive control due to sympathetic nerve injury, the location and pattern of the thermal anomalies will give important clues to the underlying pathophysiology. It is imperative that the interpreting thermographer has a strong working knowledge of musculoskeletal, arterio-venous, lymphatic, and neural anatomy, as well as the anatomical distribution of the sympathetic autonomic nervous system. An atlas of anatomy is an essential addition to any thermography reading station.

It is primarily the superficial layers of the body that will have the most thermographic relevance, while changes in the deeper muscle layers will be less visible thermographically as these layers are insulated from the skin by overlying muscles and tissues. The deepest muscles, such as the psoas, will generally not be visible to thermography. Thermal patterns will also be attenuated by a thick overlying adipose layer, sometimes to the point of being invisible to thermography. In such cases, the areas with less adipose thickness – notably the face, hands, knees, and feet – may still provide useful thermographic information.

Physiology of the hot flash

Vasomotor instability symptoms, also known as "hot flashes," are common among menopausal women; they can also occur in older men. A hot flash involves a sudden sensation of being overheated, often accompanied by sweating and vasodilation of the face, neck, and chest. Hot flashes occurring at night during sleep may generate night sweats.[151] The prevalence of vasomotor symptoms increases with obesity, anxiety, depression, higher environmental temperatures, and lower altitudes.[152]

The physiology of the hot flash involves alterations of sex hormones (lower estradiol, higher follicle-stimulating hormone, lower testosterone) as well as elevated sympathetic and diminished parasympathetic control over heart rate coinciding with vasomotor symptoms.[153] Subjects may lack a normal thermoneutral zone – the zone of core temperatures within which sweating, peripheral vasodilation, and shivering do not occur.[154] The thermoneutral zone may become so narrow that small perturbations in core temperature will trigger a heat dissipation event.

Hot flashes are only experienced when skin temperature increases.[155] Skin temperature increase occurs over about 10 minutes, after which it declines back to normal within half an hour. During this time, the core temperature drops by about 0.5°C (0.9°F).[156] Thermograms of the upper chest, shoulders, neck, and face show an overall increase in temperature of about 1°C (1.8°F).[157] Skin temperature increase may precede the actual subjective feeling of warmth by 10 to 15 seconds. Thermograms often continue to show increased skin temperature elevation for several minutes after the sensation of the flush has subsided.

Curiously, a person experiencing a hot flash may show signs of peripheral vasoconstriction (cool hands or feet) during the episode. Further research may offer insights into the mechanisms underlying the effects of hot flashes on specific regions of the body.

Physiology of the blush

Blushing is a complex psychophysiological phenomenon manifesting as a reddening of the cheeks and forehead that can also extend to the ears, neck, and upper chest. Blushing is an involuntary vasodilation on being embarrassed or praised. Darwin devoted considerable attention to the blush, which he believed occurred when "thinking about what others think of us."[158]

Physiologically, the increased skin blood flow results from the combined influence of NO, bradykinin, and histamine, along with circulating epinephrine acting on vascular β-adrenoceptors and cervical sympathetic vasodilator discharge.[159] This leads to an increase in vasodilation in the face, which is richly endowed with cutaneous blood vessels.[160] The blushing response involves elevations in cheek and forehead temperatures together with rapid fluctuations in blood flow and blood volume accompanying each heartbeat.[161]

When examined thermographically, peak facial temperatures during blushing are substantially delayed from the vascular reaction. While peak facial blood flow occurs within 20 seconds of the blush stimulus, skin temperature peaks about a minute and a half after the stimulus.[162] As blushing causes definite changes in skin temperature, situations that might induce blushing during a routine thermographic examination should be avoided.

SIDEBAR 5.4 A THERMOGRAPHIC MYSTERY

The "rule" that superficial tendons appear cool in thermal images has a frequently-seen exception: the hamstring tendons behind the knee along with the posterior plane of the knee joint often appear warmer than the adjacent muscles in subjects acclimatized in a standing position (Figure 5.17). Often the semimembranosus and semitendinosus tendons are warmer than the more lateral biceps femoris, creating a J-L pattern when both posterior knees are imaged. If the biceps femoris tendon is also visibly warm, a U-U pattern is created. A possible L-J pattern with the biceps femoris tendons being prominent is encountered less often.

Why these tendons often appear warm remains a mystery. There are no nearby vessels, muscles, or other metabolizing tissues to account for these patterns, and the large vessels in the popliteal fossa are located in the midline of the joint, away from the tendons. Subjects displaying these patterns generally have normal knee function and do not complain of posterior knee or upper leg pain. Studies investigating this thermographic enigma are needed to elucidate these findings.

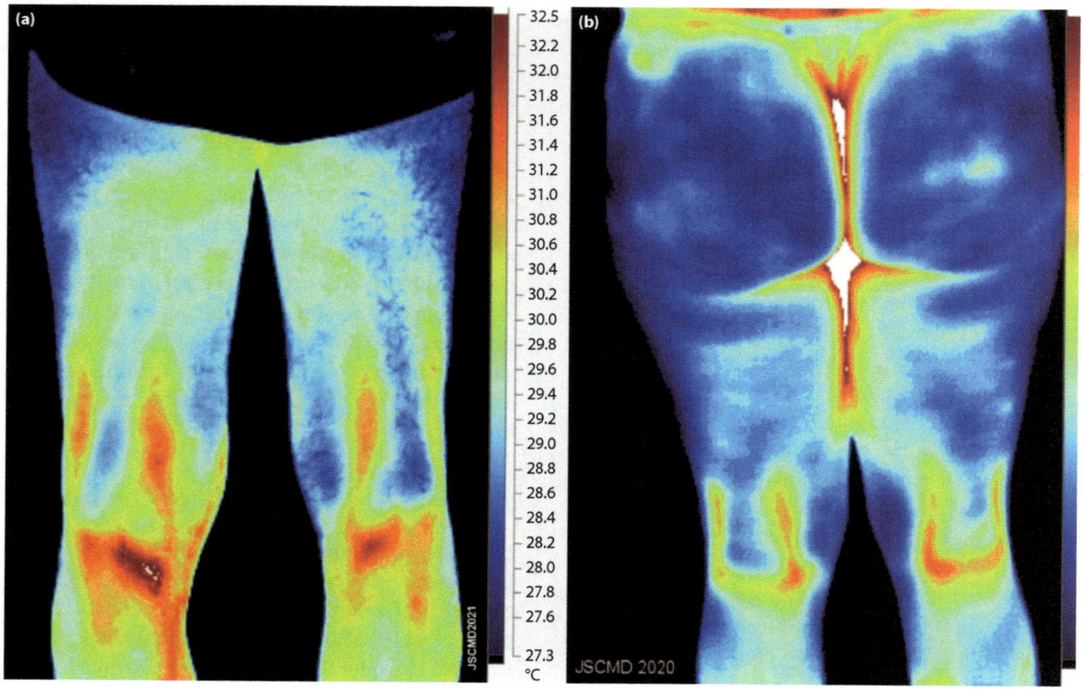

FIGURE 5.17 Posterior knees views showing a U-U pattern which corresponds anatomically to the location of the hamstring tendons and posterior plane of the knee joint. (a) 65 yoM. (b) 48 yoF.

Notes

1. Protsiv M, et al., eLife 2020; PMCID: PMC6946399. Note: Absolute Temperatures reported by different researchers may vary. Diurnal timing of temperature sampling must be considered.
2. Sund-Levander M, et al., Scand J Caring Sci. 2002; PMID: 12000664.
3. Inamasu J, et al., Ann Emerg Med. 2002; PMID: 12140503.
4. Mallet ML, Q J Med. 2002; PMID: 12454320.
5. Tarlochant F, Ramesh S, Biomed Eng Appl Basis Commun. 2005; Doi: 10.4015/S1016237205000251
6. Lepock JR. Int J Hyperthermia 2003; PMID: 12745971.
7. Al Mahri S, et al., Handb Clin Neurol. 2018; PMID: 30459024. See also: Qing Song, et al., Mil Med Res. 2016; PMCID: PMC4704265.
8. As derived from the Second Law of Thermodynamics. See: Boregowda SC, et al. Hum Perf Extrem Environ. 2001; PMID: 12182196.
9. Quesada JIP, et al., Chapter 3. In: Application of Infrared Thermography in Sports Science, Quesada JIP, editor. Springer Pub, Switzerland, 2017.
10. Stewart, JT, et al., Cardiovasc Res. 1993; PMID: 8221759.
11. Taylor NA et al., Eur J Appl Physiol. 2014; PMID: 25011493.
12. Tansey EA, et al., Adv Physiol Educ. 2015; PMID: 26330029.
13. Shilco P, et al., J Therm Biol. 2019; PMID: 30784492.
14. Romanovsky AA, Am J Physiol Regul Integr Comp Physiol. 2007; PMID: 17008453.
15. Data extracted from: Guyton AC, Hall JE, Textbook of Medical Physiology, 12th Ed, Elsevier, NL. Chap. 48. ISBN-13: 978-8131227046. See also: Tansey EA, Johnson CD, Adv Physiol Educ. 2015; PMID: 26330029.
16. Höfler W, J Appl Physiol. 1968; PMID: 5687355.
17. Mackowiak PA, et al., JAMA 1992; PMID: 1302471.
18. Quesada JIP, et al., Chapter 2, p. 43. In: Application of Infrared Thermography in Sports Science, Quesada JIP, editor. Springer Pub, Switzerland, 2017. ISBN-13: 978-3319474090.
19. Johnson JM, Scand J Med Sci Sports 2010; PMID: 21029188. See also: Gonzalez-Alonso J, et al., J Physiol. 2008; PMCID: PMC2375553.
20. Guyton and Hall Textbook of Medical Physiology, 12th Ed, UNIT XIII, Chap. 73. ISBN-13: 978-8131227046.
21. Castellani JW, Young AJ, Auton Neurosci. 2016; PMID: 26924539.
22. Glatte P. et al., Front Neurol. 2019; PMCID: PMC6746903.
23. van Beaumont W, et al., Science 1963; PMID: 13995960.
24. Fregly MJ, Blatteis CM (eds.), Handbook of Physiology. Section 4. Oxford University Press, New York, 1996. ISBN 978-0-19-507492-5.
25. Tanda G, J Phys Conference Series 2015; Doi: 10.1088/1742-6596/655/1/012062
26. Charkoudian N, J Appl Physiol. 2010; PMCID: PMC2963327. See also: Gagge AP, et al., Mechanisms of Heat Exchange: Biophysics and Physiology. Comprehensive Physiology. John Wiley & Sons, Inc, 2010; Doi: 10.1002/CPHY.CP040104
27. Tansey EA, Johnson CD. Adv Physiol Educ. 2015; PMID: 26330029.
28. This occurs when the wet-bulb temperature goes above 35°C.
29. Diagram courtesy of NOAA, the US National Oceanic and Atmospheric Administration/National Weather Service.
30. Anbar M, Quantitative Dynamic Telethermometry in Medical Diagnosis and Management, 1st Ed, CRC Press, New York, 1994. ISBN 9780849344091.
31. Johnson PC, Overview of the microcirculation. In: Handbook of Physiology: Microcirculation, 2nd Ed, Tuma RF, et al. (eds.). Elsevier/Academic Press. Cambridge, MA, 2008; ISBN-13: 978-0123745309.
32. Roustit M, et al., Trends Pharmacol Sci. 2013; PMID: 23791036. See also: Hill MA, et al., Trends Pharmacol Sci. 2009; PMID: 19541373.
33. Joyner MJ, et al., Circ J. 2009; PMCID: PMC3760385. See also: Andersen P, et al., J Physiol. 1985; PMCID: PMC1193029. See also: Armstrong RB, et al., J Appl Physiol. 1985; PMID: 4055609.
34. Johnson JM, Kellogg DL Jr, Local thermal control of the human cutaneous circulation. J Appl Physiol (1985). 2010; PMCID: PMC2963328.
35. Walsh JA, et al., Anaesth Intensive Care. 1985; PMID: 3977062.
36. Ibid 30.
37. Johnson JM, et al., J Appl Physiol. 1995; PMID: 7775340.
38. Illustration from: Wheater's Functional Histology, 6th Ed, Young B, O'Dowd G, & Woodford P., Eds.; Chap. 9 – Skin; Elsevier Pub, Amsterdam, 2014. Used with permission. Text added for clarity by jscmd.
39. The AVA glomus bodies in the skin bear no relation to the glomus cells of the peripheral sensor cells in the neck arteries.

40. Walløe L, Temperature 2016; Doi: 10.1080/23328940.2015.1088502
41. Winsor T, Karpman H, Angiology. 1958; Doi: 10.1177/000331975800900402
42. Ibid 42.
43. Chemical structure from The Wikipedia entry for norepinephrine as confirmed by The Merck Index, 15th Ed., entry 6784 – norepinephrine; The Royal Society of Chemistry, Cambridge, UK, 2013.
44. Image Source: acetylcholine.png, Wikipedia, Yohan 2004. Chemical structure confirmed by The Merck Index, 15th Ed., entries 80 & 81; The Royal Society of Chemistry, Cambridge, UK, 2013.
45. File:Nitric-oxide-3D-vdW.png. Model of nitric oxide. by Benjah-bmm27,Wikipedia 2007. File:Nitric oxide.svg by Yikrazuul (2008) as modified by Officer781, Wikipedia 2019. File:Nitric-oxide-2D.svg. Structural formula of nitric oxide by YinY, Wikipedia 2017.
46. Johnson JM, et al. Compr Physiol 2014; PMID: 24692134.
47. National Institute for Occupational Safety and Health (NIOSH). Nitric oxide. https://www.cdc.gov/niosh/npg/npgd0448.html
48. Thomas DD. Proc Natl Acad Sci U S A. 2001; PMCID: PMC14594.
49. Liew FY, et al., Immunol Today 1991; PMID: 1712593.
50. Bruch-Gerharz D, et al. Arch Dermatol Res. 1998; PMID: 9879832.
51. Kellogg DL, Jr, et al. J Appl Physiol 1999; PMID: 10194201. See also: Minson CT, et al. J Appl Physiol 2001; PMID: 11568143.
52. Kellogg DL, et al., J Appl Physiol. 1998; PMID: 9729553. See also: Shastry S, et al., J Appl Physiol. 1998; PMID: 9729554.
53. Gooding KM, et al., J Vasc Res. 2005; PMID: 16498265. See also: Johnson JM, et al., Clin Physiol. 1986; Doi: 10.1111/j.1475-097X.1986tb00239.x. See also: Taylor WF, et al., J Appl Physiol. 1984; PMID: 3527533.
54. Hodges GJ, et al., J Appl Physiol. 2008; PMCID: PMC249483. See also: Houghton BL, et al. J Physiol (Lond) 2007; PMCID: PMC1780012. See also: Minson CT, et al. J Appl Physiol. 2001; PMID: 11568143.
55. Johnson JM, et al., J Appl Physiol. (1985). 2010. PMCID: PMC2963328.
56. Polhemus DJ, et al., Circ Res. 2014; PMCID: PMC3951140.
57. Hemelrijk, SD, et al., Sci Rep. 2018; PMCID: PMC5832815.
58. Nossaman VE, et al., Cardiol Rev. 2010; PMCID: PMC2885014.
59. Thomsen LL, et al., Cancer Metastasis Rev. 1998; PMID: 9544425. See also: Thomsen LL, et al., Br J Cancer 1995; PMCID: PMC2034139. See also: Anbar M. 1994; PMID: 8076360.
60. Thomsen LL, et al. Br J Cancer 1995; PMCID: PMC2034139.
61. Ibid 30
62. Anbar M, 1995. NII Article ID (NAID) 10029002337. https://ci.nii.ac.jp/naid/10029002337/
63. Fokam D, et al., J Basic Clin Physiol Pharmacol. 2018; PMID: 30375348.
64. Harms M, et al., Nat Med. 2013. PMID: 24100998. Note: True Brown Adipose Tissue (BAT) is found in newborns and does not require neural stimulation to produce heat. BAT in adults is actually Beige or "Brite" Adipose Tissue, which is induced by cold or sympathetic neural stimulation to produce heat. As both tissues produce heat by activating UCP1, this book will refer to the adult tissues as "BAT" to avoid confusion.
65. Ammer K, Ring F, The Thermal Human Body - A Practical Guide to Thermal Imaging, 2019. Jenny Stanford Publishing, Singapore. ISBN 9789814745826.
66. González-García I, et al., J Physiol Biochem. 2020; PMID: 31845114.
67. Søberg S, et al., Cell Rep Med. 2020; PMCID: PMC8561167. See also: Law J, et al. Temperature (Austin). 2018; PMCID: PMC6209420.
68. Yoneshiro T, et al., Ann Med. 2015; PMID: 24901355. See also: Saito M. Endocr J. 2014; PMID: 24401694.
69. Klepac K, et al., Mol Aspects Med. 2019; PMID: 31283940.
70. Hanssen MJ, et al., Nat Med. 2015; PMID: 26147760.
71. Fernández-Verdejo R, et al., Mol Aspects Med. 2019; PMCID: PMC7112661.
72. Ouellet V, et al., J Clin Invest. 2012; PMCID: PMC3266793. See also: Bartelt A, et al., Nat Med. 2011. PMID: 21258337. See also Chen KY, et al., Cell Metab. 2016; PMCID: PMC4981083.
73. Haq T, et al., Sci Rep. 2017; PMCID: PMC5607277.
74. Oreskovich SM, et al., J Endocr Soc. 2019; PMCID: PMC6855213.
75. Hall JE, Guyton AC, Guyton and Hall Textbook of Medical Physiology. 13th Ed, Saunders, Saint Louis, US, 2014. ISBN-13: 978-1455770052. Cited in: Haq T, et al. Sci Rep. 2017; PMCID: PMC5607277.
76. Jimenez-Pavon D, et al., Obesity (Silver Spring). 2019; PMCID: PMC6899990.
77. Nirengi S, et al., PLoS One 2019; PMID: 31449537 PMCID: PMC6709909.
78. Note: The skin over the medial face is also enervated by parasympathetic fibers.
79. Source: OpenStax College, File:1501, Connections of the Sympathetic Nervous System.jpg in Wikipedia entry for Sympathetic nervous system. Created: 24 May 2013. CC BY 3.0.
80. Image from Wikimedia Commons, File:Songboythermal.jpg; Author: Songboy1234. Image date: 2004.
81. Raj, P, Editor. Textbook of Regional Anesthesia. Section IV, Ch12 – Monitoring in Regional Anesthesia p. 196. Elsevier Science (USA), Pub. 2002; ISBN 0-443-06569-1.
82. Hausmann JS, et al., J Gen Intern Med. 2018; PMCID: PMC6258625.
83. Illustration: Gray384.png of Wikipedia in the Public Domain. Source: Henry Gray (1918) Anatomy of the Human Body. Illustrator: HV, Carter. Vein and artery color and image title added by jscmd.
84. Illustration: Gray417.png of Wikipedia in the Public Domain. Source: Henry Gray (1918) Anatomy of the Human Body. Illustrator: HV, Carter. Vein and artery color added by jscmd.
85. Illustration: Gray432.png of Wikipedia licensed with PD-Gray's Anatomy plate, PD-US. Marshall Strother 2010.
86. Bunton GL, Fluid Balance Without Tears, 2nd Ed., Lloyd-Luke LTD, London 1966. ISBN-13: 978-0853241249.
87. Walløe L. Temperature (Austin). 2015; PMCID: PMC4861183.
88. Robertson D, ed., Primer on the Autonomic Nervous System, 3rd Ed, Academic Press, New York, 2012. ISBN:978-0-12-386525-0.
89. Shibasaki M, et al., J Appl Physiol. 2006; PMID: 16614366.
90. Baker JS, et al., J Nutr Metab. 2010; PMCID: PMC3005844.
91. González-Alonso J, et al., J Physiol. 2000; PMCID: PMC2269891.
92. Note: The biceps femoris, semitendinosus, and semimembranosus muscles comprise the "hamstring muscles."
93. Ibid 30
94. Martin HL et al., J Appl Physiol. 1995; PMID: 7559234. See also: Rooke GA, et al., J Appl Physiol. 1994; PMID: 7961221.
95. Minson CT et al., J Appl Physiol. 2002; PMID: 12381749. See also: Drummond PD. J Auton Nerv Syst. 1998; PMID: 9696264.
96. Aliò J, Padron M, Ophthalmic Res. 1982; PMID: 7099534.
97. Kenney WL, Munce TA. J Appl Physiol. 2003; PMID: 14600165.
98. Crowe JP, et al., J Physiol. 1974; PMID: 4818516. See also: Inoue Y, et al., Eur J Appl Physiol. 1995; PMID: 7729440. See also: Fennell WH, et al., J Physiol. 1973; PMID: 4720930.
99. Moreira DG, et al., J Phys Educ Sport 2017; Doi: 10.7752/jpes.2017.04286
100. Chudecka M, et al., J Therm Biol. 2014; PMID: 24956951. See also: Neves EB, et al., J Therm Biol. 2017; PMID: 29108552.
101. Antonios TF, et al., Hypertension. 1999; PMID: 10523342. See also: Levy BI, et al., Circulation 2001; PMID: 11489784.
102. Kurz A, et al., Anesth Analg. 1995; PMID: 7864426.
103. Cramer MN, Jay O. Auton Neurosci. 2016; PMID: 26971392.
104. Table entries derived from the Tissue Thermal Conductivity Database of The Foundation for Research on Information Technologies in Society (IT'IS), https://itis.swiss/virtual-population/tissue-properties/database/thermal-conductivity/ 2019.
105. Neves EB, et al., J Therm Biol. 2017; PMID: 29108552.
106. Salamunes ACC, et al, J Therm Biol. 2017; PMID: 28477901.
107. Neves EB, et al., J Therm Biol. 2017; PMID: 29108552.
108. Lazzer S, et al, Obesity (Silver Spring) 2010; PMID: 19478787.
109. Ibid 30, See also: Salamunes ACC, et al., J Therm Biol. 2017; PMID: 28477901.
110. Ring F, J Diabetes Sci Technol. 2010; PMCID: PMC2909517. See also: Marcinkowska-Gapińska A, et al., Clin Hemorheol Microcir. 2006; PMID: 17148846.
111. Balbinot LF, Clinics 2012; PMCID: PMC3521805.

112. Thiruvengadam J, et al., Biomed Tech (Berl). 2018; PMID: 28675748. See also: De Cesaris R et al. Drugs Exp Clin Res. 1985; PMID: 3836858.
113. Strangi T, et al., Int J Cardiol. 1989; PMID: 2620997. See also: Tham TC, et al. J Hum Hypertens. 1990; PMID: 2370647.
114. Charkoudian N, et al., Clin Auton Res. 2017; PMID: 28488202.
115. Hessemer V, et al., J Appl Physiol. 1985; PMID: 4077798. See also: Grucza R, et al., Eur J Appl Physiol Occup Physiol. 1993; PMID: 8223544. See also: Stephenson LA, et al., Med Sci Sports Exerc. 1982; PMID: 7132643.
116. Ibid 30.
117. Ewing KL et al. Ohio Journal of Science. 1973; ISSN: 0030-0950. http://hdl.handle.net/1811/21956
118. Hornyak ME, et al, Acta Physiol Scand. 1990; PMID: 2356759.
119. Oka T, et al., Adv Neuroimmune Biol. 2012; Doi: 10.1080/23328940.2015.1056907
120. Herborn KA et al., Physiol Behav. 2018; PMCID: PMC5945995.
121. Hahn AC et al. Biol Lett. 2012; PMCID: PMC3440979.
122. Stewart M et al., J. Dairy Sci. 2010; PMID: 20965341.
123. Burggraaf J et al., Thorax 2001; PMCID: PMC1746095.
124. Allison TG, et al., J Appl Physiol. 1992; PMID: 1629061.
125. Gordon CJ, et al., Pharmacol Biochem Behav. 1988; PMID: 3413196.
126. Mannara G, et al., Boll Soc Ital Biol Sper. 1993; PMID: 8198799.
127. Ewing KL et al., Ohio J Sci. 1973; ISSN: 0030-0950. http://hdl.handle.net/1811/21956
128. Ewing KL et al., Ohio J Sci. 1973; ISSN: 0030-0950. http://hdl.handle.net/1811/21956
129. Stohs SJ, et al., Phytother Res. 2016; PMCID: PMC5067548. See also: Pandit C, et al., J Therm Biol. 2017; PMID: 28166943. See also: Crandall CG, et al. Ann Intern Med. 2002; PMID: 12044126.
130. Tipton MJ et al. J R Nav Med Serv. 1993; PMID: 8207704.
131. Diakides NA. Bronzino JD (eds). Medical Infrared Imaging, CRC Press/Taylor & Francis Group: Boca Raton, FL. 2008. Doi: https://doi.org/10.1201/9781420008340
132. Ibid 30.
133. Marshall JM, et al., J Auton Nerv Syst. 1990; PMID: 2262666.
134. Schwartz RG et al., Pan Am J Med Thermol. 2020; Doi: 10.18073/2358-4696/PAJMT.V3N1P25-31
135. Amalu WC, Conf Proc IEEE Eng Med Biol Soc. 2004; PMID: 17271894.
136. Wilkinson JD, et al., Arthritis Rheumatol. 2018; PMCID: PMC6001804. See also: Gulevich SJ, et al., Clin J Pain. 1997; PMID: 9084952.
137. Borghi C, et al., Heart Int. 2006; PMCID: PMC3184661.
138. Carnevale LN, et al., Adv Exp Med Biol. 2019; PMID: 31562632.
139. Mills DE, et al., Am J Physiol. 1990; PMID: 2260727.
140. Auger C, et al., J Cardiovasc Pharmacol. 2016; PMID: 26974893.
141. Auger C, et al., Food Funct. 2011; PMID: 21779562. See also: Alhosin M, et al., PLoS One. 2013; PMCID: PMC3606366.
142. Bratz IN, et al., Am J Physiol Heart Circ Physiol. 2008; PMID: 18390821. See also: Ku DD, et al. Clin Exp Pharmacol Physiol. 2002; PMID: 11906464.
143. Garcia JP, et al., Rev Cardiovasc Med. 2018; PMID: 31064163.
144. Ho KKY. J Endocrinol. 2018; PMID: 29895717. See also: Lev-Bari L, et al., Isr J Med Sci. 1982; PMID: 7118536.
145. Townsend KL, et al., Trends Endocrinol Metab. 2014; PMCID: PMC3972344.
146. Nagai N, et al., J Clin Endocrinol Metab. 2003; PMID: 14671150.
147. Kassis A, et al., Clin Nutr. 2019; PMID: 30269898.
148. Lund J, et al., Adipocyte. 2018; PMCID: PMC6152508.
149. Vieira-Brock PL, et al., Pharmacognosy Res. 2018; PMCID: PMC5855371. See also: Okla M, et al., Adv Nutr. 2017; PMCID: PMC5421122. See also: Silvester AJ, et al., J Nutr Biochem. 2019; PMID: 30414469. See also: Pandit C, et al., Int J Hyperthermia. 2018; PMID: 30208750. See also: Pandit C, et al., J Therm Biol. 2017; PMID: 28166943. See also: Stohs SJ, et al., Phytother Res. 2016; PMCID: PMC5067548.
150. Crozier WR, De Jong PJ (editors). The Psychological Significance of the Blush. Cambridge University Press, Cambridge, UK, 2012. ISBN-13: 978-1107013933.
151. Viera AJ, et al., Am Fam Physician. 2003; PMID: 12643362. Note: Night sweats may also be a symptom of chronic infection, certain malignancies, autoimmune diseases, endocrine disorders, psychiatric conditions, and certain drugs. Clinical evaluation may be indicated.
152. Hunter MS, et al., Climacteric. 2013; PMID: 22946508. See also: Saccomani S, et al. Menopause. 2017; PMID: 28562488. See also: Juang KD, et al., Maturitas. 2005; PMID: 16186074.
153. Thurston RC, et al., Menopause. 2010; PMCID: PMC2866826. See also: Thurston RC, et al., 2012; PMCID: PMC3292670. See also: Thurston RC, et al., Menopause. 2016; PMCID: PMC4844776. See also: de Zambotti M, et al., Menopause. 2013; PMCID: PMC3713094.
154. Freedman RR, Semin Reprod Med. 2005; PMID: 15852197.
155. Sturdee DW, et al., Climacteric. 2017; PMID: 28379074. See also: Meldrum DR, et al., Am J Obstet Gynecol. 1979; PMID: 495671. See also: Haas S, et al., Obstet Gynecol. 1988; PMID: 3357653.
156. Ibid 30.
157. Sturdee DW, et al., Maturitas. 1979; PMID: 502877.
158. Drummond PD, et al., Psychophysiology. 2004; PMID: 15032993.
159. Jawad F, J Pak Med Assoc.1982; PMID: 6808181. See also: Mellander S, et al., Acta Physiol Scand. 1982; PMID: 6291328. See also: Drott C, et al., Br J Dermatol. 1998; PMID: 9640370. See also: Drott C, et al., J Cosmet Dermatol. 2002; PMID: 17147709.
160. Gonzalez G, et al., J Neurosurg. 1975; PMID: 1095694. See also: Ryan, TJ, Structure pattern and shape of the blood vessels of the skin. In: Jarret A, ed. The Physiology and Pathophysiology of the Skin. Vol. 2, The Nerves and Blood Vessels, Academic Press, New York, 1973. ISBN 13: 9780123806017.
161. Brummelman E, et al., Psychophysiology. 2018; PMID: 29876926. See also: Voncken MJ, et al., Biol Psychol. 2009; PMID: 19428972.
162. Ibid 150.

6

ENVIRONMENTAL CONDITIONS AND PATIENT PREPARATION

In human thermographic imaging, set and setting are extremely important. *Set* concerns the preparation of the patient for the exam, and *setting* encompasses the thermography room, personnel, procedures, positioning, and environment for the patient during the exam.

This chapter focuses on the basic environmental conditions and protocols required for clinical human thermography; the design of the thermography room will be explored. Patient positioning and necessary equipment are reviewed. Then the guidelines for preparing subjects for infrared imaging are considered. Lastly, factors leading to inadequate imaging interpretation and reporting are discussed. Careful consideration of the guidelines and recommendations laid out in this chapter should provide a solid foundation for the optimal acquisition of thermal images.

Design of the thermography room

The physical principles and imager technology that underpin modern human thermography provide the basis of the biomedical designs outlined in this chapter. Relevant factors include ambient temperature, humidity, convection, conduction, radiation, and patient positioning. The layout, dimensions, and environmental conditions of the imaging room must conform to basic requirements for effective human thermography, and may depend on the type of thermal imager used. The design of the thermographic experience as it affects the patient is also of prime importance in the acquisition of diagnostic images.

The thermography room should be large enough to maintain a consistent, steady ambient temperature. A room that is too small will have ambient temperatures that are too easily altered by the warmth of human bodies and other heat sources, such as a desktop computer. Sufficient space must be allowed for the furniture and equipment. Dimensions of the room should take into account freedom of movement for the subject, technician, and any additional personnel; the room must provide enough space for subjects of all sizes to be positioned correctly. To meet these requirements for general thermography, a minimum room size of 3 × 3.7 meters (10 × 12 feet) with a ceiling height of 2.4 meters (8 feet) is recommended. For breast examinations taken with a lens Field of View (FOV) of 25°, a patient-to-imager distance of 0.9–2.4 meters (3–8 feet) is considered adequate.[1] The room may have to be larger if single-frame full-body (head-to-toe) musculoskeletal imaging is to be done, as is now practical with 640/480-pixel imagers. A room length of about 5.5 meters (18 feet) is necessary to provide adequate distance to image a standing adult with an imager having an active FOV of 25 degrees.[2]

Although the size of the room does not alter the quality of thermal images, very large rooms can be drafty and tend to be less comfortable for the patient.[3] Ambient temperatures can be difficult to maintain in large spaces. Airflow in the area where the subject is positioned should be barely discernible, with airspeed 0.2 meters per second (0.66 fps) or less.[4] The patient area should be carpeted in order to insulate the patient from the cold floor. In medical settings where carpeting is not allowed, an impervious, washable insulated mat can be used.

Furniture items include two chairs (and/or a stool), along with a padded exam table and positioning pillows. Aside from specialized thermographic protocol needs (cold water, towels, etc.), no other large objects should be needed in the room. As patient comfort is important, relaxing artwork or posters may be placed on the walls, and pleasant music provided. The room should also have hooks and hangers for clothes, a small container to store jewelry during the exam, and a full-length mirror for dressing after the exam. The mirror should be located away from the imaging area.

When using a fixed-position imager, it is more convenient and efficient to have the tripod-mounted thermal camera linked via a cable directly to the computer so that all images are quickly transferred to the hard drive for processing and storage. The control and interpretation computers are best located in an adjacent room where they will not affect the thermographic exam conditions. The computer desk may be strategically placed so that the technician has an unobstructed window view of both the imager and subject.

If a battery-powered, hand-held imager is being used, a wire connection might be inconvenient. In this case, the image files may be stored in the camera for downloading after the thermography session using a wired connection. Some hand-held devices can automatically transfer the image to a nearby computer via Wi-Fi, thus avoiding the inconvenience of wire transfer.

Other parameters for the exam room are as follows:

- Walls, floor, and ceiling should have a matte finish and, if possible, should be insulated. The infrared imager can be used to survey the walls, floor, and ceiling of the room for any hot or cold spots that might affect the images.
- A room internal to the building without windows is recommended. Sunlight through a window can reflect off human skin. If windows cannot be avoided, all glass areas should be covered with metal foil. Windows should also have full insulating drapes or internal shutters to block infrared radiation and reflections from the metal foil or glass.
- Strong infrared sources such as incandescent (hot filament) lights must be avoided. Use only LED or fluorescent lights in the thermography room.
- No mirrors or glass are to be placed in the camera's field of view, as such surfaces reflect infrared radiation and may alter measurements.
- A calibrated thermometer/hygrometer should monitor the room temperature and relative humidity (RH). If wall-mounted, the instrument should be fastened with insulating stand-offs so as to be less affected by the wall temperature.

Temperature and air conditioning requirements

Air conditioning is essential for establishing and maintaining the desired air temperature within the exam room. It is imperative that the temperature remains steady, not varying by more than one degree Celsius (1.8°F) during the exam. Room temperatures may range from 18 to 28°C (64–82.4°F) during

DOI: 10.1201/9781003281764-7

thermographic evaluations, with 20–21°C (68–70°F) being the most commonly used equilibration temperature.[5] The chosen ambient temperature for routine examinations must not alter the patient's core temperature to the point of perspiring or shivering.

To meet these goals for ambient temperature, a fully functional Heating/Ventilating/Air-Conditioning (HVAC) system is a worthwhile investment for a thermography practice. If the building's HVAC is used to control the thermography room temperature, a separate heating/cooling zone thermostat should be installed for local control of the room's temperature, and the system should be able to both heat and cool the room at any time of year. The HVAC vents should not blow incoming air onto the patient.

If a room air-conditioner/heater (ACH) is used to control the room temperature, it is best positioned behind a screen or partition, and patients should be advised to avoid any airflow from the ACH vents. Room ACH exhaust air must be ducted outside the room, either into another room, the hall, the dropped ceiling space, or outdoors (Figure 6.1). The exhaust duct may be insulated to avoid heat reflection from the patient's skin, but this is usually not required as the duct does not generally reach temperatures over 38°C (100°F), and most of the duct can be located behind a screen. Care must be taken to ensure that the room air intake vent does not direct incoming air onto the subject. Window-mounted air conditioner/heaters can also be used if the thermography room has an outside wall. Less floor space is used by a window-mounted unit, but a screen may still be needed to deflect any air currents away from the subject.

As human non-glabrous skin is warmer than the exam room air, environmental moisture will not accumulate on it. Glabrous skin, however, often equilibrates to the room temperature when cooled. Fingers and toes may become cooler than the air temperature due to insensitive evaporative heat loss. The dew point in the room must be kept low enough so that humidity does not condense in the air, on the room equipment, or on the glabrous skin of the subject. Water condensation in the air can attenuate radiant infrared energy. Water condensation *adds* heat to a surface, though the thermographic appearance of this has not been explored. Evaporative water loss makes the skin appear cooler; the subject must be sufficiently dry and cooled prior to imaging. The relative humidity of a thermography room should be between 40% and 70%.[6] A dehumidifier is recommended in areas with higher humidity.

SIDEBAR 6.1 TROPICAL THERMOGRAPHY

In tropical countries where air conditioning may not be available, it has been suggested that cooling may not be necessary for breast exams and can be mathematically corrected up to a point.[7] However, higher ambient temperatures leave less thermal "headroom" below the body's core temperature to display abnormal findings, and normal breast skin is about 5°C (9°F) below core temperature, leaving even less headroom. In addition, glomus AVAs do not stay fully closed above a nominal 22°C (72°F) ambient temperature. To provide valid thermographic exams in rural locations, portable modules built into standard shipping containers or recreational travel trailers insulated and fitted with HVAC units can be deployed (see Figure 12.2, page 211).

Factors supporting the patient's comfort

As psychological stresses can affect the thermal image, the patient's comfort, convenience, privacy, and confidentiality are all paramount when performing clinical thermography.[8] Here are some basic guidelines for meeting these goals:

- The undressed patient should never be visible from outside the thermography and control rooms. If video monitoring is in use, the patient should be informed and assured of medical privacy. People should be able to enter the exam room without the patient being seen or glimpsed from outside areas (Figure 6.2).[9]
- One other person of the patient's choice may be allowed in the exam room; however, that individual must stay out of

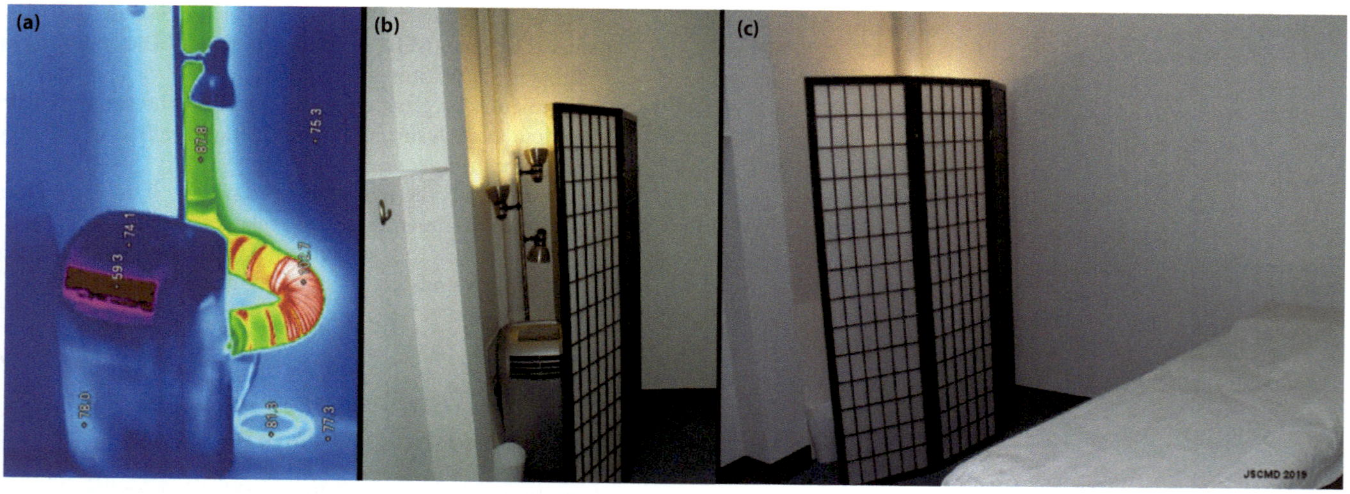

FIGURE 6.1 (a) Infrared image of a 120 V AC room air conditioner/heater (ACH). The vertical pipe exhausts warm air into the dropped ceiling space. Note that the LED lights are cool. (b) The ACH unit is located behind a screen. The room air inlet is behind the ACH unit. Patients are instructed not to stand in the ACH air outlet. (c) The screen isolates the ACH unit from the exam area. Only a small portion of the ACH exhaust pipe is exposed to the subject, minimizing reflective thermal artifact.

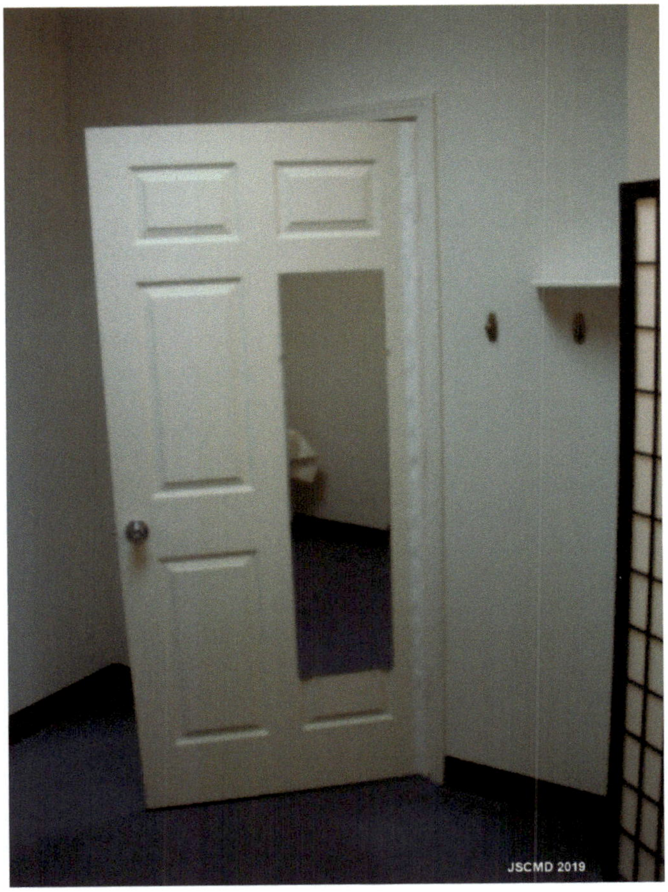

FIGURE 6.2 A thermography room door designed to allow entry while keeping the subject private. This view is taken from the patient area. Note the cloth strip covering the door hinge opening to assure privacy. The dressing mirror, hangers, and jewelry shelf are also shown.

the way during imaging and should not touch the subject. Any talking should be minimized.

- Lights in the thermography room should be diffuse and moderate; overly bright light levels may be uncomfortable for some patients.
- If the technician is of the opposite sex from that of the patient, a same-sex chaperone – either a member of the thermography practice or an acceptable chaperone of the patient's choice – should be present during the exam.
- A dressing area with clothes hooks and hangers, a place to put jewelry and valuables safely during the exam, and a full-length mirror (placed outside the imaging field) to aid in dressing after the procedure should be part of the thermography area or located in an immediately adjacent room.
- Relaxing music can be helpful for calming the patient during the temperature equilibration period. Televisions should be avoided as they become warm when on, and could effect the thermographic patterns if disturbing images are shown. Suitable artwork and posters on the walls and on the ceiling above the patient table may help the patient relax during the temperature equilibration time.

The equilibration period

Control of room temperature is essential to obtaining accurate thermograms. Changes in ambient temperature alter the amount of heat conducted through the skin.[10] Considering only radiative heat loss, an unclothed human is in thermal balance at about 25°C (77°F).[11] However, a warmer environment is required to make up for conductive and convective heat losses. An unclothed adult human in a closed room at an ambient temperature of 27–28°C (80.6–82.4°F) can sustain thermal equilibrium for long periods without shivering or sweating.[12] This is within an accepted thermoneutral zone for unclothed humans of 23–30°C (73.4–86°F).[13] Clothing and thicker subdermal fat (obesity) reduce the thermal equilibrium temperature range to 20–25°C (68–77°F) by providing increased insulation.[14]

Within the thermoneutral range of ambient temperatures, the sympathetic nervous system maintains the vasomotor tone of the skin vasculature; minute changes in skin blood flow can evoke substantial and thus easily measured changes in heat dissipation. The core temperature is maintained while *average* skin temperature is stable. *Instantaneous* skin temperature may vary slightly over 15–30 second cycles due to the pulsed sympathetic control of the glomus AVAs. Within the thermoneutral zone, AVAs play a major role in core temperature control. For this reason, thermography room temperatures are typically set below the thermoneutral zone at 18.3–21°C (65–70°F). At that temperature, the intradermal AVAs and arteriolar shunts normally stay fully closed and nitric oxide becomes the major skin vasodilator.

The three thermography equilibration temperatures

Most routine thermographic exams require that the subject be cooled to the point of full dermal vasoconstriction without shivering. However, certain special exams to observe active autonomic system functioning or arterial blood flow are best performed at warmer temperatures.

1. **Cooling**: The room temperature is set at 20–21.1°C (68–70°F), sometimes as low as 18.3°C (65°F). This temperature range elicits full autonomic vasoconstriction and is used for breast and general neuromuscular exams where muscle-generated warmth, blood vessels, inflamed tissues, and aberrant vasodilation patterns (due to NO, nerve injury, etc.) need to be visualized. The glomus AVAs normally remain closed at these temperatures.
2. **Intermediate Cooling**: The room temperature is set at 22.2–23.9°C (72–75°F). Here the subject's autonomic temperature control is in mid-range, able to raise or lower the skin temperature over the areas of interest. This intermediate temperature is useful for evaluating Complex Regional Pain Syndrome (CRPS) and nerve injury. At these temperatures, glomus AVAs normally close and open simultaneously in all limbs at intervals as directed by the hypothalamic central nervous system.
3. **Warming**: The room temperature is set at 24.4–25.5°C (76–78°F), and sometimes as warm as 27–28°C (80.6–82.4°F). At these temperatures, the subject is warmed to a point near full adrenergic sympathetic vasodilation. Sweating indicates activation of the cholinergic sympathetic system. The glomus AVAs remain mostly open

but continue to close briefly on sympathetic command at intervals of 30 seconds or longer. Local warming up to 43°C (109°F) has little, if any, effect on autonomic control of the AVA constriction timing, though dilation of the local arterioles may occur.[15] Warm equilibration is used for the detection of arterial insufficiency and abnormal vasoconstriction. Controlled warming is also useful to determine finger temperature recovery time after cold water hand immersion when evaluating Raynaud's disease and other vasospastic conditions.

Temperature equilibration typically lasts 15 minutes to provide sufficient time for the body to attain a state of thermodynamic equilibrium before the images are obtained. If the subject is to be cooled to the point of vasoconstriction, the hands and face can be quickly checked with the thermal imager to observe whether the fingers or nose are cool before taking the exam images. Subjects cool at different rates, with 10 minutes being suitable for some, while others may require 20 minutes or more for full vasoconstriction. Cooling times longer than 30 minutes may create instability of the skin surface temperatures and possibly some undesired shivering.

During equilibration and subsequent imaging, the area of the body to be scanned should remain completely bare, not covered by any article of clothing or compromised by large or constrictive jewelry. Even loose-fitting gowns should be avoided as they restrict the natural convective heat loss from the skin surface in unpredictable patterns. For maximum patient comfort and to create an atmosphere of safety, female imaging should ideally be done by a female technician. Some centers record the entire equilibration period and exam on video (with audio) to document that equilibration and exam protocols are followed, and to assure that proper professional boundaries between thermographer and subject are maintained. Video monitoring may be important for CRPS or other special exams where legal, economic, or substance use issues may be at stake. Any video records obtained are to be handled and observed under strict medical privacy rules.

Positions for temperature equilibration and imaging

The position in which the subject equilibrates to the thermography room temperature must be decided on an individual basis, depending on the body areas to be imaged, the physical limitations of the patient, and the location of any pathology or symptoms. The major limitation to examining the entire body surface without artifact is the problem of gravity. Some portion of the body must be in contact with the floor, chair, table, or other objects at all times. That body portion will sustain thermal artifacts from heat transfer differences at the contact points as well as rebound hyperemia in the areas with restricted blood flow from the force of gravity. In addition, any muscle tension that must be sustained to offset gravity or provide active balance may need to be minimized by using a particular position. Human thermography under microgravity conditions has yet to be explored. Body positioning may have significant gravitational effects on the skin temperature of the limbs. An arm will be cooler in a raised position compared to a dependent position, mainly due to drainage of venous engorgement in the raised limb. This surface temperature difference may be as large as 4–5°C (7.2–9°F), and may take as long as 5 minutes to reach a maximum difference as the veins drain or fill. The surface temperature of the leg and foot respond similarly to position change.[16] A limb that warms rapidly in a dependent position may have valvular insufficiency causing venous reflux.

This section will cover patient equilibration positions for general and special thermographic exams. Equilibration positions for breast thermography are covered in Chapter 9.

Standing Position. The majority of general thermal imaging examinations are done with the subject equilibrated either in a standing position or slowly walking. For maximum skin surface cooling, the legs should be slightly separated and the arms held away from the trunk so that the inner thighs and axillae are exposed to the ambient air. The hands should be open, not clenched. Only the soles of the feet cannot be imaged in the standing position. The skin over the leg muscles as well as the upper back muscles that support the head may appear warm due to heat conduction from the underlying muscle metabolism required to maintain balance. The standing position has been used with the subject standing on a rotating platform. Rotation may be tolerated by well-trained athletes, but older subjects or those with balance difficulties will need to be braced, or will need to use their hands to hold onto a support. Balancing aids may induce thermal artifacts, especially if the hands are used for balance.

In order to conveniently image the lateral and medial surfaces of the body, left and right views may be obtained using the "Egyptian pose," so named because such poses mimic the human figures seen in Egyptian hieroglyphics (Figure 6.3). For the left Egyptian pose, the subject stands with the right arm forward and slightly down, with the radial (thumb) side toward the camera, and the left arm forward and slightly upward with the ulnar (pinkie) side toward the camera. The right foot is placed forward, and the left foot back. For the right Egyptian pose, the arm and leg positions are reversed.

Sitting Position. The head, neck, arms, chest, spine, quadriceps, lower legs, and dorsum of the feet are suitable targets for infrared imaging after sitting equilibration. If the back is to be imaged, sitting equilibration should be done on a stool. Leaning on a chair back will produce posterior thermal artifacts, and a chair with arms will affect the forearm ulnar appearance. The patient's arms should be held away from the trunk so as not to warm the flanks. If the feet are placed flat on an insulated surface, muscle tension in the tibialis anterior and calf muscles is minimized, allowing better evaluation of anterior leg and knee conditions. The posterior muscles of the neck remain under tension similar to standing, however.

Supine Position. This equilibration position (body horizontal with face up) may be used if the region of thermal interest is limited to the anterior of the face, neck, body, legs, and feet (including the soles). Images of the entire posterior body portion from scalp to heels (including the Achilles tendons) will be compromised due to the table affecting heat losses. If the arms distal to the elbow are extended off the side of the table and the hands relaxed, those exposed portions may be imaged with the negligible artifact. The supine position allows the subject to relax fully during equilibration, especially if a pillow is provided and a bolster is placed under the knees.

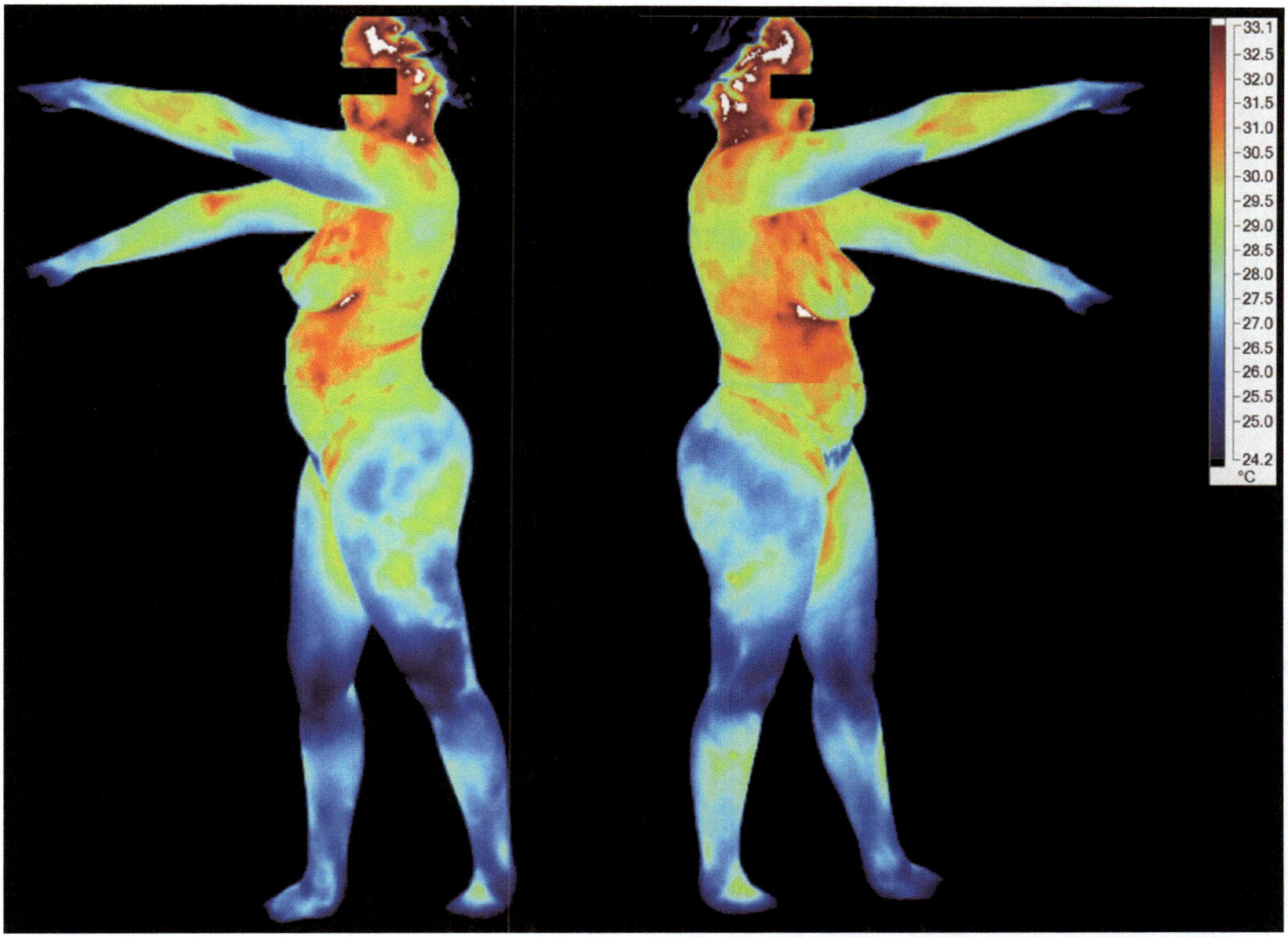

FIGURE 6.3 Composite isothermal images illustrating the "Egyptian pose" technique to obtain the lateral body views.

Prone position

Equilibration in this position (horizontal, face down) is rarely used clinically, but is useful to relax the back, neck, and posterior leg muscles. This reduces heat conducted from tense, superficial musculature and allows better evaluation of underlying inflammation. A bolster or support placed under the anterior ankles helps relax the hamstring and gastrocnemius muscles. A facial cradle such as found on massage tables allows the subject to hold the neck in a straight position, and an arm support sling can minimize the tension of the trapezius, rhomboid, and paraspinal muscles (Figure 6.4). Alternatively, the arms can be placed alongside, but not touching, the trunk.

Cranium, face, and neck

The head is best imaged when the subject is in a sitting position, which offers convenient views of all portions of the face and cranium, including the apex. Alternatively, a standing position may be utilized, with the subject bending forward for the image of the cranial apex. If the subject has long hair, it should be pulled back and tied up off the face, neck, and ears to facilitate imaging those areas completely. Side views are important to evaluate the temporal-mandibular joints, or TMJs, and can detect tympanic membrane temperatures in some subjects. The subject should be asked not to blink while an image including both corneas is taken. Inhalation and exhalation views can detect unilateral or total nasal blockage. The subject should extend the neck up about 30 degrees for the anterior and oblique neck and thyroid views. An image of the posterior neck should be taken with the neck flexed forward about 30 degrees.

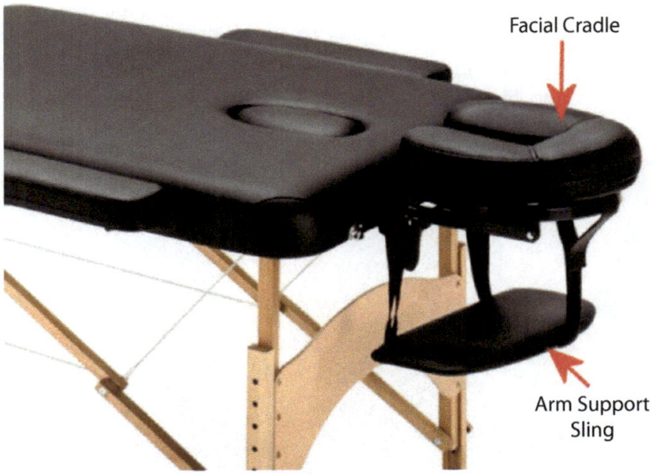

FIGURE 6.4 A patient table showing a facial cradle and arm support for relaxing the cervical and trapezius muscles using a prone position.[17]

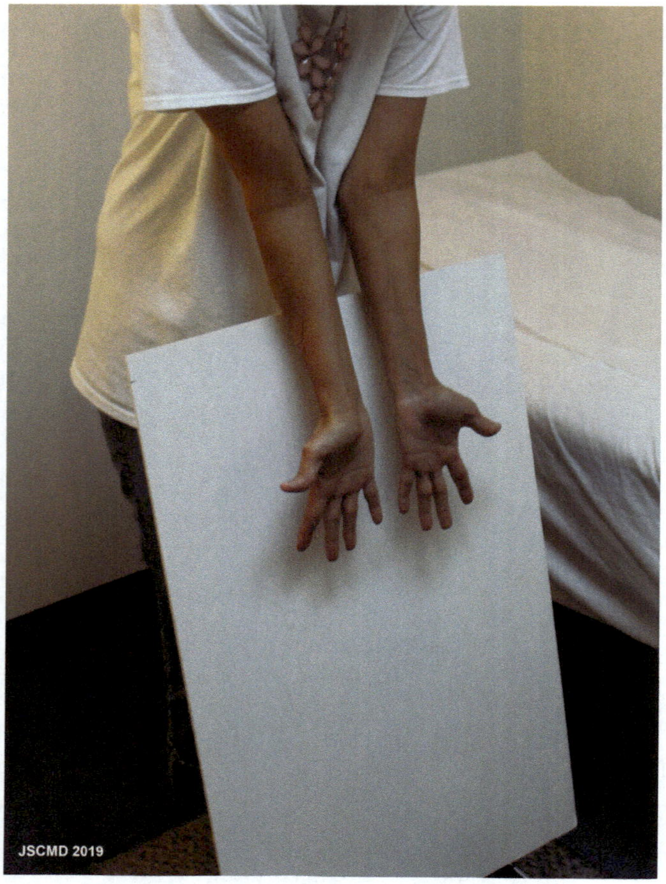

FIGURE 6.5 Imaging the hands – Palmar view. Foam-core matte-finish artboard of any color may be used as a background. The hands should not touch the board to prevent leaving thermal artifacts.

Hands

During equilibration and imaging, the hands should remain open in free air and not be clenched. Generally, both hands are imaged together to facilitate the evaluation of thermal symmetry. The subject may be in a standing or sitting position. A rigid, matte-finish board behind the hands allows an uncluttered picture of the smaller structures involved (Figure 6.5). Three views – palmar, dorsal, and radial (thumb side) – are routinely obtained at close range. Simultaneous ulnar-side views require full internal rotation of both arms, a position difficult for some subjects to assume.

Feet

Five views are required to fully evaluate one foot and ankle; seven to perform a bilateral exam using Dorsal, Lateral, Medial, Achilles, and Plantar views (Figure 6.6). The first four may be obtained with the patient equilibrated in a standing or sitting position. The plantar surface is best imaged if the subject is equilibrated in the prone or supine positions with the feet and ankles extending off the end of the table. Then, after obtaining all desired images in that horizontal position, the subject may sit or stand for the other foot views. If the subject is equilibrated in a standing or sitting position, plantar images are obtained after they have been placed in a supine or prone position for at least 5 minutes to allow the plantar surfaces to adjust to room temperature.

Some infrared imaging systems may utilize patient and equipment positioning software for each body area being imaged. Coordinated positioning of the equipment and the patient is useful in performing repeat thermal imaging. Thermography software may provide an outline of the patient's body based on the preceding set of thermographic exams so that the patient can be positioned to fit that previous outline as viewed through the thermal imager in real time. Laser-based imager-to-patient distance measurements also help with precise camera placement. These features may facilitate the positioning process, but even with software aids, session-to-session alignment of thermographic images remains a problem and must be taken into account by the interpreting thermographer. Identical patient imaging alignment is especially difficult if the images are taken at different centers using different equipment.

In certain cases, the entire upper body or lower body is scanned in order to analyze sagittal temperature symmetry as well as the thermal patterns over the ROI. Thermal symmetry is best captured with a single image including the ROI and its sagittal opposite, when possible. If two images are required, the imaging angle and camera distance must be kept the same to acquire comparable views. When visually comparing multiple images, their temperature-to-color spans must be identical to avoid display bias. Analysis software that allows equalizing the span of multiple images at one time facilitates this process. Images adjusted to the same temperature span are referred to as *isothermal images*.

Various kinds of physical stress studies or "stress tests" can be used for more specialized applications, specifically as a diagnostic test for Raynaud's disease and CRPS. This aspect of infrared imaging may entail cold or warm stimuli and is usually performed

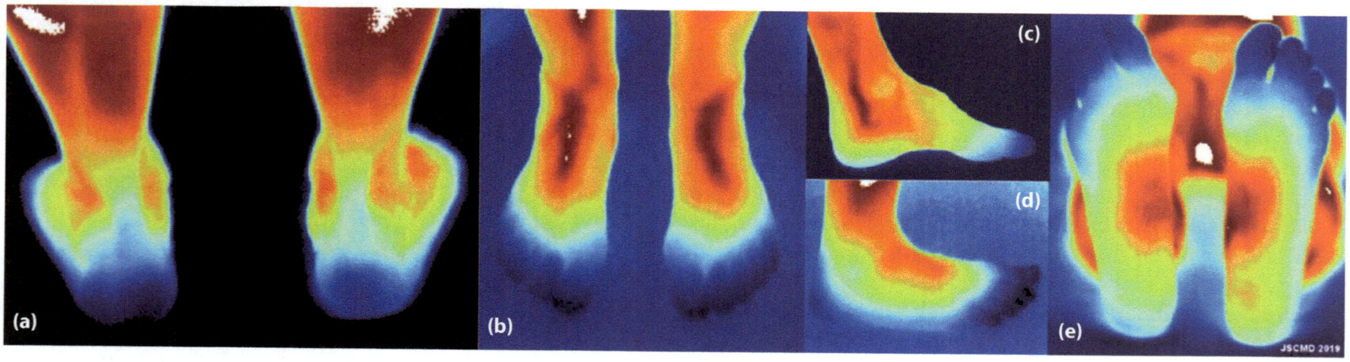

FIGURE 6.6 Imaging views of the left foot. Five views are required for a complete exam. (a) achilles view, (b) dorsal view, (c) medial view, (d) lateral view, and (e) plantar view.

following baseline thermographic imaging. It is best to follow the temperature challenge protocols outlined in valid studies of the condition being imaged. Cold-stress and ice-water stress testing have no part in routine breast or general-body examinations, however; they should be reserved for special tests of autonomic or vascular function.

Depending on the individual case, a clinical examination may be performed after thermal imaging to correlate specific findings. This may include visual inspection, palpation, percussion, auscultation, and other special examinations (neurologic, orthopedic, vascular, etc.) as deemed appropriate by the interpreting clinician. Performing this examination before infrared imaging may create thermal artifacts, thus it is best delayed until after imaging. An initial read of the thermographic images may help direct this post-imaging examination.

Pre-thermography patient instructions

It was learned early in the history of clinical thermography that the subject to be imaged had to abide by certain pre-examination preparations to avoid creating thermal artifacts. Earlier pre-exam requirements listed avoiding "sun exposure, stimulation or treatment of the breasts, cosmetics, lotions, antiperspirants, deodorants, exercise, and bathing before the examination" without stating any time period to these requirements.[18] Other thermographers listed similar proscriptions to be avoided within three to 6 hours of an exam.[19] Surprisingly, these early rules did not include avoidance of nicotine, alcohol, or medications that are now known to affect skin blood flow and thermographic appearance. Over time, pre-exam preparation instructions have grown to include a more inclusive list of what to avoid and for how long prior to a thermographic exam.

In preparing for the exam, the guidelines listed below are applicable to the vast majority of thermography scenarios. Adhering to these guidelines can help prevent thermal artifacts by minimizing the possibility of affecting blood flow and abnormal neural stimulation to areas of concern.

Although the instructions for preparing for an infrared imaging exam vary widely from center to center, the following guidelines are often advised. Though many of these instructions are based on clinical studies, there is little scientific evidence for other recommendations, and they must be assumed to be based on common sense. These instructions should be conveyed to the patient well in advance of the exam date:

- **Five Days Prior to Infrared Imaging.** Refrain from prolonged sun exposure (sunbathing or sun tanning) as well as any tanning booth activity. Thermography should be postponed if there is evidence of sunburn damage (erythema, blistering, and peeling) over the area to be imaged.
- **Within 48 hours of Imaging**. Abstain from heavy drinking or excessive alcohol consumption and getting drunk. Being under the influence of alcohol, or having a hangover, increases skin temperature and alters the thermal pattern.[20] Also, women undergoing breast thermography should avoid getting a mammogram as the mammography procedure may result in significant residual inflammation of the compressed breast tissue. If mammography is planned around the time of infrared imaging, it should be performed *after* the thermography session.
- **Within 24 hours (Beginning the Midnight before Imaging)**. Keep skin stimulation to a minimum. It is generally best to avoid any skin circulatory-related interventions such as massage, chiropractic treatments, physical therapy, nerve stimulation (TENS), electrical muscle stimulation (EMS), acupuncture, therapeutic ultrasound, and either hot or cold applications, especially if these procedures involve the area to be imaged. Also, abstain from strenuous physical activity, which may cause residual inflammation or skin circulation changes.
- **On the Day of Imaging.** Refrain from wearing heavy jewelry and tight-fitting clothing. Loose-fitting clothing is preferable because it facilitates normal, unrestricted blood circulation. Imaging might have to be delayed until skin impressions or irritations from tight-fitting clothing have subsided. Women undergoing breast thermography should not wear an underwire bra on the day of the scan, and some thermographers request that no bra be worn for several hours before the exam. To minimize irritation of the skin, both men and women should not shave the area to be imaged. Refrain from applying lotions, creams, antiperspirants, deodorants, liniments, powders, cosmetics, or perfumes to all areas of skin to be examined, as they may lower the skin emissivity or stimulate local blood flow.
- **Four hours Prior to Imaging**. Avoid getting overheated or engaging in vigorous physical exercise (e.g., running, cycling, or other workouts). Refrain from ingesting *any* alcohol, caffeine, and pungent spices such as cayenne or ginger. Do not smoke tobacco or use any nicotine-delivery products such as "vaping," snuff, gum, or patches.[21] If possible, do not take prescription blood pressure medications or vasodilators (especially nitrates) before the exam. Amphetamines and cocaine may reduce skin circulation and temperature. Avoid taking any non-prescription medicines, especially cold remedies (oral pseudoephedrine, nasal decongestants), aspirin, ibuprofen, other anti-inflammatories, and niacin.
- **Two hours Prior to Imaging**. Vigorous exercise should be avoided due to its effects on blood circulation, core temperature, and skin temperature patterns. Strong sunlight should be avoided. Do not take a bath or shower or use a hairdryer before the imaging session.
- **One hour Prior to Imaging**. If the patient eats or drinks anything, it should be bland and at room temperature or lukewarm, i.e., nothing spicy, icy, or hot. Lactating mothers: postpone breastfeeding or expressing (pumping) breast milk until after the exam.
- **Within 15 minutes of Imaging**. Use the restroom to avoid having to "go" during the 15-minute temperature acclimatization time. Nothing to eat or drink. No gum chewing. *Refrain from any cell phone use*. Turn your cell phone off or keep it out of the exam room. Microwaves are warming! Earphones and earbuds should not be used until after the exam as they affect the thermal appearance of the ear and ear canal.

Suggestions for a successful thermographic exam

For patients coming to thermography for the first time, it is helpful to offer the following statements regarding the experience of infrared imaging: "Obtaining a thermographic image is much

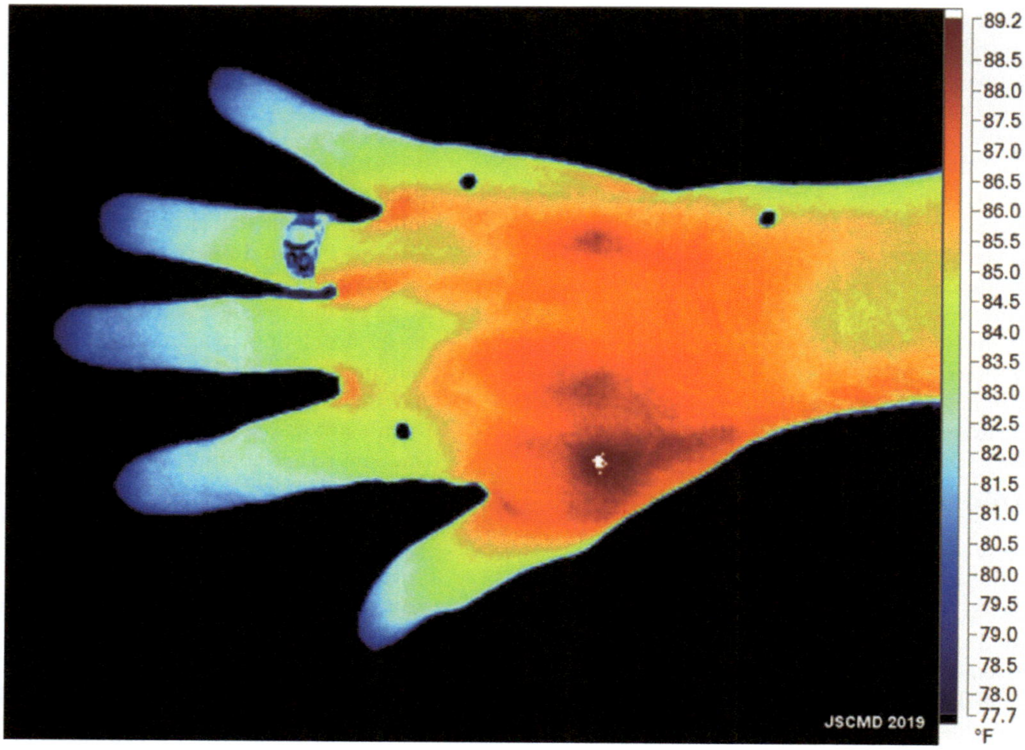

FIGURE 6.7 Small pieces of shiny metallic tape may be used to provide thermally-visible fiducial markers on the skin. They appear cool because the IR emissivity of a polished metal surface is about 5% that of skin.

like having your picture taken with a regular camera. There's no direct contact between you and the imager, nor is there any injection, radiation exposure, or dyes that must be given. Typical exams take between 15 and 30 minutes to perform, during which time you will be in a private, temperature-controlled thermography room."

The individual being imaged should share any medical conditions or disorders with the thermographer, in case one or more of these may affect skin blood flow and temperature readings. Any pains, aches, or recent injuries (potential areas of inflammation) should be reported, and all prescription medicines and supplements reviewed and recorded. The patient's weight, core temperature, and pulse oximetry may be obtained without affecting the thermal image. Blood phlebotomy and occlusion-cuff blood pressure measurements should be delayed until after the exam as they may create thermographic artifacts.

For efficiency's sake, patients should be encouraged to arrive a few minutes early to their appointment to avoid the stress of being rushed. For breast exams, the subject may disrobe only from the waist up. For full-body scans, once in the thermography room, the patient disrobes down to underwear. Briefs, thongs, or speedo-type undergarments are preferable for full-body imaging. Total nudity may be required if the condition involves the genitals or pelvic area.

In addition to removing all heavy jewelry, long hair should be pinned up to expose the neck and upper chest. If rings cannot be easily removed, they may be left in place. The mechanical stresses of trying to remove a tight ring may cause local thermographic artifacts. To show locations of symptoms, masses, skin neoplasms, or other anatomical points in the infrared image, small pieces of reflective metal tape may be placed on the subject's skin as fiducial markers before thermal equilibration (Figure 6.7).

SIDEBAR 6.2 COMMON PROBLEMS LEADING TO SUBSTANDARD THERMOGRAPHY

Clinical thermography is just being introduced into mainstream medicine. As yet, there are no official standards or regulations. Unfortunately, not every thermographer is using the best technology and technique. Technicians may be poorly trained. Even FDA-registered thermal systems may give very poor images. Here are a few things to look for when evaluating human thermal images:

Images have poor image resolution (taken out of focus or from too far away) or poor thermal resolution (not enough color differentiation to detect small thermal differences) – see Figure 6.8. Some images acquired are so poor as to be useless for diagnostic purposes.

Images have no color-coded temperature scale included alongside each picture. Without such a scale or area temperature measurements added to the image, the temperatures that the colors (or gray shades) represent cannot be determined.

Thermographic reports do not include the images. Even a long-winded report dictated by an "expert" cannot convey the information present in good thermal images. Because thermographic images of a person should remain fairly stable through the years, it is important to save the

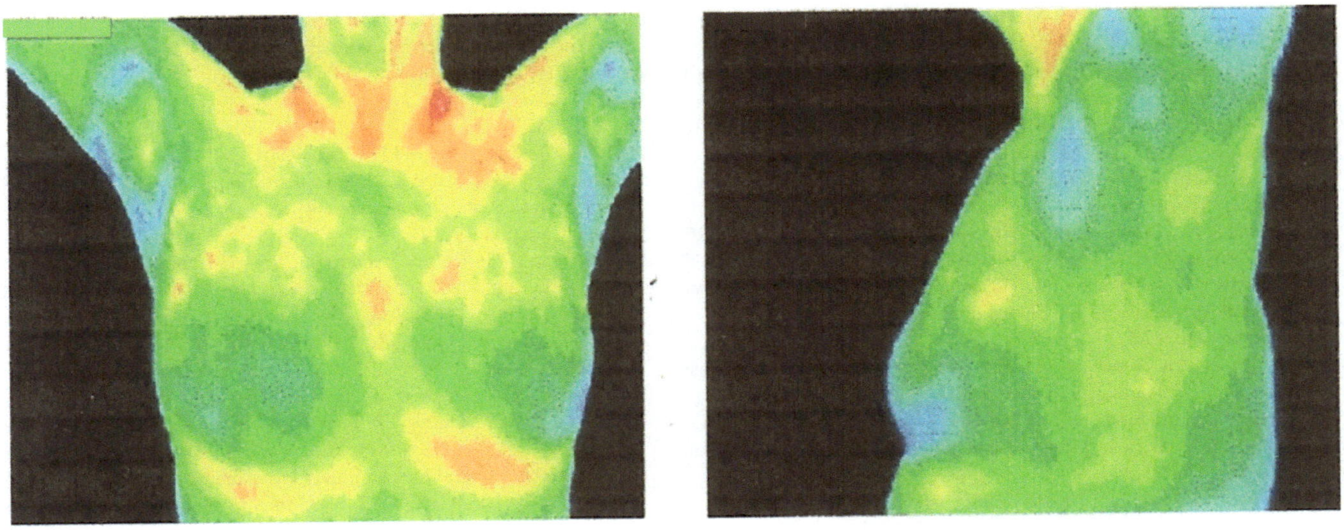

FIGURE 6.8 Examples of thermal images with poor thermal and spatial resolution and no temperature color scale.[22]

images for comparison over time. Patients should get a copy of their images, either digitally or in print.

Failure to cool down the subject before images are taken. Thermograms obtained from a warm subject do not show AVA or arteriolar constriction. This constriction is *absolutely necessary* for the detection of breast cancer, body inflammation, infection, and nerve injury. An uncooled breast thermogram is generally of no use in the detection of breast pathology.

The areas of the body to be imaged are clothed or covered during the cool-down period. Wearing any exam gown or drape over the ROI during cool-down will distort the infrared image because the cloth or paper touching the skin will affect the local surface temperatures.

All angles of the ROI are not imaged. Infrared radiance is maximum at right angles to the skin surface, and minimum in the same plane as the surface. Significant thermal findings may be hidden; a cancer in the lower portion of the breast may not be detected (Figure 6.9). It is important for the thermographer to perform a complete imaging series of all ROI surfaces.

One must beware of poor thermograms and the factors that promulgate substandard thermography. Until full DICOM standardization and accrediting of clinical thermography comes about, it is up to each thermographer to be sure that the procedure is done properly and the images taken are of the best quality.

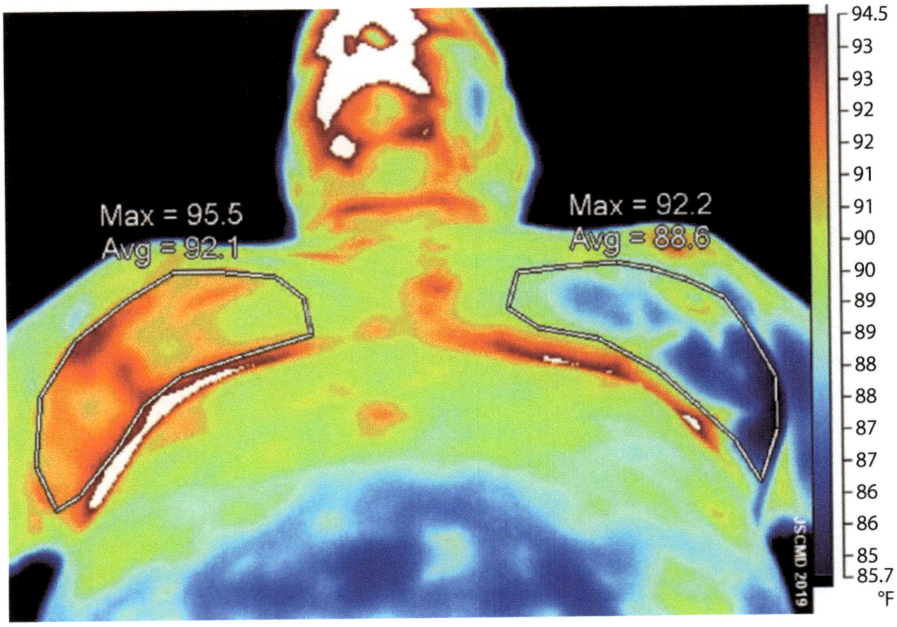

FIGURE 6.9 Abnormal underside of right breast imaged with the subject cooled supine. All the other images were normal. Biopsy positive for BrCA; Lumpectomy performed. – 67 yoF.

Notes

1. The American Academy of Thermology, Guidelines For Breast Thermology, Examination Guideline 3.1, 2018.
2. Although a 25° Field of View requires only 4.1 meters (13.5 ft.) to image a 1.8 meter (6 feet) tall individual, the room should be longer to allow both thermographer and patient to move about, unconstrained by walls or furniture.
3. Diakides NA, Bronzino JD (eds), Medical Infrared Imaging, CRC Press/Taylor & Francis Group, New York, 2008. Section 22.3.3.1.
4. The American Academy of Thermology, Guidelines For Breast Thermology, Guideline 3.3: Environmental Controls. 2018.
5. Ibid 3 Section 9.2.3.
6. The American Academy of Thermology, Guidelines For Breast Thermology, Examination Guideline 3.4, 2018.
7. Souza GA, et al., Einstein (Sao Paulo). 2015; PMCID: PMC4878624.
8. Moliné A, et al., J Investig Psychol Offender Profiling 2018; Doi: 10.1002/jip.1505
9. Robinson LJ, et al., Exp Physiol. 2016; Doi:10.1113/EP085642
10. Johnson JM, Exercise Sports Sci. Rev. 1992; PMID: 1623893.
11. Anbar M, Quantitative Dynamic Telethermometry in Medical Diagnosis and Management, 1st Ed, CRC Press, New York, 1994, p. 28.
12. Kirsch KA, In Applied Thermology: Thermologic Methods (Eds JM Engel, et al.), VCH, Weinheim, Germany, 1985, pp. 1–9.
13. The boundaries of the human "Thermoneutral Zone" vary depending on the research protocol. *See:* Pallubinsky H, et al., J Therm Biol. 79, Jan 2019; PMID: 30612680.
14. Ibid 3, Section 6-3.
15. Walløe L, Temperature 2016; PMCID: PMC4861183.
16. Shilco P, et al., J Therm Biol. 2019; PMID: 30784492.
17. Image courtesy of Dr. Lomilomi, Paramount, CA, USA, Used with permission. Annotations added by JSCMD.
18. Ibid 3. Section 9.2.3.
19. Cabrera IN et al., Chapter 4, Thermography Techniques, in Rehabilitation Medicine and Thermography. Lee MH and Cohen JM, editors. Impress Publications, Wilsonville OR, USA, 2008.
20. Ewing KL, et al., Ohio J Sci. January, 1973; 73(1): 55–58. http://hdl.handle.net/1811/21956
21. The half-life of smoked nicotine in the body is about 2 hours (see Goodman & Gilman's The Pharmacological Basis of Therapeutics, 8th ed, Pergamon Press, New York, USA, 1990, p. 546). Smoking just prior to thermographic exam may lower breast surface temperature by 3°C (see Ewing KL 1973). Cotinine, a weak but active metabolite of nicotine, has a half-life of 20 hours, and effects endothelial-dependent relaxation. See Conklin BS et al., J Surg Res. 2001; PMID: 11120631.
22. Anonymous images taken at another imaging center from a patient file of JSC, MD.

7

FORMATTING AND ANALYSIS OF THERMAL IMAGES

In 1994 thermologist Michael Anbar stated: "It seems that the days of qualitative (visual) thermology are gone for good." His pronouncement of its passing was premature, however, as he was making it based on the limited visual displays and printouts of the electromechanical thermal scanners available at that time. Over the next decade, uncooled microbolometer imagers would convert the complicated numerical analysis of quantitative thermology into full-color, high-resolution, calibrated radiometric images. Finally, the thermographer could see the qualitative thermal patterns in detail and obtain calibrated temperatures from the images as well. Today, qualitative and quantitative image analysis work together to make human thermography both clinically useful and scientifically valid.

This chapter focuses on how to format thermal images to maximize the qualitative visual information available to the human eye, and how to perform quantitative thermal measurements on the image guided by these qualitative findings. Additional information on image measurement and interpretation is offered in subsequent chapters.

Three types of thermographic evaluation and interpretation

There are three basic imaging methods for thermographic interpretation: (1) a single unilateral image, (2) images showing bilateral thermal symmetry, and (3) serial imaging over time, which also includes videothermography. What follows is a discussion of each of these approaches along with their advantages and disadvantages.

Single-image interpretation

A single image is the simplest to take, yet the least effective way to interpret a thermogram. Unilateral infrared images considered in isolation yield very limited data, providing a single snapshot in time of a constantly evolving condition (Figure 7.1a). The single image can be misleading unless compared to the surrounding areas of the body and evaluated in terms of thermal symmetry.

Nevertheless, single-image interpretation still can be used to help identify and assess certain conditions. Given the limited information afforded by one image, it is important for the thermographer to assess the entire image, not just the region of interest (ROI). "Incidental" findings such as an area of inflammation outside the ROI are important to detect and report. A well-trained thermographer should be adept at pattern recognition and able to apply that skill to the entire image or image series.

Thermal symmetry

Thermograms yield more information when sagittal symmetry information is included. The human thermoregulatory system is normally sagittally symmetrical, both qualitatively and quantitatively.[1] Thermal symmetry evaluation is based on contralateral comparisons, as when comparing the right and left limbs. In a breast study, contralateral regions of each breast are compared, such as the lower outer quadrants of the two breasts (Figure 7.1b). Temperature comparison to adjacent skin is the second type of symmetry evaluation. Absent an anatomical reason, local and symmetrical skin temperatures are normally similar.

Symmetric comparisons are especially useful in identifying various inflammatory, neurological, and vascular conditions. Different pathological processes may present with similar thermographic findings, however. For example, if the right foot is cooler than the left, this could indicate a significant neuropathy or inflammatory process on the left. It could also indicate arterial insufficiency on the right. For this reason, clinical evaluation and diagnostic tests are brought in to ascertain the underlying condition. Thermography can supply a list of differential diagnoses.

Serial imaging

A third approach to thermographic interpretation entails making comparisons of a series of images over time (Figure 7.2). Two or more infrared imaging studies are performed, with a reasonable period of time between the studies depending on the condition and its severity or risk status. The serial thermograms are then evaluated, with changes or differences between the images being identified and analyzed.

One of the advantages of serial imaging is that it takes into account the physiological and biochemical individuality of each patient. The "normal" thermal patterns corresponding to each area of an individual's body are similar to a fingerprint, with each patient having a particular infrared map of the ROI that provides a baseline. Any alteration of that infrared map on serial imaging may signal an abnormality that merits further investigation. Physiological changes discerned on serial thermograms may precede—sometimes by months or even years – any detectable anatomical changes. If pathology is suspected, the thermal information can be used to recommend further diagnostic testing.

Because of the diagnostic and prognostic power of serial imaging, it is imperative that the patient have full access to their thermal images in the event that they move or otherwise use a different thermography center. It is often best to provide the subject with high-resolution, properly formatted images that they can archive for future comparison.

Serial imaging includes radiometric thermal videography, which can provide real-time thermally-calibrated images at 9 frames per second (fps) or more. This technology allows the capture of fast temperature changes of the skin from thermal challenge testing such as cold-water immersion. Although thermal frame rates of 60 fps or more are possible, skin temperature changes occur relatively slowly, affected mainly by the arterial pulse rate at approximately one pulse per second. In addition, the thermal time constant of a microbolometer leaflet is between about 5 and 12 milliseconds (ms), depending on the imager chip. This means the time it takes each pixel to reach 99% of a sensed temperature change is typically 25 to 60 ms (5 time constants), supporting a maximum frame rate between 40 and 16 fps, respectively, for thermally calibrated videothermography.[2]

Though a frame rate of 9fps seems slow, it provides nine temperature measurements per second, fast enough to capture any surface temperature changes modulated by the pulse. Faster frame acquisition is usually not necessary for clinical thermography,

DOI: 10.1201/9781003281764-8

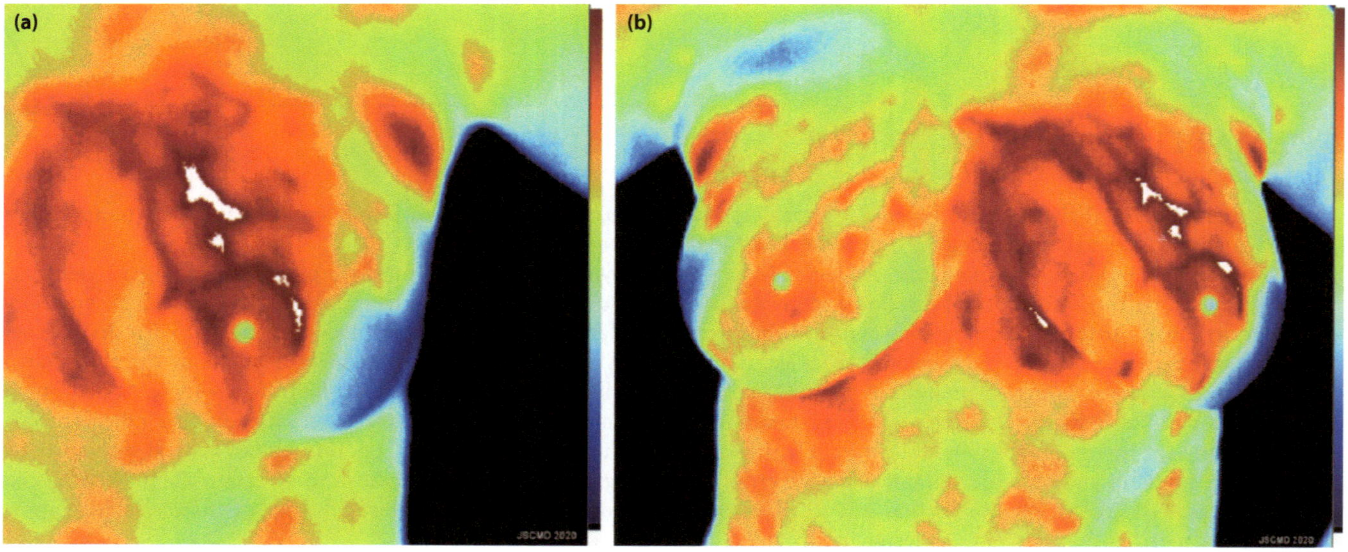

FIGURE 7.1 (a) A single, unilateral thermal image of the left breast only. (b) A bilateral thermal image of the same subject yields much more information than the unilateral image. Thermal asymmetry between the breasts can be readily detected.

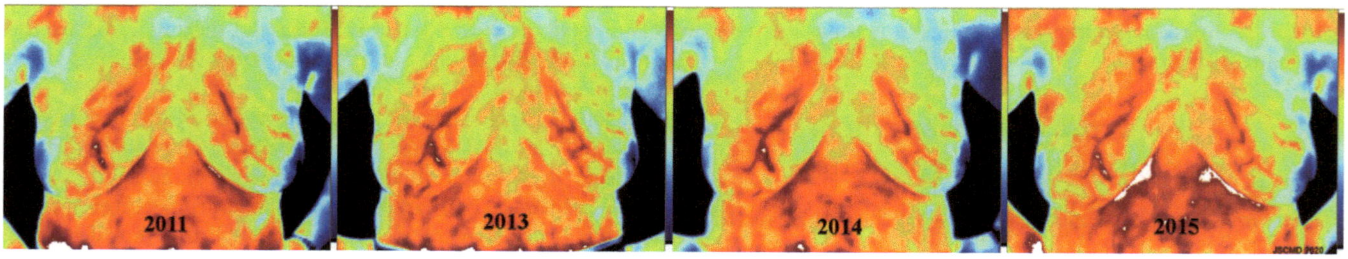

FIGURE 7.2 Serial thermograms taken over four years' time. Image comparisons over time help evaluate the stability of the thermal pattern.

and moreover may overwhelm the imaging system's memory space and interpretation algorithms with excess data. For slower imaging frame rates, many imagers can be set to take individual images at a set time interval – that is, several seconds to several minutes – thereby reducing the data that must be analyzed later.

Qualitative and quantitative analyses in thermography

The optimal interpretation of thermal images combines both qualitative and quantitative analyses. As the qualitative analysis is essentially descriptive and provides a visual representation of what is being thermally detected, this step logically precedes the quantitative analysis. The numerical data provided by quantitative measurements are essential for consistent and reliable comparisons with subsequent thermograms.

SIDEBAR 7.1 THE ART AND SCIENCE OF THERMAL IMAGING

Interpretation of a human infrared image requires two distinct analytical steps:

Qualitative Analysis. Qualitative thermography involves properly adjusting the color span over the ROI to maximize the thermal information available to the human visual system. The formatted image is then visually analyzed. Qualitative analysis may be accomplished with non-radiometric images as long as the microbolometer thermal response is linear. Once the thermographer has anatomically defined the ROI, *full-span* or *fixed-span* color scaling can be performed for human visual analysis.

Quantitative Analysis. Measurements of detected temperatures are the only way to obtain objective information for a complete image analysis. This step utilizes manual or automatic software tools to display the maximum, average, minimum, and differential temperatures of areas selected from the qualitative image analysis. Quantitative analysis requires *calibrated* radiometric images. For reliable quantitative measurements, verification of camera calibration is essential.

Comprehensive interpretation of a thermal image is a blend of art (qualitative visual analysis) and science (quantitative temperature measurements). Both methods are necessary for a full evaluation of the thermogram. Although *qualitative* image analysis depends on the visual color palette used and the thermal color span applied to the image, *quantitative* image analysis of a thermogram is independent of both these variables, requiring only radiometrically-calibrated infrared images for accuracy.

Qualitative thermographic analysis

Qualitative analysis entails properly adjusting the displayed color span over the ROI and then visually analyzing the image. This analysis may be accomplished with non-radiometric images and typically relies on a quasilinear rainbow-spectrum palette extending from blue/cool to red/warm. Training and skill in pattern recognition are important for an interpreting thermographer. Moreover, as qualitative thermal analysis relies heavily on color vision, thermographers should be evaluated for color blindness.[3] Thermographers with color blindness can interpret grayscale thermograms without difficulty; special color palettes may be required to accommodate those with such visual limitations.

Qualitative visual analysis is a quick way to determine the need for quantitative measurement of a particular area. Precise temperature measurements cannot be made by observing colors. Instead, scaled qualitative color or grayscale images can indicate where to select area, line, or point temperature measurements on radiometric images for reporting clinically significant temperatures. These quantitative temperature measurements placed over an image are much more precise than color evaluation.

To reduce visual confusion during qualitative image analysis, quantitative measurements should generally not be superimposed on the thermal image. The quantitative measurements are added later. Many software programs allow the quantitative markings to be turned off temporarily to expedite qualitative visual analysis.

As can be seen in Figure 7.3, selecting the correct color span when displaying an image for qualitative analysis is of utmost importance. Whereas too large a span will obscure the subtle thermal features of an ROI, too small a span will obliterate significant areas by pushing them off-scale. Many imaging systems will automatically adjust the thermal span of an image using the warmest and coolest pixels in the image to determine the upper and lower temperatures to be displayed. This may set the span too wide, however, as the background room temperature, not the lowest skin temperature over the ROI, will set the lower span limit. Colors over the ROI will then appear "washed out" unless the span is manually corrected.

Effective qualitative analysis requires imaging the radiance from a ROI, then digitally translating it into a temperature spectrum visible to the human eye with the least possible loss of information from the translation. The thermographer must select the ROI, and then set the color span to match the maximum and minimum temperatures within the ROI. See Figure 7.4.

Image display palettes

The three basic display options for thermographic imaging are (1) grayscales, (2) color palettes, and (3) stepped gradient palettes. What follows is a basic overview of each of these approaches.

Grayscale palettes

Grayscale imaging is visually limited because human vision detects color differences better than grayscale differences. Grayscale infrared images generally have 10-bits (1024 shades) or more of digital resolution per pixel, yet the human eye can only discern about 720 to 900 different values of gray under optimum medical display viewing conditions. Much poorer grayscale resolution occurs when viewing non-calibrated displays such as standard computer monitors.[4] Realistically, the average viewer can only detect about 30 values of gray (5-bits).[5] In comparison, a standard full-color image is a 24-bit file with 8 bits of red, 8 bits of green, and 8 bits of blue information, resulting in 16,777,216 color combinations per pixel, of which the normal human visual system can detect ten million or more.[6]

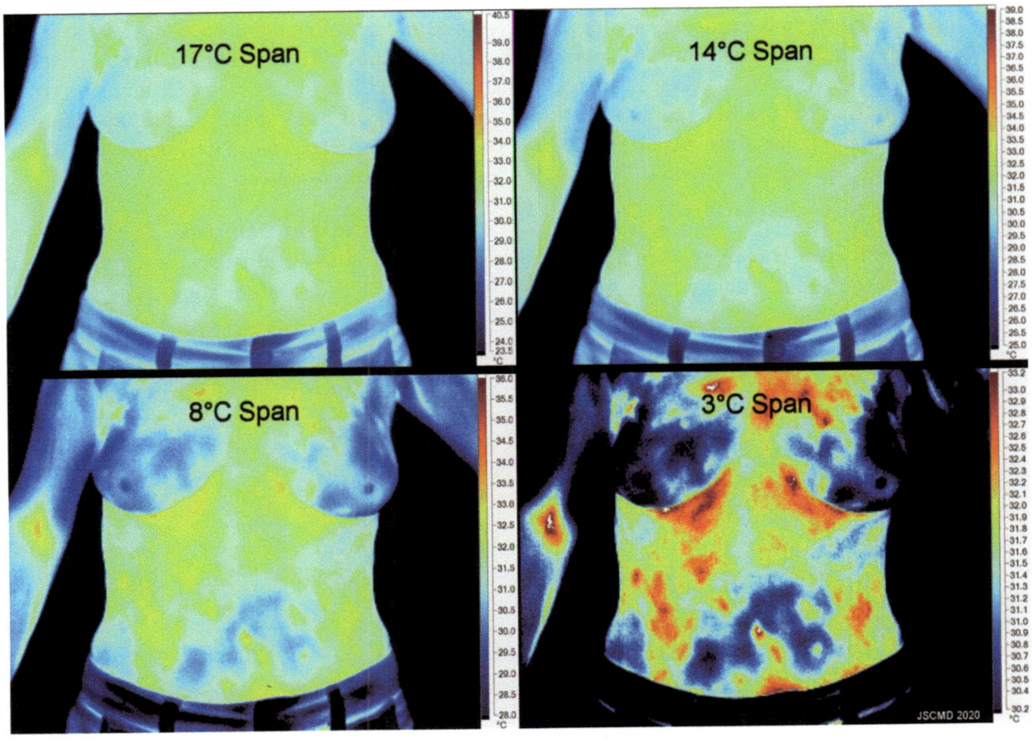

FIGURE 7.3 Effect of color span on qualitative image interpretation. All spans are centered at 32°C with the abdomen being the ROI. The lower right image was adjusted using the full-span scaling technique to provide the greatest color information for human visual analysis.

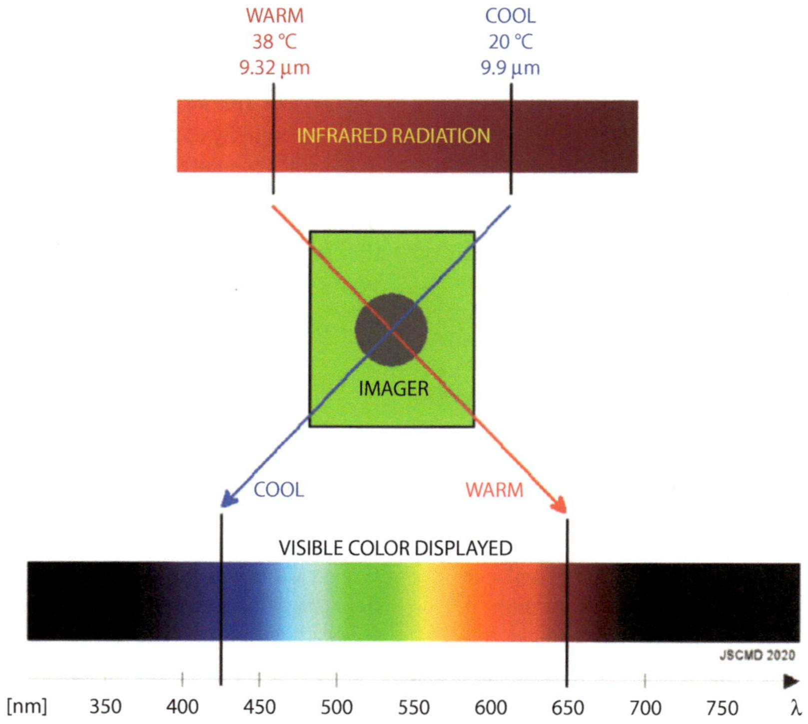

FIGURE 7.4 Schematic diagram of an infrared imager translating skin surface temperatures into visible information. Maximum information is transferred when the thermal span of the detected surface temperatures is adjusted to match the spectral bandwidth visible to the human eye. The shorter (warmer) infrared wavelengths are represented by longer visual wavelengths to accommodate the human custom that red is a "warm" color and blue is a "cool" color.

For these reasons, grayscale and reverse (negative) grayscale thermal images are now mainly of historical interest, though they are still found in research publications. Grayscale is also useful for manual focusing during image acquisition. Ironically, from a physics standpoint, all infrared images are grayscale (one analog value per pixel) and must be assigned "false colors" to be best analyzed by the human visual system. When displaying grayscale images, it is important to generate them from the original radiometric thermal image file. A blue-red spectral color thermogram printed as grayscale will give ambiguous gray values, as shown in Figure 7.5.

Color palettes

Color palettes offer a more effective way of representing thermal gradients if the colors are properly chosen and scaled. A gradient "rainbow" visual spectrum with red representing warm and blue indicating cool is intuitive to the human visual system. This palette has become an industry standard and a preferred method of thermographic representation in international medical journals (see Figure 7.6).[7] Historically, thermal palette colors have been left up to the thermographer's personal preferences, but this has led to difficulties when sharing or comparing images among thermography centers. Standardization of thermal palette colors will be needed if thermography is to gain wider acceptance.

Stepped gradient palettes

This third display option discards a great deal of clinically important thermal information. Stepped palettes are confusing to the

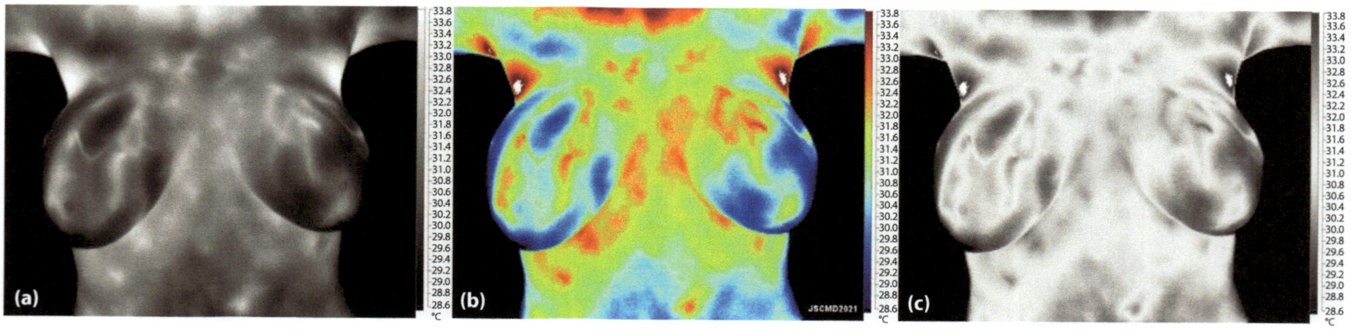

FIGURE 7.5 True grayscale thermal images must be generated from the radiometric image file, *not* from the color image converted to grayscale. (a) Grayscale image generated from the radiometric image. Note the linear grayscale. (b) Standard red-blue spectral color image generated from the same radiometric image. (c) Grayscale image generated from the spectral color image. The resulting scale is nonlinear, with light shades in the middle and darker shades at both ends, creating a confusing image where warm areas cannot be distinguished from cool areas.

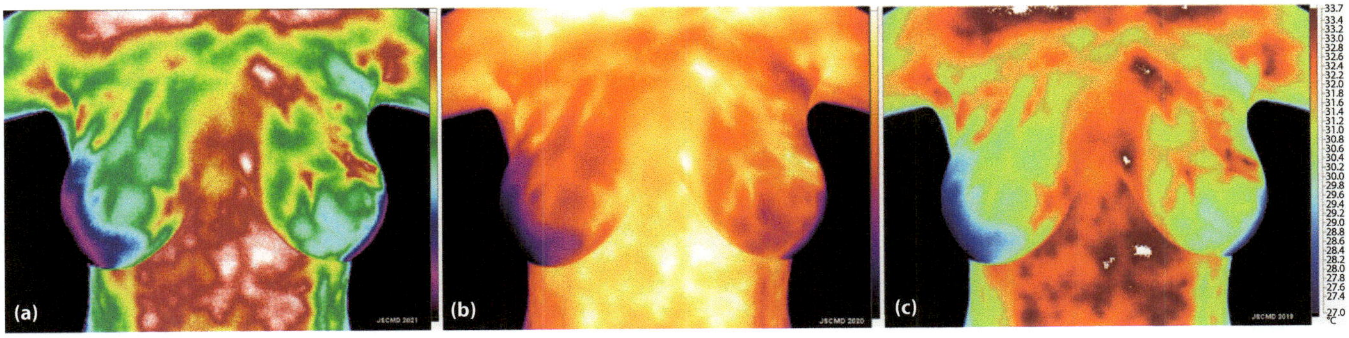

FIGURE 7.6 A full-span radiometric thermal image shown in different isothermal color palettes: (a) A "high-resolution" red-violet spectral palette with "soft" off-scale transitions. (b) A violet-yellow gradient "ironbow" color palette. Red, green, and blue are omitted from this palette, reducing the thermal information available to the eye. (c) The international standard red-blue spectral color palette with "sharp" off-scale transitions.

human eye and should be phased out of clinical thermography now that modern thermographic systems provide better thermal resolution for qualitative analysis (Figure 7.7a). This is especially true if the palette colors are not spectrally intuitive, with a white-red-orange-yellow-green-blue-black gradation. Stepped color palettes may have a place in specialized studies, but even there a fully-gradient color palette can provide the same information with much finer detail.

Stepped palettes are a result of the older infrared scanners before the year 2000 having a thermal display resolution of only ½ to 1°C, resulting in a large loss of thermal-to-visual information. Though the cryogenically-cooled sensors in these earlier scanners could detect changes of 0.1°C or less, the grayscale facsimile (FAX) printouts and early color-limited computer display terminals that presented the image for qualitative analysis were restricted to 5 to 16 values.[10] This technical constraint limited the visual interpretation of results in earlier thermographic studies.[11] Interpretation protocols made with these stepped images set the 20th-century thermographic display standards that stubbornly persist to the present day.

A variant of the stepped-gradient palette is to display adjacent ½ to 1°C temperature steps as black alternating with white, thereby producing an image that resembles zebra stripes (see Figure 7.7b). This distal thermal gradient display method is quite confusing and omits all the fine details of the image. Use of such "zebra stripe" images should be phased out of clinical use.

With the advent of calibrated, low-noise microbolometer imagers coupled to 24-bit color display technology, the stepped palette restricting each pixel to three to four bits (i.e., eight to 16 different shades or colors) makes little sense. The diagnostically -important fine thermal details required for breast thermography and other studies are largely obscured in the stepped-palette display. Interpretations of breast thermograms based solely on stepped palette images have become substandard and incomplete now that full-spectrum display technology is widely available. Full-spectrum color gradient thermal images should be considered the standard for 21st-century human thermography.

Formatting the image for qualitative interpretation

Qualitative image interpretation requires proper formatting to maximize the skin surface temperature display for detection by the human visual system. Humans have excellent color vision which, in satisfactory light conditions, surpasses the ability to

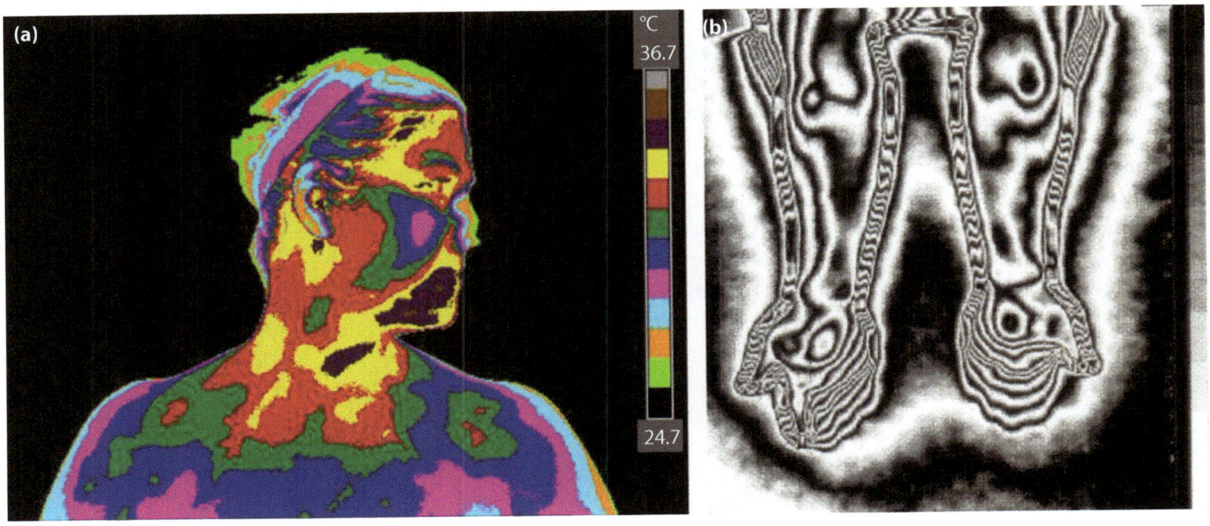

FIGURE 7.7 (a) A 12-level stepped palette infrared image using non-spectral colors with a 12°C fixed span (1°C per step).[8] (b) A monochrome "Zebra stripe" image showing the volar forearms and hands.[9]

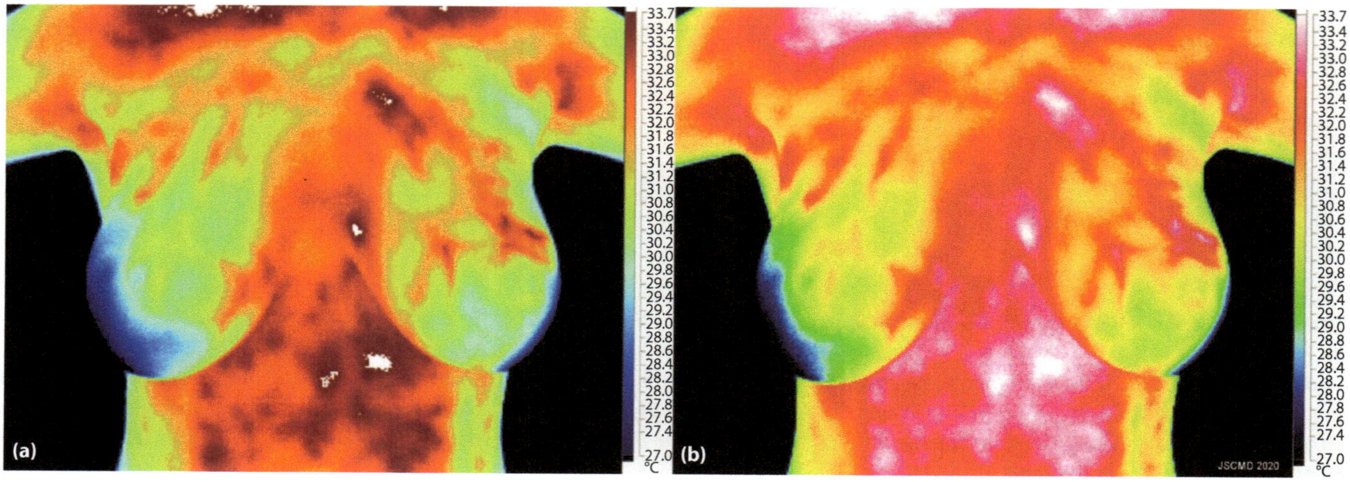

FIGURE 7.8 (a) Sharp off-scale color transitions have precise visual boundaries. (b) Soft off-scale color transition blurs the off-scale boundaries, reducing the visual precision of their location and shape.

detect shades of gray. Thus, thermal-to-visual palettes in full color are preferable. The human visual system is also excellent at edge detection, thus edge blurring or interpolation is not a desirable feature in the qualitative thermal image.[12] This section highlights the best ways to maximize the thermal-to-visual information available in human infrared images.

Color span out-of-range indicators

To provide the greatest visual impact from the thermal energy radiating off a subject, the entire visible color spectrum from deep red to deep blue must be spread out to cover the desired ROI from its coolest to warmest surface temperatures.[13] The thermal spectrum extends well beyond this visual spectrum, however, requiring "off scale" indicators to show where any thermal value exceeds the limits of the visual color scale. These out-of-range indicators are also known as saturation indicators or saturation colors (Figure 7.8).

International thermographic standards recommend that the off-span high (warmer) saturation indicator be represented by white, and the off-span low (cooler) be represented by black. This is in agreement with the grayscale standard. Other out-of-range indicator colors may be distracting or hard to detect on an image during adjustment of the color span by the thermographer.

In order to provide the best visualization of the shape and location of the warmest and coolest portions of the ROI, the cold and warm saturation color transition edges should be sharp, not "soft" or blurred. The human eye is best at detecting sharp image transitions, so blurring of these edges reduces the available acuity. The exact location and shape of the warmest spots over an ROI may be important in detecting the nature of the warmth. The coolest spots on an image are often small polyps or moles, which could be missed by a blurred cool transition. Imager software usually provides a choice of saturation indicators. It is recommended that the thermographer choose the sharp option.

Full-Span color scale technique

The *full-span color scale* technique adjusts the entire visual color span to cover the anatomic ROI temperatures without going off-scale. This technique spreads out the "active" blue-to-red spectral color scale over the ROI, maximizing the color contrast detected by the human eye. The quantitative temperature span of the ROI can then be calculated by subtracting the minimum scale value from the maximum scale value. The thermal gain of the imager must be calibrated for this measurement to be accurate.

The disadvantages of this method are as follows. The visual scale range is adjusted for each area of interest and may not color-match with other images unless isothermal adjustment methods are utilized. Also, the span may be too wide if the ROI includes the hands/feet and trunk together. This is because the fingers or toes may be at 20°C (68°F) and the trunk at 34.4°C (94°F) – a 14.4°C (26°F) span. Such a large color span may obscure small temperature differences important for image analysis (see Figure 7.9). In order to avoid this color dilution effect, full-span ROI images usually include only the hands and feet, or only the trunk and proximal limbs. A similar large-span problem also occurs when imaging the face, as bringing a very cold nose or ear into the visual span may obscure other fine details of the facial image (see Figure 13.3).

Adjusting the full-span color scale

Adjusting the color scale range for a *Full-Span* color image maximizes the thermal-to-visual information (Figure 7.10). A typical thermal display program utilizes calipers to set the span: a "top caliper" sets the upper span limit and a "bottom caliper" adjusts the lower span limit. A "handle" in between the calipers allows moving both calipers up and down simultaneously to adjust the thermal scale over the ROI without changing the set span.[14] Other software packages may have a different appearance, but the controls explained here should work in a similar fashion. Software programs that do not allow adjusting the displayed color span while observing the effects on the image are not clinically useful. Thermographers are referred to the instructions supplied with their specific software application for more details.

To set the calipers correctly for a Full Span image, first set the upper caliper so that the warmest spots over the ROI are just beginning to turn white. Then set the lower caliper so that the coolest regions over the ROI are just beginning to turn black (this should not affect the temperature position of the upper caliper), as shown in Figure 7.11. The white areas should remain the same, though some minor changes may occur as the software recalculates the span. The image is now ready for qualitative viewing. If using a

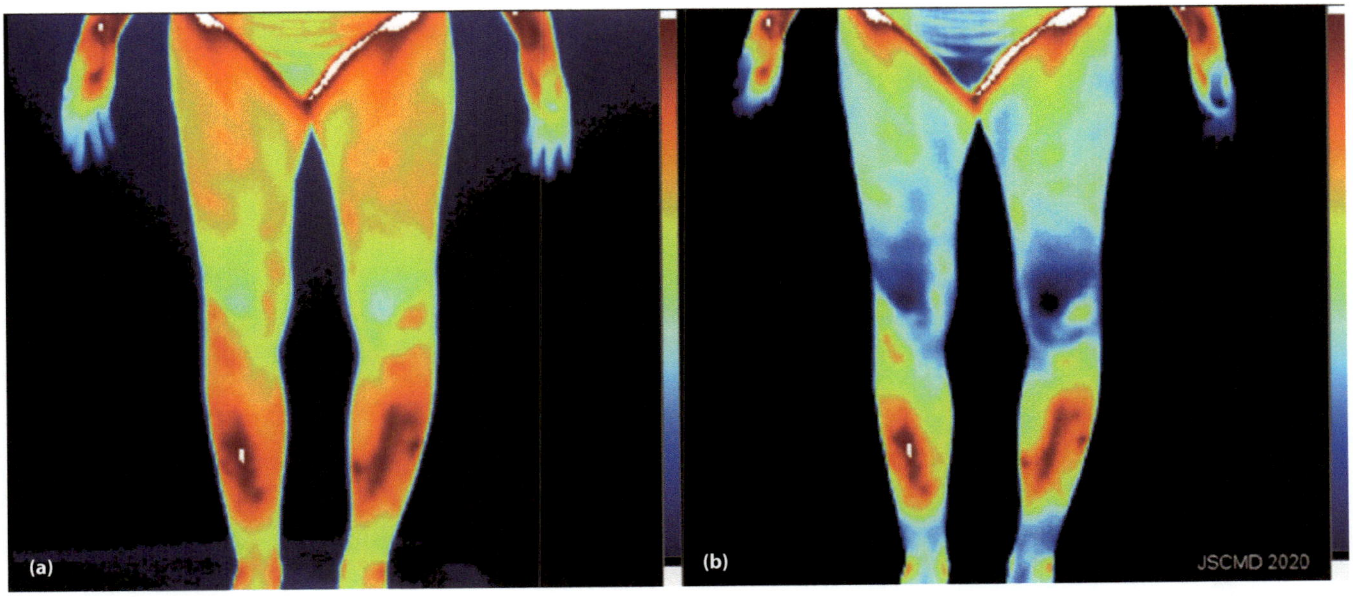

FIGURE 7.9 (a) Including cold fingers and toes in the color span may reduce visual temperature information over central-body ROIs by setting the temperature span too wide. (b) Here, the color span is maximized for the legs, revealing better thermal detail over the ROI; portions of the hands are off-scale low. Hands and feet are usually imaged separately for this reason.

calibrated imager, the temperature span of the ROI can be calculated by subtracting the lower scale value from the upper value. Areas or points requiring quantitative analysis can be visually located on this full-span scaled image.

Fixed-Span display technique

The fixed-span technique sets the caliper span to a fixed value. This technique may be used for both color and greyscale images. The fixed span is usually set to 8°C (14.4°F) for breast exams. Neuromuscular exams typically use a 10°C (18°F) span, while sports science thermography may require a 14°C (25.2°F) fixed span.[15] This fixed span is then moved up or down the radiometric temperature scale to best visualize the ROI. Fixed-span formatting techniques can be traced back to the older infrared scanner technology, but are still used for clinical studies as well as research reports. See Figure 7.12 to set up a moveable Fixed Span Color Caliper in a typical infrared display program.

The main advantage of this technique is that visual differences appear the same in every image, provided their upper (or lower) temperatures are set to the same value. This facilitates temperature comparisons between images. The disadvantage is that the scale may be too large or too small for the regions of interest, reducing the visual information available. Fine thermal details may not be as visible compared to the Full-Span technique (see Figure 7.13).

Once set for an appropriate fixed span, the caliper pair may be adjusted up or down without the ROI necessarily going off-scale, i.e., white or black. The middle handle is used for this adjustment. Some thermographers like the *high* end of the fixed scale placed so that the warmest areas of the ROI are just turning white. Other thermographers prefer the fixed span adjusted mid-span. Additionally, some thermographers like to have the *low* end of the fixed scale placed so that the coolest areas of the ROI are just turning black. All three adjustments may appear quite different visually but are thermographically valid as long as all pertinent portions of the ROI remain on-scale.

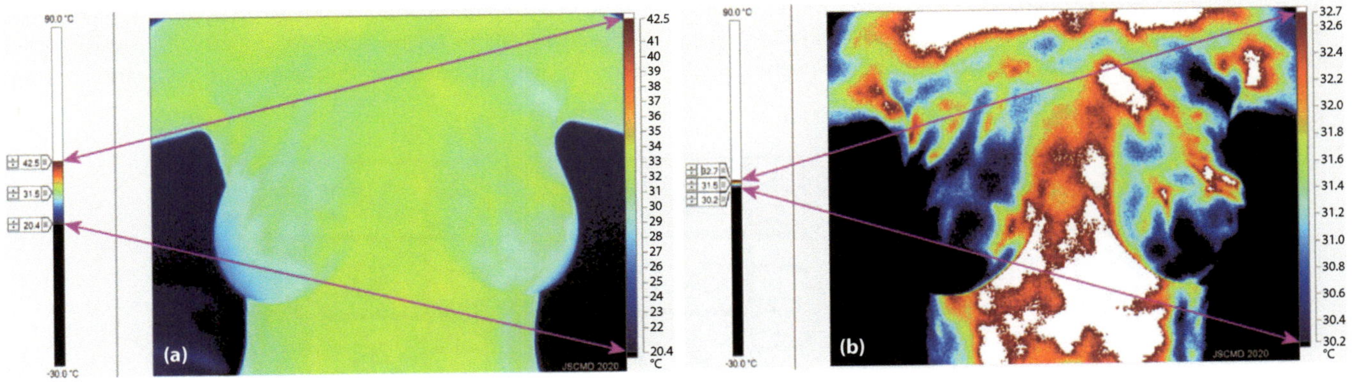

FIGURE 7.10 (a) Temperature calipers set too wide. The color span over the ROI is "washed out," reducing the visual contrast available to the human eye. The image temperature span is 22.1°C (39.8°F). (b) Temperature calipers set too narrow. Large off-scale white and/or black areas appear over the ROI. The image temperature span is 2.5°C (4.5°F).

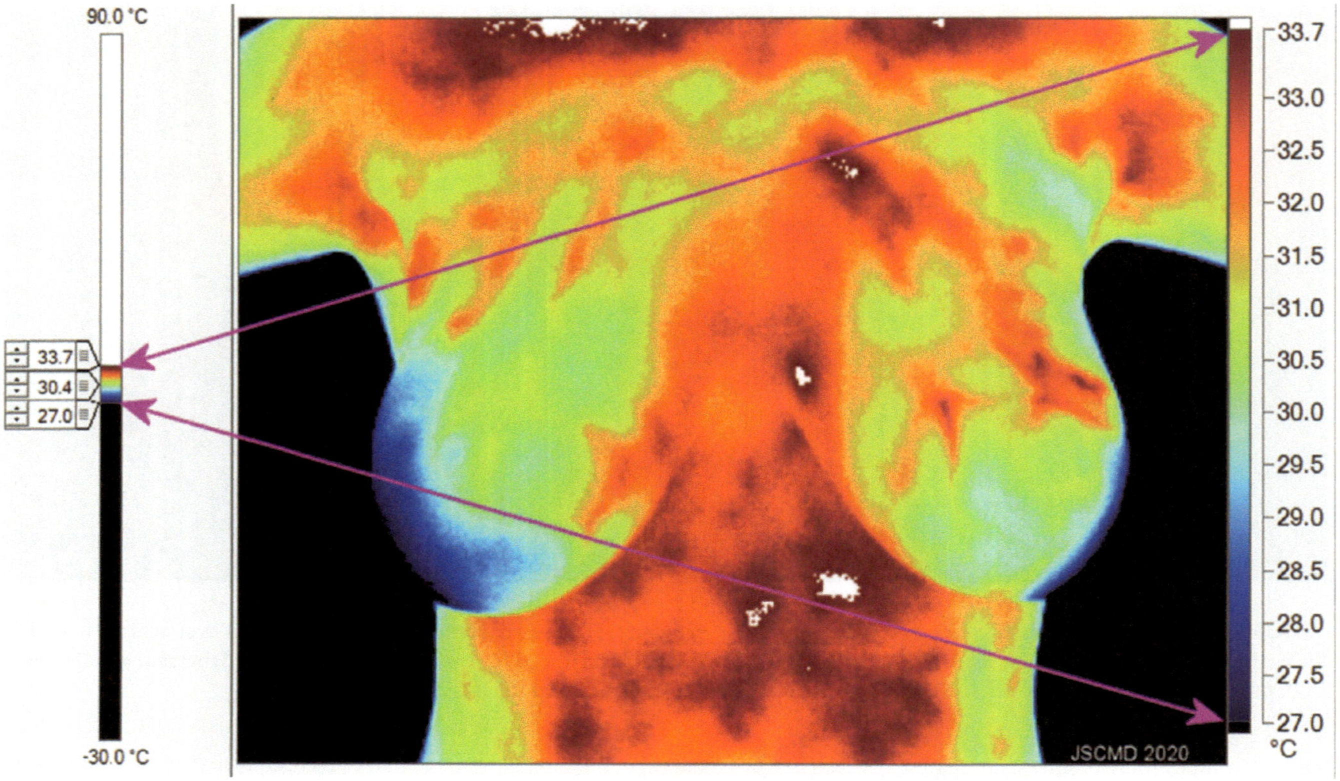

FIGURE 7.11 Temperature calipers set just right. The warmest spots of the ROI are white. The coolest spots over the ROI are turning black. The visual color spectrum is now active over the entire ROI, providing maximum thermal contrast information to the human eye. The image temperature span is 6.7°C (12.1°F).

Many thermal imagers incorporate a digital camera that provides a separate visual image taken simultaneously with the infrared image. This allows superimposing the two images. The thermographer must adjust out any parallax error between the two image axes, which may be 2.5 cm (1 inch) apart or more. With this overlay of the two image types, the patient's visual image is displayed on the thermogram.[16]

Depending on the imager, the camera, and the available software adjustments, the alignment of these composite images is more or less accurate. Applying small metallic tape "fiducial" markers to the skin of the ROI facilitates better alignment of the two images (see Figure 6.7). Specialized software is also available that overlays anatomical drawings of the skeleton, muscles, blood vessels, and lymphatics onto the thermal image (Figure 7.14). Such overlays assume that every individual is the same, however, which may not be true especially for obese subjects and when viewing venous and lymphatic anatomy.

Quantitative thermographic analysis

Precise temperature measurements cannot be made by observing colors on a qualitative image. Instead, properly spanned images direct the eye to warm or cool skin surface temperatures that require objective thermal analysis. Quantitative thermal analysis uses temperature measurements taken from calibrated radiometric images to display absolute and differential surface temperature measurements (Figure 7.15).

The first step in quantitative image analysis is to identify and define the ROIs to be measured as guided by the scaled qualitative image. To aid this, thermographic software programs

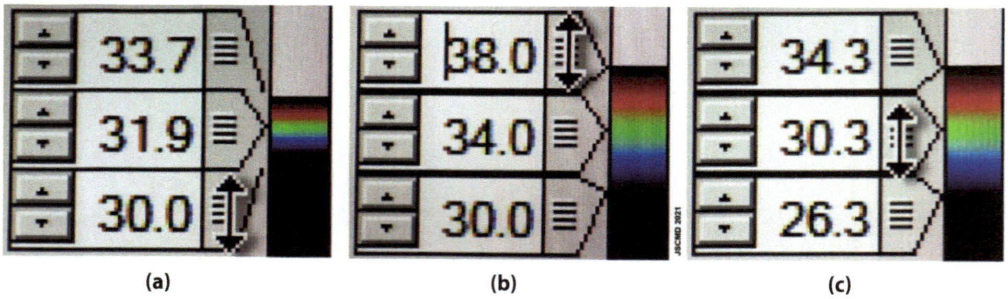

FIGURE 7.12 Setting the scale calipers for an 8°C fixed-span image. (a) Set the lower caliper to a whole number. (b) Set the upper caliper 8 degrees higher. (c) Use the middle handle to move the fixed 8°C span up and down to best view the region of interest.

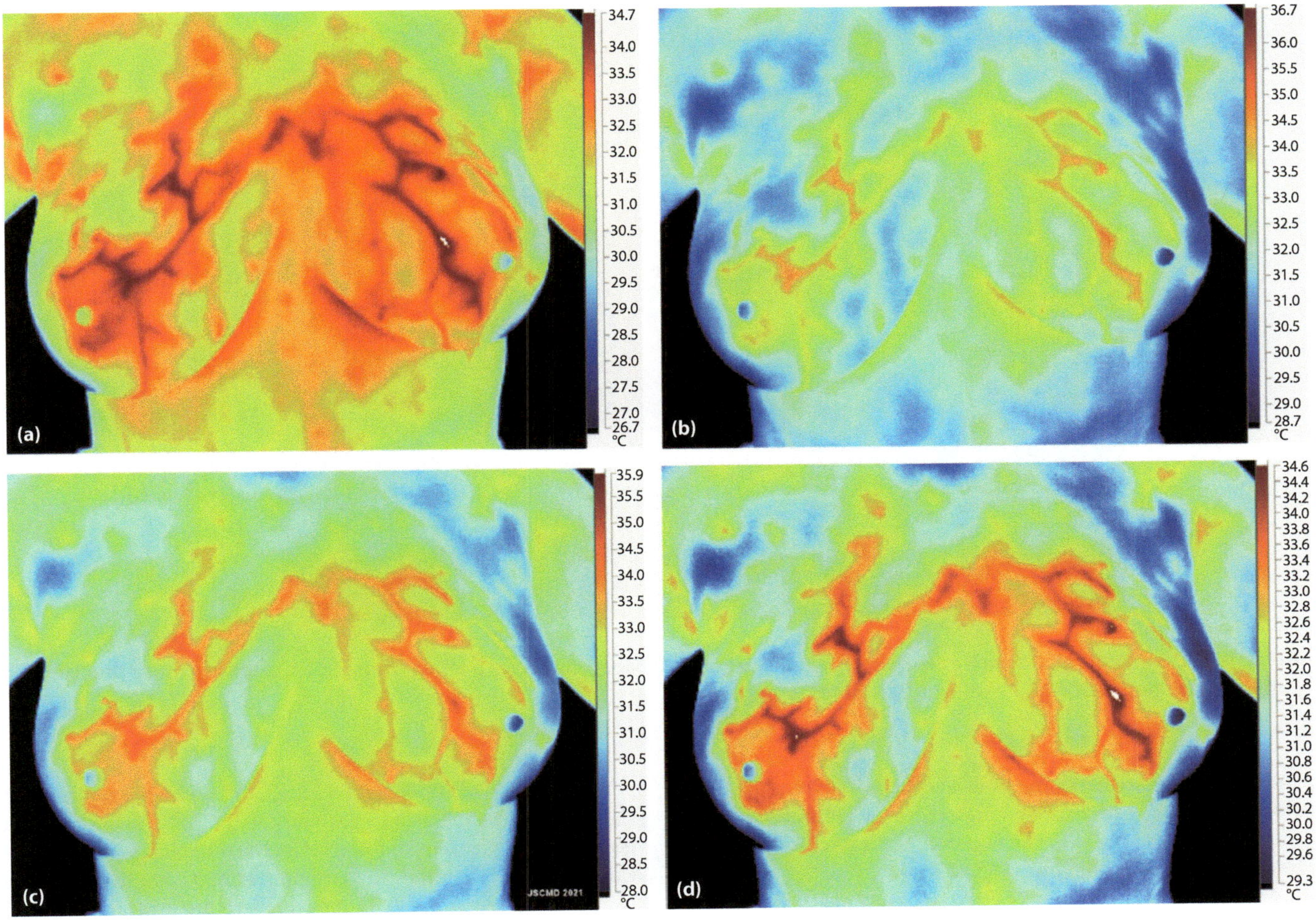

FIGURE 7.13 A radiometric image showing fixed spans versus a full-scale span image: (a) An 8°C fixed span adjusted to off-scale high. (b) The 8°C span is adjusted to off-scale low. (c) The 8°C span adjusted to the mid-span position. (d) The image with a full-scale span covering 5.3°C – 62 yoF.

use regular geometric shapes such as points, lines, squares, rectangles, circles, and ellipses. Except for points, each of these shapes can be adjusted in size and superimposed on a specific area in the image to give the maximum, average, and minimum temperatures within or along that shape. Point measurements may not be reliable as they only provide the temperature of one pixel (which may be in error) and are generally not used in formal thermographic studies, though they do provide convenient

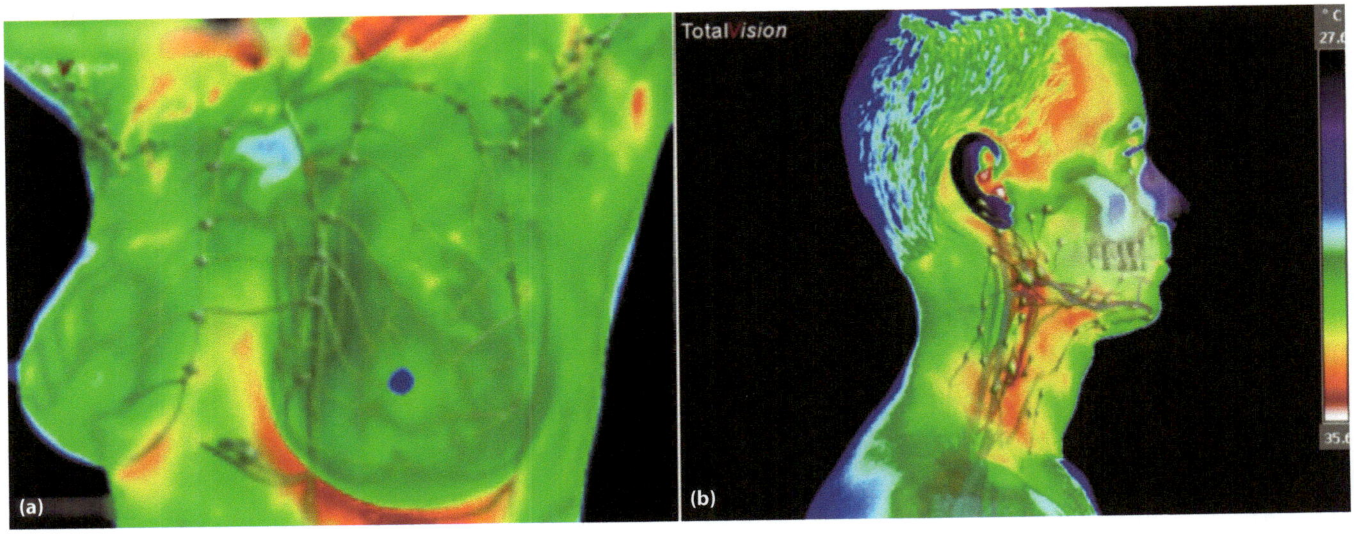

FIGURE 7.14 (a) Lymphatic anatomy superimposed over a left oblique chest thermogram. (b) An anatomy diagram over a lateral craniocervical thermal image.[17]

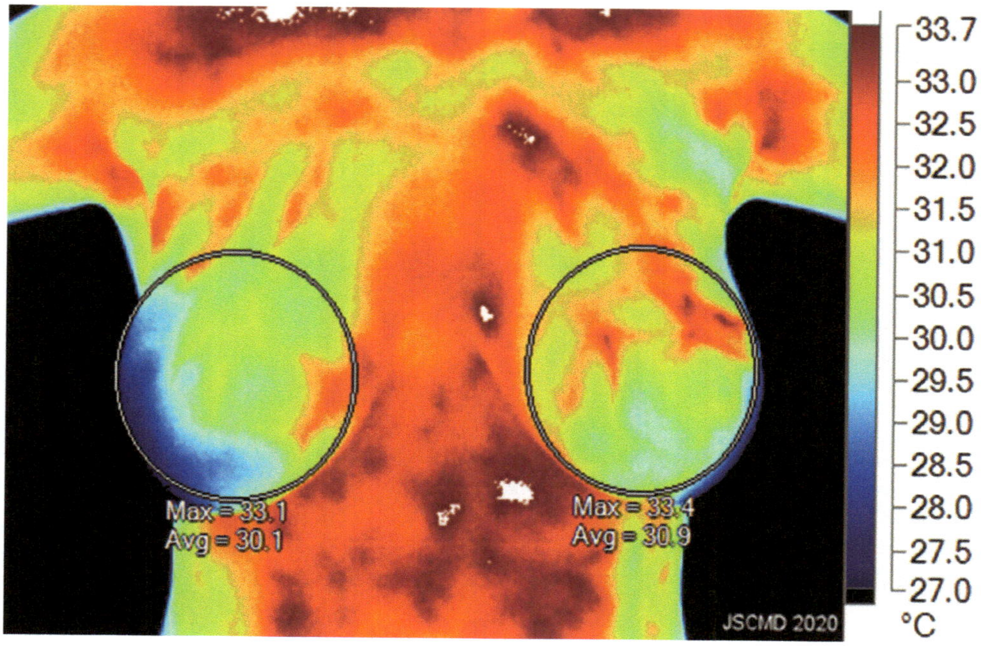

FIGURE 7.15 Area quantitative temperature measurements placed correctly over a radiometric image are more precise than color evaluation, even when using a full span color technique.

and quick measurements in clinical reports. Temperature values along a straight line may be displayed as a graph showing the thermal profile along with the maximum, average, and minimum temperatures along that line (Figure 7.16).

Manually-adjusted geometric area measurements are the most frequently used quantitative analysis tools. In some cases, the anatomical shape of the ROI does not conform to the geometric shape, which can lead to the exclusion of relevant data, or the inclusion of irrelevant data, possibly causing errors in the image analysis (Figure 7.17). Erroneously including a sliver of background temperature in an image may significantly affect the average and minimum temperature reported for that area. Analysis software that allows "free-form" drawing of irregular areas is useful in overcoming the limitations of geometrically-defined measurements.

The skin surface temperature range in an image extends from the body core temperature, nominally 36.5°C (97.7°F) (unless fever is present), down to a minimum set by the room temperature, typically 20°C (68°F) minus any evaporative heat loss; this is a span of approximately 17°C (30°F). Any temperature measurement outside these range limits must be a calibration error or artifact.

Human interpretation of a thermal image requires two steps, beginning with a qualitative assessment to determine the location of quantitative measurement sites. If thermal asymmetry or significant thermal anomalies are observed on viewing the scaled image, quantitative measurements of those areas can confirm the significance of the qualitative findings. Quantitative analysis is critical for arriving at consistent and accurate conclusions. Software should calculate the maximum, minimum, and average temperatures of the selected ROIs. Differential temperatures and

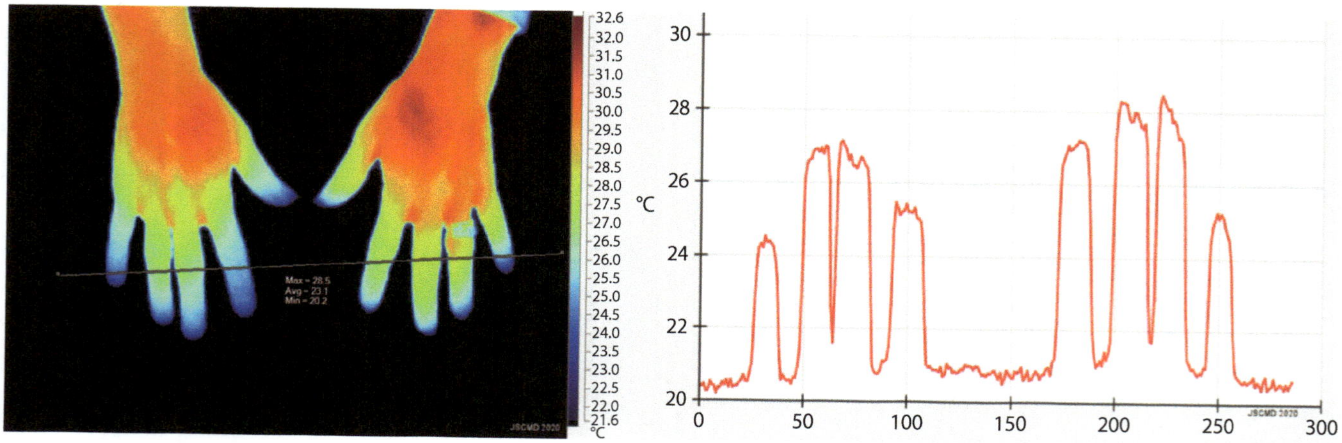

FIGURE 7.16 Transverse thermal line analysis. A line graph across an image showing mid-finger temperatures. Digits II, III, and IV on the left fingers are over 1°C warmer than the right. Line plots may facilitate quantitative measurement and documentation of thermal asymmetry.

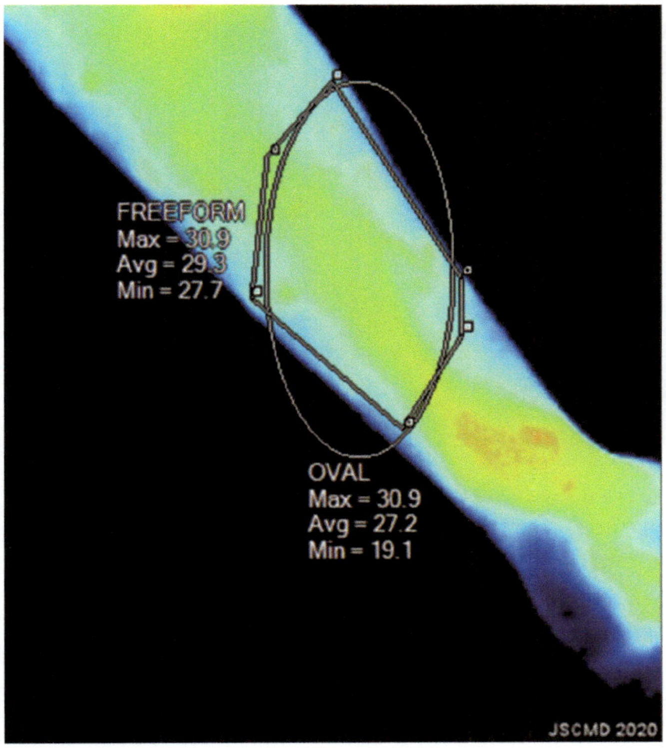

FIGURE 7.17 Quantitative measurement area error. In this example, the freeform area measurements are more accurate than the oval area measurements, which include portions of the background temperature. The minimum and average temperature results are affected, but not the maximum measurement.

standard deviation values may also be computed in the analysis software.

The ***average*** quantitative measurement is the most widely used skin temperature value in the medical literature. It can be statistically representative and reduces the effects of spurious maximum or minimum point values that can lead to errors in data interpretation. When temperature variations are large, however, the average temperature of an ROI may not provide useful information, requiring the addition of the maximum and minimum temperature values for the analysis. Subtracting the minimum from the maximum temperature detected over an area can provide the local temperature span over an ROI, useful in determining the clinical presence of underlying inflammation or other pathology.

The ***maximum*** temperature is often useful in thermographic analyses. For example, there may be a relationship between maximum temperature and traumatic injury (as well as other inflammatory events).[18] Maximum periorbital temperatures are also useful in fever detection. Closely related to the maximum temperature is the Tmax method, which enables all the measurements to have the same number of pixels for the calculation. After the thermographer chooses the ROI, the software locates the five warmest pixels with a minimum distance of pixels between each. The software selects areas of pixels around each of the pixels previously selected, and calculates the mean temperature across the pixel selection. This method can be useful in the context of comparing different patients within a group, because it helps minimize the problem of differences in the anatomical size between participants.[19]

Minimum temperature values over an area are used for two reasons. The first is to determine the temperature span detected within a measurement area. This span is calculated by subtracting the minimum from the maximum temperature value, resulting in a measurement that represents the temperature variability within that area. A low-temperature span indicates that the average temperature measurement for that area is valid. High spans indicate that the area must be reviewed qualitatively to discern the reason for the variability – small areas of inflammation, a warm superficial vein, a cool skin polyp, or other pathology.

A very low minimum temperature detected over a non-acral area may indicate that the selected area erroneously includes a portion of the background temperature.[20] This background inclusion error is corrected by adjusting the measurement area to exclude skin areas near the edge of the subject's image. Minimum temperature values may also be in error when small dots of reflective metal tape are used as fiducial location markers, as their low emissivity makes them appear cool to the infrared imager. Fiducial markers, if small, will usually have an insignificant effect on the average temperature reading.

Differential temperature measurements

Differential temperatures taken from a single image or multiple images taken at the same imaging session are more accurate than absolute temperatures because subtracting two measurements taken with the same imager will subtract out the offset error of that imager. Differential measurements remain dependent on the imager's thermal gain and gain flatness, however. Verifying these parameters is imperative to assure differential measurement accuracy (see Chapter 4).

Differences in skin temperature are often followed serially over time, often before and after an intervention. Patient preparation, equilibration conditions, time of day, and core temperature must be taken into consideration when comparing differential skin temperatures over two or more imaging sessions. Thermal offset drift between imaging sessions is canceled out of differential measurements as long as the thermal gain and image flatness are within specification (Figure 7.18). Differential temperature changes can be either positive or negative, depending on the underlying pathology. This technique has been used to test the effectiveness of anti-inflammatory agents for rheumatoid arthritis.[21] In vascular surgery, a reduction in differential foot temperature is seen due to warming of the ischemic foot after the restoration of arterial flow.[22]

A second type of differential temperature measurement focuses on the sagittal symmetry of a subject. For valid comparisons, the symmetric ROIs should be similar in shape and size, and similarly positioned in the images (Figure 7.19).[23] Using older infrared scanners, the human body was found to be thermally symmetric to within 0.24°C (0.43°F).[24] More recent studies using calibrated radiometric microbolometer images, however, have shown that the face is statistically warmer on the right side, with the average maxillary temperatures being 0.33°C (0.60°F) warmer on the right.[25] Further microbolometer-based studies of the average thermal symmetry over other body areas are needed.

Thermal symmetry can also aid in the evaluation of musculoskeletal issues. For example, asymmetries higher than 0.5–0.7°C (0.9–1.3°F) are associated with either musculoskeletal dysfunction or increased risk of injury.[26] Automated differential temperature measurements between two ROIs can be a great time-saver in quantitative image analysis and may be found in advanced imaging software applications.

Assessments of sagittal symmetry are useful in breast thermography, both qualitatively and quantitatively.[27] Longitudinal

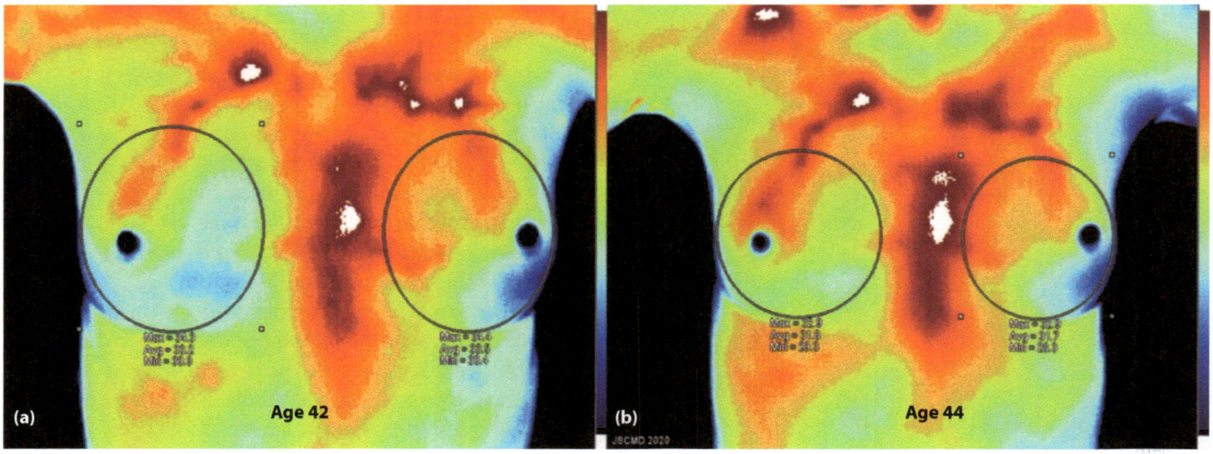

FIGURE 7.18 (a) and (b) Serial differential quantitative images of the breasts over time. The temperature spans (max minus min) over each breast have remained similar over time, while the average breast temperatures decreased bilaterally by about the same amount. This may be due to different patient equilibration, different imaging times (diurnal changes), or thermal offset changes.

thermal analysis of a horizontal line on a frontal breast thermogram can be useful in quantifying sagittal symmetry (Figure 7.20). If the line passes through the nipples, ductal versus areolar temperatures can also be compared.

A third type of differential temperature measurement involves the display of temperature differences within the ROI. An example is the forearm-to-finger skin temperature gradient, which may be considered an index of peripheral circulation and vasomotor tone during rest as well as during steady-state exercise.[28] Linear thermal measurement graphs are useful for this analysis if the line is placed along the axis of the limb or digit (Figure 7.21).

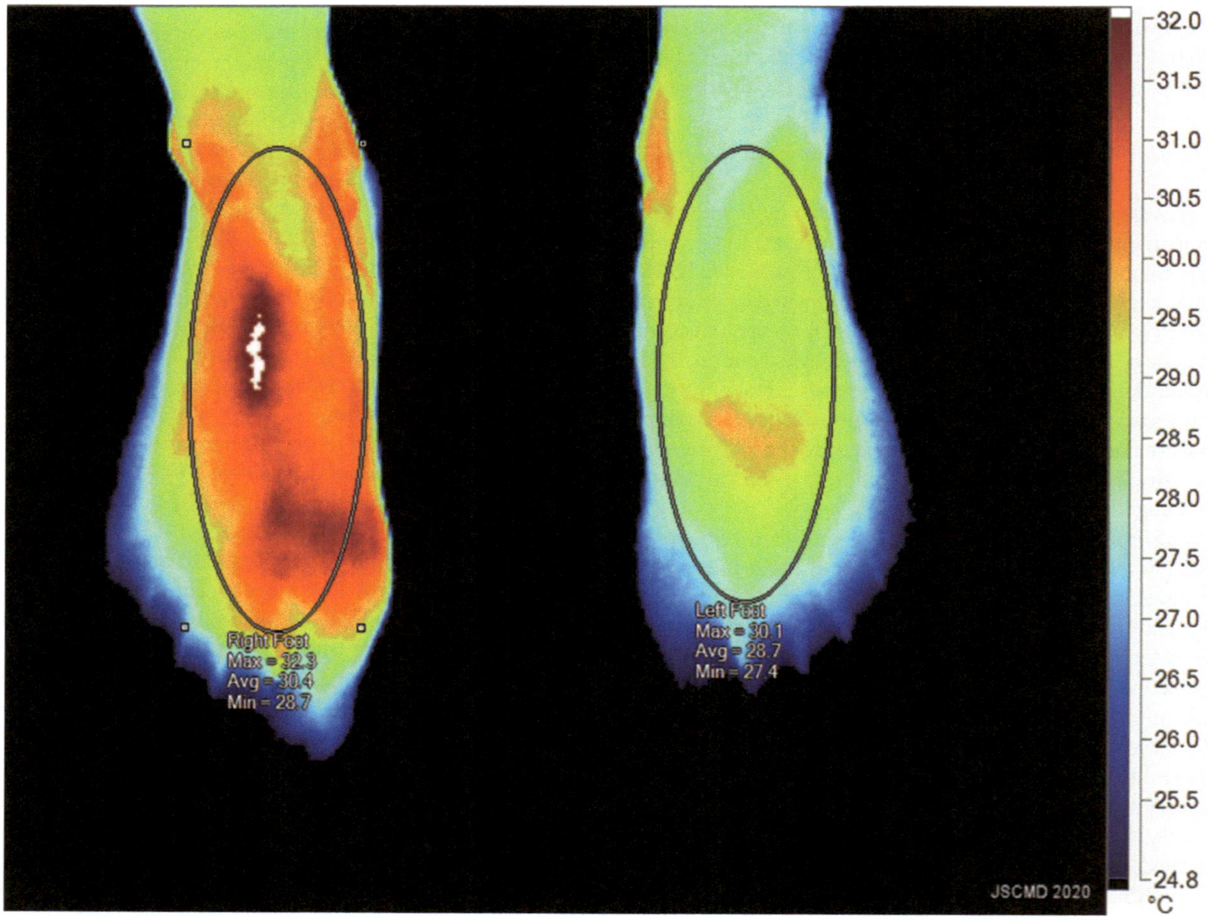

FIGURE 7.19 Elliptical differential measurement areas over the dorsum of both feet documenting clinically significant warmth on the right.

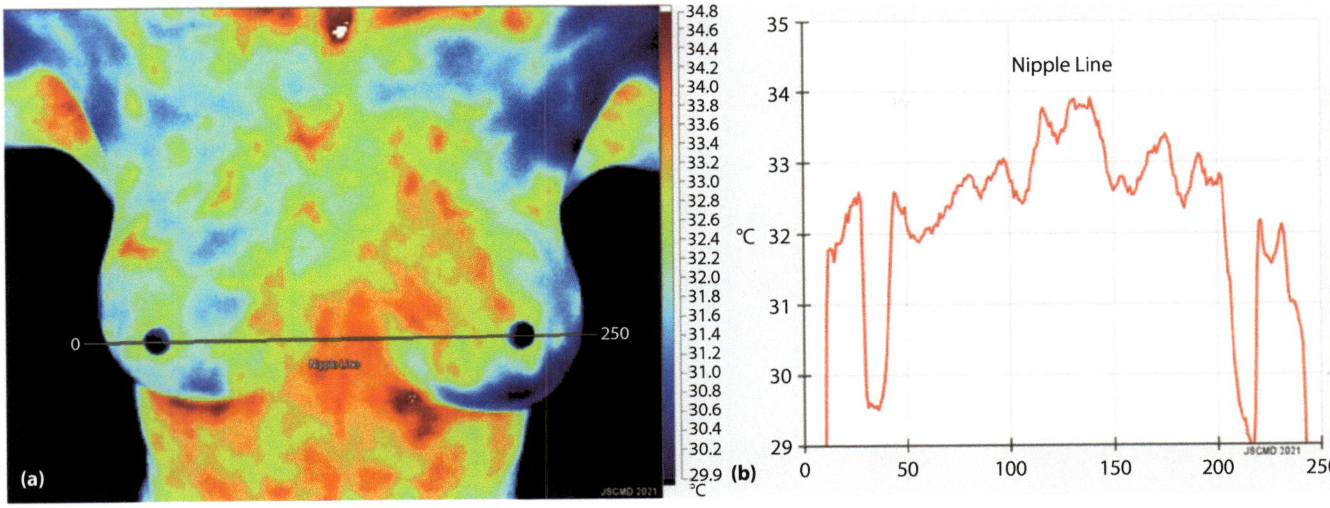

FIGURE 7.20 Graphic presentation of temperatures along a line through both nipples showing moderate asymmetry of the medial portions of the breasts. (a) The temperature asymmetry seen over the upper inner quadrant of the left breast has been stable for 7 years – TH3S, 69-year-old female. (b) The line graph shows that the sagittal symmetry of the medial breasts varies less than 1°C. The linear 0–250 scale is arbitrary and for location reference only.

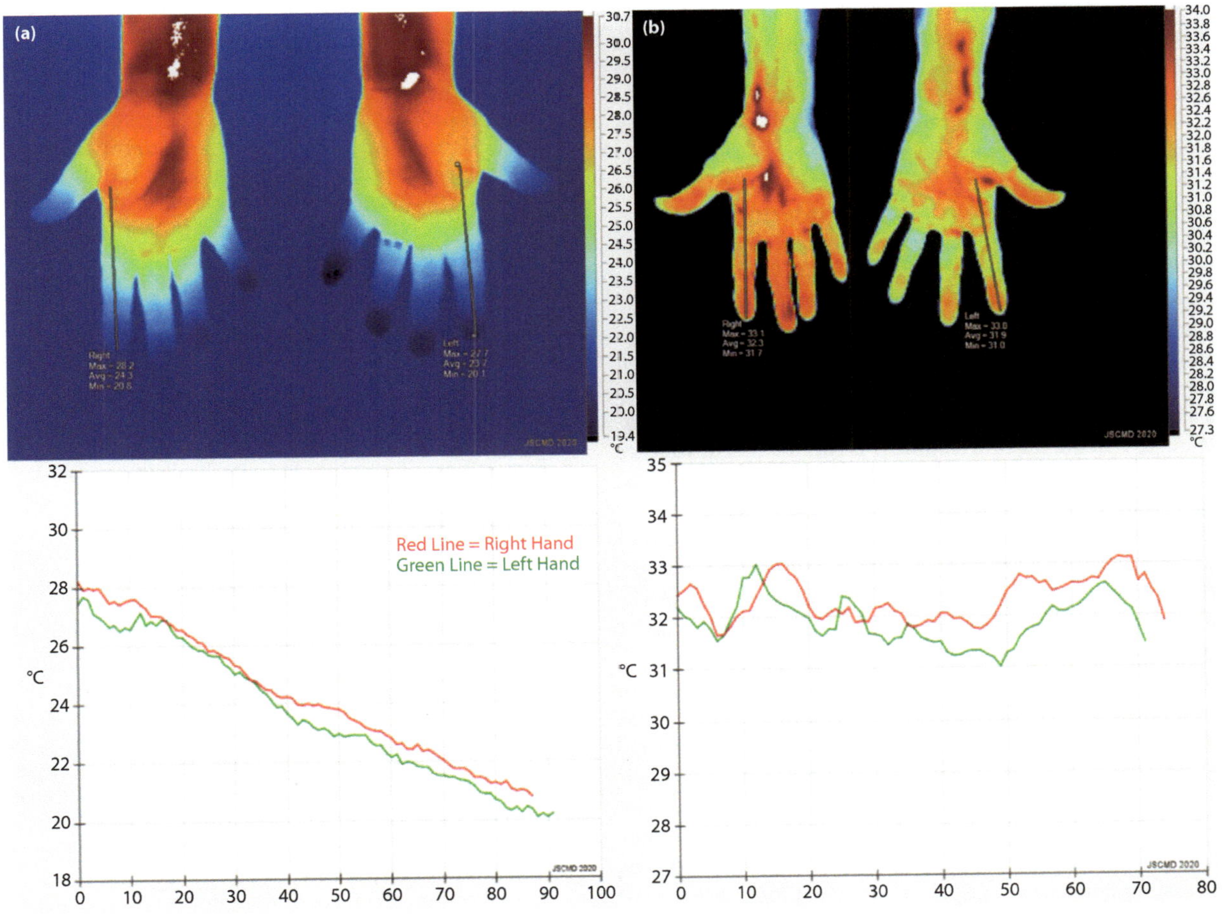

FIGURE 7.21 Longitudinal thermal line analysis. (a) Normal hands have an almost linear decrease in longitudinal finger temperatures. (b) These hands show the blotchy pattern of diffuse glomus AVA dilation. No longitudinal decrease in temperature is present, and the plots show the uneven temperature variations in the longitudinal section.

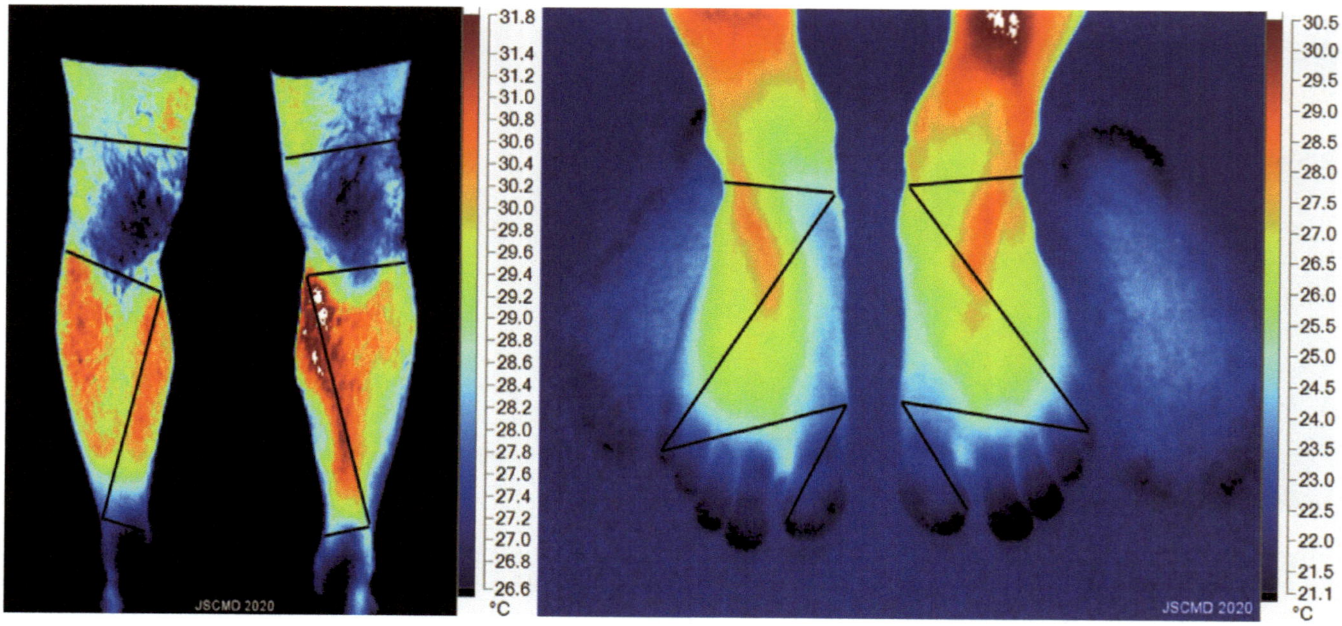

FIGURE 7.22 Images showing ROI segmentation to facilitate computerized interpretation. Anatomic structures and compartments may not be delineated by segmentation, but computer analysis can still detect normal versus abnormal infrared information if "trained" with machine learning algorithms.[31]

To exclude irrelevant data within the selected ROIs, image segmentation algorithms are being developed (Figure 7.22).[29] These algorithms automatically extract temperature data, first by distinguishing the body ROI from the background in the thermal image, then identifying pixels that comprise that body section. The segmentation process involves the demarcation of an object on an image using object-level or pixel-level properties. These properties can include the object's shape, size, texture, edges, orientation, and pixel intensity variation. Segmentation can be especially useful for finding thermal asymmetries.[30]

The purpose of the automated segmentation process is twofold: (1) to deconstruct an image into regions for subsequent analysis, and (2) to alter the representation of an image for improved analysis.[32] Segmentation techniques can be applied to optimize the measurements within the ROI.[33] Nevertheless, accurate segmentation is still subject to technical errors in image capture such as an improper viewing angle, viewing distance, or suboptimal positioning of the subject. To reduce positioning errors, the Glamorgan Protocol defines 24 body views and 90 regions of interest with the intent of maximizing inter-operator consistency of thermal images. Though following the protocol increases the reproducibility of the temperature readings, variations due to body type or positioning remain a problem.[34]

In summary, both qualitative and quantitative approaches are necessary for the professional analysis of a thermal image. Visual assessment of a gradient color or grayscale image pattern complements the measurement of temperature differences. Although quantitative analysis of a thermal image is independent of the display palette used and the thermal span of the image, qualitative image analysis is absolutely dependent on these variables, but independent of quantitative offset or gain when using a full-span color scale. Visibly selecting the appropriate areas for numerical measurements is contingent upon a well-scaled qualitative image; the quantitative measurements provide calibrated physical confirmation of the visible areas of concern.

Notes

1. Niu HH1, et al., Zhonghua Yi Xue Za Zhi (Taipei). 2001; PMID: 11720145.
2. A. J. Syllaios, et al., Proc. SPIE 5783, Infrared Technology and Applications XXXI, 2005; Doi: 10.1117/12.603153. See also: Chistokhin I, et al., Proceedings of SPIE – The International Society for Optical Engineering 2005. Doi: 10.1117/12.628888. See also: URL: https://www.flir.com/support-center/Instruments/what-is-the-response-time-for-flir-microbolometer-cameras-thermal-time-constant/, Accessed on 1 October 2021.
3. Use of the Ishihara Color Tests are useful in detecting the several types of color "blindness."
4. Kimpe T, et al., J Digital Imaging 2007; PMCID: PMC3043920.
5. Wilson C, Can You Actually See 50 Different Shades of Grey? (a self-test) Time Magazine, 8 February 2017. *Also see:* Diep F. Humans Can Only Distinguish Between About 30 Shades of Gray. Popular Science, 19 February 2015.
6. Source: How Humans See In Color. By: Reena Mukamal, Am Acad Ophthalmology Website 2017. Accessed at: https://www.aao.org/eye-health/tips-prevention/how-humans-see-in-color
7. Ring F, Jung A & Zuber J (eds.), Infrared Imaging – A casebook in clinical medicine. IOP Publishing LTD, Bristol, UK, 2015. pp. 1–6. Section 1.5.1, ASIN : B01MXPQ2K4.
8. Image courtesy of Robert Schwartz, MD. Used with permission.
9. Source: Diakides NA & Bronzino J (eds.), Medical Infrared Imaging. CRC Press, Boca Raton, FL, 2008. Chapter 18, Table 18.3. Used with permission conveyed through Copyright Clearance Center, Inc.
10. Dummer GWA, et al. (eds.), Medical Electronic Laboratory Equipment 1967–68. Pergamon Press, 1967. p. 530. ASIN : B01DSRU326.
11. Chamberlain DP, et al., Anesthesiology 1986; PMID: 3740502.
12. Shapley RM, et al., J. Physiol. 1973; PMCID: PMC1350218.
13. Because deep violet is hard to distinguish from deep blue or black, it is often omitted from this display spectrum.
14. The adjustment techniques shown in the full-span and fixed-span illustrations are derived from screenshots of SmartView thermal imaging software from Fluke Corporation, Everett, WA, USA.
15. Quesada P, et al., Application of Infrared Thermography in Sports Science, Springer, 2017, p. 71. ISBN-13: 978-3319474090.

16. Schaefer G, et al., Conf Proc IEEE Eng Med Biol Soc. 2006; PMID: 17946430.
17. Images courtesy of Med-Hot Thermal Imaging, Lakeland, FL, Used with permission.
18. Cooke WH, et al., J Appl Physiol. 1985; PMID: 21940851.
19. Ludwig N, et al., Infrared Phys Technol. 2014; Doi: 10.1016/j.infrared.2016.12.009
20. Thermographically, "acral area" refers to the fingers, toes, nose, and ears.
21. P A Bacon, Agents Actions Suppl. 1980; PMID: 6787856.
22. Sturgeon D, et al., (2019). Thermographic Imaging in Diabetic Patients with Critical Limb Ischemia Undergoing Endovascular Revascularisation. ScholArena (www.scholarena.com). J Angiology and Circulatory System, 1(1):1–8.
23. Vardasca R, et al., Thermol Int. 2012; 22:53–60.
24. Uematsu S, J Neurosurg. 1985; PMID: 2985769.
25. Campbell JS. Fact or Fiction? Exploring Two Beliefs about Oral-Systemic Thermology. Presented at the American Academy of Thermology Annual Meeting, Atlanta GA, USA, September 2019.
26. Nowakowski AZ, Conf Proc IEEE Eng Med Biol Soc. 2004; PMID: 17271896. See also: Nowakowski AZ, Brain 2006; Doi: 10.21611/qirt.2006.101. See also: Sanchis-Sánchez E et al., AJR Am J Roentgenol. 2014; PMID: 25247955.
27. Ramya Devi R, et al., J Med Syst. 2019; PMID: 31011830.
28. Keramidas ME, et al., Clin Physiol Funct Imaging. 2013; PMID: 23701282.
29. Herry CL, et al., Conf Proc IEEE Eng Med Biol Soc. 2006; PMID: 17946429.
30. Macianskyte D, et al., Dentomaxillofac Radiol. 2019; PMCID: PMC6592584.
31. See: Vardasca R, Quantitative InfraRed Thermography (QIRT) conference 2014; Doi: 10.21611/qirt.2014.089
32. Duarte A, Carrão L, et al., Procedia Technology 2014; Doi: 10.1016/j.protcy.2014.10.178
33. Barcelos EZ, et al., Sensors (Basel). 2014; PMCID: PMC4279571.
34. Ammer K, Thermol Int. 2008; 18:125–144.

8

THERMOGRAPHY REPORT GENERATION

The preceding chapter focused on image formatting and an approach to thermographic interpretation. It is critically important that such interpretation is done by a well-trained and experienced practitioner who has the following skills:

- Understanding of the applications, physics, and physiology of thermal imaging
- Hands-on skills in performing complete, high-quality infrared imaging studies
- Proficiency in thermographic pattern recognition, analysis, and interpretation
- Maintaining data integrity, standards of care, professionalism, and ethics

The technical aspects of capturing, processing, and formatting of infrared images should be performed by individuals that have the proper training. Such technical training should be provided by experienced practitioners of thermography. This book is written to be a guide; it is not intended to be a substitute for actual hands-on clinical thermography training. What follows are the technical aspects of human thermal imaging reporting based on seven years of thermography practice as guided by the American Academy of Thermology.

Once the thermography technician has qualitatively formatted and added pertinent quantitative temperature measurements to an infrared image, interpretation, and reporting are the next steps.

Thermographic data can be viewed, organized, and modified through a computer screen interface. In addition to modifying images, the thermographer can comment on each image in a special field defined during template creation. These comments briefly describe key features of the image; the comments can be stored for subsequent reports. Text "boilerplate" entries for thermography reporting are useful for facilitating rapid report generation. If frequently used phrases are stored as text, they can easily be displayed by artificial intelligence (AI) for the thermographer to choose. After this step, the images are exported into a linked word-processing file where the final report will be written before the thermographer's sign-off.

The final thermography report is the product expected by the patient and their referring practitioner. A high-quality report will demonstrate the scientifically valid information that human thermography can provide. For this reason, all elements of the report must be carefully considered, and the final document should be timely, clear, informative, and comprehensive without being overly technical.

Generation of the examination report

The simplest thermographic report is a short clinical note of the findings along with any pertinent images inserted in the patient's digital or hard-copy chart. Such a simple report assumes that the provider has taken the thermal images using a proper thermographic protocol in their facility where the subject is a patient. This "quick and easy" report keeping is similar to a clinic that incorporates X-ray capabilities. Many general medical facilities using ultrasound imaging also record their patient's imaging report in a similar manner.

When the subject for a thermographic exam is referred to the clinic by another practitioner, or when the patient is being referred to another center, a formal thermographic report needs to be generated. Moreover, without a formal report, third-party reimbursement for thermal imaging may be denied. If breast thermography or other critical thermal imaging is performed, the patient should always be provided the images in a universal format for later thermal pattern comparison. People move, clinics close, and records may be lost. Thermal images may not be available for comparison in the future if the patient does not keep a copy in his or her possession.

Formal professional thermography reports are similar to other medical imaging reports. They should adhere to a format that contains several key sections. As DICOM-compatible thermal images become standard, these formats will be defined in the image metadata. The imaging report should include one or more pertinent infrared images. At this time, however, many medical practitioners have little understanding of human thermology and may only wish to receive a clear and concise text report. Also, as many medical offices still rely on grayscale FAX technology to receive imaging reports, a full-color image will not reproduce well. For these reasons, the first page or two of a complete thermography report should consist of concise text. Any color images not to be included in the FAX are best placed on subsequent pages.

Certain practitioners may wish to see the complete report as a digital file, not a printed hard copy or FAX message. This reporting method will increase in the near future because thermal images do not convert well to office-printed images and are better viewed on a full-color flat-screen display. Standard Portable Document Format (PDF) files provide a reliable transmission method for text and color images.

The information contained in a report should provide guidance for taking appropriate follow-up action. Because thermography often detects medical issues at an incipient stage, much of the information provided can lead to strategies for prevention. The report may include recommendations for further testing as well as suggestions for disease management or therapeutic interventions.

For a complete thermography report, the following elements are considered essential:[1]

1. **Name, address, and contact information of the thermography center**. It is important to identify where the images were taken and analyzed. The center's logo and motto may also be included for branding and professional purposes.
2. **Report title identifying the type of thermographic exam performed**. Examples of suitable titles include Breast Thermography Report, Neuromuscular Thermography Study, Full-Body Thermography Report, Hand Thermography Study, and Regional Pain Study.
3. **Date and time of the thermal exam**. Time may be a relevant factor when circadian-hormonal issues are taken into account. Although published studies on this topic are lacking, attending to the time of day may help optimize the practice of breast thermography.

DOI: 10.1201/9781003281764-9

4. **Patient identification and demographics**. At a minimum, this should include the patient's name and date of birth. Other demographics may include the patient's clinic number, address, or contact information. Social security numbers and other financially sensitive information should be omitted.
5. **Conditions under which the examination was performed, including patient preparation, equilibration, and clothing**. Standard thermographic room details include the following: (1) equilibration temperature; (2) patient positions during cool-down and imaging; (3) type of imager used and its infrared bandwidth; (4) any procedures performed during imaging; and (5) how the images were post-processed and reported. Any problems during the imaging session should be stated. To simplify this section, standards for common examination procedures should be written. This section can then reference these standards, saving considerable writing and report space. Having these standards freely available on the clinic's website may increase patient awareness of the thermography procedure.
6. **Indications for performing the examination and pertinent patient history**. Any patient symptoms, diagnoses, problems, or referrals should appear here. Examples include: (1) initial thermographic breast screening; (2) chronic post-traumatic pain; and (3) patient referred for a full-body thermal health screen. A brief summary of the patient's significant medical history should be presented. Details related to pertinent tests, surgeries, treatments, trauma, lifestyle habits, prescription and non-prescription drug use, alcohol use, caffeine ingestion, and other health-related factors should be documented.
7. **Thermographic findings.** Pertinent visible or measured features in the images should be listed here, including both abnormal and pertinent normal findings. When a prominent feature on the images points strongly to a known disease or problem, such impressions are to be listed in Sections 8 or 9. The thermographic findings are sometimes entered by the technician during initial image formatting and report preparation. Technician-entered findings should always be reviewed by the interpreting thermographer.
8. **Thermographic impressions using the qualitative and quantitative findings**. Here the interpreting thermographer draws conclusions and lists the possible physiologic or pathologic conditions that might cause these findings, i.e., a differential diagnosis. A firm knowledge of differential thermography is imperative to complete this section. Are the thermal findings due to infection, trauma, carcinoma, or other pathology? It is not up to the thermographer to say at this point. Thermography provides only differential possibilities, not firm diagnoses. For breast exams, the "TH" status of each breast should be stated here. Thermographic impressions should only be reported by a fully trained and certified thermographer.
9. **Clinical impressions and planning**. This may be omitted in cases where the thermographic impressions are normal. In reporting abnormalities, it is best to avoid diagnostic terms. Instead, use the term "abnormal" in referring to the thermal characteristics. An actual diagnosis cannot be made on thermal imaging alone. Further diagnostic examination, tests, or imaging are necessary. These indicated tests are ordered directly or the patient's provider is advised to order them in the Thermography Report. Follow-up scheduling for repeat thermography should be included in this section, or it can be placed in the thermographic impressions section.
10. **Disclaimer and general advice.** Information on the use and limitations of thermography appears here. Thermography should never be presented as a stand-alone diagnostic or prognostic modality. Various thermography centers have approached disclaimers differently, with many including a whole page of small-print disclaimers, while others rely on a sentence or two, possibly referring patients to read about the limits of thermography on a clinic web page. A disclaimer statement is often issued at the end of a report.
11. **Professional signature.** Providing either a manual or digital signature on the completed thermography report is essential. This may be the signature of the qualified thermographer or the licensed medical provider completing the clinical impression section. The initials or sign-off mark of the technician completing the thermographic findings section may be included in the report. Some centers also require the date the report was signed, thus documenting the time between imaging and report completion.
12. **Images and annotations.** Images used for the findings and interpretations sections, along with image labels and any annotations, are placed here. This section may run for several pages and should start on a separate page from the report text sections listed above to facilitate printing only the text portion of the report. Images from the patient's present thermography examination as well as previous images from earlier exams may be included. To prevent confusion, images from previous exams should be labeled with the imaging date or time indicating when they were taken. In deference to patient privacy, it is preferable to omit simultaneous visual photographs with the infrared images unless they are necessary for clinical interpretation.
13. **Supporting data (optional)**. Some thermographic examinations require gathering of temperature data over time and then mathematically or graphically comparing the results before and after challenge protocols or other interventions. The observed changes are often not detectable by the naked eye, thus quantitative temperature data from multiple sites must be extracted from serial images and analyzed after the procedure is over. This analysis is often performed via custom-designed spreadsheet programs. Copies of these spreadsheets or graphs may be placed in the supporting data section. Other items that may be placed in this section include reports and images from other providers including surgical, pathological, radiological, and other pertinent sources.

Types of reports

Breast thermography exams

Since breast exams are anatomically limited in scope and the basic views defined, breast thermograms are well-suited for a standard reporting format as shown in Figure 8.1. A minimum of four infrared views are required. Some centers also include an anterior face view to document that the subject is properly cooled and has no fever. A facial image also provides identification of the images in the event of a possible chart mix-up. Interpretation and reporting of a thermographic breast exam may take up to 30 minutes to complete, depending on the secretarial help and software application available to the thermographer.[2]

Full-body thermographic exams

These reports, in marked contrast with breast exams, are lengthy and can be confusing to the reader. It may take thirty or more individual images to adequately perform an examination of the entire body (see Figure 8.2). Almost no adult has a perfectly

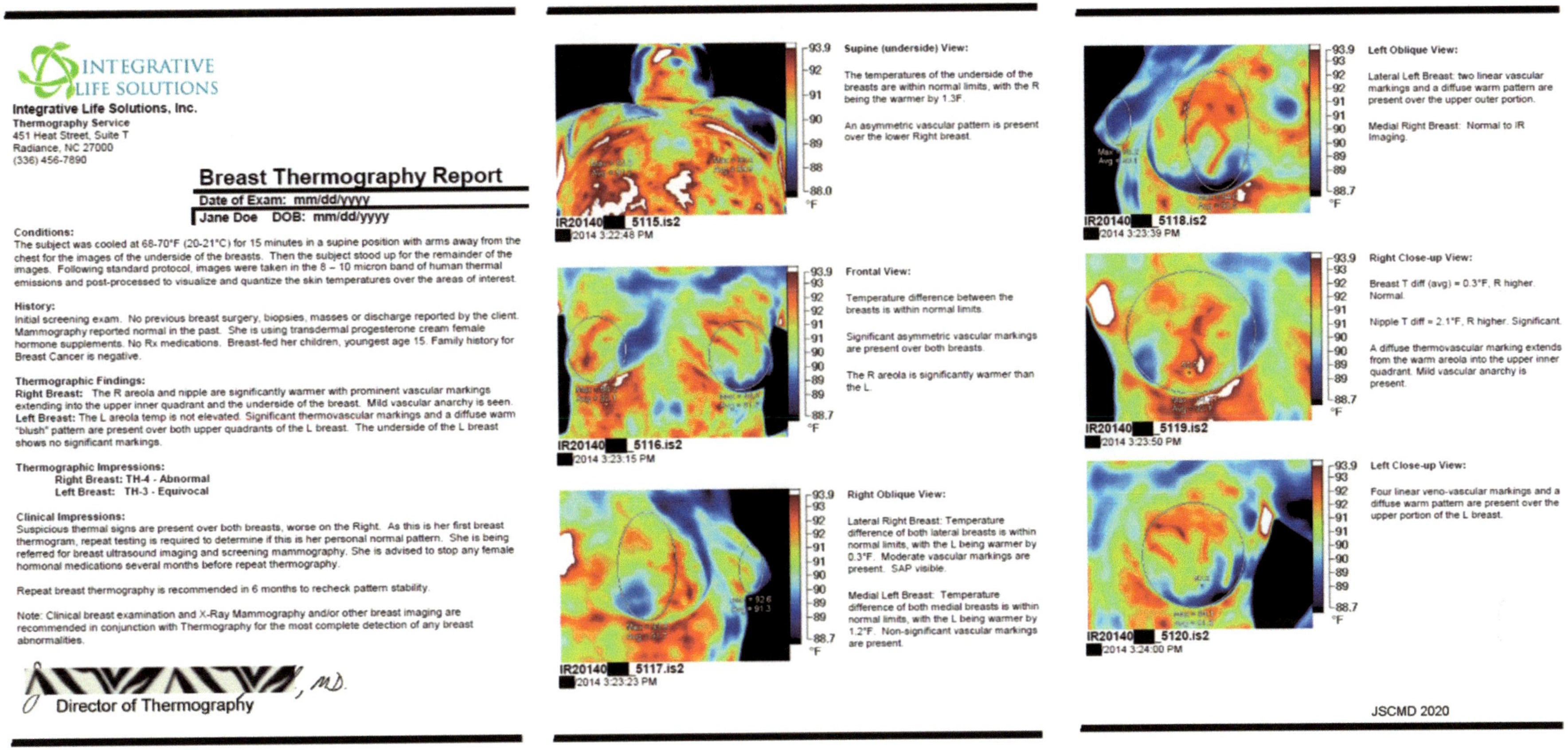

INTEGRATIVE LIFE SOLUTIONS

Integrative Life Solutions, Inc.
Thermography Service
451 Heat Street, Suite T
Radiance, NC 27000
(336) 456-7890

Breast Thermography Report

Date of Exam: mm/dd/yyyy
Jane Doe DOB: mm/dd/yyyy

Conditions:
The subject was cooled at 68-70°F (20-21°C) for 15 minutes in a supine position with arms away from the chest for the images of the underside of the breasts. Then the subject stood up for the remainder of the images. Following standard protocol, images were taken in the 8 – 10 micron band of human thermal emissions and post-processed to visualize and quantize the skin temperatures over the areas of interest.

History:
Initial screening exam. No previous breast surgery, biopsies, masses or discharge reported by the client. Mammography reported normal in the past. She is using transdermal progesterone cream female hormone supplements. No Rx medications. Breast-fed her children, youngest age 15. Family history for Breast Cancer is negative.

Thermographic Findings:
Right Breast: The R areola and nipple are significantly warmer with prominent vascular markings extending into the upper inner quadrant and the underside of the breast. Mild vascular anarchy is seen.
Left Breast: The L areola temp is not elevated. Significant thermovascular markings and a diffuse warm "blush" pattern are present over both upper quadrants of the L breast. The underside of the L breast shows no significant markings.

Thermographic Impressions:
Right Breast: TH-4 - Abnormal
Left Breast: TH-3 - Equivocal

Clinical Impressions:
Suspicious thermal signs are present over both breasts, worse on the Right. As this is her first breast thermogram, repeat testing is required to determine if this is her personal normal pattern. She is being referred for breast ultrasound imaging and screening mammography. She is advised to stop any female hormonal medications several months before repeat thermography.

Repeat breast thermography is recommended in 6 months to recheck pattern stability.

Note: Clinical breast examination and X-Ray Mammography and/or other breast imaging are recommended in conjunction with Thermography for the most complete detection of any breast abnormalities.

[redacted], MD.
Director of Thermography

Supine (underside) View:
The temperatures of the underside of the breasts are within normal limits, with the R being the warmer by 1.3F.
An asymmetric vascular pattern is present over the lower Right breast.

Frontal View:
Temperature difference between the breasts is within normal limits.
Significant asymmetric vascular markings are present over both breasts.
The R areola is significantly warmer than the L.

Right Oblique View:
Lateral Right Breast: Temperature difference of both lateral breasts is within normal limits, with the L being warmer by 0.3°F. Moderate vascular markings are present. SAP visible.
Medial Left Breast: Temperature difference of both medial breasts is within normal limits, with the L being warmer by 1.2°F. Non-significant vascular markings are present.

Left Oblique View:
Lateral Left Breast: two linear vascular markings and a diffuse warm pattern are present over the upper outer portion.
Medial Right Breast: Normal to IR Imaging.

Right Close-up View:
Breast T diff (avg) = 0.3°F, R higher. Normal.
Nipple T diff = 2.1°F, R higher. Significant.
A diffuse thermovascular marking extends from the warm areola into the upper inner quadrant. Mild vascular anarchy is present.

Left Close-up View:
Four linear veno-vascular markings and a diffuse warm pattern are present over the upper portion of the L breast.

JSCMD 2020

FIGURE 8.1 Sample of a breast thermography report. The first page contains only text and may be sent via FAX or printed and sent to the referring clinic. Full-color annotated images are included on the remaining pages. The patient should be provided a PDF or other color digital copy of the entire report for their medical files.

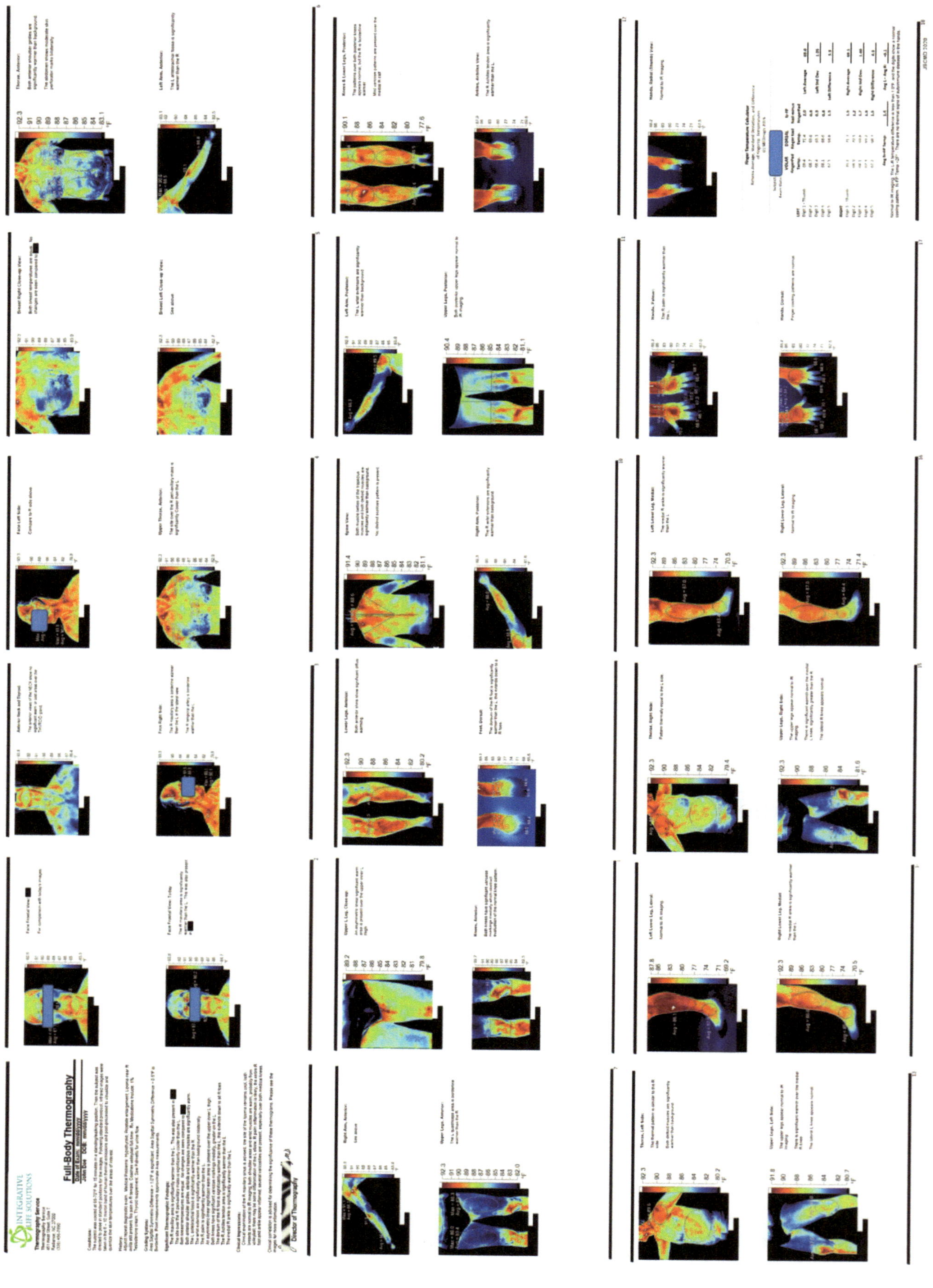

FIGURE 8.2 Example of a full-body thermography report. These reports may require 12 pages or more to complete.

normal full-body thermogram, and some subjects have many significant findings. Each abnormality may need to be described in the report unless the findings can be "bundled" into a common thermographic appearance. It is up to the individual thermographer to choose a specific approach, and the choice itself will vary depending on the subject being imaged. Even with a complex report, the text portion can usually be completed in two pages. Interpretation and reporting of a complicated full-body exam may take up to 60 minutes or more to complete. Exams with fewer significant findings may take less time, but a good qualitative evaluation of each separate image, along with comparative symmetrical analysis of the quantitative data, must never be rushed. It is often useful to insert notes describing the pertinent findings in each image before copying these notes into the thermographic findings section.

Limited regional examinations

These types of examinations are generally reported following the format for breast thermography. Studies of the face, temporomandibular joints, thyroid gland, genitals, and extremities all fall under the category of limited regional thermography. Although the report for a limited exam may be short and include relatively few thermographic images, it should include all the pertinent information required to write an adequate report (see Figure 8.3). Limited exams may need to be performed under emergency circumstances, such as thermography for testicular torsion. In these cases, thermographic conditions may not be ideal, yet they should be reported by the thermographic technician to inform the interpreting thermographer.

Thermography with challenge testing

Unlike static thermographic studies, dynamic studies must show the effects of a thermal or other challenges *over time*. The use of so-called Challenge Testing makes the internal time clock in the imaging system critically important when it comes to reporting the test results in proper sequence. If the imager does not record the time automatically on the image metafile, it is important for the thermographic technician to record all image times manually, a task fraught with potential errors. A Challenge Testing series usually begins by taking pertinent images of the region(s) of interest after the subject has equilibrated to the proper temperature for the exam. An image showing the start of the thermal challenge is strongly advised to document the type and timing of the challenge. Images of the subject are then taken at predetermined time intervals to determine the effects of the challenge.

As the effects of the challenge may not be easily observed by qualitative image recordings, careful quantitative analysis of the affected body areas must be performed. The development of a custom spreadsheet that computes the pertinent pre- and post-challenge temperatures is useful for documenting changes not readily visible. Such dependence on quantitative evaluation over time requires a stable and fully calibrated thermal imager. Thermographic reports that encompass Challenge Testing should include a statement of proper imager calibration as well as a spreadsheet copy or synopsis of the temperature changes before and after the challenge (see Figure 8.4).

Quality control to assure accurate reports

Even the most conscientious thermographic technician or thermographer may make seemingly minor mistakes that can lead to significant flaws in thermographic reporting. The most common error is a report based on images from the wrong subject. Another common error is the loss or misplacement of a patient's exam record, usually by filing it under another patient's name or deleting it by mistake. Other sources of error, such as inadequate thermal equilibration, preparation errors, and problems regarding imager calibration, have been covered in previous chapters. This section will provide advice on reducing common reporting errors using some simple techniques and protocols.

In order to keep the patient's information up to date, each client for thermal imaging should fill out a "Current Information Sheet" at every thermography session (see Figure 8.5). Different information sheets can be used depending on the thermographic study to be performed. Information sheets should be kept as brief as possible and limited to pertinent history and demographics only. It should not take over 15 minutes for the patient to complete the form. The thermographic technician should review the intake form, adding or clarifying any information and signing off on the form. As the imaging session begins, the clock time *on the imager* should be entered on the form. This step is very important should the images be misplaced later. The information sheet should be saved in the patient's individual folder at each visit.

For even stronger quality assurance, the thermography technician may keep a written list of the patient's name, the time the images were taken, and the starting and ending sequence image file numbers for each client. This will ensure the correct assignment of the thermograms to the individual clients. This list may be saved in a daily client log folder at the end of each clinic day. If it is a paper document, it should be scanned and stored for later reference in case a problem occurs.

Proper file storage, handling, and archiving are vital to a medical thermography service. The majority of filing errors occur during "handoff" of files among the thermographic technicians, the interpreting thermographers, the secretarial staff, and mail or email services. Protocols outlining these handoff procedures should be written and followed diligently by all who handle these files. Files and reports must be correctly stored for follow-up and comparison. Files must be treated as confidential by all parties to protect client privacy as required by medical privacy regulations such as HIPAA.[3] Robust password or lock-and-key protection of all data is essential. Encrypted backups at regular intervals on password-protected media are advised. Backup copies should be securely stored off-site. Clients of a thermography clinic may return for repeat scans over many years, thus all patient data should be stored in individual folders that are easily accessible and searchable. Even after a thermography clinic or center ceases operation, many jurisdictions require medical record storage for a number of years. To meet these requirements, the storage, protection, and availability of thermographic records are of utmost importance.

Post-imaging follow-up procedures

After the thermography exam, the images undergo digital post-processing, interpretation, report generation, and archiving. The images, thermographic results, and interpretation may be delivered, mailed, or emailed to the patient within a specified period. The ordering physician is sent the text portion of the report. If the patient desires, the report is sent to their chosen healthcare provider as well. It is advisable to view the images on a full-color computer monitor. Paper prints of the images will generally not be as satisfactory as a thermal image presented on a good-quality computer display.

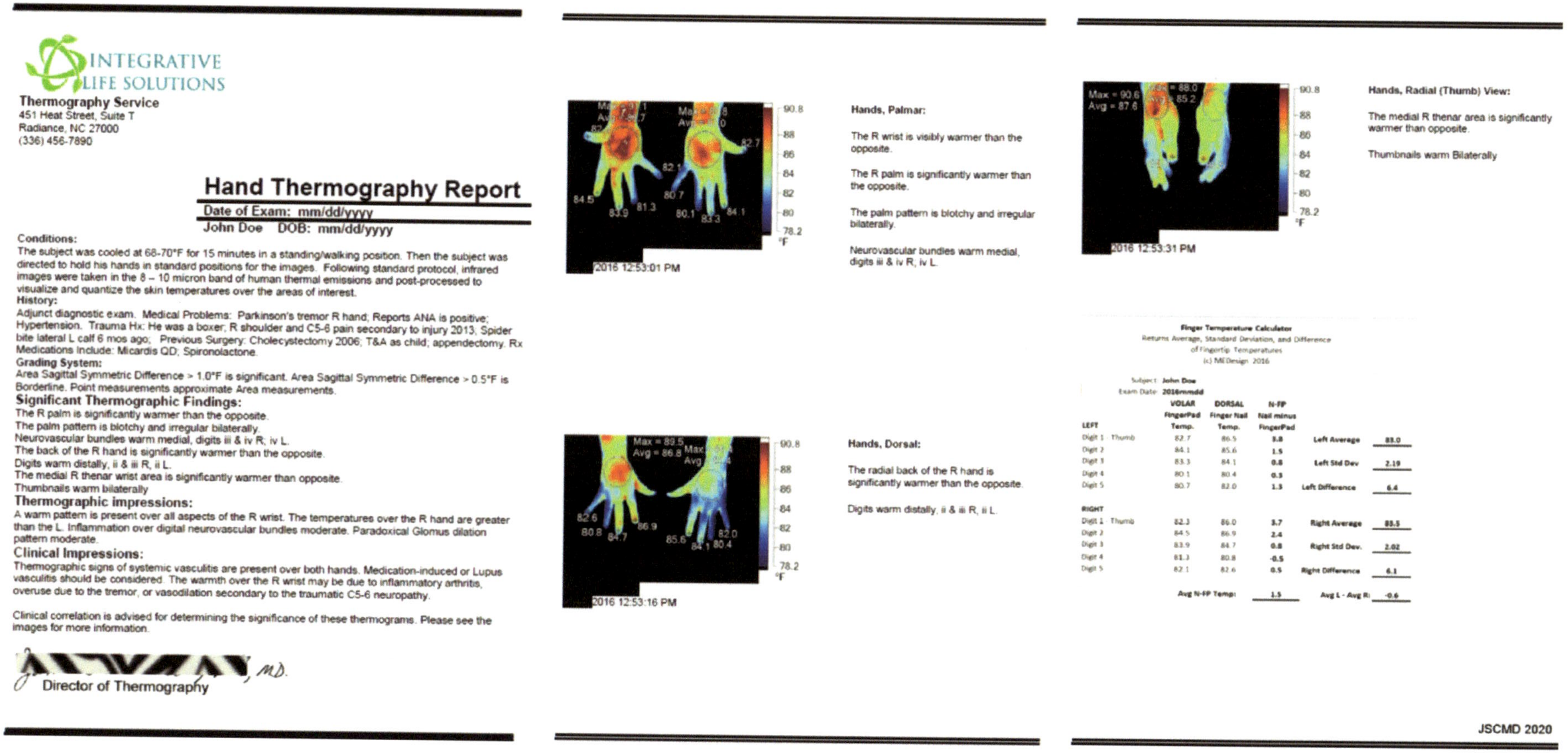

INTEGRATIVE LIFE SOLUTIONS

Thermography Service
451 Heat Street, Suite T
Radiance, NC 27000
(336) 456-7890

Hand Thermography Report

Date of Exam: mm/dd/yyyy

John Doe DOB: mm/dd/yyyy

Conditions:
The subject was cooled at 68-70°F for 15 minutes in a standing/walking position. Then the subject was directed to hold his hands in standard positions for the images. Following standard protocol, infrared images were taken in the 8 – 10 micron band of human thermal emissions and post-processed to visualize and quantize the skin temperatures over the areas of interest.

History:
Adjunct diagnostic exam. Medical Problems: Parkinson's tremor R hand; Reports ANA is positive; Hypertension. Trauma Hx: He was a boxer; R shoulder and C5-6 pain secondary to injury 2013; Spider bite lateral L calf 6 mos ago; Previous Surgery: Cholecystectomy 2006; T&A as child; appendectomy. Rx Medications Include: Micardis QD; Spironolactone.

Grading System:
Area Sagittal Symmetric Difference > 1.0°F is significant. Area Sagittal Symmetric Difference > 0.5°F is Borderline. Point measurements approximate Area measurements.

Significant Thermographic Findings:
The R palm is significantly warmer than the opposite.
The palm pattern is blotchy and irregular bilaterally.
Neurovascular bundles warm medial, digits iii & iv R; iv L.
The back of the R hand is significantly warmer than the opposite.
Digits warm distally, ii & iii R, ii L.
The medial R thenar wrist area is significantly warmer than opposite.
Thumbnails warm bilaterally

Thermographic impressions:
A warm pattern is present over all aspects of the R wrist. The temperatures over the R hand are greater than the L. Inflammation over digital neurovascular bundles moderate. Paradoxical Glomus dilation pattern moderate.

Clinical Impressions:
Thermographic signs of systemic vasculitis are present over both hands. Medication-induced or Lupus vasculitis should be considered. The warmth over the R wrist may be due to inflammatory arthritis, overuse due to the tremor, or vasodilation secondary to the traumatic C5-6 neuropathy.

Clinical correlation is advised for determining the significance of these thermograms. Please see the images for more information.

[redacted], MD.
Director of Thermography

2016 12:53:01 PM

Hands, Palmar:

The R wrist is visibly warmer than the opposite.

The R palm is significantly warmer than the opposite.

The palm pattern is blotchy and irregular bilaterally.

Neurovascular bundles warm medial, digits iii & iv R, iv L.

2016 12:53:16 PM

Hands, Dorsal:

The radial back of the R hand is significantly warmer than the opposite.

Digits warm distally, ii & iii R, ii L.

2016 12:53:31 PM

Hands, Radial (Thumb) View:

The medial R thenar area is significantly warmer than opposite.

Thumbnails warm Bilaterally

Finger Temperature Calculator
Returns Average, Standard Deviation, and Difference of Fingertip Temperatures
(c) MEDesign 2016

Subject: John Doe
Exam Date: 2016mmdd

	VOLAR FingerPad Temp.	DORSAL Finger Nail Temp.	N-FP Nail minus FingerPad		
LEFT					
Digit 1 - Thumb	82.7	86.5	3.8	Left Average	83.0
Digit 2	84.1	85.6	1.5		
Digit 3	83.3	84.1	0.8	Left Std Dev	2.19
Digit 4	80.1	80.4	0.3		
Digit 5	80.7	82.0	1.3	Left Difference	6.4
RIGHT					
Digit 1 - Thumb	82.3	86.0	3.7	Right Average	83.5
Digit 2	84.5	86.9	2.4		
Digit 3	83.9	84.7	0.8	Right Std Dev.	2.02
Digit 4	81.3	80.8	-0.5		
Digit 5	82.1	82.6	0.5	Right Difference	6.1
		Avg N-FP Temp:	1.5	Avg L - Avg R:	-0.6

JSCMD 2020

FIGURE 8.3 A report of a limited regional examination. Here the hands are fully evaluated, including an optional spreadsheet analysis of the fingertip temperatures. Only three thermal images are required for this study.

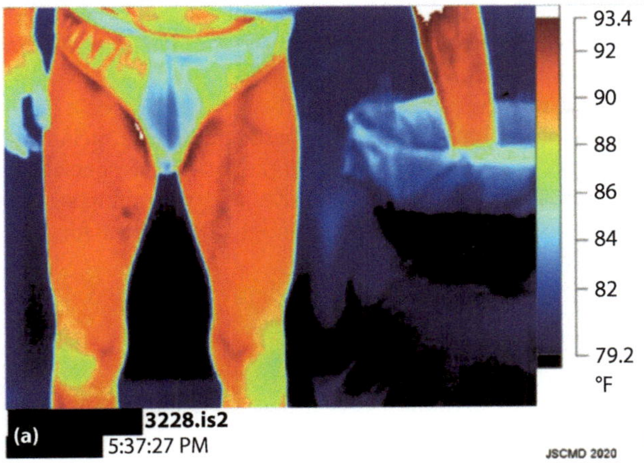

(b)

SITE	Before Cooling Left	Before Cooling Right	T-diff L minus R	Start Cooling Left	Start Cooling Right	T-diff L minus R	Post Cooling A Left	Post Cooling A Right	T-diff L minus R
Thigh Anterior	93.4	94.0	(0.6)	90.9	90.7	0.2	90.9	90.4	0.5
Thigh Posterior	91.9	91.1	0.8	91.9	91.0	0.9	91.3	90.4	0.9
Thigh Lateral	91.8	92.0	(0.2)						
Thigh Medial	92.3	93.4	(1.1)						
Knee Anterior	87.1	87.6	(0.5)				87.1	86.8	0.3
Knee Posterior	92.4	91.0	1.4	92.0	90.7	1.3	91.7	90.3	1.4
Knee Lateral									
Knee Medial									
Calf Anterior	92.1	92.7	(0.6)	90.9	91.5	(0.6)	91.2	91.5	(0.3)
Calf Posterior	89.8	89.4	0.4	91.0	90.3	0.7	90.5	90.0	0.5
Calf Lateral	91.6	92.1	(0.5)						
Calf Medial	91.0	92.1	(1.1)						
Ankle Anterior	90.4	90.8	(0.4)						
Heel Posterior	82.2	81.6	0.6	83.6	84.2	(0.6)	82.2	82.5	(0.3)
Foot Dorsum	91.5	90.7	0.8	89.8	90.1	(0.3)	89.0	89.0	0.0
Great Toe	81.5	77.0	4.5	79.7	76.4	3.3	79.5	76.1	3.4
M-P Joint Great Toe	85.3	82.7	2.6				82.4	81.3	1.1
Third Toe	77.5	77.5	0.0	76.6	77.5	(0.9)	76.2	77.0	(0.8)

FIGURE 8.4 (a) Image documenting the time of cold challenge initiation to evaluate CRPS of the right leg. (b) A portion of a spreadsheet designed to compute differential temperatures before and after the challenge.

The results sent to the patient should include the following:

- A full explanation of any problem areas and recommended follow-up or referrals. This text section of the report may be printed on a monochrome printer as a summary report.
- All full-color digital images should be provided for review and archiving.
- A printed receipt should be included with the proper medical diagnosis (ICD code) and the CPT procedure codes for insurance reimbursement.
- A written order for the thermogram from the referring medical practitioner may facilitate insurance reimbursement. As third-party payers have different policies about thermography, patients should contact their carrier for instructions.

Medical Infromation:
Show any breast problems or procedures on this diagram. Use the code letters below as a guide. Write or draw in any other important medical information. If this is a repeat exam, be sure to show any **new** changes.

Close Relative with breast cancer? [No] [Yes]
Breastfed any children? [No] [Yes]
Using *any* female hormones? [No] [Yes]
Last Menstrual Period: ____________________

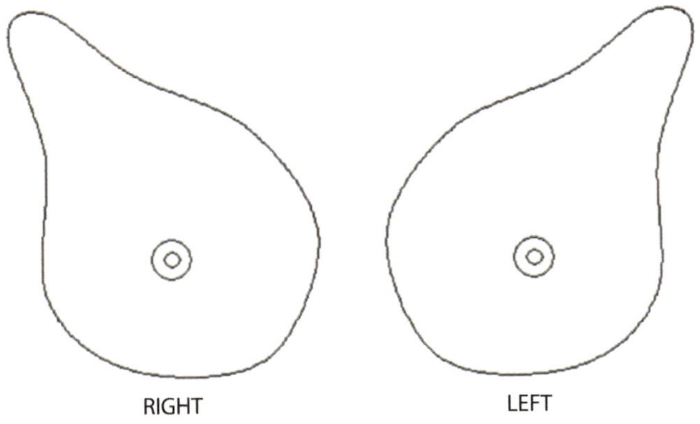

A - Abcess (state "old" or "active")
B - Bruising (fresh or fading)
C - Known sites of breast cancer
D - Dermatitis (rash or other skin changes)
G - Skin Graphics (tattoos)
I - Breast Implant(s)
L - Laceration (cuts or non-surgical scars)
M - Mass or lump (benign or unknown)

N - Nipple changes or discharge
P - Painful area(s)
Q - Piercings
R - Radiation Therapy Areas on breasts
S - Surgery sites (Lumpectomy, biopsy, etc.)
T - Blunt Trauma sites on breasts
U - Suspicious areas on Ultrasound or Mammography
X - Mastectomy (complete breast removal)

ICD: ____________________
CPT:

Tcam =
Tstd = ____________
Tcor = °F

Time of scan:	Thermographer	Interpreter

Client, please sign here: ______________________________

JSCMD 2020

FIGURE 8.5 A partial current information sheet for breast thermography. The patient demographics and general history sections are not shown here. Entries at the time of the exam may include providers' initials, ICD/CPT reimbursement information, and imager offset data (Tcor).

The results sent to a healthcare provider include:

- If digitally transmitted, a full-color file that includes the summary report and annotated infrared images.
- If FAXed, include the text-only summary report, explaining any concerns, problems, and recommendations.
- The thermographer may also send the provider all the patient's full-color digital files should it be requested.
- A printout of the text pages from the most recent exam report can be provided as a summary report if the receiving office uses paper medical files.

All the patient's files should be archived on the backup servers for future reference and comparison. Protected backups are also to be kept off-site for data preservation. Whether "Cloud Storage" is used for file backup depends on the reliability and confidentiality of the cloud service.

The patient may be given an appointment to repeat the thermographic scans, with the time interval decided as appropriate for the condition being followed. If any problems are noted on the patient's exam, the thermographer may recommend to the scheduling staff and in the summary report that the next thermogram should be obtained sooner than that for a normal exam. Repeat appointment reminders via phone call, email, or postal carrier will increase patient re-examination compliance.

Personal consultation with the thermographer-clinician may be arranged. This may be important if the patient has special concerns, or has thermograms from other thermographic services for comparison. An additional fee might be applied for these consultations.

Notes

1. The basics elements of thermographic report formatting may be found under the guidelines of the American Academy of Thermology (AAT). *See* https://aathermology.org/organization-2/guidelines/
2. This reporting time required is based on the author's experience (jscmd). Reporting time for breast exams is not stated in Guideline 6: Exam Time Considerations at https://aathermology.org/organization-2/guidelines/guidelines-for-breast-thermology/
3. HIPAA – The United States Health Insurance Portability and Accountability Act of 1996 as amended.

9

BREAST THERMOGRAPHY

Breast cancer (BrCA) is the most prevalent cancer among women living in developed countries and the most common cause of cancer death for women worldwide.[1] For over 100 years, early detection has been the goal of BrCA screening, and various imaging techniques have been developed to help find tumors before they enlarge. The main modalities today are digital X-Ray mammography, ultrasound scans, magnetic resonance imaging (MRI), and thermography. X-Ray mammography is the dominant screening tool, while ultrasound and MRI are used mainly for confirmatory purposes.[2]

Despite claims that mammography screening has achieved a 30% reduction in BrCA mortality, the best designed studies indicate smaller gains.[3] Screening mammography may be no better at reducing death from BrCA than clinical breast examination.[4] Improvements in the treatment of BrCA, not screening mammography, account for the major share of reductions in BrCA mortality in Europe and North America.[5]

The improved resolution of microbolometer-based infrared imagers provides a powerful adjunct to screening mammography. Breast thermography can now image thermal changes associated with NO vasodilation, lymphatic inflammation, and venous proliferation.[6] Abnormalities in this thermal information help detect BrCA. See Figure 9.1.

Breast thermography reveals abnormal conditions that may indicate not only cancer or precancerous growths but also other problems such as cysts, local infections, soft-tissue inflammation, or recent trauma. These areas emit different heat patterns over the affected regions of the breast. Abnormal patterns can be followed over time without radiation risk or physical distortion of the breasts.[7] If thermal instability or asymmetrical patterns arise, ultrasound, mammography, and MRI can be used to characterize a mass and to determine whether further procedures are warranted.

Since the advent of microbolometer-based thermal imagers, thermography has reemerged as a valuable clinical tool for BrCA prevention and management. This chapter will introduce the basic applications of breast thermography, address comparisons between thermography and other imaging procedures, and provide practical guidance for effective infrared imaging of the breast.

Potential roles of breast thermography

Breast thermography has been used to detect, assess the risk of developing, and determine the prognosis of BrCA. Infrared thermal imaging of women with dense breasts is an especially important since mammography performs poorly when evaluating dense breasts. Mammography is also not advised for younger women because of ionizing breast radiation, which potentially increases tumor development.[8] As themography involves no ionizing radiation or mechanical trauma, it may be used at any age. Infrared imaging can monitor patients with *in situ* breast lesions and patients who have undergone breast conservation therapy (lumpectomy).

Early breast cancer detection

Cancer screening aims to detect cancer before symptoms appear, when the disease is easiest to treat. *Sensitivity* is a quantitative measure that reflects the ability of a test to identify all people who have a disease or condition. It is the most critical factor for predicting the impact of screening on BrCA mortality. A screening tool with high sensitivity means that very few women with BrCA will go undetected. As long as the sensitivity remains high, *specificity* can be more modest, particularly if the test is to be used as a preliminary screen for identifying persons requiring further investigation or diagnostic planning.

Since 2000, clinical studies of breast thermography have demonstrated a sensitivity consistently exceeding 95%.[9] This sensitivity is also seen in women with very dense breasts.[10] A study of 1008 females (ages 20–60) with no previous diagnosis of BrCA, showed a thermographic sensitivity of approximately 98%, specificity of 99%, a positive predictive value of 84%, and a negative predictive value of 100%.[11]

With mammography, tumors are frequently missed because of dense breast tissue, which basically has an X-ray masking effect. Approximately 50% of all women have dense breasts.[12] Thus, many breast tumors are invisible to mammography until the tumor becomes sufficiently large to be detectable. This limitation also applies to digital breast tomosynthesis, the newer "3D" screening mammography tool.[13]

Breast density has direct biological relevance. The percent of mammographic density (PMD) is a well-established risk factor for BrCA; the risk increases proportionally with increasing PMD.[14] In addition, tumors associated with denser breasts tend to have a poorer prognosis.[15] Unfortunately, dense breasts are far more prevalent among younger women, a group that should not be screened with mammography.[16]

Fortunately, the sensitivity and specificity of thermography are unaffected by breast density. To the contrary, the specificity of thermography is statistically *improved* in dense breast tissue compared to fatty breast tissue.[17] Performed alternately with biennial mammography, thermography may detect the small, faster-growing tumors that are hidden from mammography.

SIDEBAR 9.1 WHO CAN BENEFIT MOST FROM SCREENING THERMOGRAPHY?

Specific subgroups of women for whom annual breast thermograms may be particularly helpful include the following:

- Younger women with established risk factors (e.g., BRCA mutations, obesity, frequent exposure to thoracic radiation at an early age).
- Postmenopausal women considered to be at very low risk.
- Women with dense breasts.
- Older postmenopausal women with a higher breast cancer risk (e.g., multiple first-degree relatives with breast

DOI: 10.1201/9781003281764-10

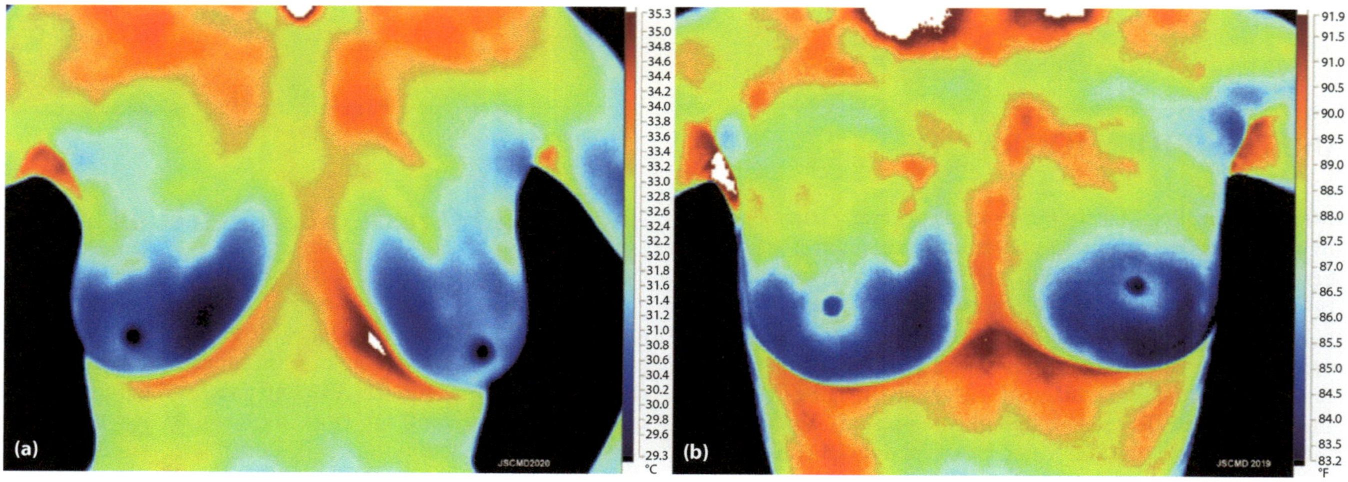

FIGURE 9.1 (a) Normal breasts TH1 bilaterally – 63 yoF. (b) Micro-calcifications found on mammography are present in the upper outer right breast. Thermographic findings of lymphatic markings with NO blush over that area are present, but subtle – 49 yoF.

cancer, family history of early ovarian cancer, and inherited genetic mutations such as BRCA1, BRCA2, and TP53).

- Women in areas where breast mammography may not be available.

Risk-based assessment for guiding prevention

Risk assessment refers to the determination of whether a woman is at low, average, or high risk of developing BrCA during her lifetime. (Note: male breast cancers are extremely rare, and have their own risk factors.[18]) An abnormal thermogram carries a heightened risk of BrCA, and may be considered an *independent* risk factor for BrCA.[19]

Breast thermography can detect BrCA as much as eight years before mammography.[20] The presence of an otherwise unexplainable abnormal infrared pattern of the breasts predicts a ten-fold increased risk of a woman getting BrCA.[21] Mammography and ultrasound are generally unable to detect the minuscule tumors (2–5 mm in diameter) that may show up on an abnormal thermogram. Only an MRI can confirm the presence of such tiny tumors. As thermography can indicate the presence but not the location of an otherwise undetectable tumor, thermography is often "too right too early."

Monitoring disease progression after DCIS

An abnormal thermogram can help identify the early stage of an invasive tumor's development. However, infrared imaging may be less helpful detecting growths that are at the pre-invasive stage, including Ductal Carcinoma in Situ (DCIS), as shown in Figure 9.2. DCIS is a noninvasive precursor neoplasm that, in many cases, will not progress to invasive BrCA. Low-grade DCIS represents an indolent disease in the majority of mammographically detected cases.[22] Based on the best available evidence, about one-third of DCIS cases will become an invasive disease, and most of those cases have a favorable prognosis.[23]

Early DCIS apparently does not generate enough NO to be detectable via thermography. During the epithelial-mesenchymal

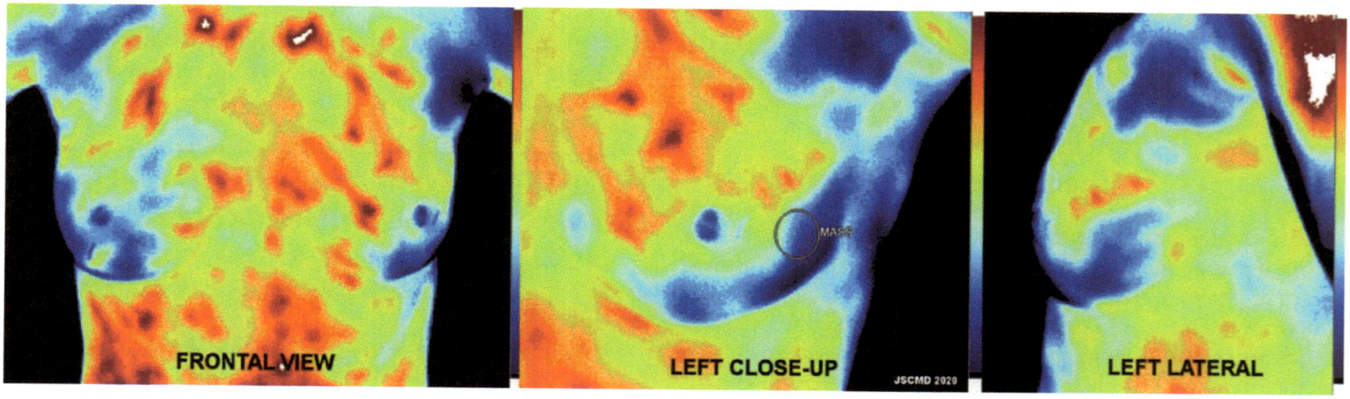

FIGURE 9.2 53-year-old female with an invasive 1.5 cm ductal adenocarcinoma at three o'clock in the outer left breast. The left close-up view shows the location of the palpable tumor. Extensive DCIS accompanied the tumor. The cool area over the mass suggests that NO was not being generated. An asymmetric, indistinct vascular pattern is present over the upper inner breast quadrant. Perineural but not lymphatic tumor invasion was seen in the lumpectomy specimen.

transition from DCIS to invasive carcinoma, however, there is a surge in NO production inside DCIS cells.[24] This surge in NO will result in an increase in overlying skin blood flow, providing the physiologic basis for using thermography as a monitoring tool for detecting malignant change in indolent DCIS.

Due to concerns about overtreatment of DCIS, postponing treatment for low-risk cases has been suggested, especially in older women for whom other competing causes of death pose a more pressing concern.[25] In such cases, surgical treatment would be postponed, and the patient would be monitored by *active surveillance*. Breast thermography can be useful in this surveillance. Because of the ubiquity of mammography and the calcifications associated with DCIS, most cases are initially seen on a mammogram and are less discernible on a thermogram.[26] Once a malignant process begins to unfold, thermography may offer the best possible alert system for the presence of invasive disease.

Assessment of disease potential and prognosis

Thermal imaging offers a window into the invasive behavior of the BrCA. Breast thermography detects the inflammatory processes accompanying tumor angiogenesis, growth, invasion, and metastasis.[27] Active BrCA with a less favorable prognosis generates a stronger thermal signal, indicating more aggressive disease behavior.[28]

Breast thermography can be a prognostic tool for predicting tumor growth and survival in BrCA patients. Node-negative patients with an asymmetric thermal pattern have a significantly increased risk of mortality. The temperature difference between the cancer site and the contralateral control site correlates with cancer-specific mortality.[29] Abnormal thermograms are strongly correlated with the Ki-67 proliferative index and other prognostic indicators; markers for faster-growing tumors that are more likely to recur and/or metastasize.[30] Human epidermal growth factor receptor-2 (HER-2) levels are correlated with the increased local skin temperature seen in BrCA patients. HER-2-overexpressing breast cancers tend to have more aggressive disease potential.[31]

BrCA patients with lymph node metastases have significantly worse disease survival if they have thermographically "hot tumors" compared to "cold tumors."[32] The prognostic ability of an abnormal thermogram may be most consistent for younger patients.[33] Additional research is needed to monitor disease progression in BrCA patients.

Post-operative monitoring for local and regional recurrences

Infrared imaging helps detect early signs of local-regional recurrence following treatment of BrCA (Figure 9.3). During breast-conservation surgery to remove a primary tumor, tiny "rests" of cancer cells may remain after the operation. Recurrences can occur where the cancer was originally (local recurrence) as well as in the lymph nodes (regional recurrence). Thermography may be used to monitor changes in the temperature pattern over the chest area that may presage the return of cancer.

Postoperative radiation may, unfortunately, preclude the use of thermography to detect BrCA recurrence. Following radiotherapy, the irradiated breast becomes hyperthermal; this increased inflammation can continue for 6 months to a year.[34] Therefore, it is recommended that at least 6 months elapse before thermal imaging due to the residual inflammation. Postoperative radiation "burns" should decrease in time, while signs of BrCA recurrence will not. See Figure 9.29 on page 112 for an example of post-radiation hyperthermia of the breast.

Artificial intelligence in thermal BrCA detection

Infrared imaging cannot actually diagnose cancer; it only indicates the presence of an abnormality. Like mammography and ultrasound, thermography is an *adjunctive* diagnostic technique. Only a biopsy or surgical excision can provide a definitive diagnosis. Imaging is used to help identify a possibly malignant mass. Recent advances in artificial intelligence (AI), however, have led to refinements in thermographic pattern analysis. AI requires "teaching" or "transfer learning" by comparing clinical outcomes and tissue pathology to thermographic findings involving thousands of patients.

In 2018, researchers examined various AI methods for BrCA detection and concluded that Support Vector Machines (SVM) offered the greatest diagnostic accuracy. When applied to the various imaging technologies, SVM detected 93% of tumors with digital mammography, 96% using ultrasound, and 100% with thermography.[35] Until large, long-term studies are carried out on DICOM-standardized images, however, widespread acceptance of AI-based thermographic interpretation will be difficult.

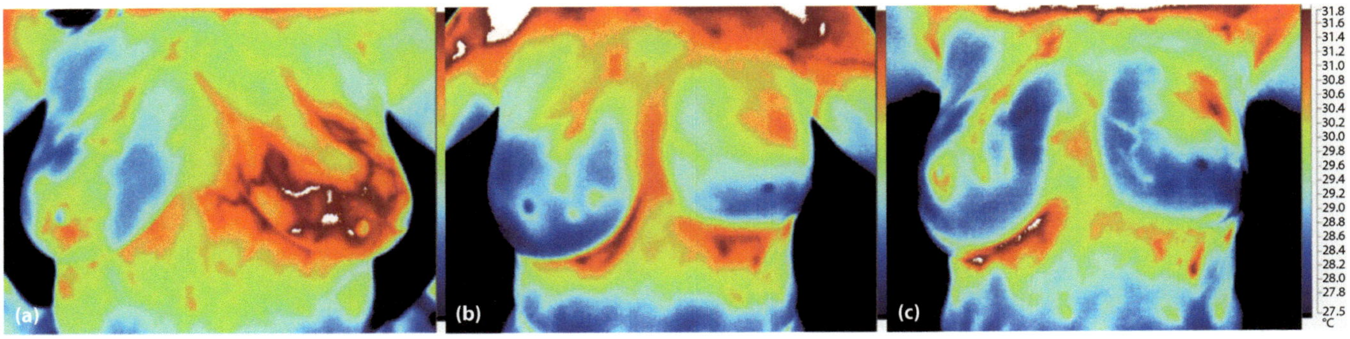

FIGURE 9.3 Pre- and post-op thermograms of carcinoma of the left breast – 66–69 yoF. (a) February 2014: Initial thermogram TH-5 on the left. Previous mammography reported normal. (b) June 2016: S/P left mastectomy with reconstruction done August 2015. Diagnosis: Carcinoma stage 2B, estrogen and progesterone positive. (c) February 2017: Follow-up thermogram shows a localized warm area over the upper outer quadrant, which may be a postoperative ligamentous strain pattern or BrCA recurrence.

SIDEBAR 9.2 THE FALSE POSITIVE CONUNDRUM

An abnormal thermogram may indicate the presence of a small active tumor that is undetectable by mammography or ultrasound imaging. This abnormal thermogram may be classified as a "false positive" when a subsequent diagnostic mammogram is read as normal. However, the mammogram may well be a "false negative." Thermographic efficacy in the detection of BrCA cannot be determined by short-term studies. A long-range follow-up observation period of eight to ten years is needed to determine a true false-positive rate.[36]

Studies have confirmed that thermography is able to detect occult tumors missed by mammography. Thirty percent of breast cancers will likely be missed by mammography without thermography.[37] The disparity in detection rates between mammography and thermography is most pronounced in women with dense breasts.

Bottom Line: An abnormal breast thermogram should always be followed closely despite a negative diagnostic mammogram.

The anatomic and pathologic basis of breast thermography

To interpret a set of properly-scaled breast thermograms, the thermographer compares the temperature and thermal patterns of the two breasts, and evaluates any sagittal asymmetry between them, using the underlying anatomic structures as a guide (Figure 9.4). This involves two steps: qualitative pattern recognition of the heat patterns, and quantitative comparison of the actual temperatures of the breasts.

Thermography can visualize three basic signs of BrCA: (1) venous proliferation, (2) lymphatic inflammation, and (3) skin arteriolar vasodilation from local NO production (Figure 9.5). What follows is a description of the appearance of these three processes. (Note: perineural invasion by malignant cells may also affect breast thermographic appearance, but this has not been adequately studied.[39]) Although the areas of the breast involved and thermal signs generated will vary from case to case, the underlying pathological mechanisms remain the same. By combining these three signs with anatomical considerations, the presence and rough location of the underlying disease may be determined.

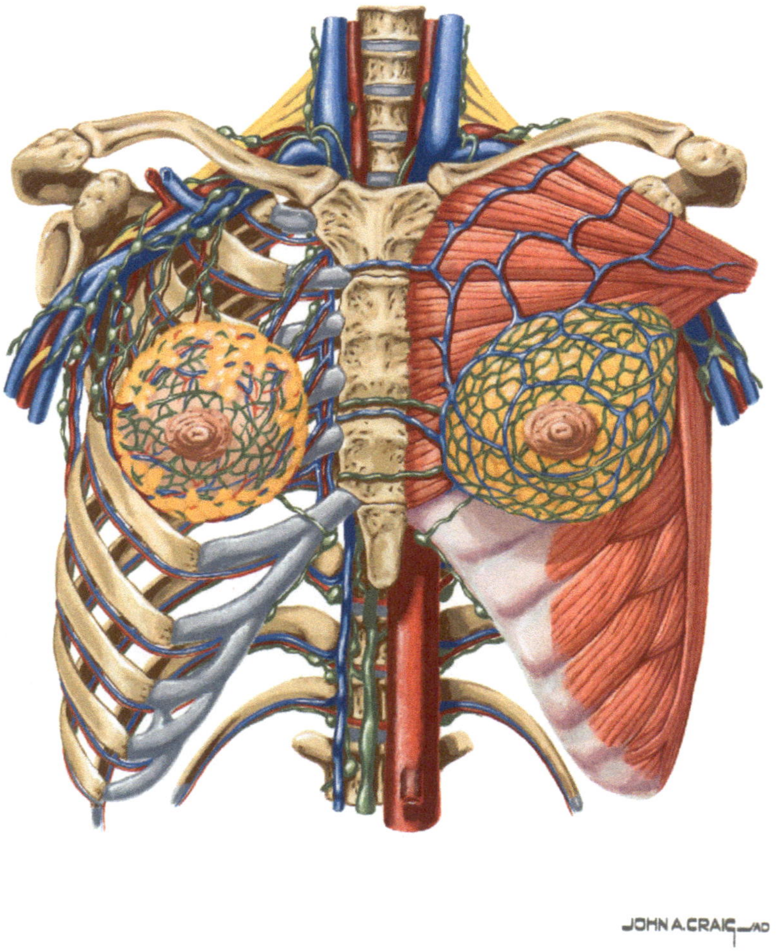

FIGURE 9.4 Frontal view of the female chest wall showing the arterial (red), venous (blue), and lymphatic (green) vessels.[38]

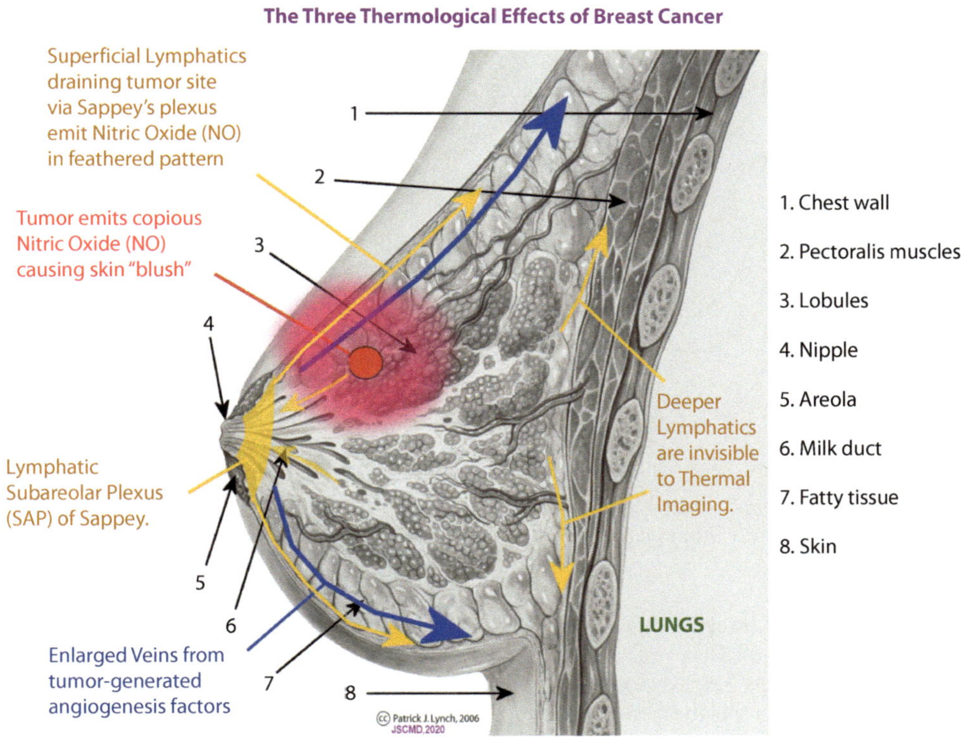

FIGURE 9.5 Sagittal section of the female breast showing the three qualitative thermal signs of breast cancer: Venous proliferation (blue), lymphatic inflammation (yellow), and nitric oxide-induced vasodilation (red).[40]

Lymphatic inflammation

Anatomically, the lymphatic vessels draining the parenchymal mammary lobules and milk ducts flow anteriorly into the subareolar lymphatic plexus of Sappey (SAP). The SAP then drains through the superficial lymphatic plexus of the breast toward the axillary, subclavicular, and parasternal lymph nodes (Figure 9.6). Lymph vessels may also extend from the inferior portion of the breast downward, where they can be visualized crossing the ribs below the breast (Figure 9.7). Lymph vessels may be seen draining the breast without inflammation of the SAP. The lymph vessels of the deeper stromal breast structures (suspensory ligaments and adipose tissue) close to the chest wall may be invisible to thermal imaging as they drain into the deep lymph system of the submammary space.

The nipples of the breast are normally cool bilaterally except in cases of breastfeeding, infection, trauma, or tumor. As a general rule, the differential nipple temperature measurement

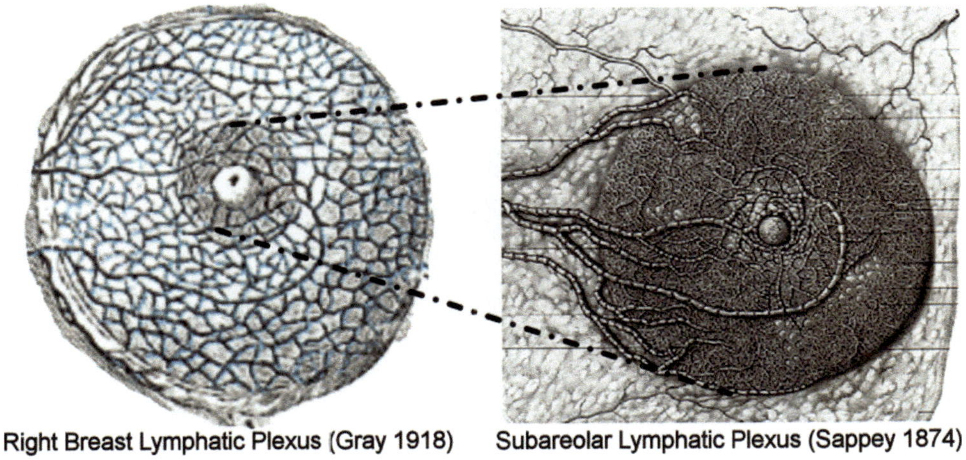

FIGURE 9.6 The superficial lymphatic plexus of the right breast showing the relation to the subareolar lymphatic plexus of Sappey. Most of the lymphatics in the breast lobules drain anteriorly into Sappey's plexus.[41]

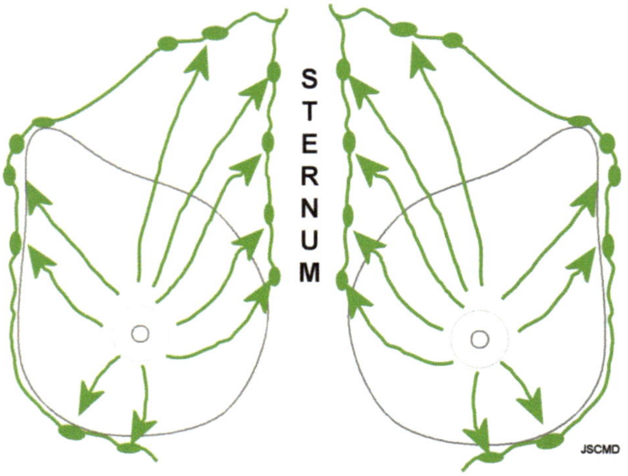

FIGURE 9.7 General flow directions of the superficial lymphatic plexus of the breasts as they drain Sappey's plexus.[42]

should not exceed 1.0°C (1.8°F); however, this quantitative guideline may be less important than qualitative analysis of both the nipple and the areolar appearance.[43] A warm nipple associated with a normal areolar temperature is indicative of a ductal inflammation. In Figure 9.8a, the warm right areola, along with a warm nipple and inflamed draining lymphatics, points toward a ductal neoplasm; the warm areola and cool nipple shown in Figure 9.8b is indicative of a lobular neoplasm without ductal inflammation. Pathologic confirmation of these thermographic findings is needed.

As the superficial lymph drainage system over the breast consists of a fine reticular network of communicating vessels, when inflamed, it takes on a wispy, feather-edged, "cirrus" look and may form small loops or whorls.[44] Thus, lymph vessels often can be visually differentiated from the thermal appearance of veins. When both types of vessels are present, however, it may be difficult to distinguish between the two. The terms "vascular markings" and "vascular anarchy" may be used to refer to a mixed venous and lymphatic thermal appearance.

Venous dilation and proliferation

The superficial veins of the breast extend radially out from a loop centered about the areola called the *circulus venosus*.[45] The veins form irregular circumferential anastomoses as they progress toward the axilla, clavicle, and parasternal areas. Some of these anatomical branches and anastomotic loops can be seen in Figure 9.4. When visible thermograhically, venous loops are generally larger than lymphatic patterns (Figure 9.9). The vein edges also appear straighter and less feathery than lymphatics. A nulliparous woman may show no venous pattern. Breast veins are normally enlarged and complex in the pregnant or breastfeeding woman. These dilated veins decrease in size and number after lactation, but often remain visible to infrared imaging – see Figure 13.11, page 233. This venous pattern normally remains stable and unchanged for many years, though it may decrease after menopause. Varicose veins may form over the breast, but these varicosities are rare.[46] Under the influence of angiogenic substances emitted from certain breast tumors, as well as increased venous blood flow through the area of the tumor, the breast veins may enlarge, proliferate, and become quite complex.

Nitric oxide "blush"

Many, if not most, malignant breast tumors and tumor-associated immune cells emit nitric oxide, or NO, a gas that freely diffuses in all directions through body tissues (with the exception of bone). If a small breast tumor is close enough to the skin surface, the surrounding "cloud" of NO prevents the normal

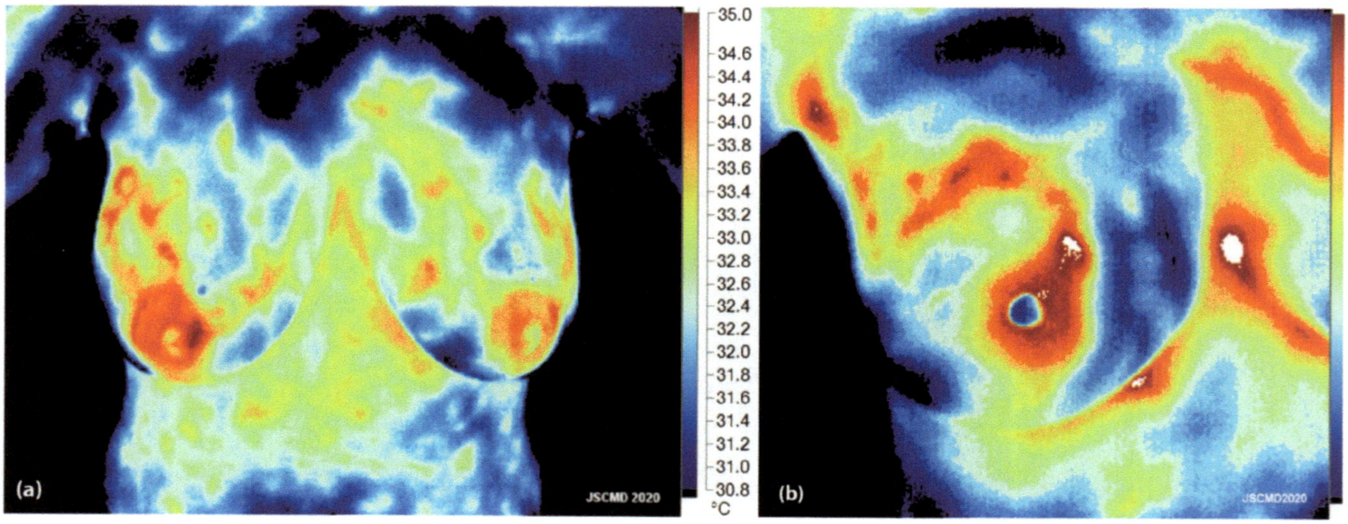

FIGURE 9.8 (a) Both sub-areolar lymphatic plexuses are warm; three superficial lymph drainage patterns are present on the right. The nipples are also warm bilaterally, greater on the right; no history of breast surgery – 47 yoF. (b) 10-year history of a non-tender mass lateral to the right nipple; MRI-guided biopsy diagnosed invasive lobular carcinoma. Note the cool nipple despite the warm subareolar lymphatic plexus – 51 yoF.

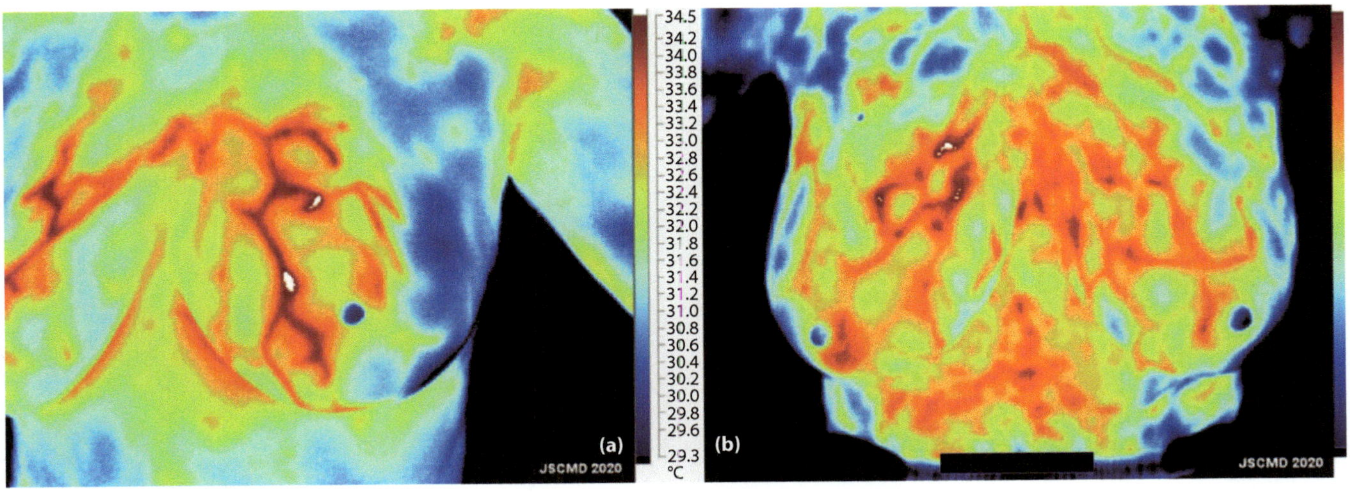

FIGURE 9.9 (a) Venous thermal markings, moderate, over medial left breast – 62 yoF. (b) Venous thermal markings, complex, bilateral. Etiology unknown; mammography normal – 57 yoF. Note also a small mole over the upper right breast.

sympathetically-controlled vasoconstriction from occurring in a cooled subject. Thus, the area over the tumor appears warm because the overlying skin arterioles cannot vasoconstrict (Figure 9.10). Arterial blood continues to flow in these dilated vessels, warming the overlying skin. In some cases, this tumor "blush" is not accompanied by venous or lymphatic signs, and is the only clue to the underlying tumor. Other causes of inflammation, such as infection, injury repair, or autoimmune conditions also emit NO and may appear similar to the thermal pattern of a breast malignancy.

Inflammatory breast cancer

Invasive Inflammatory Breast Cancer (IIBC) is an aggressive BrCA in which malignant cells block and inflame the lymph vessel plexus in the skin of the breast. This type of BrCA is called *inflammatory* because the breast appears red and swollen, and is usually tender to the touch (Figure 9.11). Most inflammatory breast cancers are invasive ductal carcinoma, developed from cells that line the milk ducts of the breast. This type of cancer is rare, accounting for only one to 5% of all invasive breast cancers in the United States. IIBC may also occur in males but tends to strike younger women, especially obese women, women of color, and women with dense breasts. Sometimes mistaken for infectious mastitis, IIBC is a diffuse disease that produces rapid swelling and redness of one-third or more of the involved breast. In untreated cases, the lymphatic edema of the breast may cause a clear drainage, usually from the lower portion of the breast. In most cases, there are no discrete masses or other signs that appear on X-ray mammography, though the inflammation shows up dramatically on breast thermograms. Early detection of IIBC is important because the disease tends to run a rapid course and metastasize quickly, with preferential sites of metastasis including the bones, liver, lungs, brain, chest wall, or distant lymph nodes.[47]

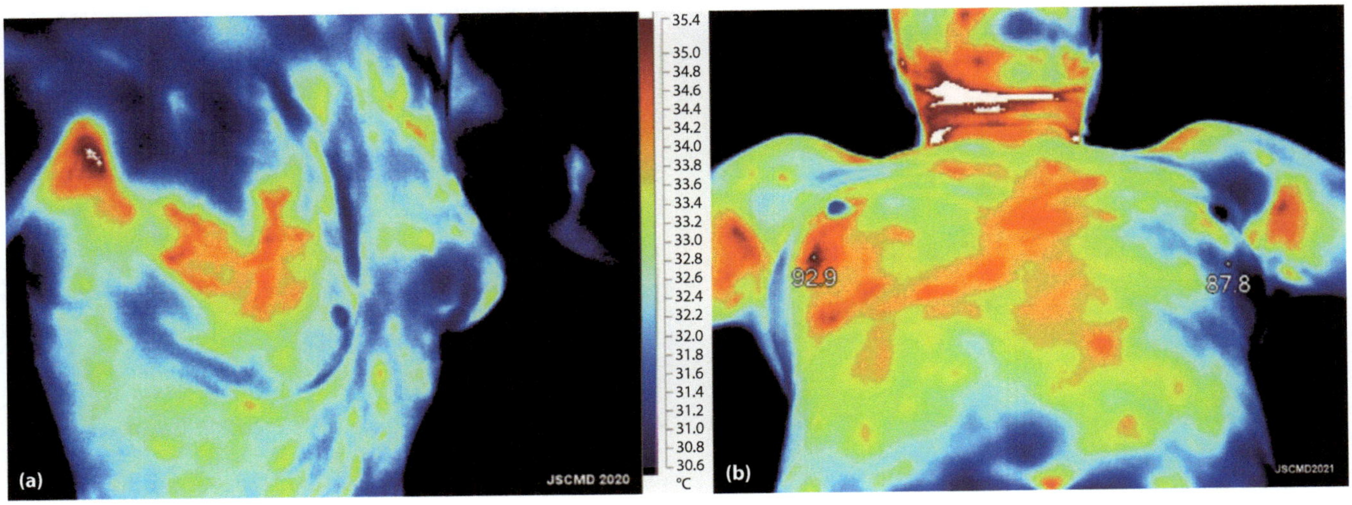

FIGURE 9.10 (a) Nitric oxide "blush" associated with a diffuse lymphatic pattern over the upper outer quadrant of the right breast in a 45 yoF. (b) Nitric oxide "blush" under right breast, 51 yoF.

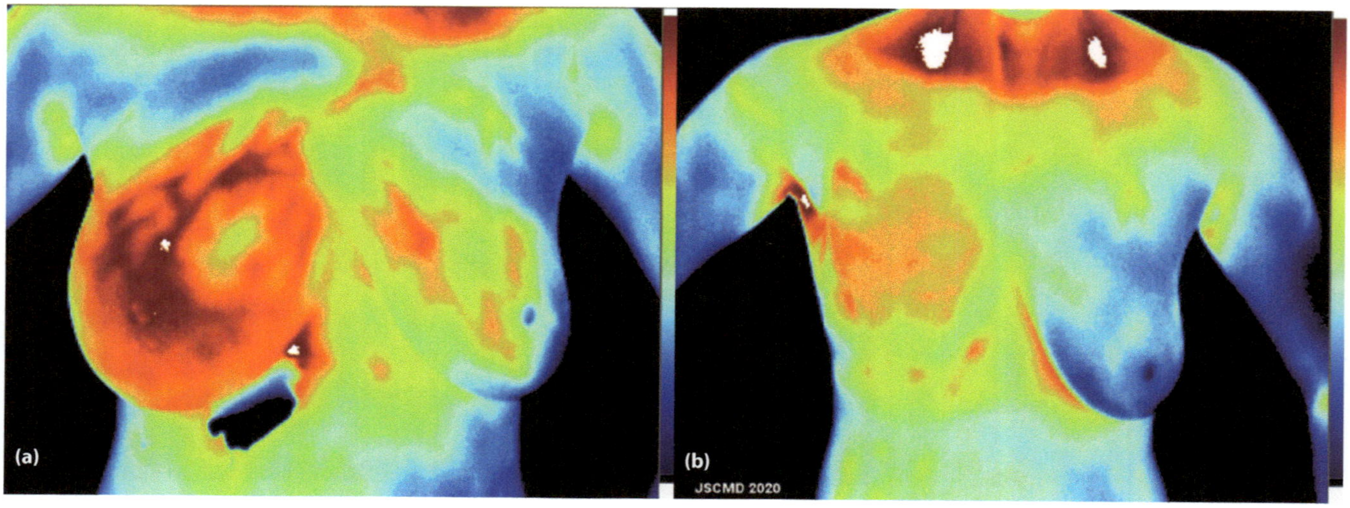

FIGURE 9.11 Advanced inflammatory breast cancer in a 37-year-old female. (a) Preoperative image. Note that the dressing to absorb the lymphatic drainage from the swollen right breast appears cool due to liquid evaporation. (b) Post-mastectomy image.

Breast cysts

Breast cysts are non-metabolizing fluid-filled sacs with thermal insulating properties. Thus, they often appear as a cool oval or round area on thermal imaging (Figure 9.12). Multiple cysts might mask the presence of an underlying tumor; therefore, it is prudent to repeat the thermogram two weeks after aspiration of the cysts. Fresh needle punctures may affect the thermographic image. If the repeat thermogram comes back normal, more confidence can be had in the results. Upon cytological analysis of an aspirated cyst, any indication of cellular abnormality would indicate the need for further investigation.

Interpretation and classification of thermal breast findings

Among the various standards and methods for interpreting breast thermograms, the most concise and established is the Ville-Marie (V-M) Infrared Grading Scale.[48] First reported in 2001, this interpretation scale may be due for an upgrade. The older-generation infrared scanner used for the V-M study had poor spatial and thermal display resolutions (see Figure 1.9 on page 9). With a thermal display resolution of only 0.5°C to 1.0°C, the thermal step size delineating the abnormal signs was assigned a size of 1.0°C. With modern microbolometers having excellent spatial resolution and a 20-fold increase in thermal display resolution, both

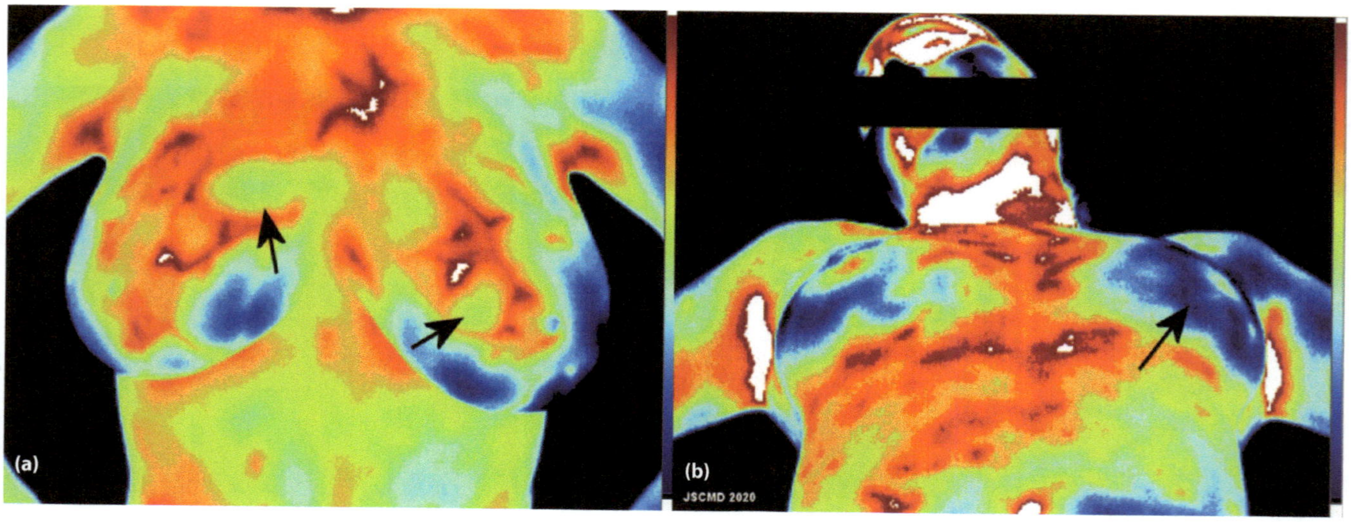

FIGURE 9.12 Thermographic appearance of breast cysts. (a) History of multiple breast cyst aspirations. The cool oval areas (arrows) indicate possible locations of superficial cysts – 56 yoF. (b) Large cyst in lower L breast (arrow) confirmed on ultrasound. The area is cooler than the opposite breast – 39 yoF.

the significant "abnormal" temperatures and the qualitative criteria listed here must be re-evaluated with these improvements in mind. Nevertheless, the V-M Infrared Grading Scale remains a valid method of interpreting breast thermograms with this caveat: Abnormal-appearing qualitative breast images should not be interpreted as normal just because the quantitative temperature differences in the V-M scale are not fully met.[49]

Abnormal signs with the V-M infrared grading Scale*

1. Significant area of vascular asymmetry or visible intermammary temperature difference in a properly scaled gradient color image. Nipples not symmetrically cool.[50]
2. Vascular anarchy, i.e., unusual tortuous or serpiginous vessels that form clusters, loops, abnormal arborization, or other aberrant patterns. This includes unusual venous clusters and lymphatic inflammation patterns.[51]
3. A 1°C (1.8°F) focal increase in temperature (ΔT) when compared to the contralateral site *and* when associated with the area of clinical abnormality, such as a palpable mass or retracted (or warm) nipple.
4. A 2°C (3.6°F) focal ΔT versus the contralateral site, without a clinical abnormality.
5. A 3°C (5.4°F) focal ΔT versus the rest of the ipsilateral breast when not present on the contralateral site.
6. Global breast ΔT of 1.5°C (2.7°F) versus the contralateral breast.

*Unless stable over 3–6 months' time period (minimum) or due to known non-cancer causes (local infection, recent benign surgery, radiation, trauma, bruising, sympathetic imbalance, etc.).

V-M Breast Infrared Grading Scale (Figures 9.13-9.17):

TH-1 = Absence of any vascular pattern to mild vascular symmetry (**Normal**).
TH-2 = Significant but symmetrical vascular pattern to moderate vascular asymmetry, particularly if stable (**Normal Vascular**).
TH-3 = One abnormal sign (**Equivocal**).
TH-4 = Two abnormal signs (**Abnormal**).
TH-5 = Three abnormal signs (**Severely Abnormal**).

V-M thermography conditions

Infrared imaging takes place in a draft-free, thermally controlled room maintained between 20°C and 21°C (68°F and 70°F) after a 15-minute equilibration period during which the subject is disrobed above the waist with hands and arms held away from the sides. Subjects are asked to refrain from alcohol, coffee, smoking, exercise, deodorant, and lotions prior to imaging. Jewelry near the chest is to be removed. Cell phones and microwave devices are not permitted near the client during the cooldown or the exam.[52]

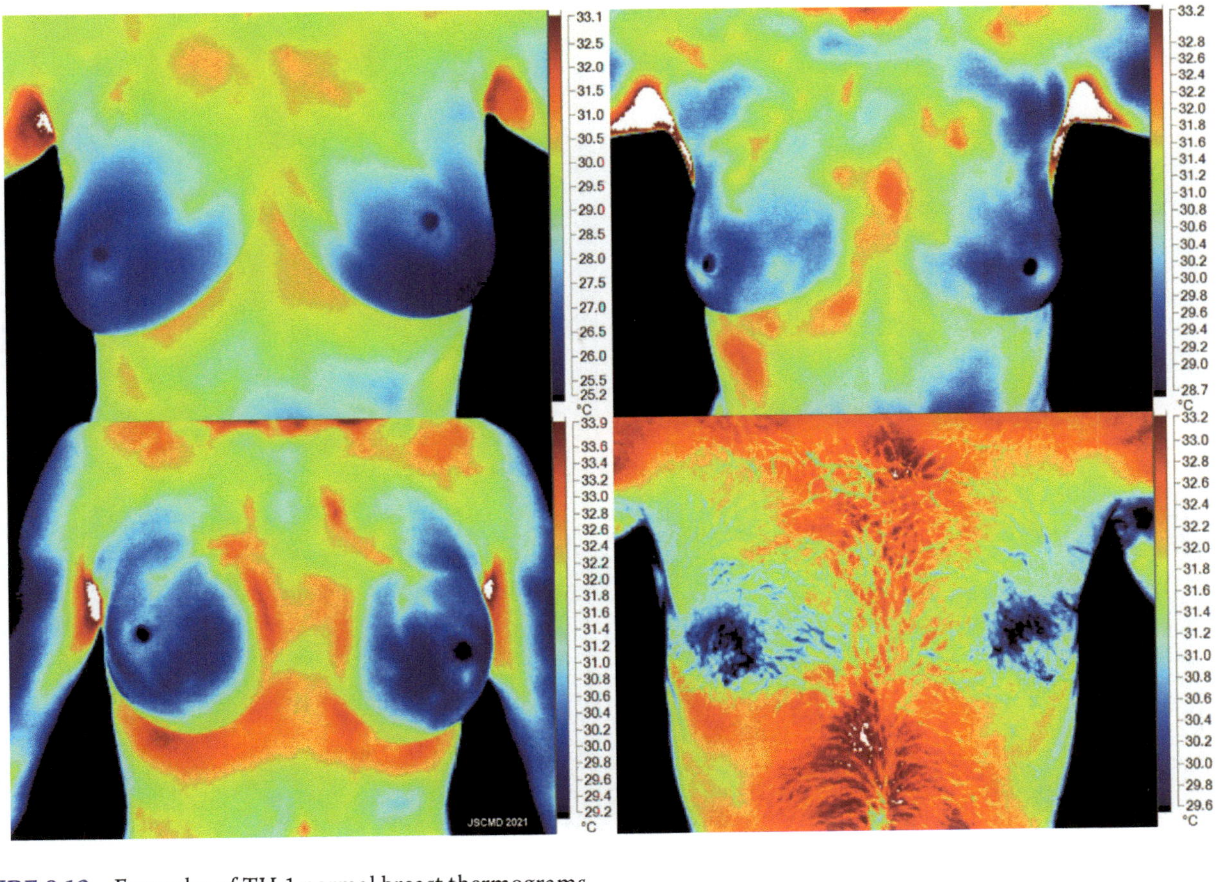

FIGURE 9.13 Examples of TH-1 normal breast thermograms.

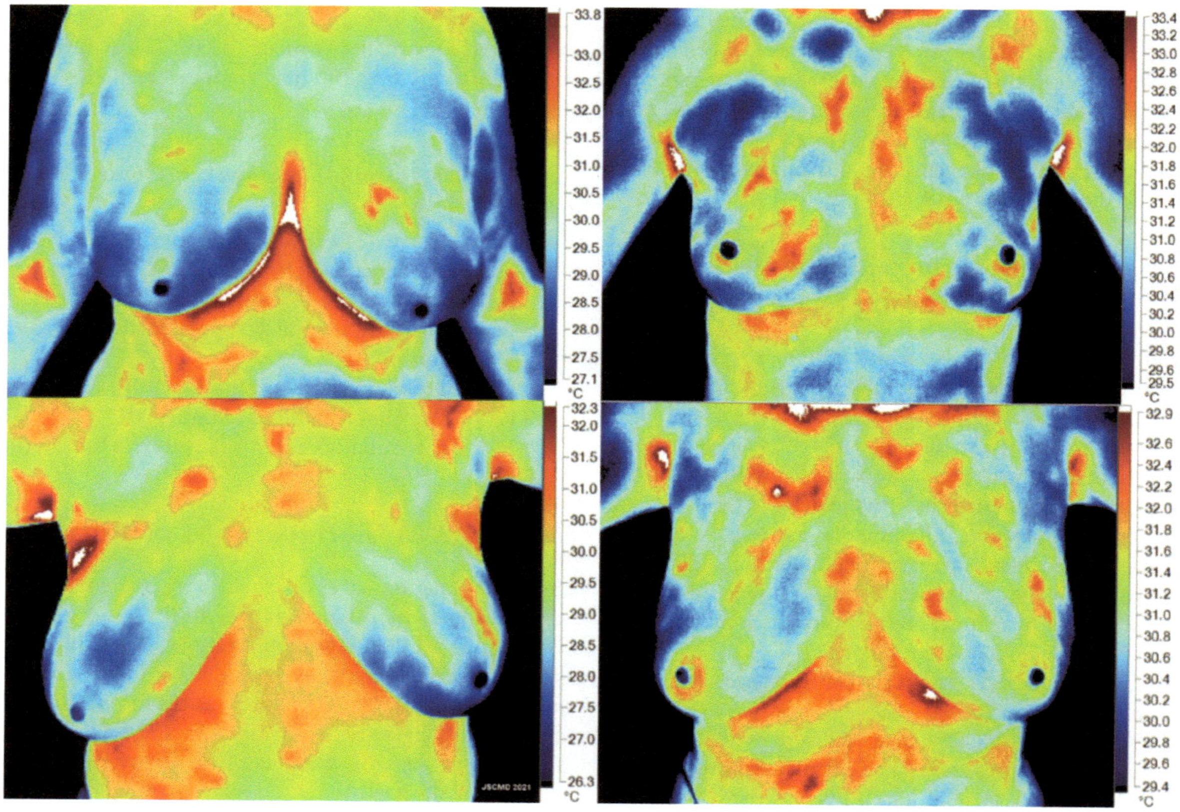

FIGURE 9.14 Examples of TH-2 normal-vascular breast thermograms.

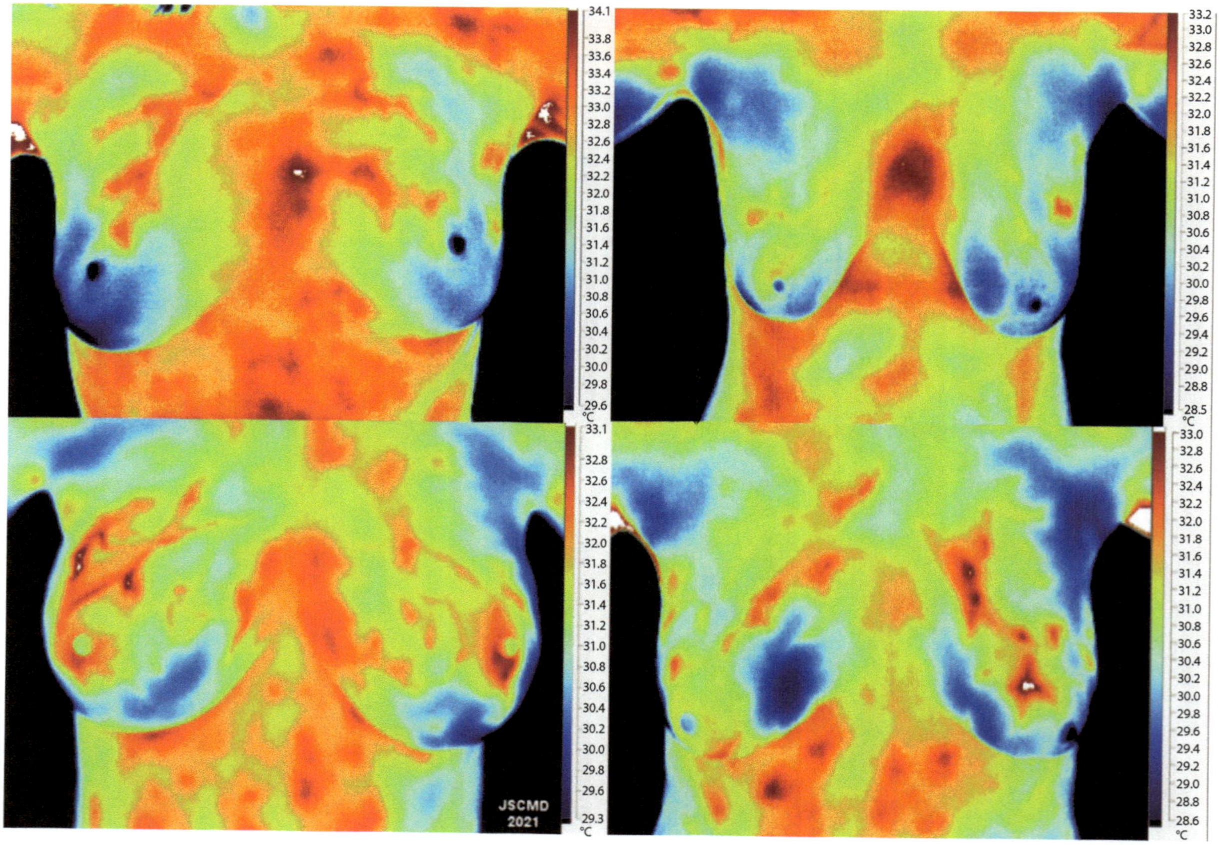

FIGURE 9.15 Examples of TH-3 equivocal thermograms. These patterns must be stable over 6 months, minimum, to be considered normal and re-classified as TH-2 (some centers use the classification TH-3S).

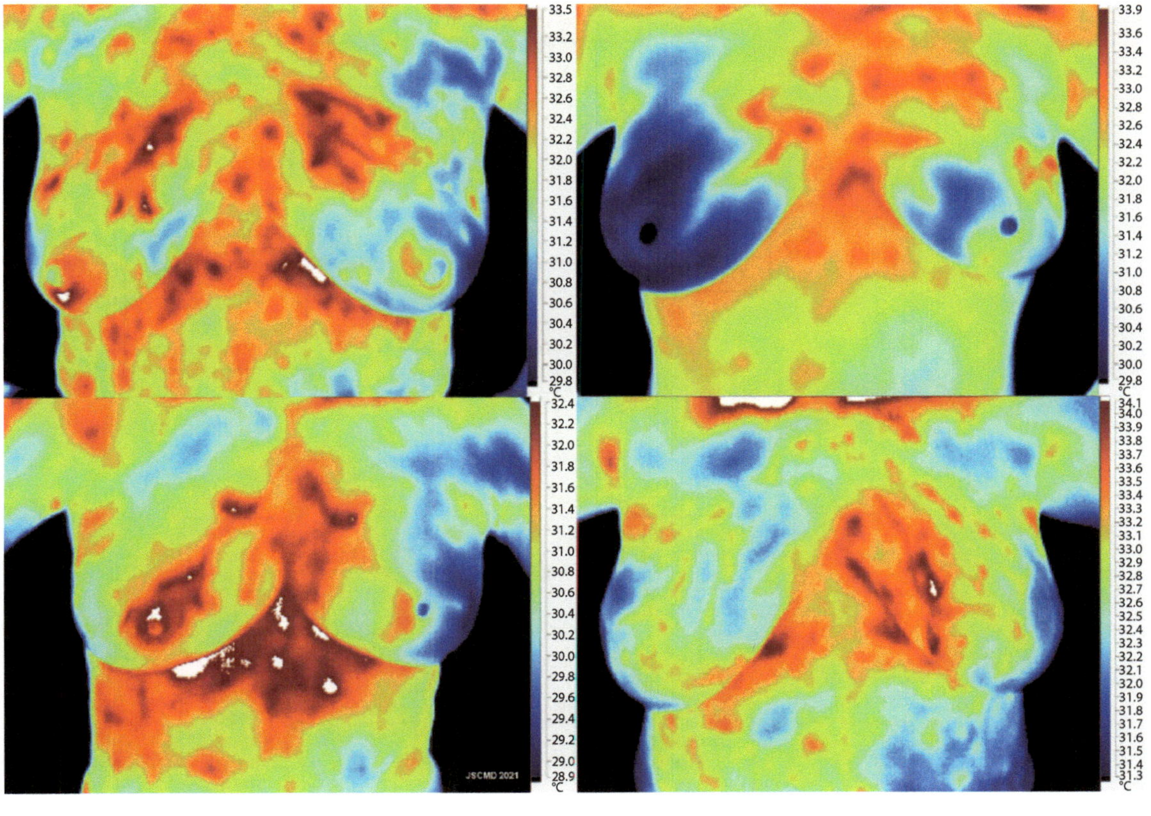

FIGURE 9.16 Examples of TH-4 abnormal thermograms.

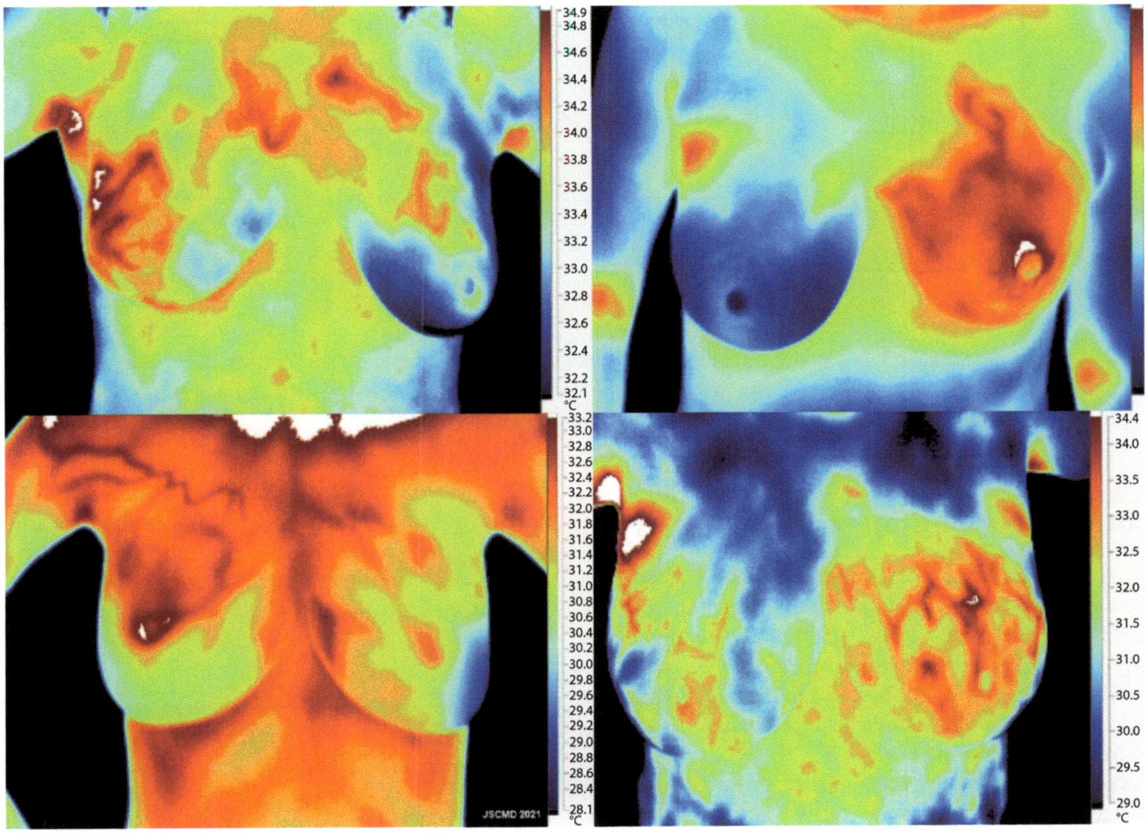

FIGURE 9.17 Examples of TH-5 severely abnormal breast thermograms.

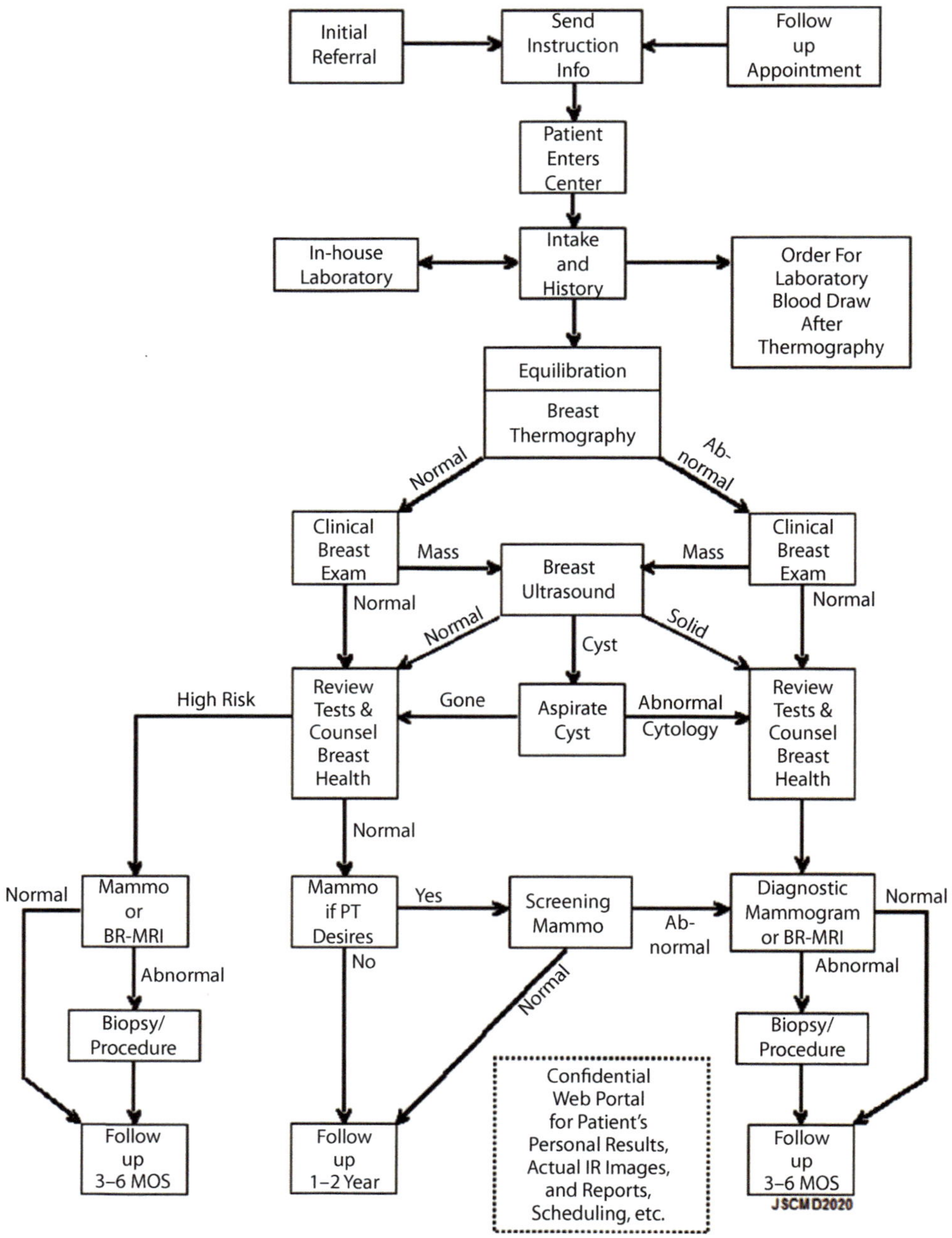

FIGURE 9.18 Basic flow diagram of a proposed breast health center utilizing breast thermography, clinical examination, and breast ultrasound as the primary screening tools. X-ray mammography and/or MRI are added for abnormal cases, high-risk cases, or if the subject requests. Biopsy and other procedures are performed as indicated.

Breast thermography procedure

The properly performed and interpreted breast thermogram makes a powerful adjunct to stand-alone mammography in the detection of BrCA. The thermogram itself must be obtained with a calibrated thermal imager on a properly prepared and vasoconstricted subject under controlled thermal conditions; it should be interpreted as a gradient full-scale color image using the criteria delineated in the V-M Grading Scale.

The process of procuring a thermogram from the individual varies from one thermography facility to another. What follows is a discussion of good practices, most of which have been embraced by the American Academy of Thermology, International Academy of Clinical Thermology, and other reputable organizations. See Figure 9.18 for a flow diagram of a proposed breast health clinic incorporating thermography in the testing protocol.

SIDEBAR 9.3 PRE-BREAST IMAGING INSTRUCTIONS

In order to obtain high-quality thermograms, certain pre-imaging requirements must be met. (See Chapter 6 for more details on pre-thermogram Environment and Protocols.) In this variation, the patient should agree to avoid or abstain from the following activities:

- Hot environments or baths, massage, strenuous exercise, or physical therapy for at least 3 hours prior to the exam
- Consuming hot spicy food or strong caffeine-containing coffee or teas within one hour of the visit
- Gum chewing at the time of the cooldown or exam
- Smoking for at least 2 hours before the infrared imaging exam
- Applying lotions, creams, powders, or makeup on the breasts the day of the exam
- Using underarm deodorants or antiperspirants on the day of the exam
- Shaving the chest, armpit or underarm area on the day of the exam
- Bathing within 1 hour of the exam (this means a short shower; a hot bath is not allowed)
- Physical stimulation or treatment of the breasts, chest, neck, or back for 24 hours prior to the examination, with treatment such as chiropractic, acupuncture, massage, physical therapy, TENS, electrical muscle stimulation, ultrasound, or ice or heat use)
- Prolonged sun exposure or sunbathing (especially if accompanied by sunburn) the day before as well as the day of the exam
- Prolonged use of a cell phone (more than 2 minutes, with the phone held up to the side of the head) within 30 minutes of the exam

Scheduling a breast health exam

The process generally begins with a referral coming either from a health care professional or by self-referral. This is followed by contact between the patient and the clinic staff, either in person, by phone, or using digital means. Upon scheduling a thermography procedure, the patient should be sent or instructed to download an information packet and pre-imaging instructions from the clinic. The instruction packet is important, so the patient understands what to expect regarding the exam process for this first clinic visit. It is also important that the thermography clinic has a warm, welcoming atmosphere and feels like a peaceful, healing environment.

Arrival and labs

The patient is encouraged to arrive 15–20 minutes before the imaging exam to check-in and complete any forms. The patient is invited to use the restroom to provide a urine sample if needed and to empty their bladder before the cooldown period. If blood samples are ordered, they should be drawn *after* imaging to avoid affecting the thermographic results. The patient's ability to tolerate the procedure (e.g., cooling, positioning) and any contraindications to the procedure will need to be assessed at this time, and the imaging protocol adjusted and documented if necessary.

History taking

Collection of a relevant medical history is necessary prior to the performance of the exam. This process should be computerized and made part of the patient's record which can be updated from time to time. The interpreting thermographer should refer to this history to aid qualitative analysis and locate quantitative measurements.

A Patient History centered on breast health might include the following:

- Review of compliance with the thermography pre-imaging instructions
- Menstrual history, i.e., date of the last menstrual period (LMP) or postmenopausal status
- Any breast plastic surgery procedures, including breast implants, lifts, or reductions
- All medications and supplements (especially hormones, niacin, vasodilators, etc.)
- Breast pain, lumps, discoloration, or other symptoms. A breast diagram is useful to describe sites of masses, pain, surgeries, etc.
- Type of breast support garments used, such as an underwire bra
- Breastfeeding history, especially if recent
- Recent chest/breast trauma, bruises, and especially rib fracture
- Any BrCA/DCIS diagnosis with basic details, including stage, grade, hormone receptor status, and location
- Date and result of most recent mammogram, if any, along with details of any previous abnormal mammograms or call-backs
- Date and result of most recent breast ultrasound, if any, and the specific region of the breast studied.
- Date of most recent breast MRI, if any, and main findings
- Any previous breast biopsies: dates, diagnoses, and applicable sites
- Breast conservation surgery (lumpectomy or wide local excision) with surgical site, the year it was performed, and diagnosis (benign or malignant)
- Mastectomy and breast reconstruction with dates of both
- Breast radiotherapy specific as to the site and approximate treatment timeframe (first and last radiation sessions)
- Administration of chemotherapy, antiestrogens, or other pharmacologic agents for breast cancer
- Complementary and alternative cancer therapies

The patient should provide a list of *all* medications and supplements to the thermography technician at the time of the exam. In most cases, this will be part of the intake process, as it is important to have an up-to-date list upon entering the thermography center. The patient may continue taking most prescription medications; however, she should inform the technician as to whether niacin, nitrates, vasodilators, or beta-blockers are among the medications recently taken.

The equilibration period

After disrobing, the patient should stay in the thermography room for about 15 minutes to acclimate and allow sympathetic vasoconstriction to occur. The temperature in the room should be 20–21°C (68–70°F) with calm air. To facilitate the cooling process, and to prevent creating any thermal artifacts, the patient is asked to keep arms and hands away from the chest wall and not to touch, rub, or scratch the breasts or the surrounding skin (Figure 9.19).

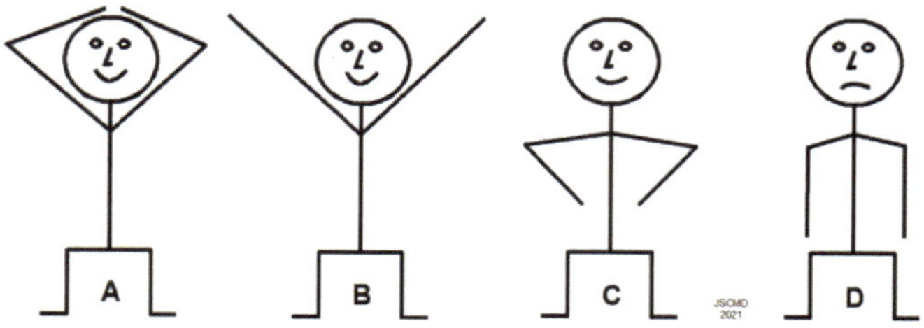

FIGURE 9.19 Arm positions during thermal equilibration and imaging: (a) Good. Axillae and breasts fully exposed for imaging. (b) Good. May be more strenuous than (a). (c) Acceptable. Axillae are cooled but not easily imaged. (d) Poor. Arms are at sides. Axillae not cooled or exposed. Lateral breasts not fully cooled.

Standing equilibration

A simple method for cooling down involves having the patient stand or walk slowly around the room, with arms and hands away from the torso, thus allowing cool air to reach the axillae. Any air drafts from the air conditioner or air vents should be avoided. During the last part of acclimation, the patient is asked to raise her arms and maintain this posture while the thermal images are taken. The images may be obtained using either an adjustable fixed-position or a hand-held camera technique.

Sitting equilibration

A second cooling method involves the subject sitting in a chair, leaning forward with each elbow on the corresponding knee. This allows space between the arms and the body so that all sides of the breasts, including the undersides, are exposed to the cool air. Arms are raised during the actual imaging. This sitting position is convenient for a fixed-camera thermal imager.

Supine equilibration

A third option is to have the patient lie supine (face up) on a padded table with her arms away from her sides. Pillows under her head and knees may be used for comfort, and the patient may nap or just relax. At the completion of the cooldown period, the patient is advised to lie still. The thermographer stands at the foot of the table and takes an image of the underside of the subject's breasts first. Then the subject stands up with arms held away from her sides or above her head for the remainder of the images. A hand-held camera technique is best for this protocol.

Prone equilibration

A fourth equilibration method presently under development has the subject lie prone (face down) on a padded table with the anterior chest extended over an opening so the breasts can hang down through the aperture. All surfaces of both breasts are thus exposed to one or more small infrared imagers underneath the table. If only one imager is used, it is rotated around the breasts, imaging all surfaces. Alternatively, five or more fixed-position imagers can take views of both breasts simultaneously, thus reducing the mechanical complexity of the device. A single-imager prone equilibration system called MAMRIT (Mammary Rotational Infrared Thermographic system) has been patented by Tuscano Systems.[53] A limitation to prone position imaging is that the axillary areas may be difficult to image. Whether the infrared appearance of breasts imaged while prone will correspond to breast images taken in other positions remains to be explored.

The imaging procedure

The imaging protocol is designed to detect and measure infrared emissions from all surface areas of the breasts at an imaging angle of 45 degrees or less; this requires imaging from a minimum of four directions. The four images in the top row of Figure 9.20

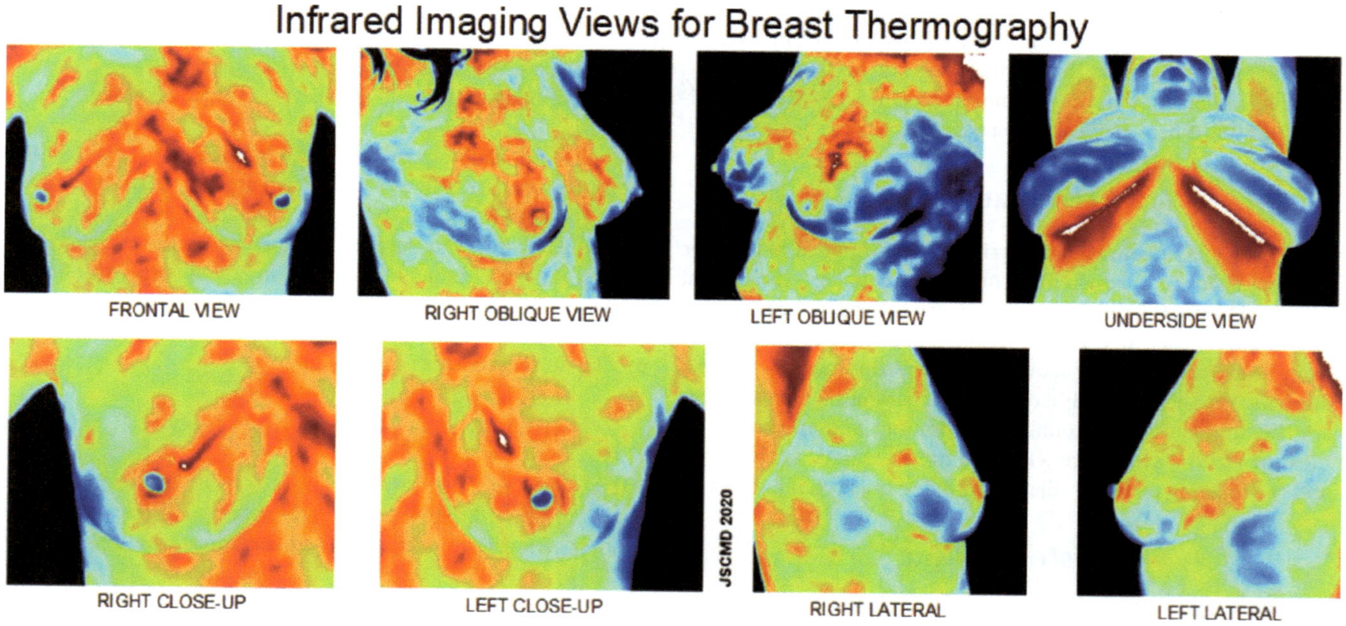

FIGURE 9.20 The eight common imaging views for qualitative breast thermography. The four views on the top row are required to image all aspects of both breasts. The four views on the bottom row may be done in addition, but are not required for a complete thermal examination.

visualize the entirety of both breasts and comprise a complete breast thermogram. The other views (lower row), as well as other special views, may be taken in addition if needed at the discretion of the thermographer.

The primary image is a frontal breast view, which provides the baseline impression of both breasts. Right and left oblique views (at approximately 45 degrees lateral to the sagittal plane) provide views of the lateral and medial surfaces of both breasts. An underside view is performed with the imager directed up and the woman leaning backward, arms stretched up and back. This provides a view of the underside of the breasts, which is particularly important for large-breasted women. (Note: if the patient is acclimatized in the supine position, this underside view is done first and does not need to be repeated standing.) This basic series of four imaging directions takes into account the infrared emission from curved surfaces and allows an accurate qualitative and quantitative analysis of all surface areas of both the breasts. Other views may also be taken as the individual case requires.

To detect any autonomic asymmetry, the subject's shoulders, lower neck, and chest wall may be included in the frontal view. Asymmetry can also be observed by imaging the upper back. A frontal face view is also useful for image identity confirmation and to document that the patient is properly vasoconstricted (cold nose and ears) and has no fever, as assessed by the maximum periorbital temperature.

The positioning of the patient for imaging depends on the chosen protocol. Having the patient seated at the same distance from the camera enables consistent thermal imaging from one year to the next. Having the patient stand makes for uncomplicated positioning for the four breast views. Supine acclimatization allows the subject to relax during cooldown and facilitates the underside image. Each positioning method has its own advantages and limitations. It is up to the thermographer to select the most appropriate position, taking into account the goals of the examination and the physical condition of the patient.

Cold challenge stress testing

The once-common practice of taking a second set of thermal breast images with the woman immersing one or more limbs in cold (or even ice) water is not supported by thermographic evidence. This purposely stressful as well as uncomfortable procedure has not been found to enhance the detection of "occult" cancers as was previously theorized. Nor was it found to affect the clinical decision-making process during thermographic interpretation. In light of these negative findings, a thermographic breast exam should not be judged incomplete or substandard if the imaging protocol omits Cold Challenge Stress Testing.[54] The routine use of Cold Challenge Stress Testing in breast thermography is to be discouraged as an unnecessary, uncomfortable, and possibly harmful impediment to women wishing to monitor their breast health using thermal imaging.

Image quality check

After the images are taken, the thermographer will check the quality of the images and transfer them to the patient's file folder. This typically takes only a few minutes. Meanwhile, the patient can get dressed and put her jewelry back on. If the images are found to be inadequate, the subject must disrobe and be cooled again for at least five to ten minutes before repeat images are taken.

Thermography results and follow-up

After the thermograms go through digital post-processing, qualitative interpretation, quantitative measurement (Figure 9.21), report generation, and archiving, the results are mailed or emailed to the patient and her healthcare provider within a timeframe established by the clinic.

Patients should be encouraged to come back for regular thermograms at least biennially. The initial thermogram only offers a

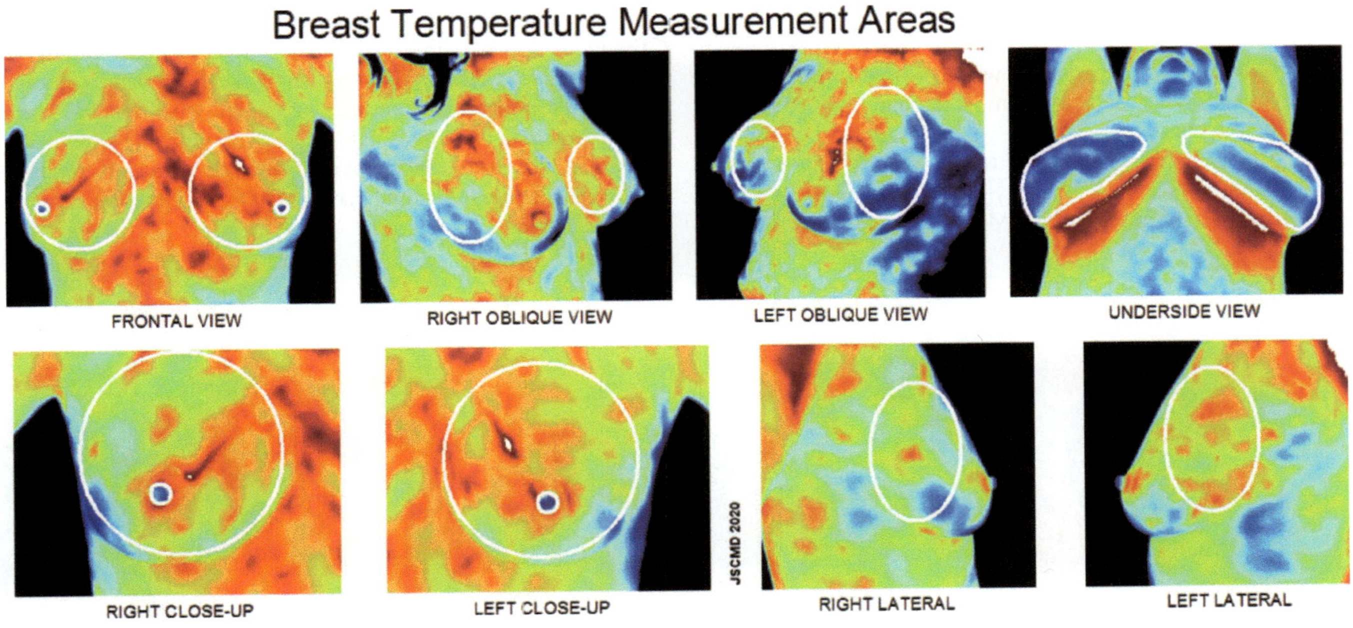

FIGURE 9.21 Areas of temperature measurement for quantitative breast thermography. The upper ten area measurements are necessary to evaluate both breasts completely. Nipple temperatures should not be overlooked. The lower row of measurements may provide additional thermal information, but these are not required for a complete breast thermogram series.

"snapshot" of the breast's condition and may reflect physiological processes that may worsen, stabilize, or even improve on future images. Obtaining thermograms over an extended period enables the thermographer to determine whether a possible abnormality (TH-3) is stable. Stability can only be determined with repeat infrared imaging. If a TH-3 image is unchanged in 6 months or longer, then it can be classified as stable and be designated as TH-2 or TH-3S.

The thermographic monitoring process for a low- or average-risk case:

- Annual thermography and manual breast exam starting at approximately age 25.
- If a breast mass is palpated, perform breast ultrasound.
- Aspirate ultrasound-confirmed masses or cysts using fine-needle method (FNA).
- Send samples to the lab for cytologic diagnosis of cyst aspirates or cells.
- If any tests are abnormal, or if the patient requests, add further imaging such as mammography or breast MRI, as indicated.

The thermographic monitoring process for a *high-risk* case:

- Annual thermography and manual breast exam starting age 21
- Breast ultrasound to detect and assess any existing mass found on exam
- Cytologic evaluation of aspirates from any cysts or masses
- Mammography in women (age 40 or older) without dense breasts
- Breast MRI if indicated in high-risk women with dense breasts

SIDEBAR 9.4 BREAST THERMOGRAPHY LIMITATIONS

As with mammography, infrared thermal imaging of the breast has limits in its ability to detect breast tissue abnormalities. The following constraints should be kept in mind:

1. Thermography works less well in women with very large breasts when detecting tumors deep in the breast, close to the chest wall.
2. Thermography cannot be used to anatomically localize a tumor or lesion. This is typically done with ultrasound, mammography, or breast MRI.
3. Thermography generally will not be helpful in detecting dormant, quiescent, or inactive tumors.
4. If both breasts have very high vascularity, they may be less likely to show temperature asymmetry if cancer is present.
5. Compared to mammography, thermography is poorly suited for detecting microcalcifications in early DCIS.[55]

Breast thermography artifacts

Breast implants

Though not often considered breast artifacts, both silicone and saline breast implants cause major distortion of the breast images (Figure 9.22). As the implants are placed behind the breast glands and ducts, these structures are pressed forward into full view for infrared monitoring. Any NO vasodilation, venous hypertrophy, or lymphatic inflammation should show up well. Skin over an implant appears cool due to the large breast surface area exposed to the environmental temperature, reduced skin blood flow due to pressure from the implant, and the thermal insulation of the implant material. X-rays used in mammograms cannot go through silicone or saline implants well enough to show the breast tissue on standard views, so special X-ray views (said to be painful) have been developed. Of major concern is possible implant rupture during mammography.[56] Some centers have patients sign a waiver saying the clinic is not responsible should the implant rupture or shift during mammography. Thermal imaging in conjunction with manual breast examination may be the preferred screening method for breasts with implants.

Cooper ligament strain

A common artifact that causes a markedly warm area over the upper anterolateral chest wall in women with large breasts is due to inflammation of Cooper's ligaments, also known as the fibrocollagenous septa (Figure 9.23). Attached to the pectoral fascia, these ligaments are strong connective tissue bands that suspend the breast against gravity and maintain its structural integrity. Strain-induced "Cooperitis" is usually seen bilaterally, though it may be unilateral, especially in women with unequal breast sizes. When the Cooper's ligaments are chronically stretched or strained, this may suggest that a better bra is needed. It could also indicate that the individual may benefit from reduction mammaplasty if other therapies fail.

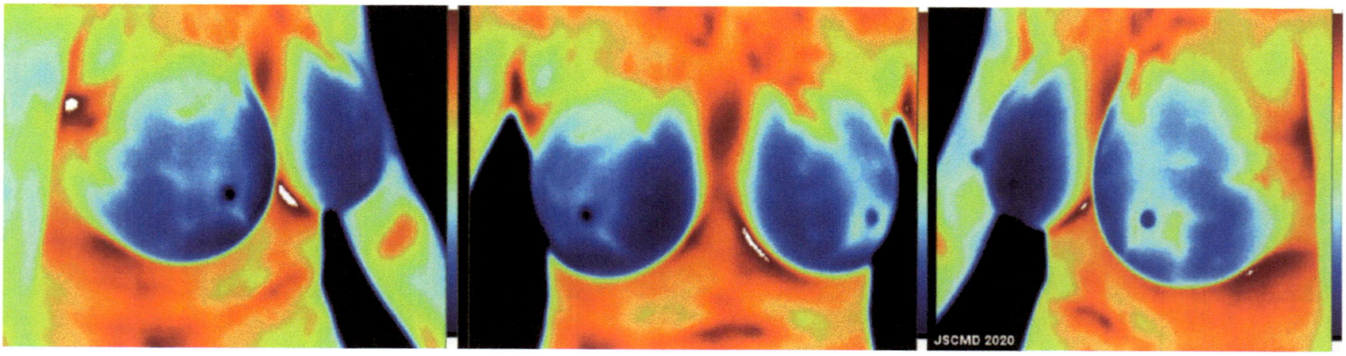

FIGURE 9.22 Breast implants, normal, 53-year-old female.

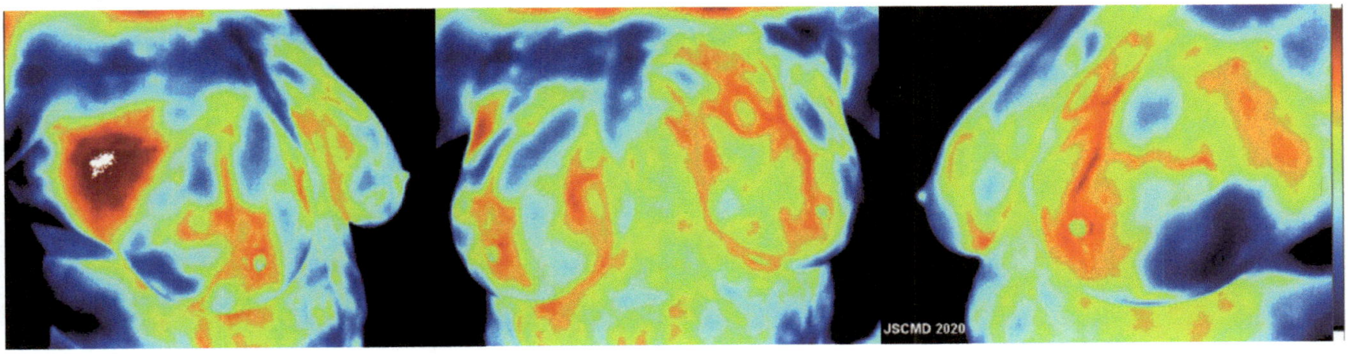

FIGURE 9.23 Inflammation of the breast suspensory ligaments of Cooper, worse on the right. Note the asymmetric positions of the breasts in this 51-year-old female with no history of breast surgery, masses, or hormone use.

Chronic radial inflammation of the breast (CRIB)

Another occasionally encountered artifact has been attributed in the past to "costochondritis"; however, the thermal markings of this condition do not agree with the anatomy or orientation of the costal cartilages or pectoral muscle fibers. The markings are usually located over the upper inner quadrant of the breast and may be unilateral or bilateral. They appear warmest or most pronounced along the lateral borders of the sternum, progressing downward and lateral at an angle of approximately 45 degrees. They are sometimes branched. Often, they appear to originate near the nipple, extending off the breast in a radial direction (see Figure 9.24).

A review of anatomical structures with this physical orientation reveals one major possibility: the lymphatic vessels draining the breast. These superficially located vessels empty into lymph nodes located between the costal cartilages at the border of the sternum, where the warmest portion of this thermal marking is seen. Nonetheless, since it has not yet been shown that these patterns are due to, or correspond with, lymphatic inflammation,

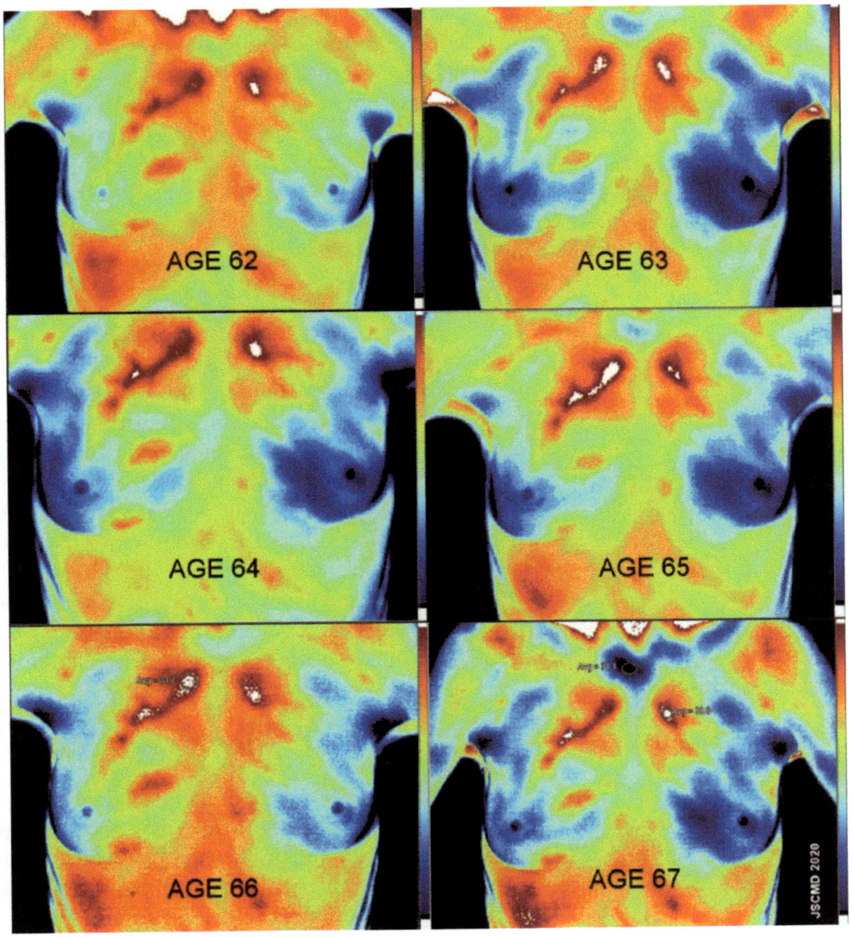

FIGURE 9.24 Chronic radial inflammation of the breast (CRIB), bilateral and stable over 5 years in a 62–67-year-old female. No breast or chest wall symptoms reported.

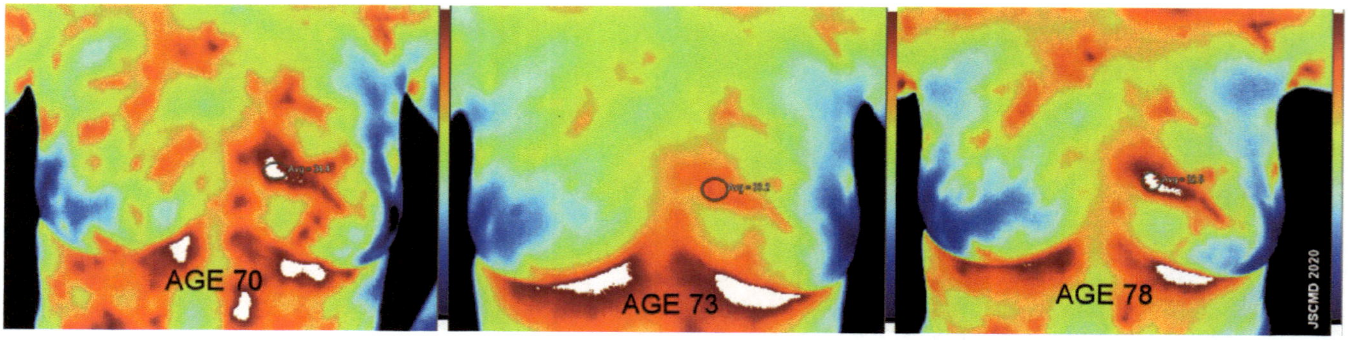

FIGURE 9.25 Chronic radial inflammation of the breast (CRIB), unilateral on left and stable over 8 years in a 70–78-year-old female. Diagnostic mammogram reported normal.

they will be referred to generically as CRIB patterns. These markings occur singly, in groups, bilaterally, or in several separated locations. They may create an alarm when seen on an initial thermogram, as they resemble the lymphatic inflammation seen with carcinomas, but they often remain thermographically stable for many years (Figure 9.25). Breast masses are usually absent on physical exam, though the affected areas may be tender to pressure. A diagnostic mammogram will generally come back negative. More research is needed to investigate this thermal anomaly. Why would lymph vessels and nodes draining the breast be chronically inflamed? Does this indicate a pre-cancerous condition? For the present, thermographers should be aware of this condition and follow it closely at first, then more routinely if no changes in the pattern are seen over time.

Nipple de-enervation artifact

Surgical procedures for reduction mammoplasty involve transplanting the areola and nipple for a better appearance post-surgery. If the nerves to the nipple and areola are not carefully preserved during surgery, these areas will have no sympathetic fibers to initiate vasoconstriction. The denervated areolae and nipples will remain warm (Figure 9.26). More advanced plastic surgery techniques now preserve the areolar nerves, retaining the nipple vasoconstriction reflex. An alternative procedure is to remove the areola and nipple completely, tattooing faux areolae on the breast and constructing "nipples" by bunching skin with a special suture technique. The tattoos, once healed, generally cannot be visualized in thermographic images.

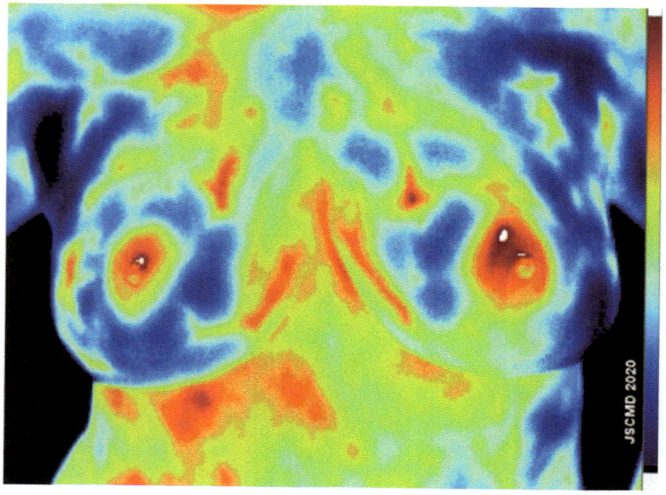

FIGURE 9.26 Areolar denervation. This 50-year-old woman underwent breast reduction surgery one year earlier. Note the warm areolae and nipples bilaterally.

Underwire bra pressure neuropathy

An underwire bra can cause irritation and pain under the breasts. This is due to not only to local skin irritation but also chronic pressure on the intercostal nerves, resulting in a local neuropathy. Upon imaging, the condition appears as a red line or groove under the breast, coincident with the painful area (Figure 9.27a). Physical examination reveals the breast fold skin to be dry and not macerated, though itching and rash may occur if dermal allergy to the metal wire is present. In such cases, the patient should be advised to stop wearing the underwire bra. The discomfort should subside quickly. The type of bra a patient uses should be determined during the intake process.

Intertrigo

A breast condition that appears thermologically similar to underwire bra irritation is Intertrigo. This condition usually appears in women with pendulous breasts where the skin under the breast fold remains occluded, warm, and moist for long periods (Figure 9.27 b&c). A mixed growth of fungi and bacteria propagate in these conditions, irritating and inflaming the skin. This problem may be worse in patients with diabetes mellitus. The warm pattern in the fold of the breast can be clinically differentiated from underwire bra irritation in that it is a moist condition, whereas underwire bra irritation is usually dry.

Glomus AVA dilation effects

The physiology of glomus bodies, also known as arterio-venous anastomoses (AVAs) is discussed at length in Chapter 5. Normally closed at equilibration temperatures below 21°C (70°F), glomus AVAs may open from unknown influences during processes such as autoimmune disease or the action of certain drugs. Though mostly located in the distal extremities, glomus AVAs are scattered throughout the skin surface, and thus may affect the thermal appearance of the breasts if the AVAs are open. A review of

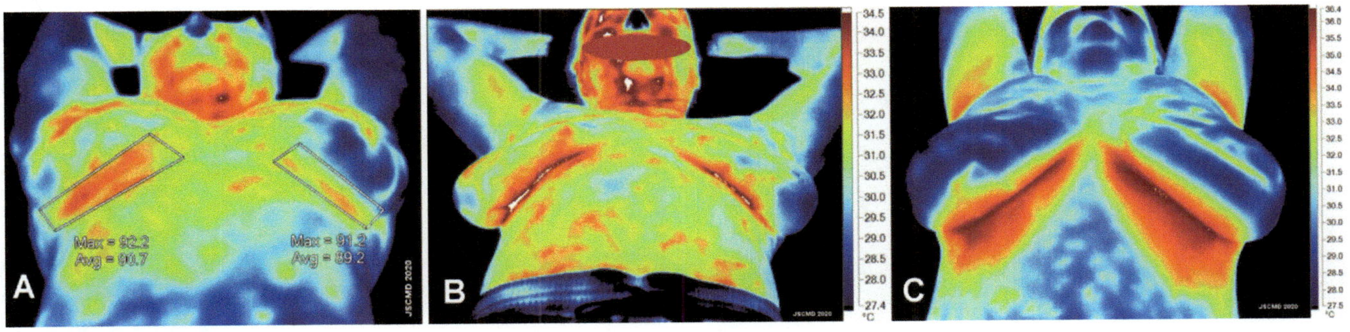

FIGURE 9.27 Inflammation under the breasts: (a) Underwire bra artifact with pain under the right breast – 45 yoF. (b) Intertrigo, chronic bilateral – 66 yoF. (c) Intertrigo, extensive – chronic moist rash under breasts, skin cracked and inflamed – 46 yoF.

properly cooled female subjects in the ILSITS database showing signs of paradoxical glomus dilation (PGD) reveals that the skin over the breast tissues shows relatively little effect from open AVAs (Figure 9.28).[57] Whether this is due to breast skin having fewer AVAs than the skin of the abdomen and upper chest or whether AVAs over the breast do not open under conditions of PGD is not known. Thermographers should be aware of the pattern of glomus dilation when evaluating both breast and body thermograms.

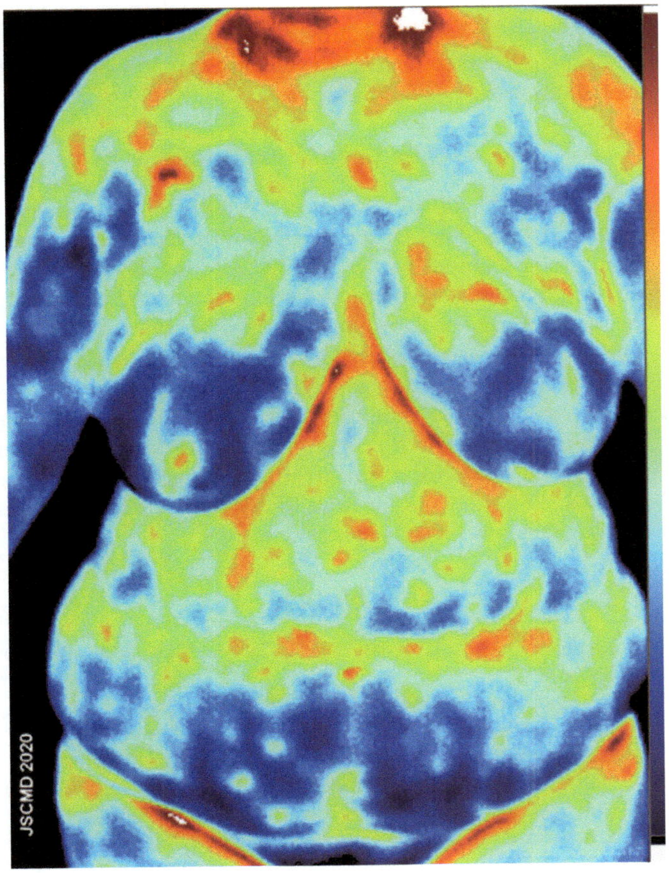

FIGURE 9.28 Typical "spotty" glomus AVA dilation pattern from systemic lupus in a cooled 56-year-old female. The upper chest wall and abdomen are affected. Note the relative sparing of the skin over the breast tissue.

Breast trauma and ecchymosis

Trauma to the breast may occur from assault or accidents, such as domestic abuse, airbag deployment, or a large dog jumping up with paws placed on the breast area. Significant trauma to the breast may result in abrasion, ecchymosis, bruising (including hematoma), and laceration. Ecchymoses and superficial bruises may not show up thermally, unlike inflammation caused by soft tissue damage. A large hematoma may appear cool. With the patient's consent, visual photographs should be taken to document the trauma. Breast screening thermography should be repeated once the trauma has healed – 1 month for a simple ecchymosis, six or more months following an underlying rib fracture.

Post-radiation treatment artifact

Radiation treatments for carcinoma involve radiating the breast with ionizing radiation strong enough to damage susceptible tissues along with the neoplastic cells. This radiation is akin to burning the tissues in a controlled fashion. Post-radiation burn artifact is seen in thermal images as a pronounced area of warmth over the treatment area, sometimes persisting for months after the treatment is over (Figure 9.29). As this post-radiation appearance may mimic local neoplastic recurrence, it may cause alarm on thermographic imaging. With time, post-radiation artifact should fade, while the thermographic appearance of cancer recurrence will tend to become worse.

Recently it has been discovered that breast thermography "artifacts" seen *during* radiation therapy are useful in determining how a tumor is responding to treatment. The researchers conclude "assessing the efficacy of radiotherapy during treatment [via repeat thermographic imaging] makes it possible to change the treatment regimen, dose, and radiation field during treatment as well as to individualize treatment schedules to optimize treatment effectiveness."[58]

Escharotic treatment artifact

"Alternative" medical treatments are not always safe or benign. The thermographer may encounter patients who have self-treated palpable breast masses with escharotic salves, on the theory that chemically burning the overlying skin will "dissolve" the underlying mass. These salves often contain bloodroot (*Sanguinaria*

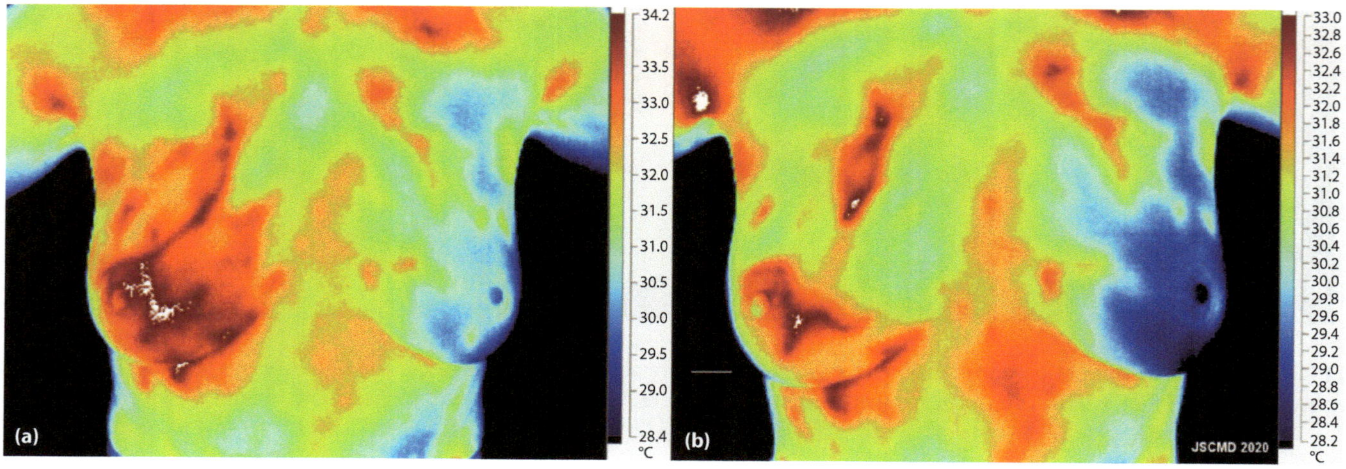

FIGURE 9.29 Radiation inflammation. (a) 64-year-old woman one-year post-lumpectomy for right ductal carcinoma. Post-surgical radiation ended 9 months previously. (b) Repeat thermogram 6 months later shows the inflammation improving.

canadensis) or other topically toxic ingredients. If used over a period of time, escharotics kill the dermis, leaving a full-thickness denuded wound that appears very warm to thermal imaging (Figure 9.30). This inflamed wound obscures any thermal findings from the underlying mass, making breast thermography useless until the area heals completely. Ultrasonography, X-ray mammography, or breast MRI may be required to determine the nature of any masses.

Artifact from breast creams and gels

The application of nonprescription creams to the breasts to improve their thermographic appearance represents a pernicious and disturbing thermographic artifact. These applications reduce the thermal emissivity of the skin and increase evaporative cooling, thus making the area appear cooler (better) on thermograms. Proprietary creams containing only water, sodium magnesium silicate, disodium phosphate, and sodium chloride have been marketed for this purpose by including serial thermal images in advertisements to demonstrate the cream's efficacy. Any apparent thermographic improvement is actually due to artifact. These applications can reduce the interpretation of a thermogram by one TH grade or more, perhaps delaying the diagnosis of an underlying malignancy. Patients should be cautioned about this thermographic scam.

NOTE: This caveat does not apply to prescription topical creams for breast applications. An experimental breast cream for DCIS containing 4-hydroxy Tamoxifen is presently being developed, and other such topical remedies are sure to follow should the therapy prove successful.[59]

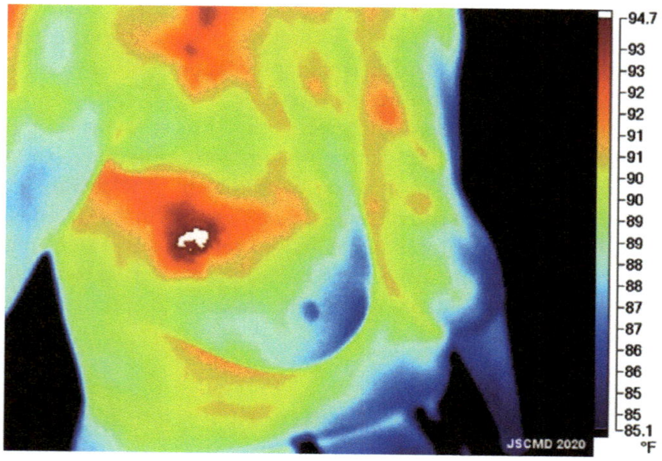

FIGURE 9.30 Skin ulcer from applying escharotic cream to treat a breast mass – 59 yoF. The nature of the underlying lesion cannot be determined by thermography due to the overlying chemical inflammation.

Other breast artifacts

Artifacts may be due to the patient's inability or unwillingness to adhere to guidelines for preparation for the thermogram, such as exercising vigorously or consuming nicotine, niacin or alcohol shortly before the imaging session. Scratching or rubbing the breasts during cooldown may create warm thermal artifacts. Touching the breasts with cold, vasoconstricted hands creates "fingerprints" of cool artifact. Pregnant or breastfeeding patients will also tend to show "abnormal" thermograms that are attributable to the physiologic effects of pregnancy or lactation. When an unknown or strange thermographic pattern is seen, check the patient's clinical history for clues or ask them directly, perhaps showing them the images to jog their memory.

Notes

1. Azamjah N, et al., Asian Pac J Cancer Prev. 2019; PMCID: PMC6745227.
2. In Digital Mammography, also called full-field digital mammography (FFDM), the X-ray film is replaced by solid-state detectors.
3. Humphrey LL, et al., Ann Intern Med. 2002; PMID: 12204020.
4. Miller AB, et al., Ann Intern Med. 2002; PMID: 12204013. See also: Miller AB, et al., J Natl Cancer Inst. 2000; PMID: 10995804.
5. Rostgaard K, et al., Acta Oncol. 2010; PMID: 20397766. See also: Early Breast Cancer Trialists' Collaborative Group (EBCTCG). Lancet. 2005; PMID: 15894097.
6. See: https://aathermology.org/organization-2/guidelines/guidelines-for-breast-thermology/. See also: Golestani N et al., EXCLI J. 2014; PMCID: PMC4464455. See also: Ohsumi S et al., Breast Cancer Res Treat. 2002; PMID: 12206513.

7. Diakides NA, et al., In: Medical Infrared Imaging. Diakides NA, Bronzino J (Eds.), CRC Press, Boca Raton, FL, 2007.
8. Lagadec C, et al., Stem Cells. 2012; PMCID: PMC3413333. See also: Puvanesarajah S et al., Cancer Prev Res (Phila). 2018; PMCID: PMC5984721.
9. Morales-Cervantes A, et al.,. EXCLI J. 2018; PMCID: PMC6295635. See also: Madhu H et al., Annu Int Conf IEEE Eng Med Biol Soc. 2016; PMID: 28268508. See also: Ramya Devi R, et al., J Med Syst. 2019. Doi: 10.1007/s10916-019-1267-8. See also: Parisky YR, et al., AJR Am J Roentgenol. 2003; PMID: 12490517. See also: Arora N, et al., Am J Surg. 2008; PMID: 18809055. See also: Kolarić D, et al., Coll Antropol. 2013; PMID: 23941007.
10. Arora N, et al., Am J Surg. 2008; PMID: 18809055. See also: Parisky YR, et al., AJR Am J Roentgenol. 2003; PMID: 12490517.
11. Rassiwala M, et al., Int J Surg. 2014; PMID: 25448668.
12. Nelson HD, et al., U.S. Preventive Services Task Force Evidence Syntheses, 2016 Jan. Report No.: 14-05201-EF-1. PMID: 26889531.
13. Østerås BH, et al., Radiology. 2019; PMID: 31407968.
14. Boyd NF. Am Soc Clin Oncol Educ Book 2013; PMID: 23714456.
15. Roubidoux MA, et al., Radiology. 2004; PMID: 14695385.
16. Melnikow J, et al., Ann Intern Med. 2016; PMCID: PMC5100826.
17. Parisky YR, et al., AJR Am J Roentgenol. 2003; PMID: 12490517.
18. Abdelwahab Yousef AJ, Semin Oncol. 2017; PMID: 29526255.
19. Wright T, et al., Mol Diagn. 2003; PMID: 14529321. See also: Head JF et al., Ann N Y Acad Sci. 1993; PMID: 8279754.
20. Ng EY et al., J Med Eng Technol. 2001; PMID: 11780767.
21. Head JF, et al., IEEE Eng Med Biol Mag. 2002; PMID: 12613215.
22. Feinberg J et al., Cancer Treat Res. 2018; PMID: 29349758.
23. Cowell CF, et al., Mol Oncol. 2013; PMCID: PMC5528459. See also: Hong YK et al., Am J Surg. 2018; PMID: 30244816. See also: Sanders ME et al., Cancer. 2005; PMID: 15884091. See also: Van Zee KJ et al., Ann Surg. 2015; PMCID: PMC4739638.
24. Monteiro HP et al., Nitric Oxide 2019; PMID: 31009708.
25. Masood S, Breast J. 2015; PMID: 26547899. See also: Harris JV, JAMA Intern Med. 2016; PMID: 27244094.
26. D'Orsi CJ, J Natl Cancer Inst Monogr. 2010; PMCID: PMC5161079.
27. Munn LL, Wiley Interdiscip Rev Syst Biol Med. 2017; PMCID: PMC5561333. See also: Todoric J, et al., Cancer Prev Res (Phila). 2016; PMCID: PMC5142754.
28. Ham M, et al., Arch Pharm Res. 2013; Doi: 10.1007/s12272-013-0271-7
29. Wu LA, et al., BMC Cancer. 2016; Doi: 10.1186/s12885-016-2602-9
30. Head JF, et al., Ann N Y Acad Sci. 1993; PMID: 8279754.
31. Davoli A, et al., Cancer Chemother Pharmacol. 2010; PMID: 20087739.
32. Ohsumi S, et al., Breast Cancer Res Treat. 2002; PMID: 12206513.
33. Fernandopulle SM et al., Pathology. 2006; PMID: 16753742. See also: Anders CK, et al., J Clin Oncol. 2008; PMID: 18612148.
34. Ulmer HU, et al., Cancer. 1990; PMID: 2340467.
35. Sadoughi F, et al., Breast Cancer (Dove Med Press). 2018; PMCID: PMC6278839.
36. Amalu WC, et al., In: Medical Infrared Imaging. Diakides NA, Bronzino J, (Eds.), CRC Press, Boca Raton, FL, 2007, Section 9.10. See also: Amalric R, et al., Bibl Radiol. 1975; PMID: 1180864.
37. Prasad SS, et al., Breast Dis. 2016; PMID: 27767959. See also: Arora N et al., Am J Surg. 2008; PMID: 18809055. See also: Kolarić D et al., Coll Antropol. 2013; PMID: 23941007.
38. Netter illustration used with permission of Elsevier Inc. All rights reserved. www.netterimages.com
39. McLelland R, Recent Results Cancer Res.1990; PMID: 2236859.
40. Original color graphic and annotations by Patrick J. Lynch displayed in greyscale. Wikipedia File: Breast anatomy normal scheme.png, 3 September 2007; Color overlays and color text by JSCMD.
41. Image sources from the public domain.
42. Drawing guided by illustrations by Memorial Sloan Kettering, Medicrux.com, Memorang, and CD Clemente.
43. Guideline for Breast Thermography, Section 9.2. American Academy of Thermology, Greenville, SC, 2018. The 1.0°C (1.8°F) cutoff criterion is based on studies using older thermal scanners that could not isolate nipple from areolar temperatures.
44. Gray H, Anatomy of the Human Body, 27th Ed, Lea & Febiger, Philadelphia, 1965, p. 809 and illustration on p. 792.
45. Gray's Anatomy of the Human Body – 27th edition. Goss CM, ed., Leas & Febiger, Philadelphia, 1959. p. 1385. This ring of veins is also called the *areolar venous plexus.*
46. Jesinger RA, et al., Radiographics 2011; PMID: 22084191.
47. Source: NIH National Cancer Institute 2019: https://www.cancer.gov/types/breast/ibc-fact-sheet
48. Keyserlink JR, et al., In Medical Infrared Imaging Principles and Practices, Diakides, Bronzino & Peterson, eds., CRC Press, Boca Raton, FL, 2013, Section 11.2.1.
49. Piana A, et al., Pan Am J Med Thermol. 2019; 1(2):93–100.
50. Criterion added by JSCMD on observing the qualitative appearance of BrCA in the ILSITS database. Exceptions include lactation, trauma, and nipple infection. Further studies are needed to confirm this criterion.
51. The infrared scanner used in the Ville Marie Study (Bales Scientific, CA) did not have the spatial resolution to determine venous from lymphatic thermal appearance, so they reported abnormal findings as "vascular anarchy."
52. *Adapted From* Functional Infrared Imaging of the Breast. In The Biomedical Engineering Handbook, Medical Devices and Systems, 3rd Ed, Ch. 26, p. 11, JD Bronzino, ed, CRC Press, 2006.
53. Lakshmi NVSSR, et al., 2015 Global Conference on Communication Technologies (GCCT), Thuckalay, India, 2015. Doi: 10.1109/GCCT.2015.7342727. See also: Hakim, A et al., J Med Syst. 2020; PMID: 32613403
54. Diakides NA & Bronzino J (eds.), Medical Infrared Imaging, CRC Press, Boca Raton, FL, 2008. Section 9.2.5.
55. Parisky YR et al., AJR Am J Roentgenol. 2003; PMID: 12490517.
56. See: https://www.cancer.org/cancer/breast-cancer/screening-tests-and-early-detection/mammograms/mammograms-for-women-with-breast-implants.html
57. ILSITS – Integrative life Solutions Incorporated Thermography Service. A single-location, single-thermographer imaging clinic which operated in Clemmons, NC, USA, from 2010 to 2017.
58. Hoffer OA, et al., J. Biomed. Opt. 2018; PMCID: PMC5933077.
59. Lee O, et al., Clin Cancer Res. 2014; PMCID: PMC4101910.

10

GENERAL THERMOGRAPHY

The use of infrared imaging to detect and evaluate thermally detectable conditions in humans is a vast and complex subject. A few practical points are worth mentioning before discussing the various thermographic applications that can supplement medical diagnosis and prognosis. Sometimes the thermographer will be interested in only one area of the human body and will concentrate the images on that site and the symmetrically opposite area. At other times, a thermal analysis of the entire body may be needed. If the human body were spherical, floating, and without appendages, only six images would be required to accomplish a general thermographic evaluation. Of course, the body is not spherical, and its complicated shape requires a variety of body positions and imaging angles for a full thermal imaging assessment. Whereas a minimal breast exam may require only four or five images, thirty or more images are typically needed to properly view the entire surface of the human body, as depicted in this collage of typical images (Figure 10.1).

Many positions are used to thermally image the human body. The specific selection of images and positioning techniques used for a thermographic exam are determined not only by the individual case but also by the clinical judgment and experience of the thermographer. In addition, the proper interpretation of each thermogram should take into account the clinical history and physical findings of the problem along with the results of any associated medical studies.

This chapter is by no means a complete listing of all the situations for which general thermography has relevance. Because there is insufficient space to cover the full range of thermally-detectable conditions, this chapter will emphasize topics of clinical importance. Significant thermographic artifacts and questionable findings will also be addressed. Thermography for specialty conditions will be reviewed separately in Chapter 11.

SIDEBAR 10.1 A TALE OF TWO IMAGERS

The original thermographic images in this book were obtained with two industrial-grade infrared imagers. One of these imagers was later found to be thermally uncalibrated, with a normalized thermal gain as low as 0.20. This means that a 1.0°C temperature difference between two points on a subject would be recorded as a mere 0.20°C difference on the thermogram. Fortunately, this poor thermal gain was linear over the physiologic temperature range, therefore, the error could be compensated qualitatively by increasing the infrared-to-visual gain using the full-span thermal caliper technique; however, any quantitative absolute and differential temperature measurements would remain in error.

For this reason, images taken with the uncalibrated thermal imager were determined to be useful only for qualitative evaluation. Those images that are exclusively for qualitative analyses are presented with a color reference scale but no numerical scale. The second thermal imager was fully calibrated over the entire physiologic temperature range; calibrated numerical temperature scales accompany the images taken with that imager. Those images can be used for both qualitative visualization and quantitative differential measurements. The calibration curves of both imagers can be seen in the section on Bucket Calibration in Chapter 4.

Moral of the story: Thermographers are encouraged to check the thermal offset and gain of their imagers to avoid erroneously interpreting uncalibrated images.

Skin findings in thermography

Besides being the body's largest organ, the skin is the organ visible to infrared analysis. Presented in this section are thermal findings pertaining to diseases, injuries, toxins, and neoplasms of the skin itself. Thermal findings coming from deeper tissues, systemic diseases, or pertaining to specific anatomical sites will be discussed in later sections.

- The skin, guided by neural input, is the major source of heat radiating or evaporating from the body.
- The skin, nails, mucus membranes, eardrums, and corneas are the only surfaces we can non-invasively visualize thermographically.
- Skin temperatures will vary based on local environmental, neural, and vascular conditions, and on the warmth of underlying organs such as muscles.
- Skin blood flow is the major source of heat transfer from the core body to the environment.
- Heat is constantly generated in deeper body tissues. The skin is normally cooler than the core, providing a thermal gradient for heat removal.
- Skin blood flow increases with the presence of nitric oxide (NO) and histamine, as well as vasodilator agents such as alcohol, niacin, hydralazine, and lisinopril.
- Skin blood flow is decreased by vasoconstrictive sympathetic neuron activity; nicotine, epinephrine, and other drugs reduce skin perfusion. Arterial insufficiency can also have a negative impact.

Thermal burns (infrared skin injury)

Burn wounds alter the skin's thermoregulatory capacity; the nature of these effects depends on the burn depth. Deep (full-thickness) burns cause subdermal arterial damage, reducing dermal blood perfusion and lowering the local skin temperature.[1] By contrast, partial-thickness burns remain perfused, and inflammation from tissue injury increases the local skin temperature. Infrared imaging can be used to determine the depth of the burn by measuring the temperatures over a burn wound.[2]

Burn wounds are usually evaluated by visual means. However, visual diagnosis of burn severity has proven inadequate for selecting appropriate treatment.[3] Burn wound "conversion" is a process in which superficial partial-thickness burns advance, causing deeper tissue necrosis. Recent studies indicate that thermography can identify which wounds will convert, thus offering an important tool for guiding burn care.[4]

Warm acute burn areas will generally heal better than cool ones. For limbs with large burns, the temperature of the washed

DOI: 10.1201/9781003281764-11

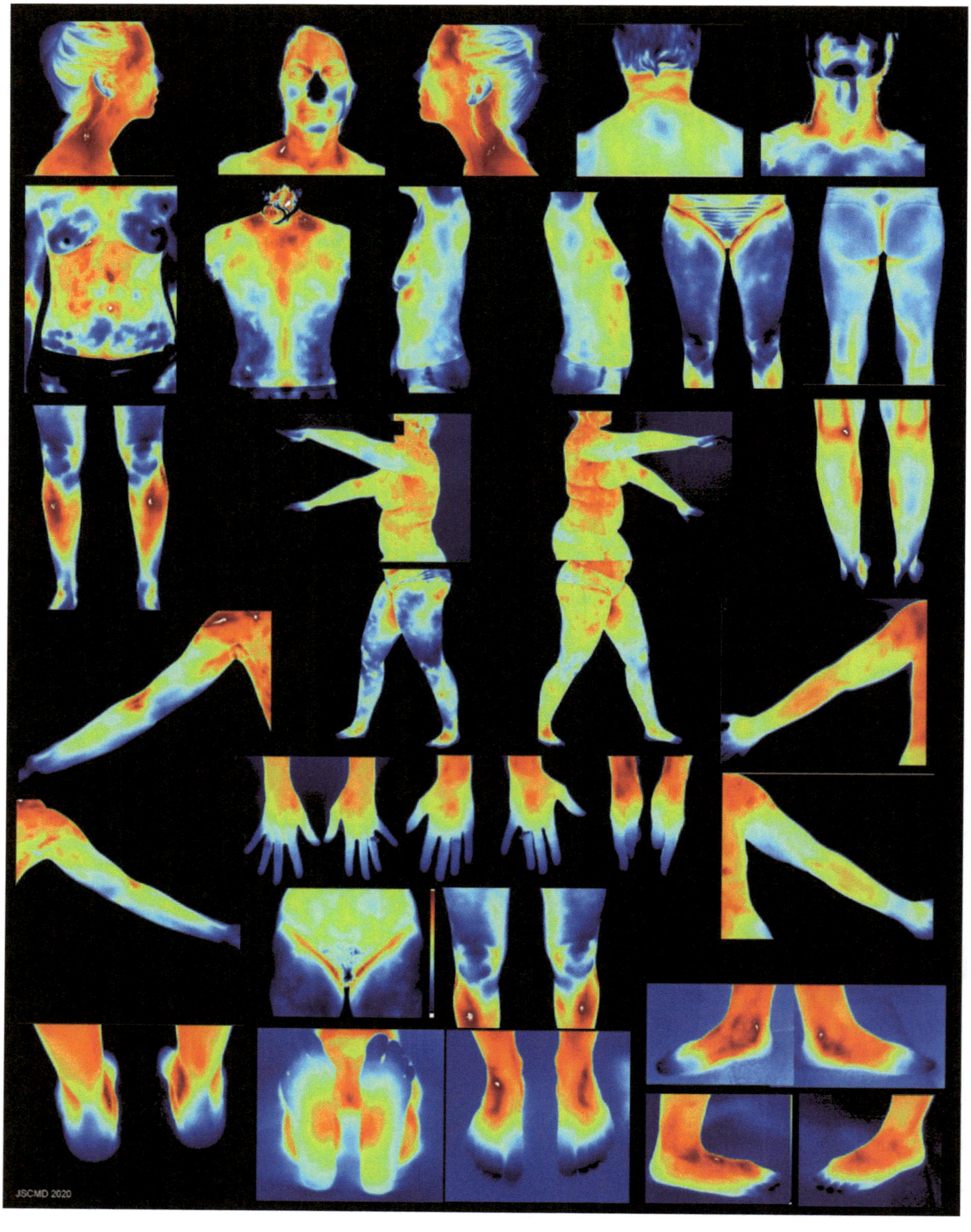

FIGURE 10.1 Some common imaging views taken in the practice of general thermography.

and debrided burn area is compared to the temperature of adjacent healthy skin (the ΔT value) to predict the clinical outcome. Limb areas showing a ΔT greater than 5°C (9°F) may require amputation. A ΔT greater than 3°C (5.4°F) predicts the possibility of successful wound grafting, while a difference less than 3°C (5.4°F) indicates the burn will re-epithelialize without surgery if kept clean and non-infected (Figure 10.2).[5]

The predictive value of thermography in burn wound assessment has been confirmed in numerous studies.[7] Thermography helps minimize the possibility of performing unnecessary surgery on burn wounds that would eventually heal on their own.[8] Smartphone-compatible thermal imagers have enabled convenient analysis of burn wounds. By correlating burn wound temperature with burn depth and progression, such technology

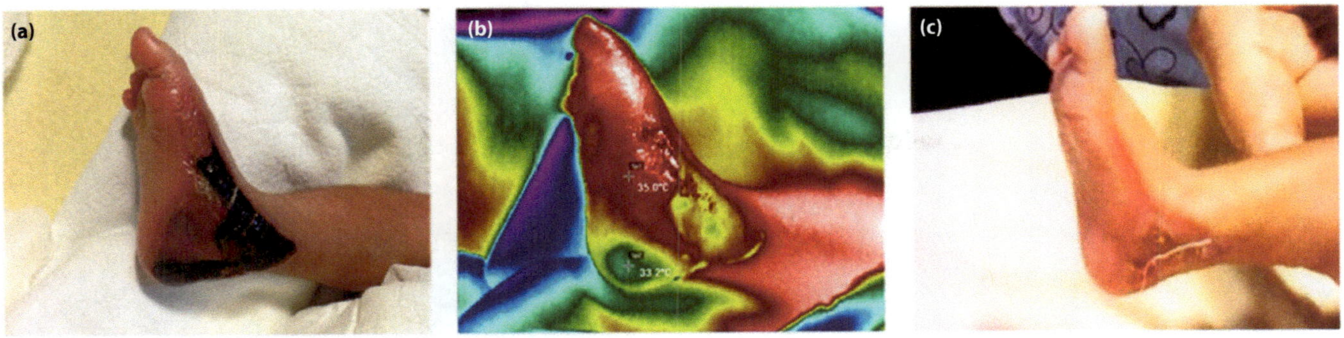

FIGURE 10.2 4-week-old infant with foot burn. (a) Photograph. (b) Infrared image. ΔT was 1.8°C. (c) The burned areas healed well after 7 days without the need for grafting.[6]

can predict the number of days needed for healing.[9] This simple bedside imaging can determine burn wound viability and severity.[10]

Sunburn (ultraviolet skin injury)

Sunburn involves a different damage mechanism, quite distinct from thermal burns. Thermal burns are caused by excess *infrared* (IR) exposure, which can penetrate deeply by conduction. Sunburn is caused by excess *ultraviolet* (UV) exposure, which does not penetrate the skin deeply or create much heat. UV exposure damages dermal cellular organelles and DNA, causing inflammation. Strong ultraviolet sources other than sunlight can also cause skin damage. Overexposure to a welding arc results in a type of UV burn that appears similar to sunburn, though the distribution over the skin is different. Like welder's burns, overexposure to UV reflecting off snow causes corneal photokeratitis ("snow blindness") and can damage anatomy not usually affected by sunburn, such as the roof of the mouth or the interior of the nostrils.[11]

Upon intensive exposure to excess UV radiation, dermal blood vessels dilate due to inflammation, increasing blood flow; immune cells are then recruited to clear away damaged cellular debris.[12] These processes cause the redness, warmth, and pain associated with sunburn. There is rarely any damage to the subdermal arterioles, which are protected by the superficial dermal layers.

Ultraviolet injury is often well demarcated by clothing or shadowed areas, and may show surface temperatures 4°C (7.2°F) higher than adjacent non-burned skin in severe cases.[13] In mild cases, thermographic findings may be minimal or nonspecific. Sunburn disrupts thermoregulation of the skin. Following immersion in cold water, sunburn raises skin temperature and can amplify heat losses.[14] Ultraviolet burns to the anterior chest area, whether from sunlight or a tanning bed, may markedly affect the breast thermogram. Thermography should be delayed until any blisters, erythema, or peeling are no longer present.

Frostbite (hypothermic skin injury)

If the thermoregulatory mechanisms of the skin are overwhelmed by exposure to intense cold, tissue injury can result. This occurs when the physiologic vasodilation seen during cold exposure is insufficient to keep the tissues from freezing. Disruption of arterial circulation and permanent loss of local thermoregulatory capacity are the results.[15] Frostbite injury can be divided into three zones: (1) coagulation, (2) stasis, and (3) hyperemia. The zone of *coagulation* is the most severe region of injury and causes irreversible tissue damage. The zone of *stasis* is the middle region and is characterized by tissue damage that may be reversible with restoration of adequate blood flow. The zone of *hyperemia* is the most proximal and least damaged region. Generally, full or partial recovery is expected and occurs over many days.[16]

In frostbite of the hands, the rewarmed fingers may initially be cold on thermal imaging of a vasodilated patient due to thrombosis of the digital arteries. After 3 months, only the distal phalanges may still be cold on imaging. With full recovery of a surviving digit, a pattern of glomus AVA dilation may be seen due to sympathetic nerve damage from the freeze injury.[17]

Chilblain, also known as *pernio*, is a superficial injury typically occurring after one to 5 hours in cold, wet conditions at temperatures below 16°C (50°F). Small erythematous papules appear on the skin, most often on the dorsal surface of the fingers, though the ears, face, shins, and feet may also be affected. The lesions are swollen, tender, itchy, and painful. Upon rewarming, the skin becomes inflamed, red, and hot to the touch, with an itching or burning sensation that may continue for several hours.[18] It is during this rewarming phase that chilblain becomes thermographically visible. Recovery from chilblain is usually complete without lasting effects.

Scars

Whenever the dermis is damaged, the body forms a scar – a matrix of fibrous connective tissue – to repair the damage. The new scar tissue has a different mechanical strength and altered local vasculature compared to undamaged skin. Temperature differences between the healing scar and the peri-scar area can be monitored using thermography.

A scar, if fully healed, is the same temperature as the surrounding skin (under steady-state conditions), as it no longer has the increased metabolism of active tissue repair and is not producing NO. Healed scars can rarely be seen in infrared images (Figure 10.3b). Dynamic cooling is usually necessary to differentiate mature scar from peri-scar tissue, with the scar area remaining thermographically cooler upon rewarming.[19] Wounds that are still healing and scars with underlying suture inflammation or infection may appear warm (Figure 10.3a). Large keloids and hypertrophic scars may first appear warm due to intrinsic inflammation, becoming cooler when mature, though definitive thermographic studies are not available.[20]

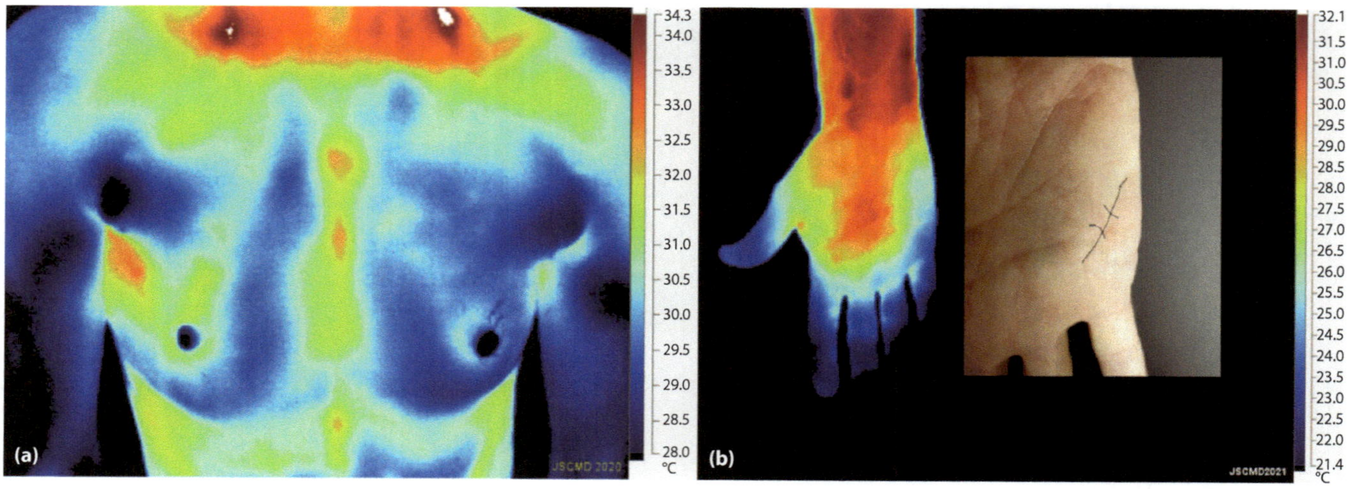

FIGURE 10.3 (a) Persistent scar inflammation from multiple thoracotomies for congenital heart valve problems. Low-grade infection or inflammation of the retained sternal sutures may be present – 49 yoF. (b) An old healed scar from a full-thickness laceration of the right hypothenar area. The wound location is indicated by black lines on the visible image – 77 yoM.

Tattoos

Tattoos are body art made by inserting ink, dyes, and pigments into the dermis to alter the observed skin color. Indelible (permanent) tattoos are rarely visible with infrared imaging. Temperature differences with surrounding tissue only appear if the tattoo is fresh (i.e., inflamed from needle punctures), infected, or otherwise inflamed due to a chemical or allergic reaction. Temporary metallic tattoos will generally appear cooler than the surrounding skin due to the low infrared emissivity of metal surfaces.

Open wounds and abrasions

Open wounds and abrasions generally appear warmer than surrounding skin. Wound surface temperatures will range between 31°C and 35°C (87.8°F and 95°F).[21] Temperatures are lower over wounds with eschars (devitalized tissue) versus wounds without eschars. Eschar is a thermal insulator and has no arterial circulation, thus it appears cooler than the surrounding wound.

Granulation tissue, consisting of an accumulation of fibroblasts and myofibroblasts, forms on the surfaces of a wound during the healing process. On a thermogram, granulation tissue appears mottled, with interspersed hot and cool areas due to uneven surface evaporation, avascular wound debris, and neovascularization (see Figure 10.4).

Bruises

Superficial hematomas experimentally induced by injecting 0.5 ml of fresh autologous blood into the dermis appear cool. Small areas of dermal ecchymosis (bruising) caused by intense manual tissue pinching appear red and 1°C to 5°C (1.8°F to 9°F) warmer than adjacent skin because the underlying tissue is inflamed by the injury.[22] Fresh blood outside of blood vessels

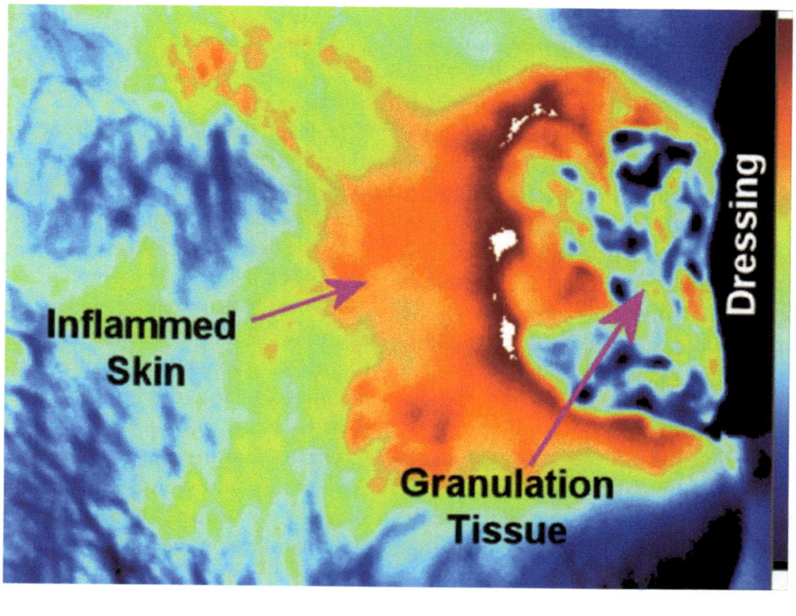

FIGURE 10.4 A large non-purulent granulating wound of the anterior upper chest wall – 35 yoM.

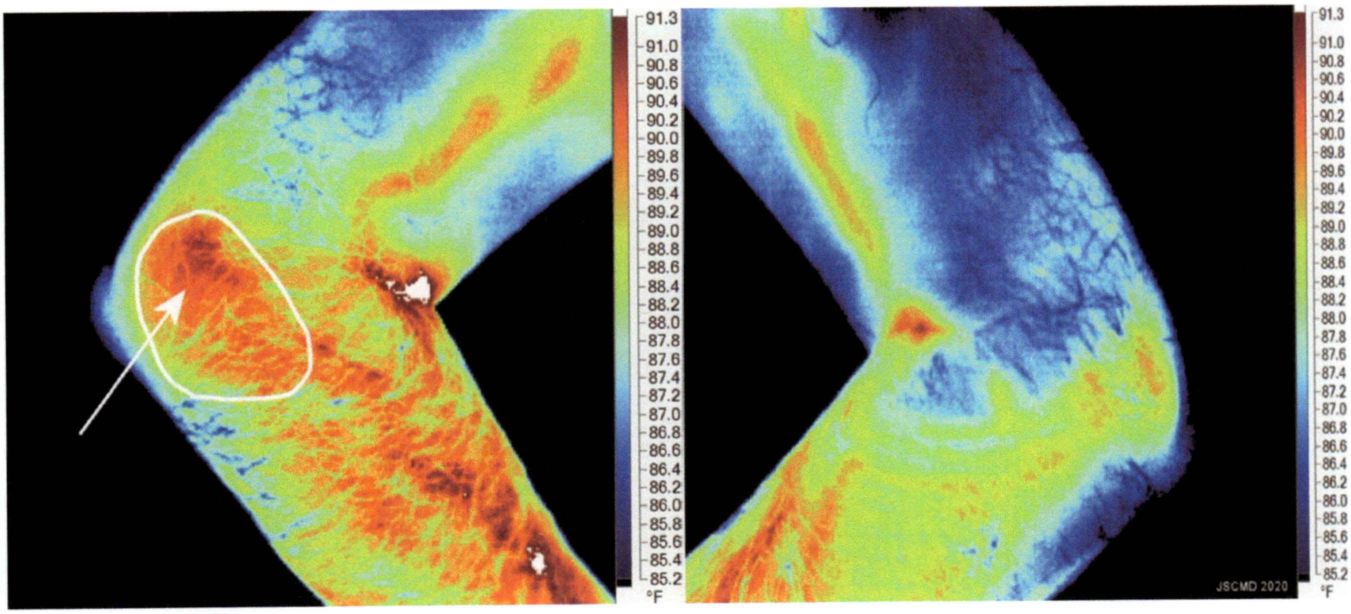

FIGURE 10.5 Isothermal images of both lateral elbows 3 hours after minor trauma to right epicondyle (arrow) with superficial ecchymosis outlined in white. The subject, a 76-year-old-male, has been cooled at 21°C for 15 minutes. Note non-traumatic warmth over wrist extensor muscles on the right and warm cephalic veins bilaterally.

attracts macrophages which emit NO as they help resolve the extravasated blood (Figure 10.5). The vasodilation effect of NO emitted around an ecchymosis is blunted, however, because extravasated hemoglobin neutralizes NO locally.[23] At times, a very large hematoma may organize into a mass surrounded by a rim of hyalinized fibrous tissue, chronic inflammatory infiltrate, and granulation tissue.[24] More research is needed into the thermographic appearance of acute and resolving hematomas.

Insect bites

Nontoxic insect bites such as mosquito, chigger, or flea bites generally produce vasodilation due to local histamine release, making them appear warm (Figure 10.6).[25] This thermal appearance should fade over several hours as itching and swelling decrease, though in some subjects, the local warmth and symptoms may last for several days.

Stings

Stings where an active toxin is injected dermally or subdermally, such as bee, wasp, or spider, may cause a spreading local hyperthermia that is thermographically visible for days after the envenomation event (Figure 10.7). As shown in Figure 10.8, scorpion envenomation may cause either hyperthermia or hypothermia. Spider bites almost always create an area of hyperthermia around the envenomation site (Figure 10.9). In addition, spider venoms that cause tissue necrosis, such as from the Brown Recluse spider

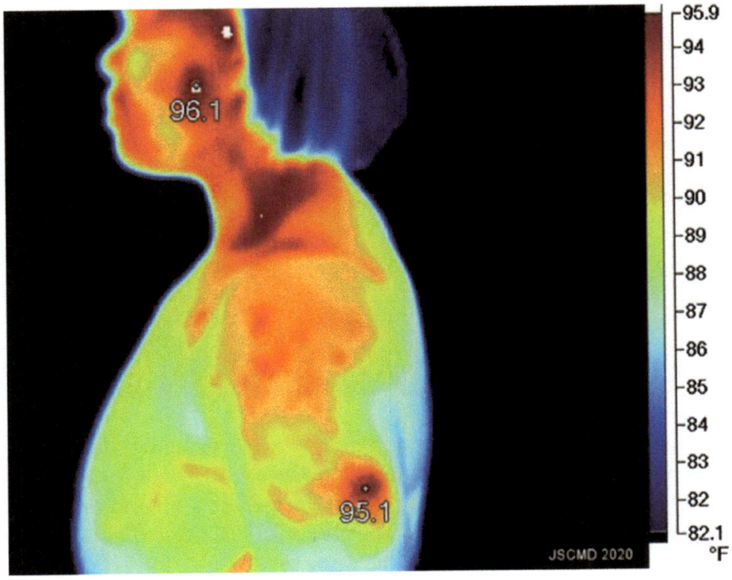

FIGURE 10.6 Mosquito bite reactions on the arm and cheek of a 12-year-old female.

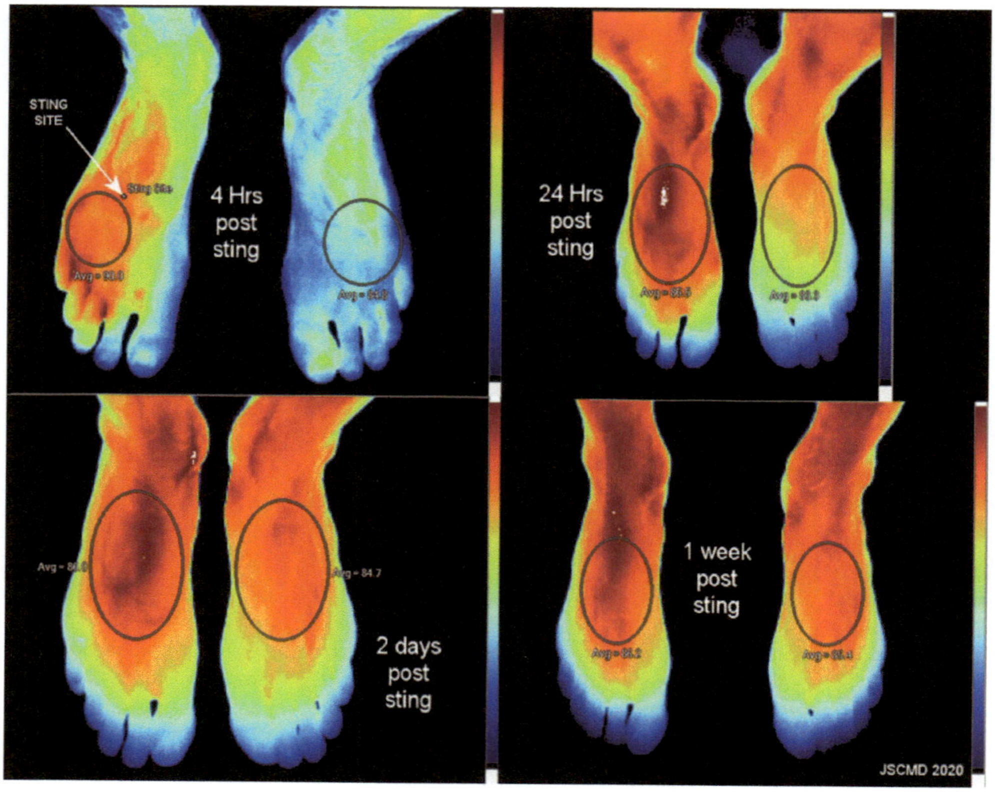

FIGURE 10.7 Hymenoptera sting progression in a 72-year-old male. The initial thermal reaction spread distally, then progressed proximally, fading over several days.

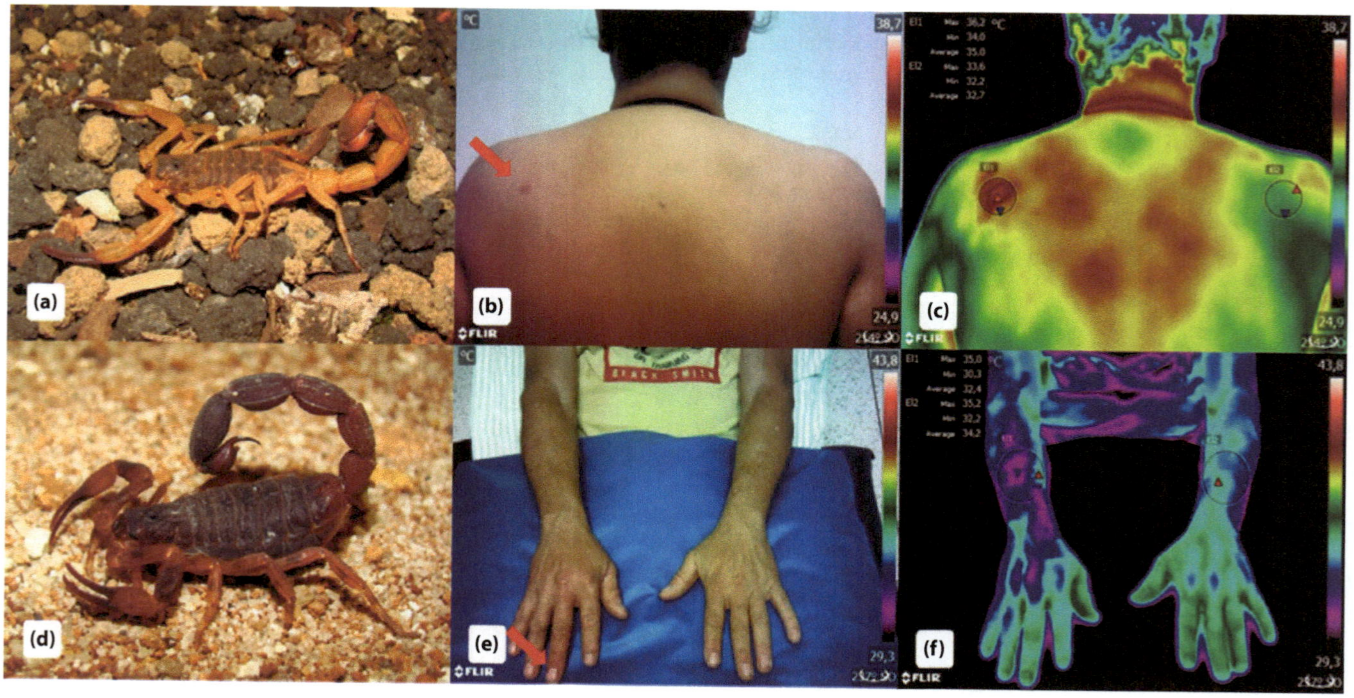

FIGURE 10.8 Scorpion stings. Case 1: A 16-year-old girl was stung by a scorpion identified as *Tityus serrulatus* (a) about 2 hours prior to admission to the hospital. Clinical examination on admission revealed a severe, localized, burning pain with a small area of erythema on the left scapular region (b). The infrared imaging (IR) performed on admission showed a significant temperature rise at the sting site ($\Delta T = 1.5°C$). (c). Case 2: A 49-year-old man was admitted with a *Tityus bahiensis* (d) scorpion sting on his right middle finger one hour before admission. He complained of local pain radiating to the whole forearm. He had a small area of erythema on the distal phalanx of the affected finger (e). The IR performed on admission showed a region with decreased temperature extending from the sting site to the elbow ($\Delta T = -1.8°C$) (f). (Images and captions thanks to Carlos Roberto de Medeiros et al., São Paulo, Brazil.[26])

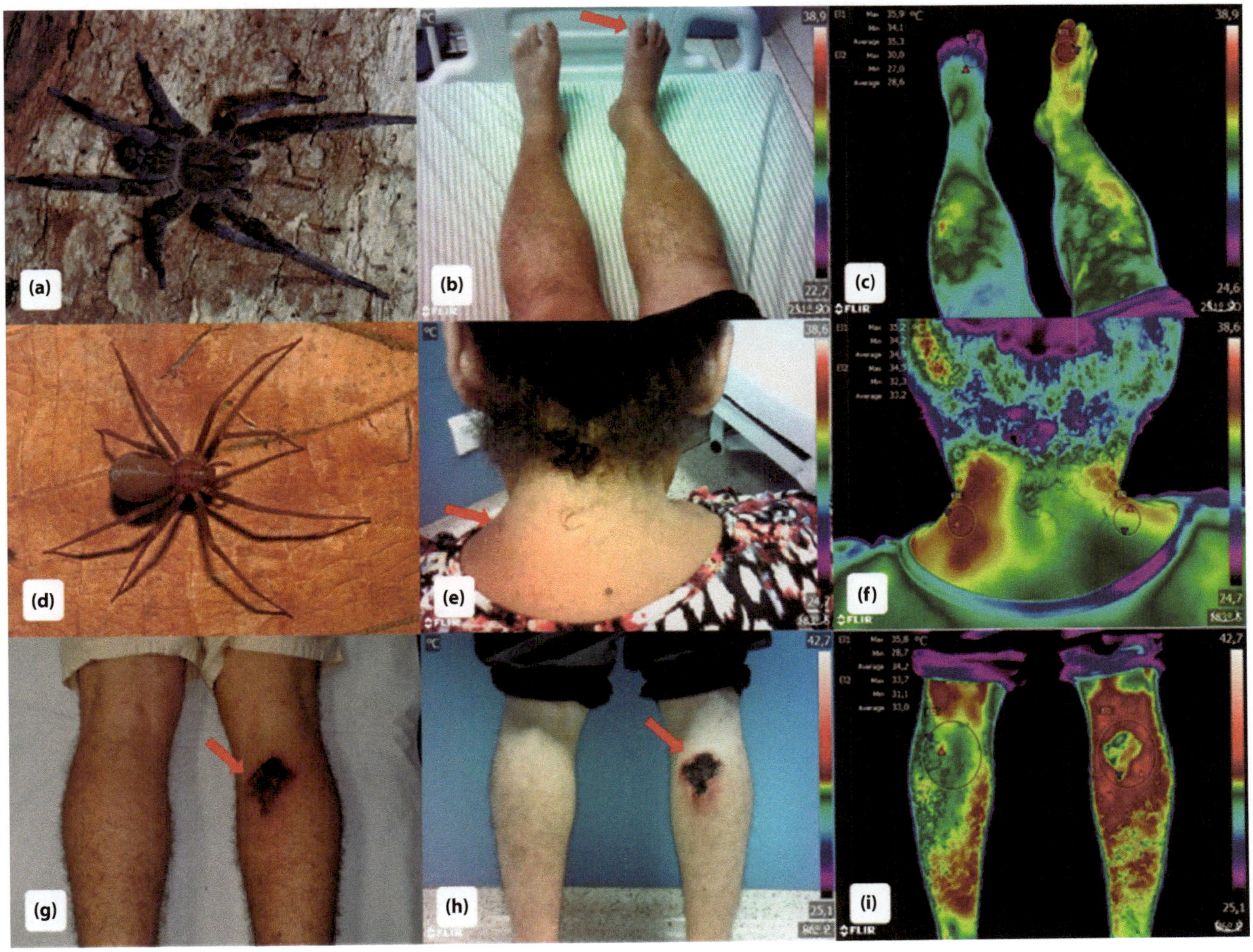

FIGURE 10.9 Spider bites. Case 1: A 56-year-old man was admitted to our hospital 2 hours and a half after being bitten on his right hallux by a Brazilian wandering spider identified as *Phoneutria nigriventer* (a). Clinical examination showed local severe burning pain radiating to the knee and a small area with erythema involving his right hallux (b). The infrared imaging (IR) performed on admission showed a region with increased temperature extending from the bite site to the knee ($\Delta T = 7.4°C$) (c). Case 2: A 71-year-old woman was bitten on her neck by a brown spider identified as *Loxosceles gaucho* (d). She visited the hospital about 19 hours after being bitten. She presented with an erythematous area of 4 × 2 cm in the right cervical region (e). There was no local necrosis. The IR performed on admission showed a significant increase in temperature at the bite region ($\Delta T = 2.2°C$) (f). Case 3: A 32-year-old man visited the hospital three days after being bitten by a brown spider (*Loxosceles* sp.) on his right popliteal region. Clinical examination showed an erythematous area of approximately 8 × 4 cm with a central brownish-crimson area of 5 × 6 cm with thin dark blisters (g). After 21 days of evolution, the wound had become a well-defined ulcer (h). The IR carried out at this time (i) showed significant asymmetry between the temperatures observed in both lower limbs ($\Delta T = 1.2°C$). In the affected leg, a central area with decreased temperature was observed, corresponding to the necrotic wound. (Images and captions thanks to Carlos Roberto de Medeiros et al., São Paulo, Brazil.[27])

(*Loxosceles reclusa*) may cause full-thickness damage to the subdermal tissues, with the destruction of arterioles to the skin. Hypothermic necrosis may be seen in such cases, similar to a full-thickness burn.

Snake bites

Snake bites and envenomation

Thermography used in the emergency room on patient arrival can determine the extent of venom diffusion from fang punctures associated with snake bites (Figure 10.10). Tissue damage can be determined and followed with subsequent thermal analysis as the hyperthermic area spreads and then diffuses. Equally important is the use of thermography to determine whether a snake bite has actually caused envenomation, in which case no significant hyperthermic reaction takes place.

Skin infections

Cellulitis

Cellulitis is a bacterial skin infection in which the skin appears red, warm, swollen, and painful to the touch. Ascending lymphangitis may also be present. Streptococci or staphylococci

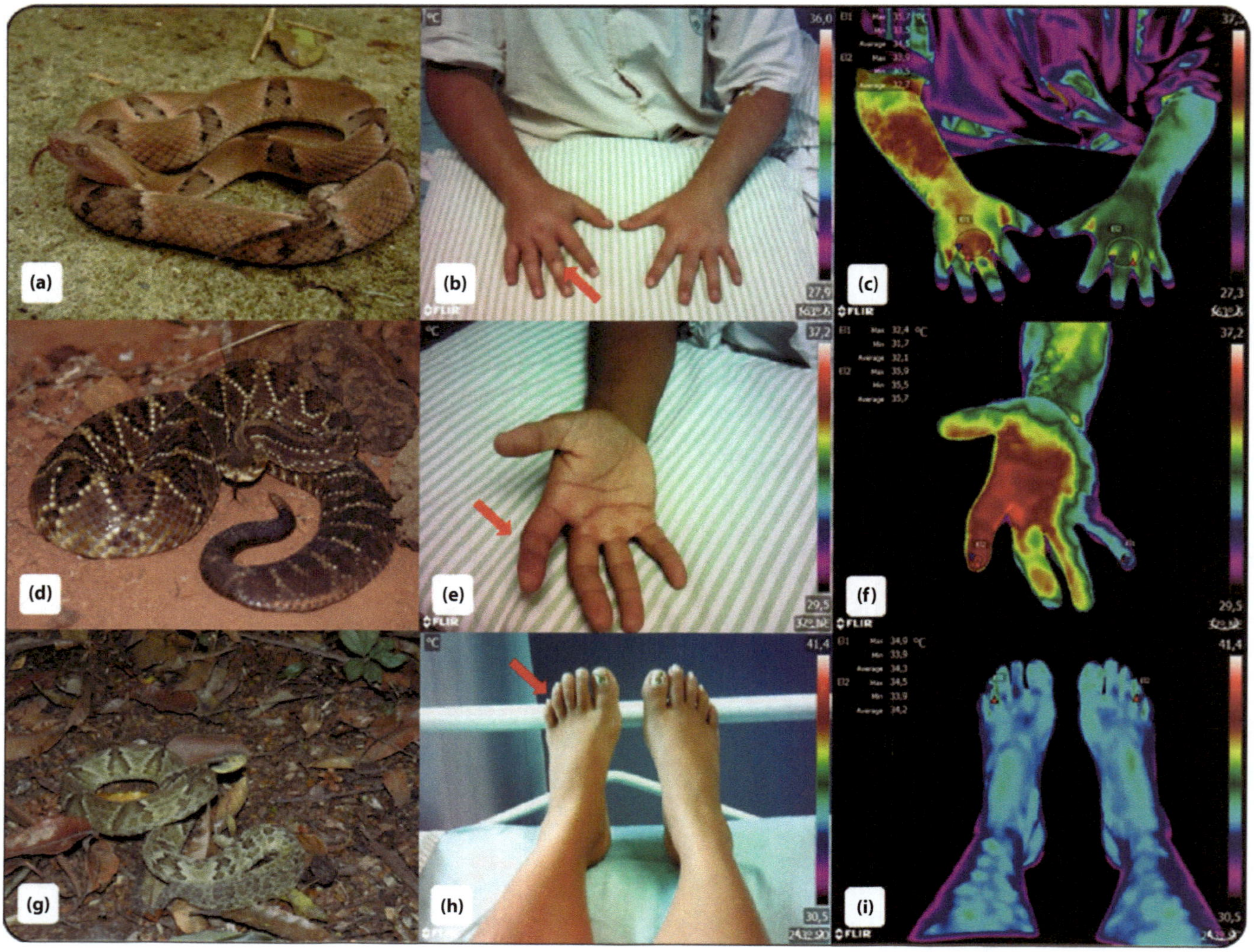

FIGURE 10.10 Snake bites. Case 1: A 28-year-old man was bitten on his right middle finger by a lance-headed viper identified as *Bothrops moojeni* (a) 15 minutes prior to arrival at the hospital. Erythema, marked edema, and two fang marks could be observed at the bite site (b). Infrared imaging (IR) conducted one day after the snakebite showed a significant asymmetry between the temperatures observed in both the bitten and the healthy upper limbs ($\Delta T = 1.8°C$) (c). Case 2: A 28-year-old healthy man was bitten by a rattlesnake (*Crotalus durissus* terrificus) (d) on his right index finger an hour and a half prior to arriving at the hospital. On arrival, he reported mild pain at the bite site, generalized myalgia, and visual impairment. He had a small erythematous lesion on his right index finger without swelling, (e) and pronounced ptosis. The IR conducted 10 hours after the snakebite showed a significant temperature rise at the bite site, as confirmed by the difference between the temperatures of the fingertips of the index and little fingers ($\Delta T = 3.6°C$) (f). Case 3: A 27-year-old woman was bitten on her left fourth toe by a lance-headed viper identified as *Bothrops jararaca* (g) about 2 hours prior to admission to the hospital. On arrival, she reported only pain at the bite site, with two localized fang marks, but without localized erythema, edema, ecchymosis, or systemic symptoms (h). Results of routine laboratory tests, including her coagulation profile, were normal. After 18 hours of observation, the patient showed no other symptoms, the diagnosis was considered to be a dry bite, and she was discharged without the use of antivenom. The IR performed at admission showed no asymmetry between the temperatures observed in both lower limbs ($\Delta T = 0°C$) (i). (Images and captions thanks to Carlos Roberto de Medeiros et al., São Paulo, Brazil.[28])

are the most likely causes. Severe cases of bacterial cellulitis can produce tissue damage, necrosis, disseminated infection, septic shock, and death. Nearly one in every three diagnoses of bacterial cellulitis is incorrect, however, resulting in the misuse of antibiotics.[29] Cellulitis must be differentiated from *pseudocellulitis*.[30] Since localized skin warmth is a characteristic feature of true cellulitis, thermography may help differentiate these conditions.

Cellulitis and pseudocellulitis can be distinguished using an infrared imager integrated into a smartphone, even in patients examined in an Emergency Department without thermal equilibration. (Note: EDs are usually kept cool to retard bacterial growth.)[31] Temperature gradients are significantly greater in cellulitis patients than in pseudocellulitis patients. Cellulitis areas show a mean maximum skin temperature 2.6°C (4.7°F) warmer than pseudocellulitis areas. Absolute temperature values should not be considered diagnostic due to the large temperature offset range of cellphone imagers.[32]

Differential temperature measurements are a more reliable indicator. True cellulitis is 3.7°C (6.6°F) warmer than the contralateral unaffected area; pseudocellulitis is about isothermal. A temperature difference of 0.47°C (0.85°F) determines true cellulitis with 97% sensitivity, detecting all of the cellulitis patients and half the pseudocellulitis patients correctly.[33] Thermography, even in ED settings, can differentiate true- from pseudo-cellulitis in most cases. Further studies using calibrated thermal imagers are needed.

Skin abscess (boils)

Bacterial abscesses of the skin exhibit a circumscribed warm zone on infrared images of a properly cooled subject (Figure 10.11). Skin abscesses can range in size from small facial pimples to large swollen lesions. Staphylococcal bacteria are implicated in most cases. As a dermal abscess matures, it becomes white in the center from the erosion of the underlying pus – "pointing." Pus is non-metabolizing debris, so pointing may appear cooler than the surrounding inflammation; thermographic studies are needed to confirm this. As the abscess resolves by either spontaneous involution or external drainage, the warm zone slowly resolves over several days or weeks as the local inflammation recedes. Fully-resolved abscesses are usually not visible to infrared imaging, although they may leave a visible scar.

Pressure ulcers (decubitus ulcers, bedsores)

Incapacitated or paralyzed patients are at high risk of developing bedsores because they tend to spend long periods in a sedentary mode, damaging the skin that overlies bony areas of the body.[34] The prolonged pressure results in local ischemia, eventually producing tissue necrosis.[35] Chronic pressure ulcers show inflammation and disruption of the collagen matrix.[36]

The early visual signs of bedsores (erythema or purple discoloration) may be missed in darkly pigmented individuals. Infrared imaging, however, can detect pressure ulcers in all patients equally. [37] Thermography is useful as a bedside technology for the early detection of pressure ulcers.[38] The ischemic tissue from pressure ulcers will appear blue (cooler) on a thermogram.[39] This qualitatively "cooler" thermogram indicates ischemia that may not be visible to the human eye.

Decubitus wound scores (0 = favorable, 16 = unfavorable) are directly correlated with wound bed temperature. As this score increases, the thermographically detected wound temperature increases.[40] Classifying pressure ulcers based on temperature can help predict healing at three weeks, even though the pressure ulcer's visual appearances may not have changed appreciably. A higher temperature in the wound site relative to the peri-wound skin may imply the presence of infection.[41]

Incipient pressure ulcers can be detected by thermography on hospital admission. Even under non-ideal thermographic conditions with room temperatures between 18°C and 29°C (64.4°F and 84.2°F) and an "acclimatization time" as short as 30 seconds, a temperature difference between a pressure area and the surrounding unaffected skin can detect possible decubiti. Differential temperatures between –2.5°C and –6°C (–4.5°F and –10.8°F) are found in ischemic conditions, while temperatures between +0.8°C and +2°C (+1.4°F and +3.6°F) indicate reactive inflammation from partial ischemia or perhaps infected skin areas.[42] In the absence of infection, decubitus-prone areas appearing hyperthermic indicate patent subdermal vasculature capable of supplying the skin when pressure is relieved. A cooler decubital area indicates damage to the subdermal vasculature and a poorer prognosis for circulatory recovery.[43]

Skin tumors

Dermal neoplasms are important to examine whether they are malignant or benign. Static thermography can determine whether a skin growth is cooler than the surrounding skin, in which case it is almost universally benign. Skin lesions warmer than surrounding skin may be due to malignancy, infection, or increased local circulation (benign A-V malformations, small skin varicosities, etc.) among other causes. Kaposi's sarcoma and infantile hemangiomas, both highly vascular skin growths, appear warmer than the surrounding normal skin.[44] Malignant lesions, however, may often appear to be the same temperature as the surrounding skin, and may not be noticeable in static images, especially if they are small (diameter under 5 mm/0.2 in.).[45]

To fully assess skin malignancy requires dynamic thermography. The basic dynamic technique is to cool the lesion and some surrounding normal-appearing skin, then stop the cooling suddenly

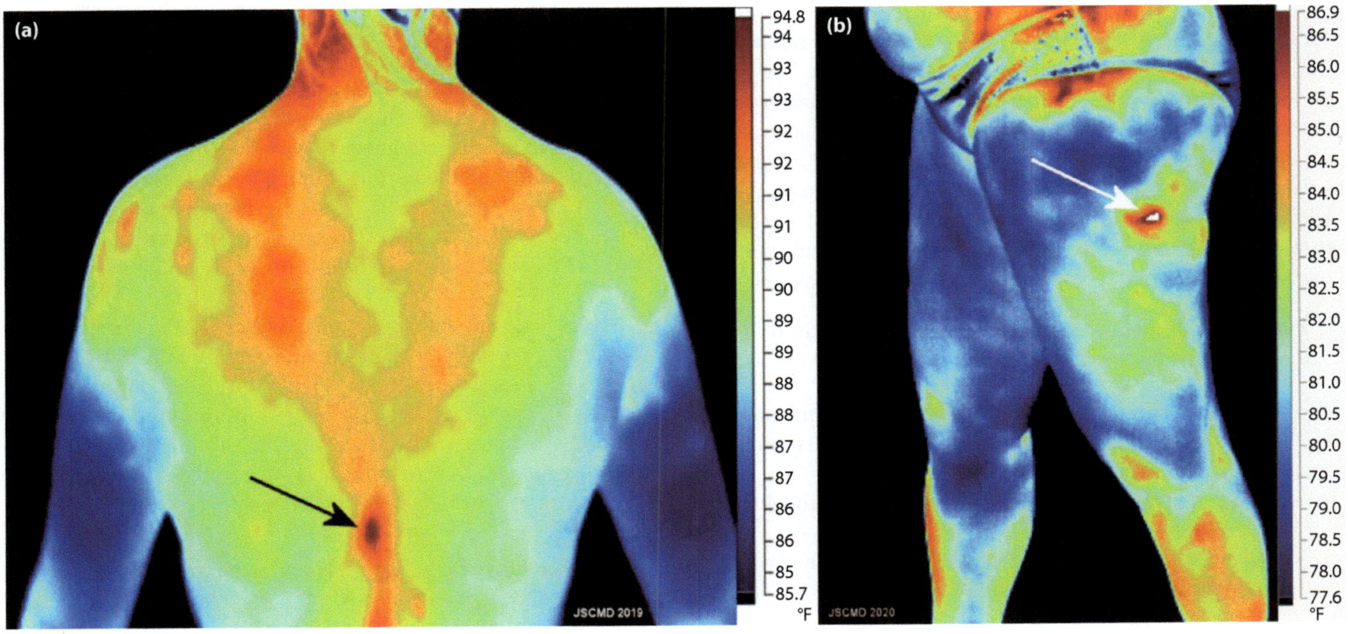

FIGURE 10.11 (a) An early abscess over lower thoracic spine. – 29 yoF. (b) A small skin abscess over the left lateral thigh. – 52 yoF.

and take multiple timed thermograms of the area as it warms back toward baseline temperature. Because malignant skin tumors generally emit nitric oxide and may have more arterial vasculature than the surrounding healthy skin, the lesions warm up significantly faster and can thus be characterized by thermography.[46]

A suspect skin tumor that appears to be the same temperature of the surrounding skin on static thermography can be further examined using dynamic thermography. Some dynamic detection methods have claimed sensitivity and specificity values greater than 99% in skin cancer detection using extremely complicated mathematical analysis. Because such esoteric approaches may be unavailable to the general thermographer, however, a simpler method for detecting malignant melanoma will be described here. As dynamic rewarming techniques have been shown to detect squamous and basal cell skin carcinomas, the protocol shown below for melanoma may also be applied to the detection of these other common skin malignancies.[47]

Malignant melanoma

Malignant melanoma is the deadliest of all skin cancer types.[48] Early detection is critical for improving survival.[49] The standard practice is to biopsy any pigmented lesion that is clinically concerning.[50] Non-pigmented melanomas, which make up two to eight percent of all melanomas, must also be anticipated.[51] Imaging methods that enable accurate detection of melanoma are needed. Thermography is a non-invasive method that can lessen the need for biopsy and offer a way to detect and monitor melanoma.[52]

Thermography can differentiate malignant melanoma from benign skin lesions. In a recent trial, 251 palpable lesions were assessed by thermography. Malignant lesions less than 15 mm in size were differentiated from benign lesions with 100% specificity and 95% sensitivity. The imaging was well tolerated and easily implemented.[53] Comparing the difference in thermal responses between healthy and malignant tissue and matching the data with biopsy results, heightened metabolic activity and increased blood perfusion of a melanoma can be detected via infrared imaging.[54]

To dynamically detect malignant dermal lesions, an approach called *Quantification Analysis of Induced Thermography* (QUAINT) has been developed. The test entails local conductive cooling to induce a known change in skin temperature over the tumor and surrounding normal skin. The cooling is then rapidly removed and the skin rewarming is monitored by thermography. The cooling period is relatively short (60 seconds); the skin surface is cooled about 10°C to 15°C (18°F to 27°F) below normal. When evaluating a melanoma lesion, a small area of skin (nominally 4 × 4 cm/1.6 × 1.6 in.) including the suspect neoplasm is actively cooled and then allowed to rewarm. The thermographer measures surface temperature differences between the lesion and the surrounding healthy tissue during thermal recovery. The procedure is as follows:

Evaluation of melanomas via the QUAINT Method

Required environment and equipment:

- This test should be done in a cool environment (20°C, 68°F) to observe skin rewarming by the lesion (and not the environment).
- The patient should be in a sympathetically vasoconstricted state.
- A small therapeutic gel pack at nominal thermography room temperature (20°C, 68°F).[55]
- Three or more small (1–2 mm) adhesive metal foil "fiducial" markers are placed around the lesion so it can be located in the thermal and visual images later.

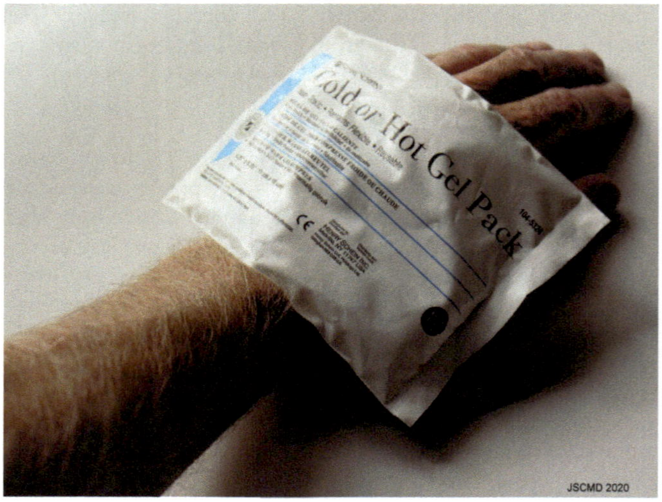

FIGURE 10.12 QUAINT dynamic thermal analysis cooling technique: A room temperature (20°C, 68°F) gel pack is applied over the suspected dermal lesion for 1 minute.

Procedure:

- An initial thermogram and a visible-light image are taken as a baseline. The lesion is usually not apparent in this static thermal image. The small foil markers should be visible in both images.
- The cooling gel pack is lightly applied to the lesion and surrounding healthy skin for 60 seconds (Figure 10.12).
- After removal of the cool pack (T = 0 sec), close-up radiometric thermal images are taken at T = 30, 40, 50, and 60 seconds.
- An active malignant melanoma will warm up faster than the surrounding healthy skin due to increased metabolism and NO production within the tumor. This can be detected and measured in the sequential images. As NO diffuses easily through tissues, the warm area may appear larger than the visible lesion.
- A rewarming lesion minus normal-surrounding-skin temperature difference (ΔT) of +0.3 to 3°C (+0.5 to 5.4°F) at 50 to 60 seconds is positive for malignancy. A properly-scaled graph of the tumor and peripheral skin temperatures can provide more confidence in the results (Figure 10.13).
- Non-malignant lesions will have the same thermal recovery, or less, than the healthy tissue; ΔT will be zero or negative.
- Caveat: Melanoma *in situ* may not respond thermally as described above. When in doubt, an adequate excision biopsy of the small lesion will diagnose and may cure at the same time.

Metastatic malignant melanoma lesions located in or just below the dermis are warmer than surrounding skin on static thermographic images (Figure 10.14).[56] This is probably due to NO production in the metastatic tumor or from immune responses by the body in its attempt to fight off the invading cells. A general thermography skin screening may pick up these metastases by detecting their pathologic hyperthermia.

Moles, warts, and other benign neoplasms

Dermal papillomas, actinic keratosis, moles, lipomas, and other benign skin neoplasms usually appear cool on static thermal images (see Figures 10.15 and 10.16) and show a similar or slower

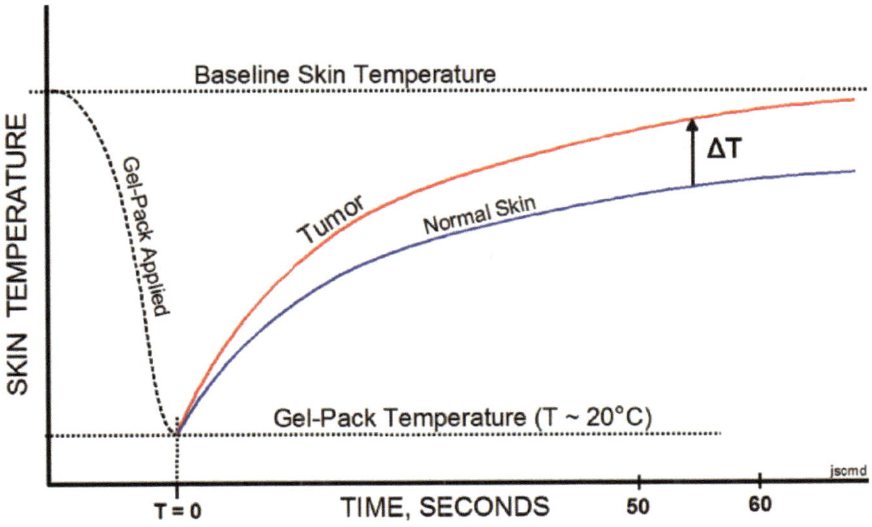

FIGURE 10.13 Graph depicting the basic principle of QUAINT dynamic rewarming thermography to detect skin malignancy. The cool gel-pack is removed from the skin surface at t = 0; ΔT is measured between 50 and 60 seconds later.

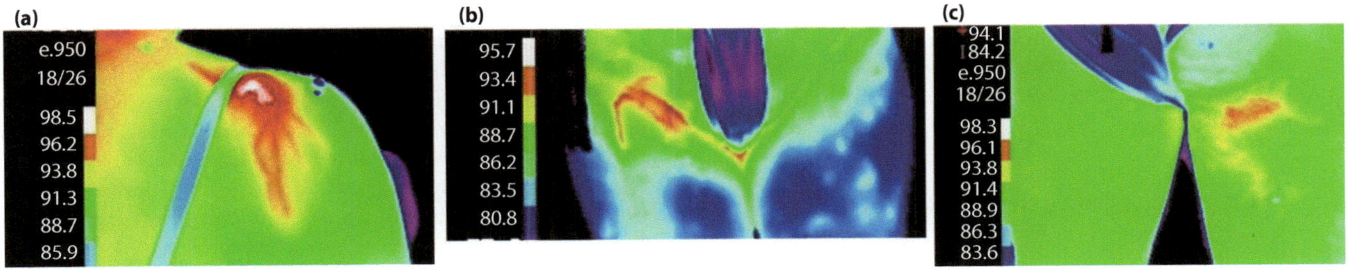

FIGURE 10.14 Examples of hyperthermic malignant melanoma metastases are shown (a) on the top of the left shoulder, (b) in the right groin, and (c) in the upper left thigh. Note the lymphatic inflammatory patterns accompanying the warm areas.[57]

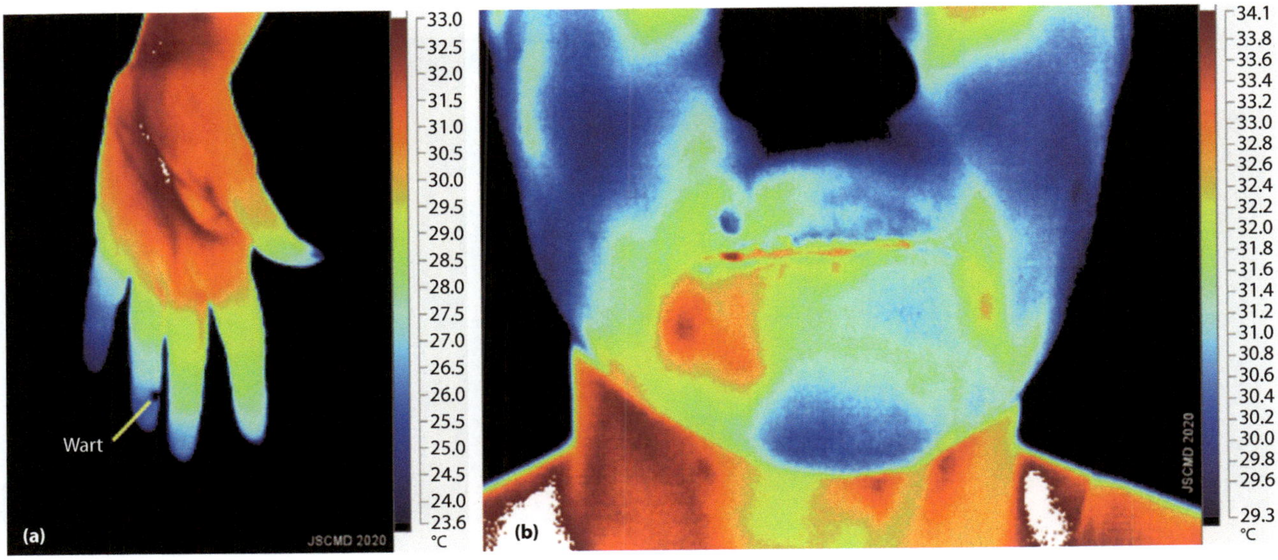

FIGURE 10.15 (a) Common warts (verruca vulgaris) appear cool unless inflamed by traumatic or escharotic attempts to remove them. – 67 yoF. (b) This hirsute mole on the right upper lip appears cool – 46 yoF.

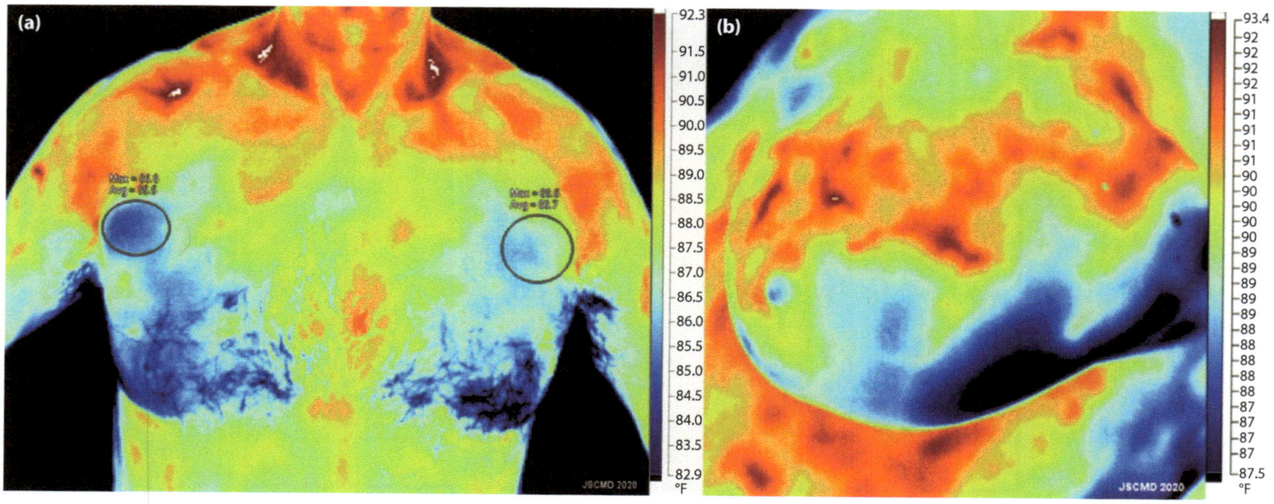

FIGURE 10.16 (a) A benign, mobile 4-cm lipoma over the right pectoralis tendon (circled) appears cooler than the left. (b) Multiple fibroepithelial papillomas in the left axilla appear as cool spots. – 57 yoF.

rewarming curve compared to normal adjacent skin when subject to dynamic techniques such as QUAINT. Thermography is a reliable non-invasive method in the detection and post-treatment follow-up of hemangiomas, vascular malformations, and vascular growth after biomaterial implants in the pediatric population.[58]

Other thermographic skin findings

Dermatographia

Dermatographia (also called dermographism or "skin writing") appears warm in infrared images. If the scratched or otherwise traumatized skin becomes red and elevated, it is called red dermographism, which is a diagnostic finding of physical urticaria. If the site becomes white, it is called white dermographism; this is usually seen in patients with atopic dermatitis.[59] Whether thermography can discern white from red dermographism remains to be studied.

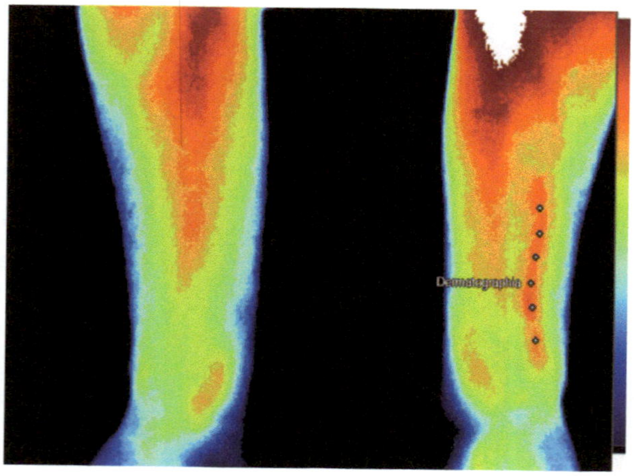

FIGURE 10.17 Red dermatographia from a fingernail scratch (marked) appears warmer than the local skin. – 57 yoM.

Glomus dilation and arterial perforators

Glomus bodies (arteriovenous anastomoses, or AVAs) are microscopic arterio-venous shunts located just under the skin surface. They are scattered throughout the skin of the body, and are most concentrated in the fingernail beds, volar fingers, and palms; the concentration of AVAs in the toenail beds is not as great as in the fingernails. AVAs are physiologically dilated after exercise (Figure 10.18). Because of their distal (acral) location, glomus bodies in the hands and feet provide excellent heat dissipation to the external environment. When sympathetic adrenergic tone is reduced post-exercise, AVAs shunt warm arterial blood into the returning veins just under the skin, where they increase dermal radiative and convective heat loss.

When the body is cooled down below 21°C (70°F) for thermographic imaging, the glomus bodies (AVAs) should close. The physiologic control of glomus dilation is not completely understood.

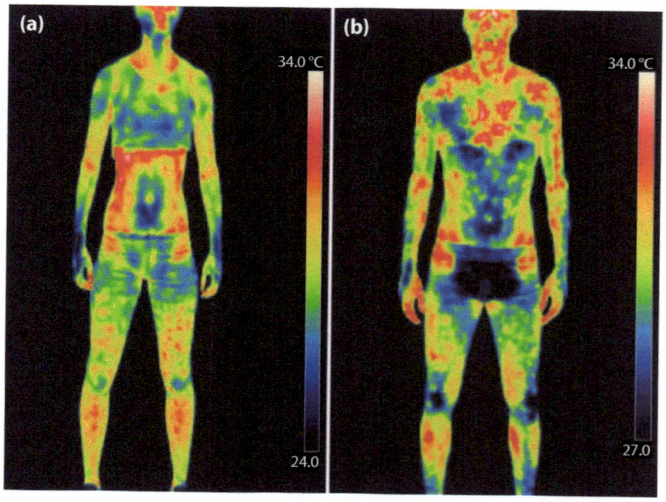

FIGURE 10.18 Post-exercise glomus AVA dilation patterns, anterior. Note the warm hands and arm veins. (a) Female. (b) Male.[60]

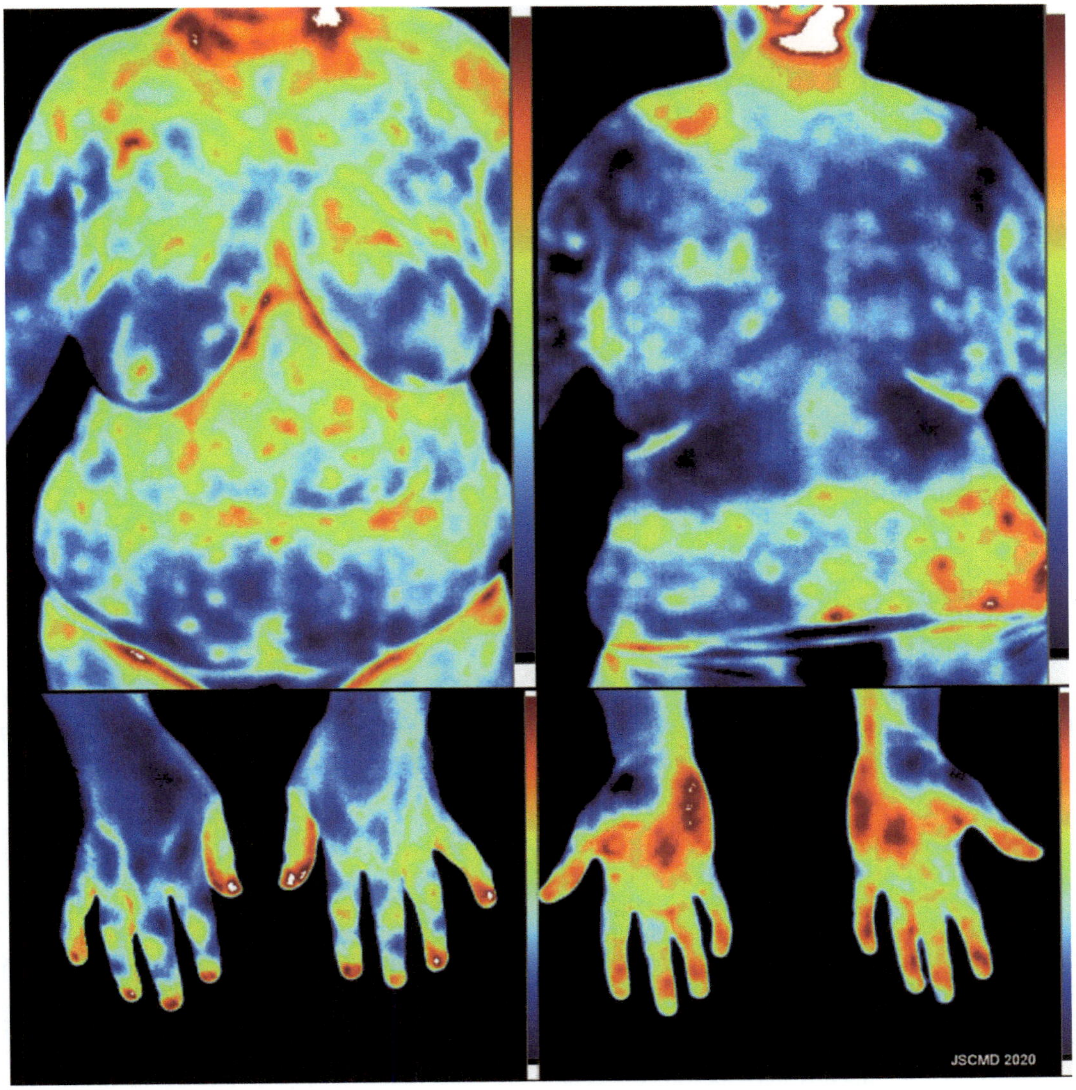

FIGURE 10.19 Extensive paradoxical glomus dilation (PGD) pattern in a cooled subject with lupus erythematosus. – 53 yoF.

AVAs can be dilated paradoxically after equilibration below 21°C (70°F) by certain disease states and medications (Figure 10.19). Increased levels of circulating NO present in autoimmune and other diseases may be implicated in this phenomenon. Glomus dilation of the trunk may or may not be accompanied by glomus dilation in the hands, and *vice versa*.

Arterial perforators are subdermal vascular bundles containing a small artery and accompanying veins. They carry blood through the body's subdermal fat layers to supply the skin. These vascular perforators are important to locate and preserve when mobilizing skin flaps in surgical procedures. The thermal appearance of arterial perforators may be hard to distinguish from a glomus AVA dilation pattern (Figure 10.20). Perforator vessel sites in the legs have been found to coincide statistically with acupuncture points.[61] Although this finding may guide practitioners in the rough location of perforator sites, static or dynamic thermography of a cooled subject combined with Doppler ultrasound imaging is recommended to confirm their actual locations. See the subsection on Plastic Surgery in Chapter 11 for more information.

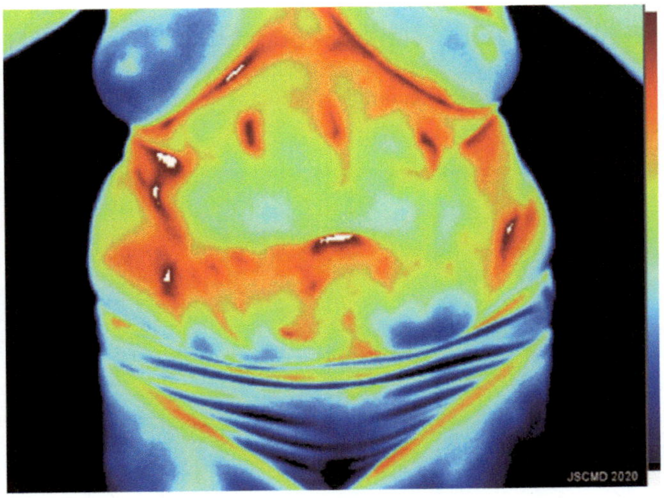

FIGURE 10.20 Abdominal vascular perforator pattern in a cooled 64-year-old female. This pattern may be confused with that of glomus AVA dilation of the abdominal wall.

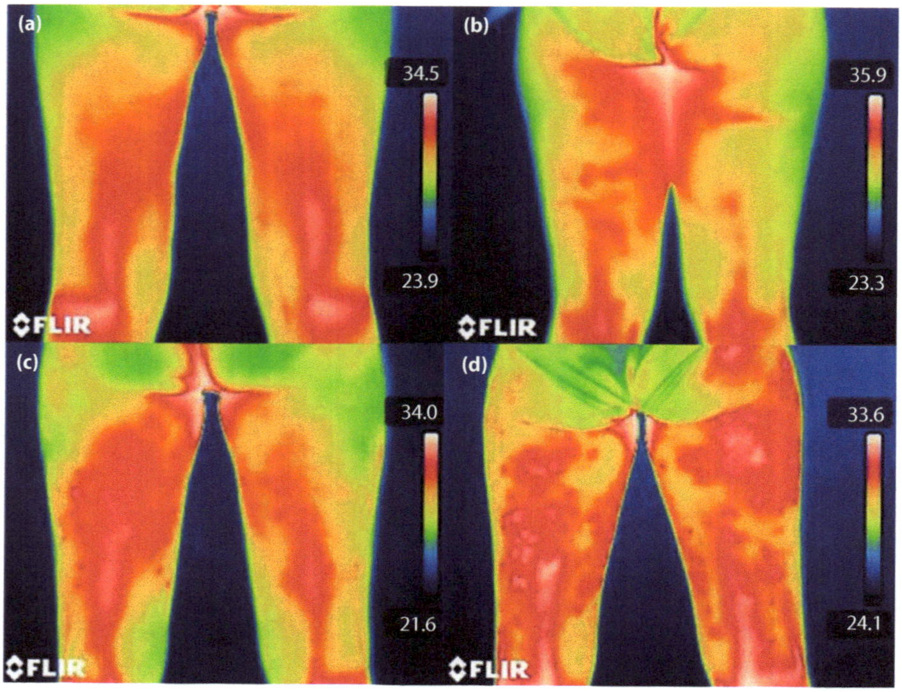

FIGURE 10.21 Stages of gynoid lipodystrophy as seen thermographically over the posterior upper legs. (a) Stage 0: cellulite-free skin. (b) Stage 1: mild cellulite. (c) Stage 2: moderate cellulite. (d) Stage 3: severe cellulite.[64]

Gynoid lipodystrophy (cellulite)

Gynoid lipodystrophy (GLD), more commonly referred to as cellulite, mainly affects females beginning in puberty, progressing with age. GLD is a structural, inflammatory, and biochemical condition affecting subcutaneous tissues, resulting in dimpling of the skin over the buttocks, legs, and abdomen, with less involvement of the breasts and upper body.[62] Due to the low-grade inflammatory component, GLD may be detected and staged thermographically (Figure 10.21).[63] The thermal appearance of cellulite may be confused with glomus AVA dilation, varicose veins, or arterial perforators.

Thermography of the head and face

The cranium is normally warmer than the face (Figure 10.22). This is likely due to the 12 watts of heat constantly generated by the brain, representing about 16% of the resting body energy.[65] Besides being carried by blood convection down the right jugular vein (in most cases), diploic veins between the two layers of the skull remove some of this cerebral heat. The cerebrospinal fluid circulation also helps remove some heat produced by the brain.[66] The remaining heat is conducted through the bones of the skull, which are in close contact with the overlying skin. The scalp may remain warm even during physiologic sympathetic vasoconstriction of the face and body.

Statistically, the face is not thermally symmetric. Although studies using older infrared scanners reported a close sagittal symmetry of face and body skin temperatures, more recent studies using thermally calibrated microbolometer imagers have shown that the right side of the face is often, but not always, warmer than the left. The histogram in Figure 10.23 shows this imbalance in maxillary temperatures. The tendency toward increased temperatures on the right is also seen in the mouth and the corneal areas.[67]

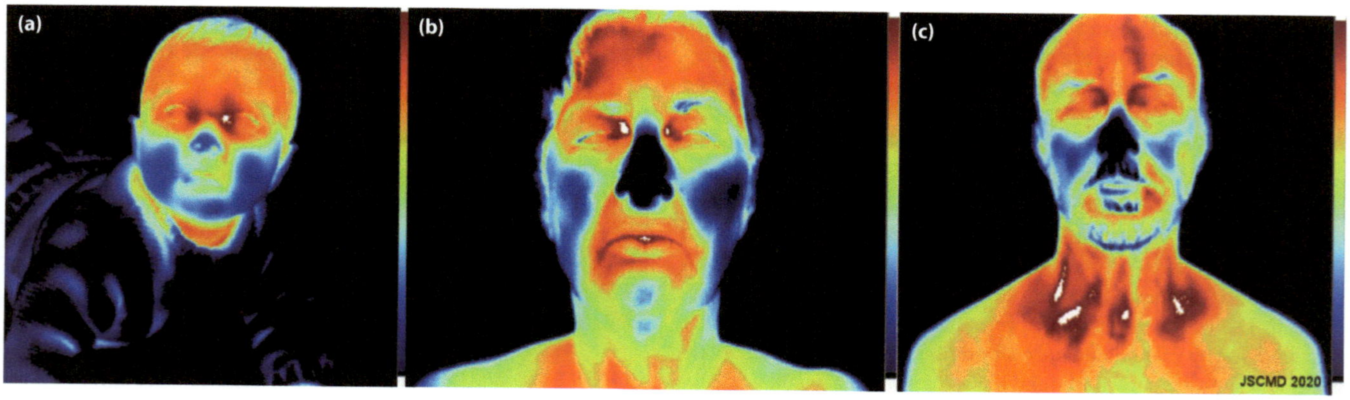

FIGURE 10.22 The cranium is normally warmer than the face. (a) 7-month-old male, (b) 72-year-old female, (c) 74-year-old male.

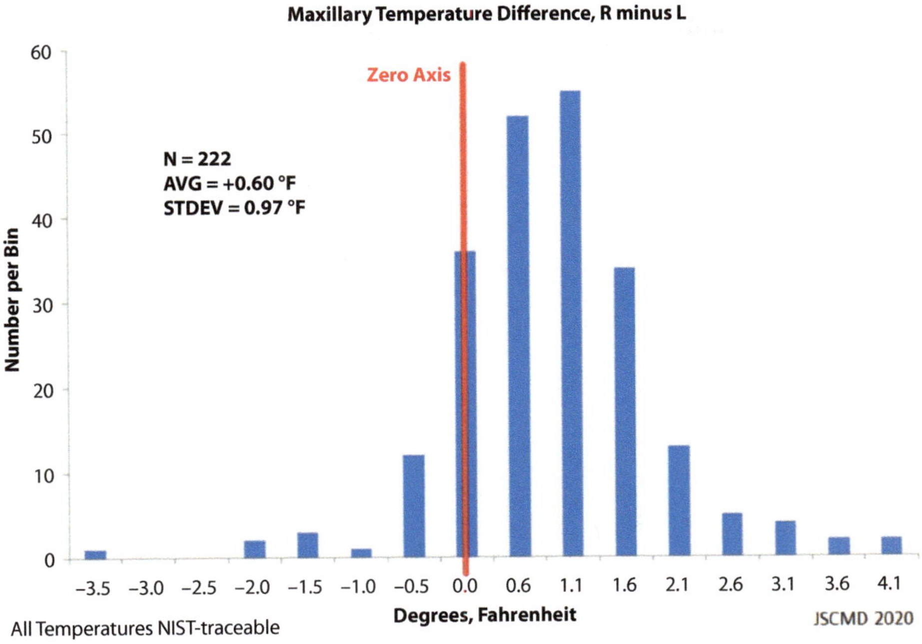

FIGURE 10.23 Histogram showing the sagittal thermal imbalance over the maxillary areas of 222 subjects undergoing routine thermographic imaging. The right maxillae averaged 0.60°F (0.33°C) warmer than the left.

Autonomic enervation patterns of the face

The face is supplied by three types of autonomic nerves, each having their own anatomic enervation area and effect on skin circulation.[68] The basic patterns of autonomic vascular control of the face are as follows:

1. **Sympathetic vasodilation** occurs all over the face except the lips and eyes (Figure 10.24). This strong mechanism brings blood to the face especially when the body is warm; it is the likely neural carrier of the blushing reaction. This effect will show up best when the subject is warm.
2. **Sympathetic vasoconstriction** of the face is usually seen in a cooled subject (Figure 10.25). It is most pronounced over the eyes, nose, lips, and ears, but it occurs over all facial skin surfaces.
3. **Parasympathetic vasodilation** occurs over the central portion of the face, and can be triggered by eating very spicy foods or otherwise irritating the eye, nose, or mouth (Figure 10.26). Other causes of parasympathetic vasodilation remain to be studied. This pattern may appear stronger on one side of the face (see Figure 10.27). Patients with clinical Rosacea may have this same thermographic appearance.[69] Whether the parasympathetic vasodilation pattern is associated with Rosacea or is a coincidental appearance requires further study.

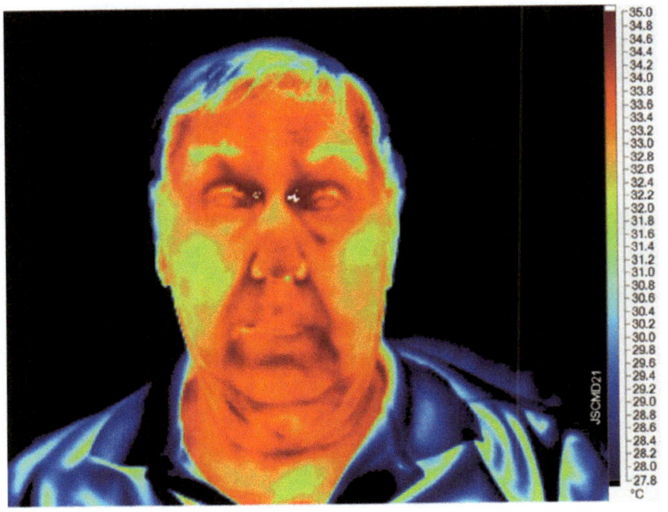

FIGURE 10.24 Sympathetic vasodilation pattern over the face of a clothed and warm subject. All skin surfaces are vasodilated by this neural stimulation, including the nose and ears. Sweat droplets are not present – 71-year-old male.

Autonomic imbalance

The autonomic enervation patterns of the body are usually bilateral, but "autonomic imbalance," due to variations in the autonomic tone of the two sympathetic nerve trunks, may occur over either side of the face and neck, perhaps from trauma, surgery, or congenital variations (Figures 10.28 and 10.29). This is an important finding and should be reported. The side that appears *cooler* has the greater sympathetic vasoconstrictor tone. This type of autonomic imbalance seems stronger than the statistical tendency toward increased temperatures over the right side of the face.

Ocular thermography

The eyes and the other structures of the orbits and surrounding skin are important to observe during thermographic imaging and interpretation. Facial images should be taken at close range to maximize ocular detail. Eyeglasses and contact lenses are best removed before temperature equilibration to avoid any thermal artifacts they may create (Figure 10.30). Subjects should be instructed to open the eyes fully during image acquisition. Additional images with the eyes closed may be useful to define certain ocular pathologies.

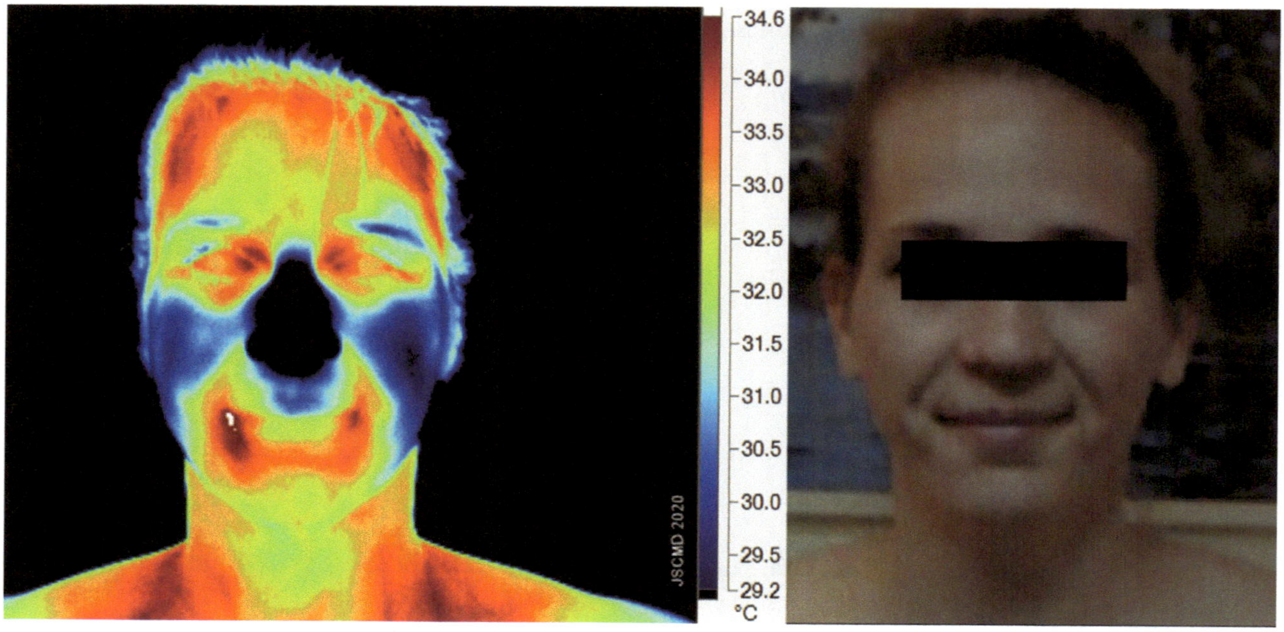

FIGURE 10.25 Sympathetic vasoconstriction pattern over the face of a cooled subject, a 27-year-old female. This is the normal facial appearance of a person properly cooled for a thermographic examination.

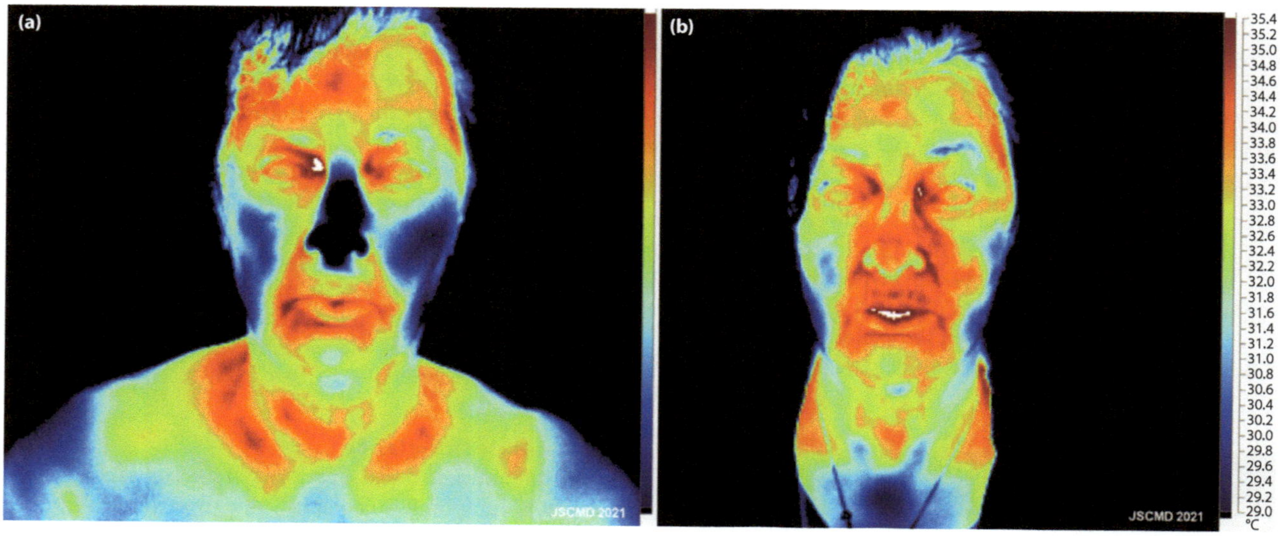

FIGURE 10.26 (a) Sympathetic vasoconstriction and (b) parasympathetic vasodilation thermal patterns of the face in the same subject about one year apart. – 77 yoF.

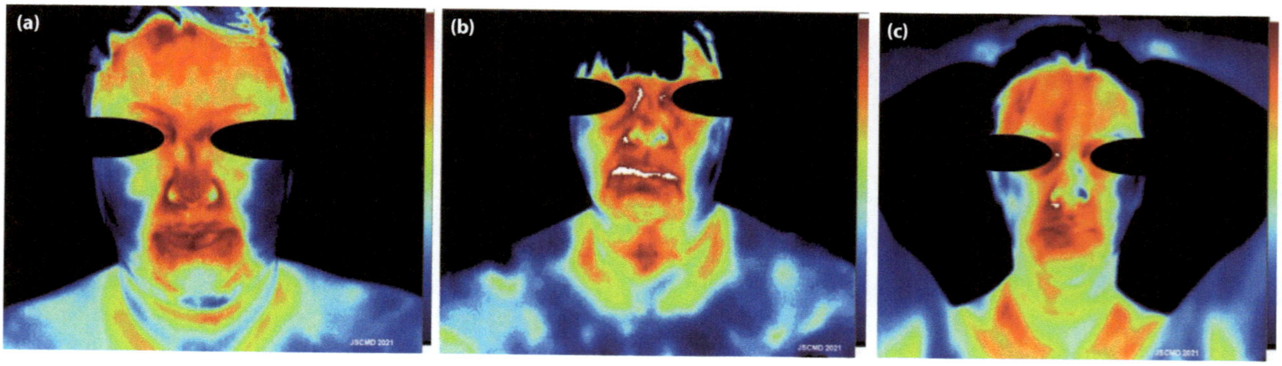

FIGURE 10.27 Parasympathetic vasodilation patterns of the face. The central portion of the face, including the nose, remains warm even after thermal equilibration at 20°C. Note that the ears are cool, unlike the pattern seen with sympathetic vasodilation. (a) 45-year-old female, (b) 63-year-old female, (c) 40-year-old female.

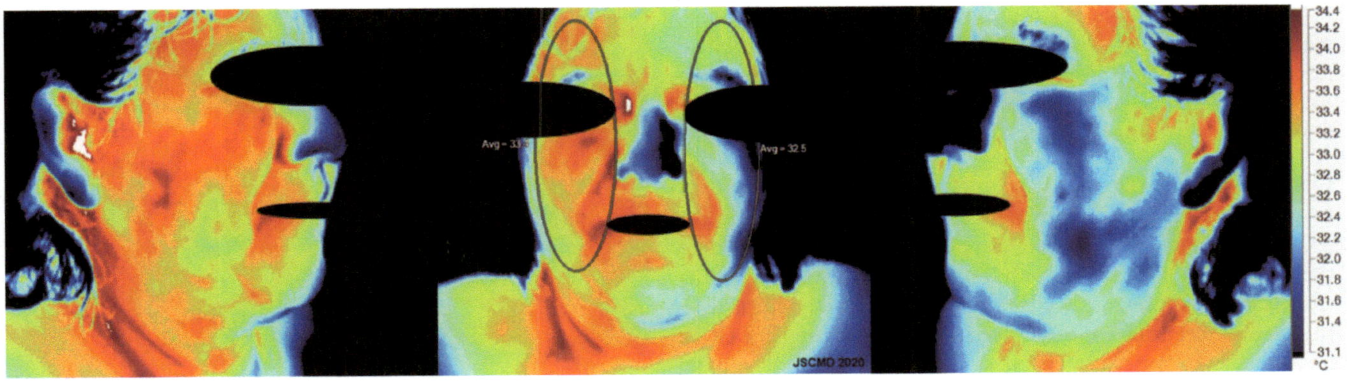

FIGURE 10.28 Isothermal views of sympathetic vasoconstrictor imbalance involving the face and neck. The sympathetic tone is greater on the patient's left. – 55-year-old female.

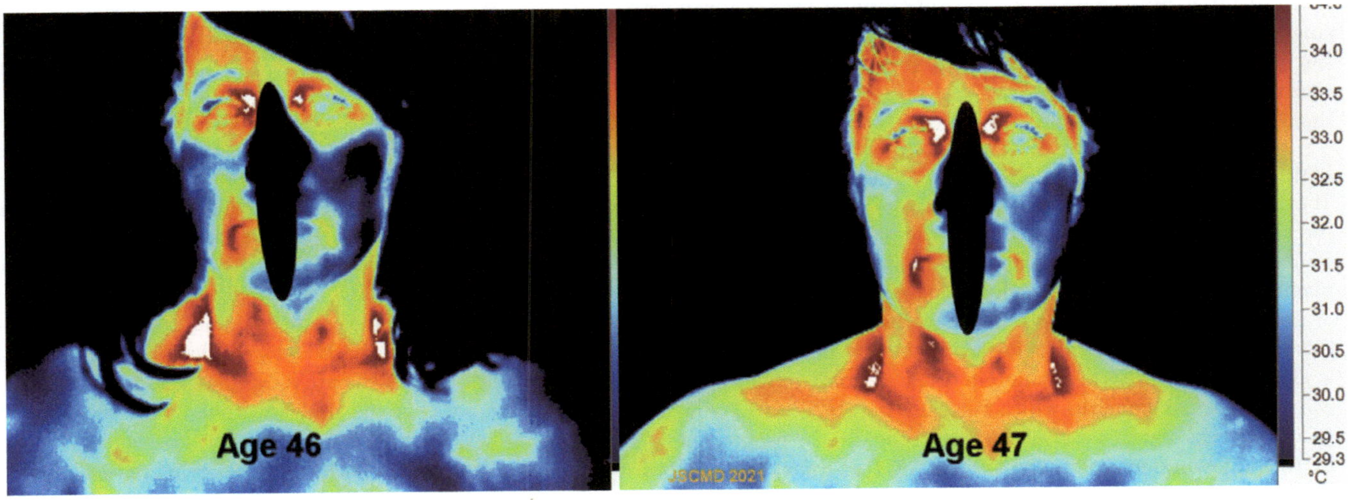

FIGURE 10.29 Sympathetic vasoconstrictor imbalance of the face. Images of the same subject. Note the corneal and mid-face temperatures. The sympathetic tone is greater on the left.

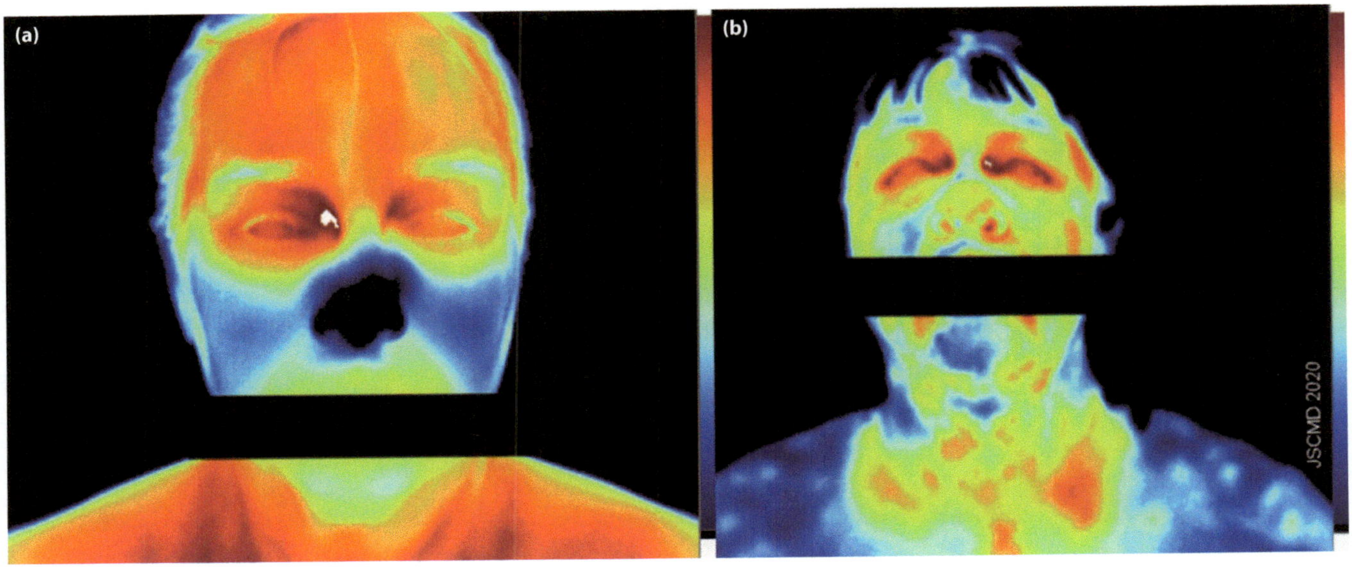

FIGURE 10.30 Eye artifact: Subjects equilibrated wearing eyeglasses; took them off just before images were taken. (a) 48-year-old female, (b) 60-year old female.

Ocular thermography is a complicated sub-specialty. If abnormalities are found on thermal imaging, the patient should be informed and referral for ophthalmic examination may be indicated. Much more detailed information can be found in the Ophthalmic Thermography section of Chapter 11.

Orbital vasculature

In the periorbital areas, the veins are larger in diameter, have less of a muscular wall, and are almost the same temperature as the arteries, so they show up well on thermograms. The supratrochlear veins (previously the frontal veins) which appear over the medial forehead are often seen in thermograms as well as photographs of normal subjects. As these veins drain the diploic veins that run within the frontal cranial bone, they may become warm with increased neural activity in the frontal lobes.[70] Local increased venous pressure from bending forward, neck occlusion, or increased intrathoracic pressure from forced vocalization or the Valsalva maneuver may cause enlargement of the supratrochlear veins, but not the arteries. The supraorbital vein is much smaller than the supratrochlear and tends to run laterally to meet the ipsilateral superficial temporal vein. It is seen only rarely on thermograms. The orbital arteries and veins are discussed further in the Neurology section of Chapter 11.

Sinusitis and sinus pain

The nasal sinuses are small, air-filled, mucosa-lined cavities within the nasal bones that each connects to the nasal airway through a small passage called an ostium. Sinuses are located within the maxilla, ethmoid, frontal, and sphenoid bones (Figure 10.31).

Sinusitis is an inflammation of the mucosa of one or more of the paranasal sinuses. *Acute* sinusitis lasts up to four weeks and is almost always of viral or allergic origin; it may develop into *chronic* bacterial sinusitis, which typically lasts at least 12 consecutive weeks and may persist for years. The disease progresses in the following manner: The ostium of the sinus becomes obstructed from mucosal swelling due to a virus or allergy. The air within the sinus is then absorbed by the mucosal surface, creating a painful *negative* pressure in the sinus. If the ostium is not reopened, a transudate fluid begins to fill the cavity, providing a medium for bacterial growth. The bacteria attract an exudate of white blood cells and serum, which creates a painful (and dangerous) *positive* pressure within the sinus.[72] Bacterial sinusitis is not a benign disease. Serious complications may arise such as periorbital infections, meningitis, and brain abscess.[73]

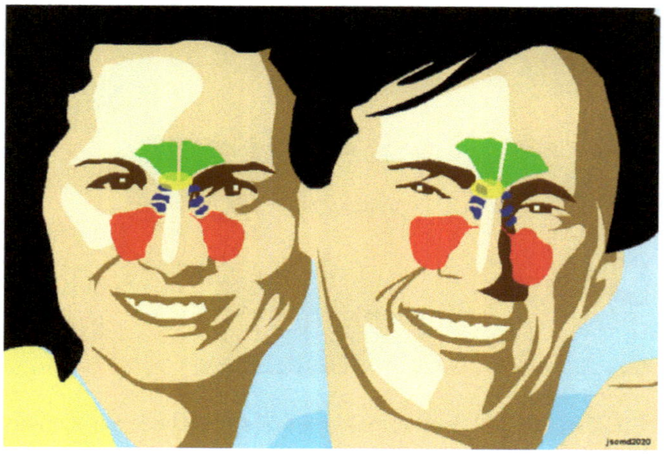

FIGURE 10.31 Scale diagram of the typical location of the paranasal sinuses in adults. Red: Maxillary sinuses; Blue: Ethmoid "air cells"; Green: Frontal sinuses; Yellow: Sphenoid sinus (too deep to be detected thermographically).[71]

Viral and congestive (negative pressure) sinusitis produce little inflammation and may not be detectable thermographically; bacterial sinusitis creates distinct inflammation (Figure 10.32). If the infection is in one of the maxillary or frontal sinuses, warmth is usually detected by qualitative thermography, though the normally warm cranium may mask abnormal heat over the frontal sinuses. The ethmoid air cells are located adjacent to the physiologically warm areas at the inner canthus of the eyes, which tends to mask any inflammatory process in those small sinuses. Nevertheless, ethmoiditis may be detected by increased warmth over the medial ipsilateral orbit.[74] Thermography fails to pick up sphenoidal sinusitis, presumably because of the deeper location of the sphenoid sinus. Therefore, thermography should be deemed unreliable as a method for identifying sphenoidal sinusitis.

Along with viral infections and allergies, chronic sinusitis can be caused by structural abnormalities in the nasal passages,

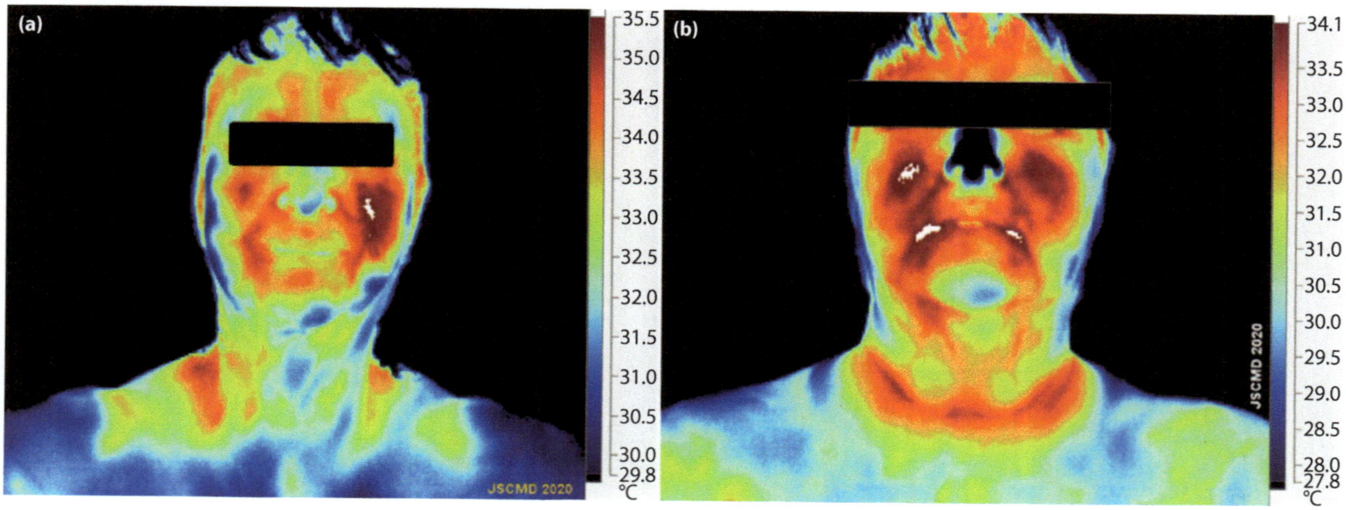

FIGURE 10.32 (a) Maxillary sinusitis, bilateral, worse on the left. Both frontal sinuses may also be inflamed. – 69 yoF. (b) Thermograph of bilateral maxillary sinusitis, warmer on the right. The cool nose differentiates this appearance from that of parasympathetic vasodilation. – 57 yoF.

a tumor, or nasal polyp that keeps the sinuses from draining normally.[75] Chronic fungal infection of the sinuses can also occur. Thermography is useful to differentiate bacterial sinusitis versus viral or congestive sinus pain. The thermographic appearance of chronic fungal sinusitis and other conditions remains to be studied.

Thermography is superior to X-rays in detecting frontal and ethmoidal sinusitis and on par with X-ray in diagnosing maxillary sinusitis.[76] Thermography may be a useful supplemental diagnostic tool for maxillary sinusitis.[77] There is some diagnostic confusion, however, caused by the definition of "sinusitis." When maxillary and frontal sinuses are thermographically assessed, regions of higher temperature are found to be in agreement with the maxillary clouding on X-ray imaging. Thermography is an effective way to differentiate individuals with significant sinusitis from those without.[78] Thermography may help reduce the need for radiographic imaging to detect and evaluate sinusitis and to gauge the effectiveness of treatment.

Other nasal findings

When cooled under thermographic conditions, most subjects show a cold nose due to sympathetically-modulated vasoconstriction. Besides the parasympathetic vasodilation pattern discussed above, an abnormally warm nose may be due to infection or other inflammation of the nasal structures such as chondritis of the nasal septum.[79] Infections such as small boils in the nasal antrum are usually unilateral. Whether nasal neoplasms are detectable via thermography remains to be studied.

Rosacea is a chronic cutaneous inflammatory condition that affects mostly the skin of the nose and cheeks, resulting in redness, pimples, swelling, and small and superficial dilated blood vessels. The etiology and pathogenesis of rosacea are not fully understood, though neurovascular dysregulation appears to play a role. Indeed, the thermal appearance of this condition is similar to that of facial parasympathetic vasodilation – a warming of the central face and nose.[80] Whether parasympathetic vasodilation conditions of the face are predictive or causative of rosacea and rhinophyma remains to be studied.

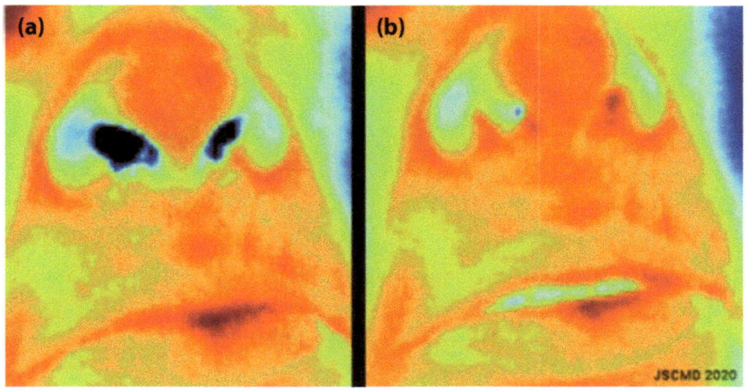

FIGURE 10.33 Thermographic respiratory monitoring by nasal imaging of a normal uncooled subject. At room temperature, the nares appear cooler on inspiration and warmer on exhalation. (a) Inspiration. (b) Expiration.

Respiratory monitoring by thermographic methods is possible as shown in Figure 10.33, but patient movement makes this difficult without specialized algorithms to follow the nasal location. Nasal respiratory monitoring can detect blockage of a nasal passage; the nares on the obstructed side will show decreased or absent cyclical temperature changes with respiration.

Ear findings in thermography

The outer ear, consisting of the pinna, tragus, and the external ear canal meatus, is readily visible on lateral thermographic images of the head. For a valid thermal evaluation, the subject should be thermally equilibrated with the hair pulled back off the ears. Under cooling conditions, the pinna generally appears cool while the tragus and meatus of the canal appear warmer. If the thermal imaging axis is aligned with the ear canal, the temperature of the tympanic membrane may be detected (Figure 10.34).

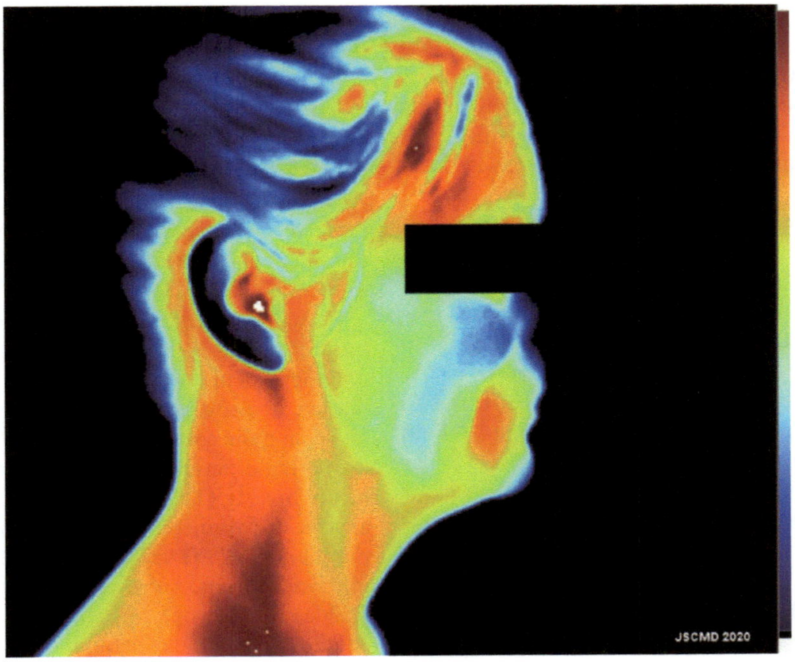

FIGURE 10.34 Normal thermal appearance of the lateral view of the right ear in a cooled subject. Note the cool pinna and the warmer tragus. The temperature of the tympanic membrane may be detected as the warmest area (white) at the meatus of the ear canal. – 45-year-old female.

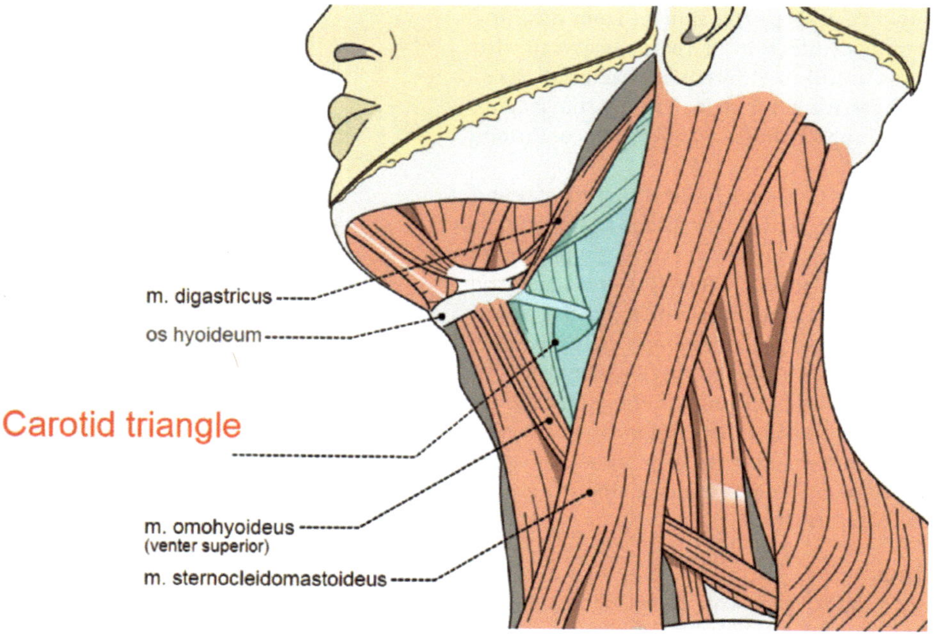

FIGURE 10.35 The carotid triangle – A portion of the submandibular area – may become warm in cases of tonsillitis and tonsillar abscess, and lymph nodes may be detected in this area.[83]

Excessive ear wax or other obstruction may obscure the tympanic membrane.

The pinna may appear abnormally warm in a cooled subject due to infection, recent injury, or other inflammation-related issues. An acute or chronic infection affecting an ear-piercing site will typically show localized warmth, while a generalized chondritis of the ear cartilage will make the entire pinna warmer than normal.

Pharyngotonsillitis

Acute tonsillitis is a rapid-onset infectious inflammation of the tonsils, situated in the lateral recesses of the oropharynx. Though tonsillitis is most frequently caused by self-limiting viral infections, bacterial infections including streptococci may cause severe febrile disease with neurological and cardiac sequelae. Complications include peritonsillar abscess. Infection of the small pockets within the tonsils (cryptic tonsillitis) may produce chronic foul-smelling, purulent discharges along with local swelling and pain.

Acute tonsillitis produces dermal hyperthermia in the ipsilateral carotid triangle (Figure 10.35). There is a strong positive correlation between the temperature of the submandibular area on the affected side and, curiously, warming in the center of the ipsilateral palm, a finding that may be due to unilateral autonomic signaling.[81] The submandibular temperature difference compared to adjacent areas typically exceeds 0.6°C (1.1°F) in acute cases, while ranging from 0.3 to 0.6°C (0.54 to 1.1°F) in chronic tonsillitis. Warm areas occur over the submandibular lymph nodes. Healthy volunteers without tonsil pathology show symmetric temperature distribution in the right and left submandibular region.[82]

Tooth and dental problems in thermography

Though much has been reported about the effectiveness of facial thermography in detecting dental disease, good-quality studies showing definite qualitative or quantitative data are lacking.[84] As the bodies of the teeth are not directly adjacent to the external skin surface, being separated from the skin by the buccal cavity and cheek, localized tooth problems such as pain from a cracked tooth or a simple cavity in the tooth surface will not cause discernible thermographic findings. Thermography has been shown to be useful in detecting major or chronic dental infections, however (Figure 10.36).[85] Persistent tooth root infection may create a minor (and often overlooked) warm area lateral to the infected area. A more developed dental abscess will cause localized soft-tissue swelling and warmth that is thermographically apparent. Herpes labialis (cold sores) may be detected in the prodromal and active stages as a warm area over the symptomatic site. Thermal findings return to normal on resolution of the viral attack.[86]

Invasive dental procedures including local anesthetic nerve blocks may cause damage to mandibular or maxillary nerves. The inferior alveolar nerve is apparently most prone to injury, showing a 0.5°C (0.9°F) higher temperature over the nerve distribution area on the damaged side (Figure 10.37). Local block of the inferior alveolar nerve with lidocaine temporarily produces the same thermographic picture and can thus be used to objectively assess a successful nerve block.[87]

Though more than one book has been published claiming that facial thermography or other dental imaging may indicate the development of breast cancer due to the effect of chronic inflammation, no definite link has been found.[88] A study of 222 women looked for any correlation between bilateral facial temperatures (including differential temperatures) and thermographic scores of the breasts (TH scores); no correlation was found between any facial parameter and the TH score of either breast.[89] The microbiome of the oral cavity can play a role in the induction of other neoplasms, however.[90] The positive correlation of dental problems and neoplasms with an unhealthy lifestyle and inadequate nutrition may confound studies that do not account for this these associations, and can lead to incorrect conclusions pertaining to the magnitude of the effect of dental disease on carcinogenesis.[91]

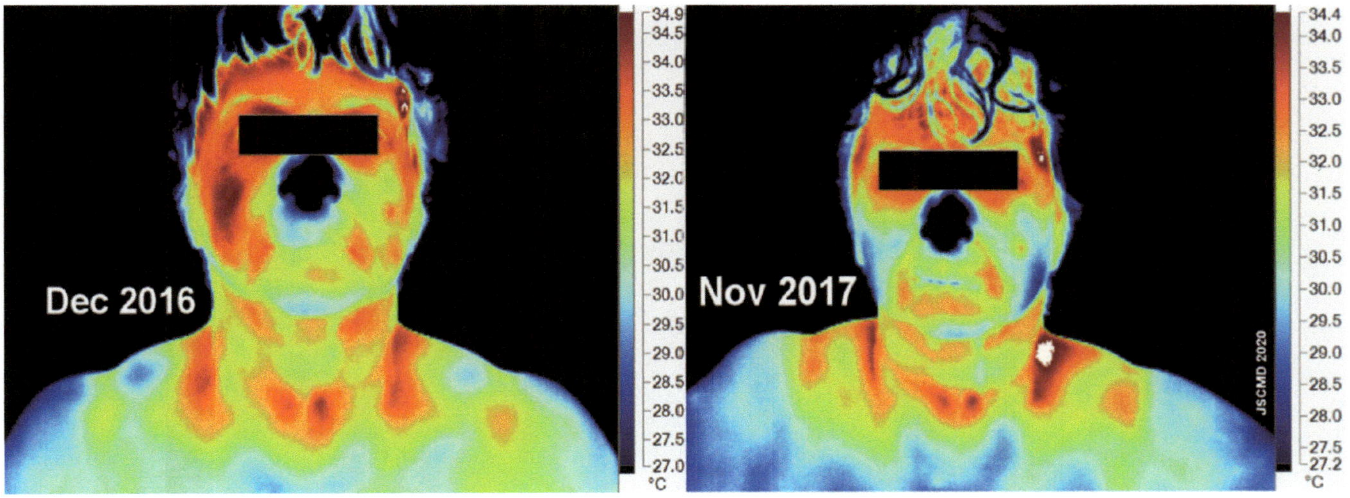

FIGURE 10.36 Thermal signs of abscess of a right upper molar tooth detected in 2016 were absent one year later. Notice how the warm pattern appears lateral to that of a maxillary sinus infection. – 66-year-old female.

Thermography of the mouth and tongue

Observation of the patient's tongue is an important part of East Asian medicine. Visual examination is used to determine "cold-heat pathologic patterns" (CHPPs). Because this method is subjective, infrared imaging of the tongue has been explored as a more objective approach. Different heat patterns over the tongue surface, such as lateral, root, or tip warmth are considered in determining the CHPPs.[92]

Problems arise because the tongue is normally moist, thus its surface temperature is affected by the constantly varying air temperature, humidity, and evaporative cooling caused by inhalation and exhalation. The average temperatures of various areas over the tongue vary about 1.6°C (2.9°F) with respiration. The qualitative thermal appearance of the tongue surface also varies considerably with respiration.[93] Still images must be taken at known points in the respiratory cycle to be comparable. Qualitative videothermography may detect shifting areas of dryness and evaporation that herald disease (Figure 10.38). More research under is needed to evaluate the medical use of tongue thermography.

Intraoral thermography has been attempted to detect infections of the teeth, gums, and other structures in the mouth. Unfortunately, due to the fairly uniform surface temperatures within the oral cavity, thermal artifacts produced by uneven liquid evaporation of saliva, and the difficulty in cooling the interior of the mouth to bring about thermal contrast, intraoral thermography has yet to become a successful imaging tool.

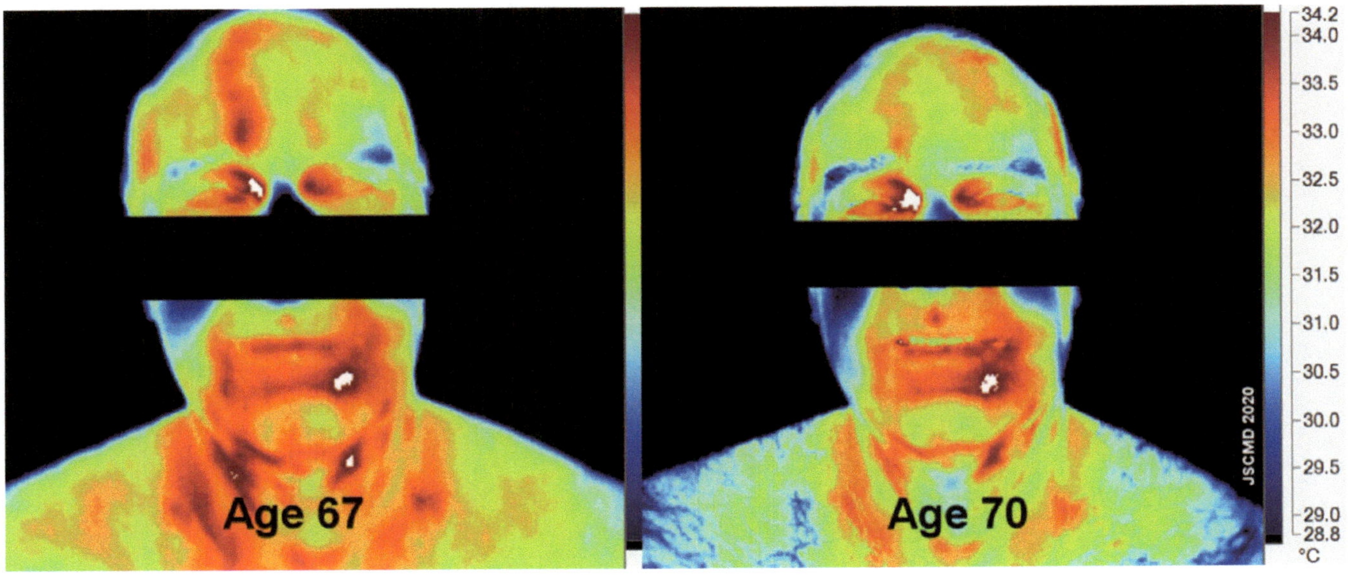

FIGURE 10.37 Persistent warm spot over the left mental foramen of the mandible, presumably due to previous damage to the left inferior alveolar nerve during a dental procedure.

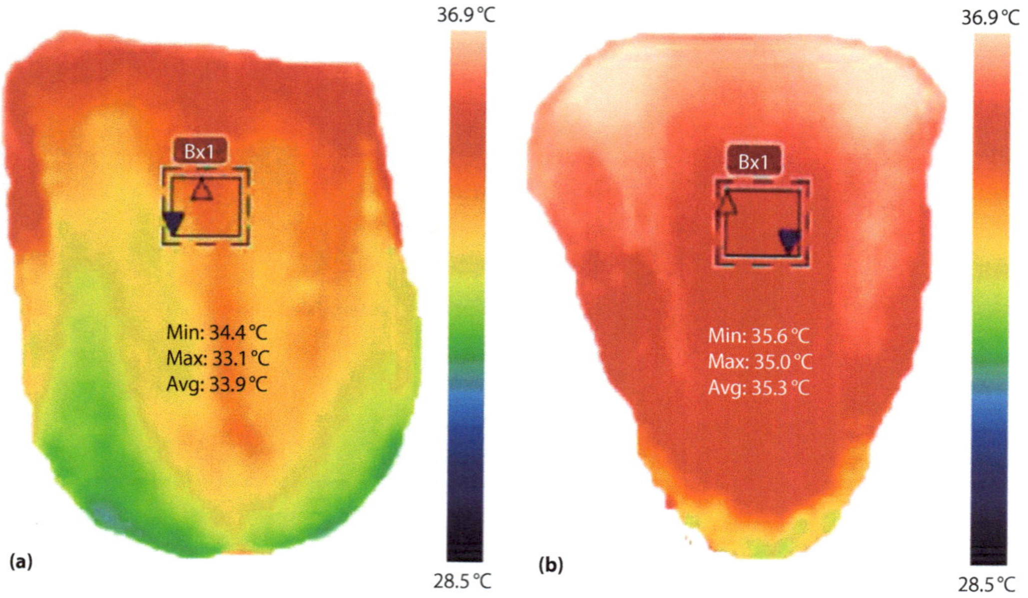

FIGURE 10.38 Thermography of the tongue to evaluate diabetes type II. Sample isothermal thermograms of the tongue. (a) Normal subject. (b) Diabetic subject.[94]

Temporomandibular joint (TMJ) disorder

The temporomandibular joints, or TMJs, are the pair of joints between the mandible and the temporal bones of the skull (Figure 10.39). Temporomandibular joint dysfunction (TMJD) is a common problem, causing pain in the involved joint, clicking noises on chewing, and restricted jaw movement. Arthritis may be a cause of TMJD. Patients with osteoarthritis or internal derangement of the TMJ, perhaps from previous trauma, often have synovitis of the TMJ.[95] This creates chronic inflammation in the synovial tissue, progressive degradation of the cartilage, and subchondral bone remodeling.[96]

The possibility of using thermography to detect TMJD has been an area of considerable medical interest.[98] One type of TMJD may be due to a compression of the joint's microscopic vessels by jaw muscle hyperactivity, resulting in a *decrease* in the local skin temperature.[99] Conversely, skin temperature over the TMJ is increased in individuals with joint pain.[100] TMJD patients show greater asymmetry in skin temperatures adjacent to the joints than individuals without this condition.[101]

There are few controlled trials to assess infrared imaging as a test for unilateral TMJ arthralgia.[102] Well-designed studies of the reliability of thermography in determining TMJD are lacking.[103] Thermography has low accuracy in detecting women

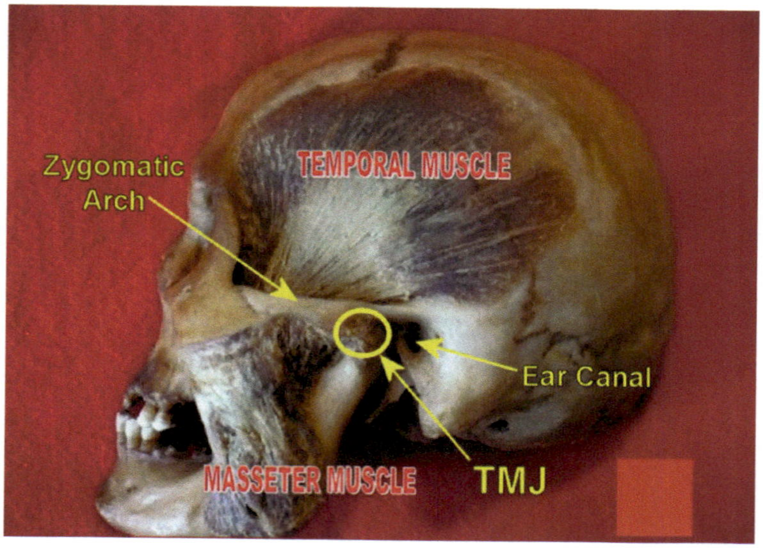

FIGURE 10.39 Anatomical location of the left temporomandibular joint (TMJ) and major surrounding structures.[97]

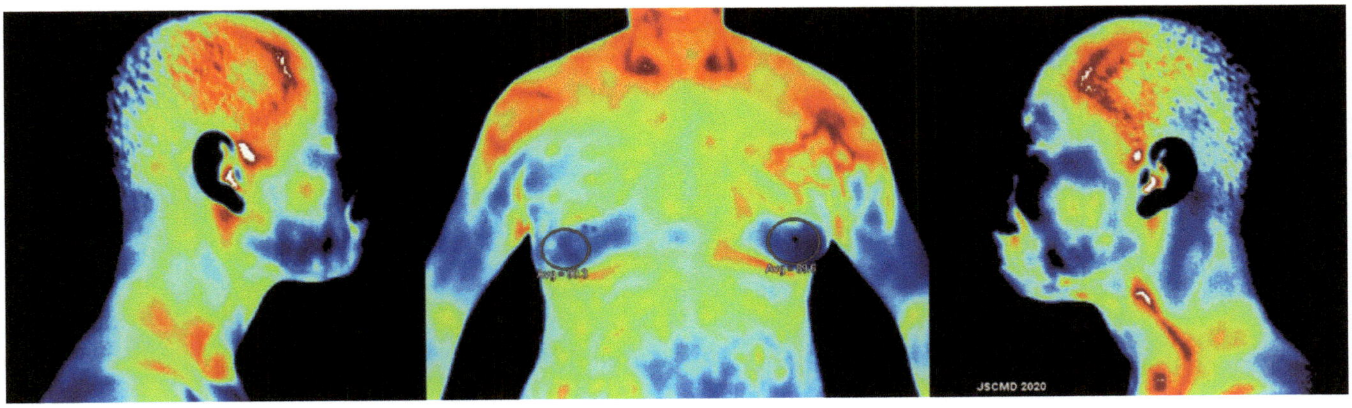

FIGURE 10.40 Thermal pattern of temporal arteritis. The scalp arteries are usually not visible due to the normal warmth over the cranium. Other signs of vascular inflammation are present – Note the unusual vascular "cape" pattern over the left chest wall, with a less extensive pattern over the right shoulder. The left external jugular vein also appears inflamed. – 58-year-old male.

with TMJD.[104] There appear to be two syndromes, depending on whether inflammation is present in the affected TMJ. When the condition is quiescent, thermograms may show no anomaly. When the joint is inflamed, the overlying area of the skin becomes significantly warmer compared to the non-symptomatic side. Inflammation of the masseter muscle or its attachment to the zygomatic arch will cause skin warmth *anterior* to the TMJ, and might be confused with TMJD. Inflammation of the ipsilateral parotid gland may also create a warm pattern anterior to the TMJ. More research is needed in this area.

Temporal arteritis (giant cell arteritis, GCA)

Temporal arteritis is an insidious but dangerous autoimmune disease that causes headache, malaise, and localized tenderness over the arteries coursing up the sides of the cranium.[105] Pain on chewing may lead to an incorrect diagnosis of TMJ pain. The disease mainly attacks the temporal, cranial, and other carotid branch arteries. The aortic arch and arteries of the upper extremity may also be involved. Venous phlebitis may accompany the arterial inflammation.[106] In GCA, NO is generated by macrophages that accumulate in all layers of the inflamed vessel wall.[107] It is this excess NO that dilates the skin arterioles near the diseased artery, creating local areas visibly warmer than the background heat of the scalp (Figure 10.40). Thermography is reported to detect this condition without resorting to biopsy of the involved arteries, and the effectiveness of therapy may be followed by serial thermograms.[108] Thermographers should promptly warn of the possibility of temporal arteritis on finding warm scalp arteries.

Facial fever detection and screening

The mobility of human populations has prompted the development of methods to efficiently detect fever and reduce disease spread.[109] Thermography offers a practical way to measure facial skin temperature as a proxy for core temperature. Thermography has been utilized for fever screening of persons with suspected infection in many international quarantine stations.[110]

Two types of infrared technology can provide viable fever screening options: (1) infrared thermal imagers (i.e., thermography) and (2) non-contact infrared thermometers (NCIT) – hand-held thermopile-based single-point surface thermometers.[111] Forehead skin temperatures, however, whether measured by NCIT or thermography, are unreliable as an indicator of fever.[112] The temperature of the spot just medial to the inner canthus of the eye is normally the warmest part of the face (Figure 10.41).[113] The inner canthus is an indicator of core body temperature.[114] These warm spots are too small to be reliably measured by NCIT, and show variable results in eyeglass wearers. A recent

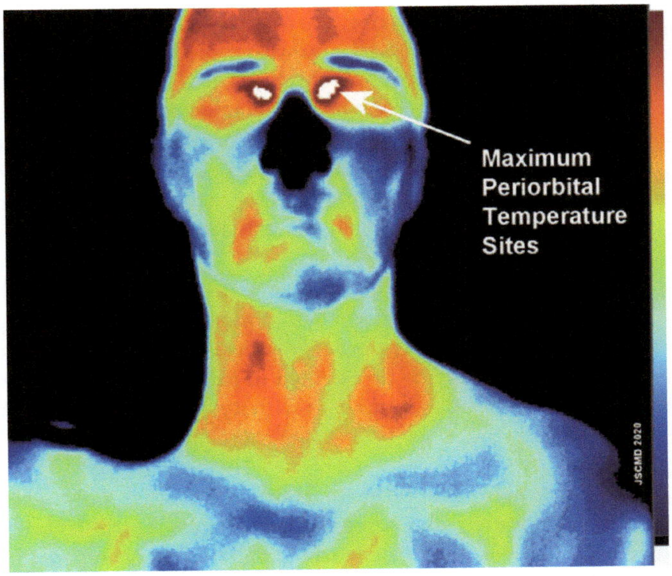

FIGURE 10.41 Thermogram showing the location of the warmest areas on the face – the inner canthus areas of both eyes. Just deep to the very thin skin at these locations run the nasal artery, the angular artery, and several veins branching from the angular vein, one of which communicates with the ophthalmic vein as it exits the skull. – 27 yoF.

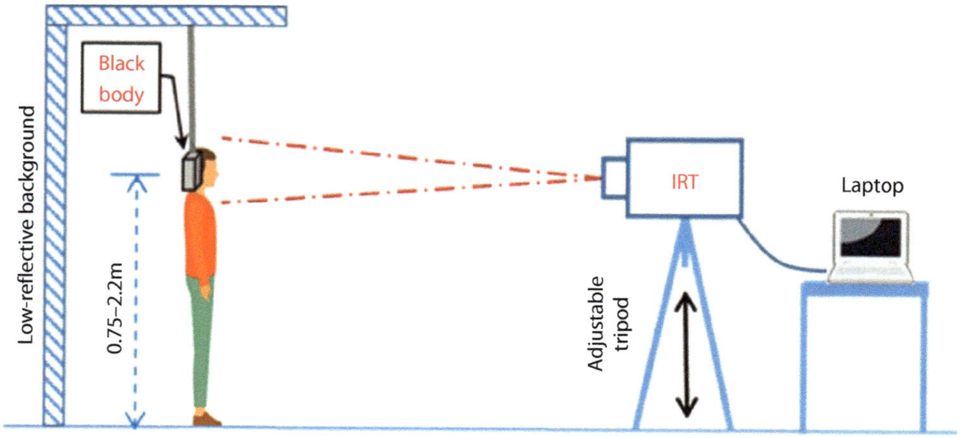

FIGURE 10.42 Recommended physical setup for thermographic facial screening to detect fever. Note the blackbody temperature standard for correcting IR background effects and imager offset.[122]

study found thermography to be more accurate than NCIT in terms of fever detection.[115]

Thermography can reliably distinguish between normal and febrile individuals by utilizing a threshold temperature alarm. 36.3°C (97.3°F) has been used as the threshold temperature. Readings that exceed this temperature trigger an alarm, at which point a contact thermometer is used to verify the person's temperature.[116] Some confusions exist, however, because a 34.6°C (94.3°F) cutoff value was suggested by the same researchers.[117] Imager offsets may account for this discrepancy. In children, thermography was reasonably accurate in detecting fever at a pediatric clinic, and proved to be a better predictor than parental report.[118]

Noncontact fever screening needs to take into account the effects of age, recent exercise, use of eyewear, ambient temperature, afebrile infection, and antipyretic medications. Infrared fever screening via thermography or NCIT is a rather inexact technology; one that can be fooled by applying cream to lower the skin emissivity, or by wiping one's forehead, eyes, and nose with a cool, damp cloth prior to getting scanned. The positive predictive value of thermographic fever screening ranges from 3.5% to 65.4%, indicating its highly variable detection of febrile individuals.[119]

To overcome the drawbacks of fever-based screening, both heart rate and respiration are being integrated into screening algorithms to bolster the screening accuracy.[120] These three vital signs are found to be elevated in influenza patients, and the method's sensitivity and specificity (85.7%, 90.1%) were higher than those of fever-based screening alone (60.7%, 86.4%).[121]

Thermography can estimate body temperature only when proper calibration and screening procedures are followed.[123] Temperature offset and gain must be calibrated and compensated at frequent intervals. Including a blackbody standard set to the fever cutoff temperature in each thermal image improves detection accuracy (Figure 10.42). At present, IEC 80601-2-59 is the international standard for performance evaluation of thermography in large-scale fever screening.[124] Standards include measuring only one person's temperature at a time and allowing time for a person to adjust to environmental changes. Additionally, the subject should not wear a hat or glasses, and hair should be pulled away from the face.[125]

In the controlled setting of a thermography room where the subjects are at rest and have been properly equilibrated to a temperature of 20°C to 21°C (68°F to 69.8°F), measurement of the maximum periorbital temperature may be more accurate. A screening cutoff of 36.3°C (97.3°F) is in agreement with data collected in a thermography room – the ILSITS Data, as shown in Figure 10.43. If less than 5% of these thermography subjects actually had a subclinical fever, then a reasonable fever cutoff temperature would be about 36.3°C (97.3°F). Note also the few subjects with very low periorbital Temperatures (below 93.5°F [34.2°C]). Testing for hypothyroidism or other hypo-metabolic conditions may be warranted in these subjects.

Thermography of the neck

Thyroid gland

The thyroid gland is an endocrine gland located anterior and lateral to the trachea in the lower neck (Figure 10.61). It is the only endocrine gland that is visible to infrared imaging. The thyroid is located close to the skin, the central part being essentially adjacent to the surface, and the lobes separated from it by three thin muscular layers. The normal active thyroid gland weighs around 15 grams and generates about 1.3 watts of heat.[126] Heat generated in the thyroid warms the overlying skin by thermal conduction. The thyroid gland's heat comes from its metabolic activity and blood perfusion, both of which increase in active thyroiditis, hyperthyroidism, and thyroid cancer (Figure 10.44b). Hypometabolic conditions such as idiopathic hypothyroidism, administration of exogenous thyroid hormone, or post-inflammatory scarring of the gland create a cool-appearing thyroid area (Figure 10.44a).

Thyroiditis occurs in the autoimmune conditions such as Hashimoto's thyroiditis and Graves' disease.[127] Subacute thyroiditis is a transient thyrotoxic state and results in temporary hyperthyroidism, generally lasting a few weeks but sometimes persisting for months (Figure 10.45).[128] Postpartum thyroiditis is a thyroid dysfunction that manifests within one year

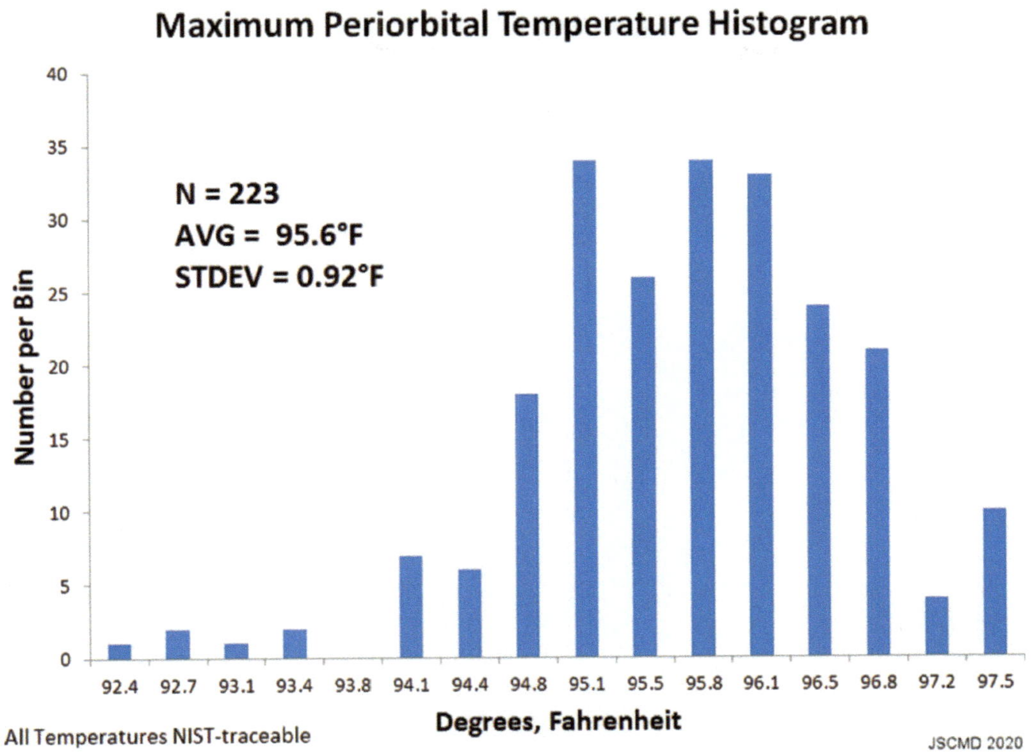

FIGURE 10.43 NIST-calibrated maximum periorbital temperature data from the ILSITS study data. All data was collected under standard thermographic conditions. An estimated fever cutoff of 36.3°C (97.4°F) fits the data.

of pregnancy. Hyperthyroidism and toxic nodular goiter are more commonly seen in older women.[129] An inflammatory component is commonly present in most if not all cancers, and thyroid cancer is no exception.[130] There may be an increased risk of thyroid cancer among patients with Hashimoto's thyroiditis.[131]

Thyroid disorders are often detectable via infrared imaging. Many inflammatory markers are associated with both benign and malignant thyroid diseases, as well as with autoimmune thyroid disease and radiation exposure to the thyroid.[132] Over-activity of the gland may appear thermographically as a warm area in the lower midline of the neck. Sometimes one of the thyroid lobes is warmer than the other (Figure 10.46). Thyroid cancer may be visible as warmth over the thyroid gland, often unilateral with other linear markings up the neck, presumably from inflamed vasculature.

Thermography can visualize cold thyroid nodules representing benign disease and warm areas representing malignancy.[133]

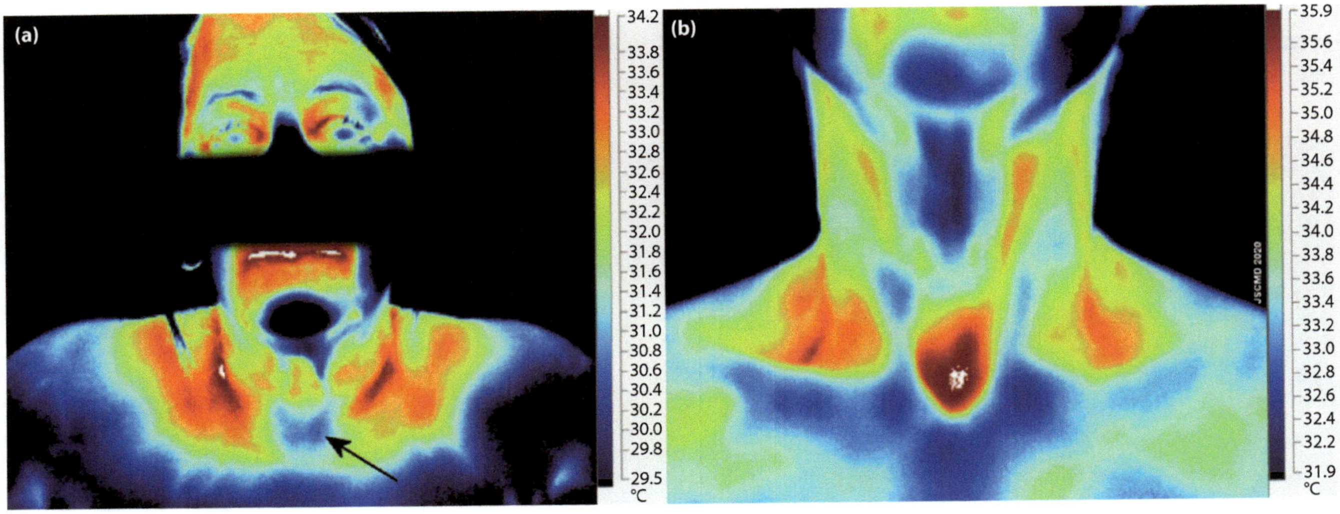

FIGURE 10.44 (a) Thermal image of hypothyroidism in a 63 yoF being treated with thyroxine. Notice the cool thyroid area (arrow). (b) The thyroid area appears unusually warm, indicating possible hyperthyroidism, carcinoma, or acute thyroiditis. – 63 yoF.

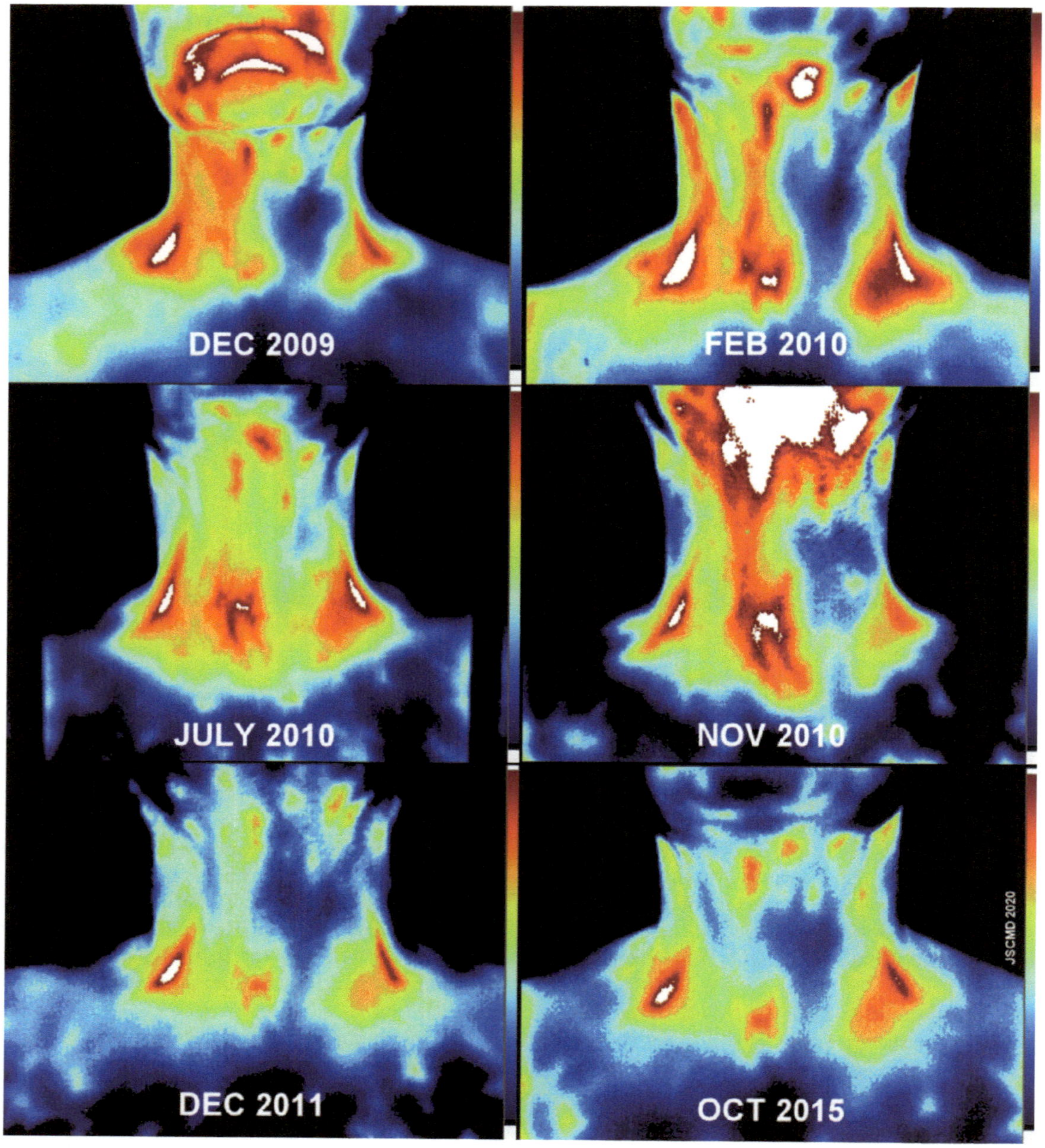

FIGURE 10.45 Six-year progression of the temperature pattern over a palpable, non-painful mass in the right thyroid lobe of a middle-aged female subject. Involution occurred without allopathic treatment or surgery, suggesting thyroiditis as the likely etiology.

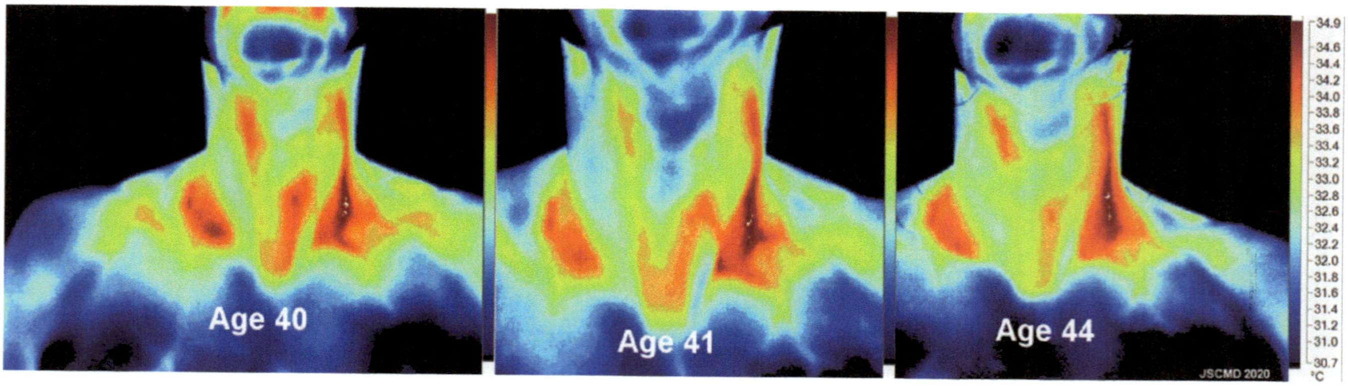

FIGURE 10.46 Warm nodule in the left thyroid lobe of a female subject, showing thermological improvement over 4 years' time. The pattern over the left external jugular vein is also persistently warm, an unusual finding.

Any nodule associated with hyperthyroidism may increase blood flow and metabolic activity, thus appearing warm.[134] Thermography is more precise than ultrasound imaging for the selection of thyroid nodules to be biopsied via fine-needle aspiration; sensitivity and negative predictive value of thermography are both 100%, compared to 95% and 17%, respectively, for ultrasound imaging.[135] On thermal imaging, malignant and premalignant tissues of the thyroid consistently exhibit higher temperatures when compared to those of surrounding tissues.[136]

Goiter refers to a swelling of the neck caused by enlargement of the thyroid gland. Whether the swelling will appear warm via thermography depends on the underlying etiology.[137] Hyperthyroid goiter appears diffusely warm, while hypothyroid goiter often shows a cool gland area. Hashimoto's thyroiditis may have variable thermal findings depending on the state of the disease process – active or quiescent. Graves' disease is characterized by a diffusely hyper-vascularized thyroid, showing high yet variable temperatures over the gland.[138] Thermography also offers an assessment tool for patients with active thyroid eye disease (TED), with good accuracy and specificity.[139] TED patients with active ophthalmopathy showed orbital temperatures around 3°C (5.4°F) higher than normal, and had eyelid temperatures above 37°C (98.6°F).[140] More severe cases of TED may present with systemic fever of unknown origin.[141]

Various methods have been proposed for detecting thyroid "hot spots."[142] The thermal contrast of the thyroid image can be increased by a cooling process during infrared imaging (dynamic thermography).[143] Local heat generation is about fourfold higher for patients with thyroid tumors compared to healthy controls.[144] Dynamic thermography is useful to detect and monitor thyroid malignancy.[145]

Thyroid thermography does not involve ionizing radiation, thus avoiding a potential threat to a fetus during pregnancy.[146] Thermography offers a reliable option for assessing thyroid nodules during pregnancy.[147] Having a safe, non-toxic monitoring tool for pregnant women with thyroid problems can complement standard medical care. When thyroid disease is left untreated during pregnancy, it is associated with an increased risk of miscarriage, placental abruption, hypertension, and growth restriction.[148]

Other thermographic neck findings

Neck veins

Blood vessel patterns are often seen in thermograms of the anterior neck. As the carotid and other arteries are too deep anatomically to significantly affect the skin temperature (see Figure 5.11a), it is the more superficial veins that are visible in qualitative thermograms of the neck. The most likely vessels to appear in thermograms are the external jugular veins. Large, warm neck veins may indicate venous congestion due to right heart failure or fluid overload. These dilated veins are best seen with the subject reclining at a 45-degree angle.

In most cases, the Right internal jugular vein drains the majority of warm blood flowing from the brain due to its connection with the superior sagittal sinus, while the left internal jugular drains the cooler facial regions.[149] The large internal jugulars are, like the arteries, too deep to be detected thermographically; however, the thermally-visible external jugulars anastomose with and run parallel to the internal jugulars, carrying much the same blood (and heat) (Figure 10.47).[150] The differential temperature of the right and left external jugular veins in healthy subjects may serve as an indicator of cerebral activity. More research is needed to clarify this finding.

Lymph node patterns in the neck

The anatomical triangles of the anterior neck are rich with lymph nodes. When enlarged and activated by infection or neoplasm, the thermal pattern of these nodes shows blotchy and uneven

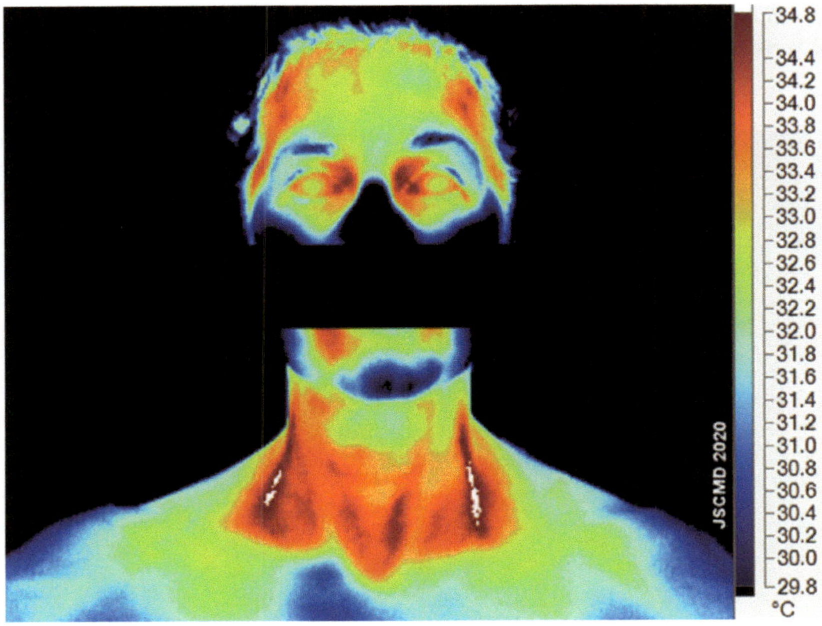

FIGURE 10.47 External jugular vein pattern, bilateral (white markings in neck), normal. – 59 yoF.

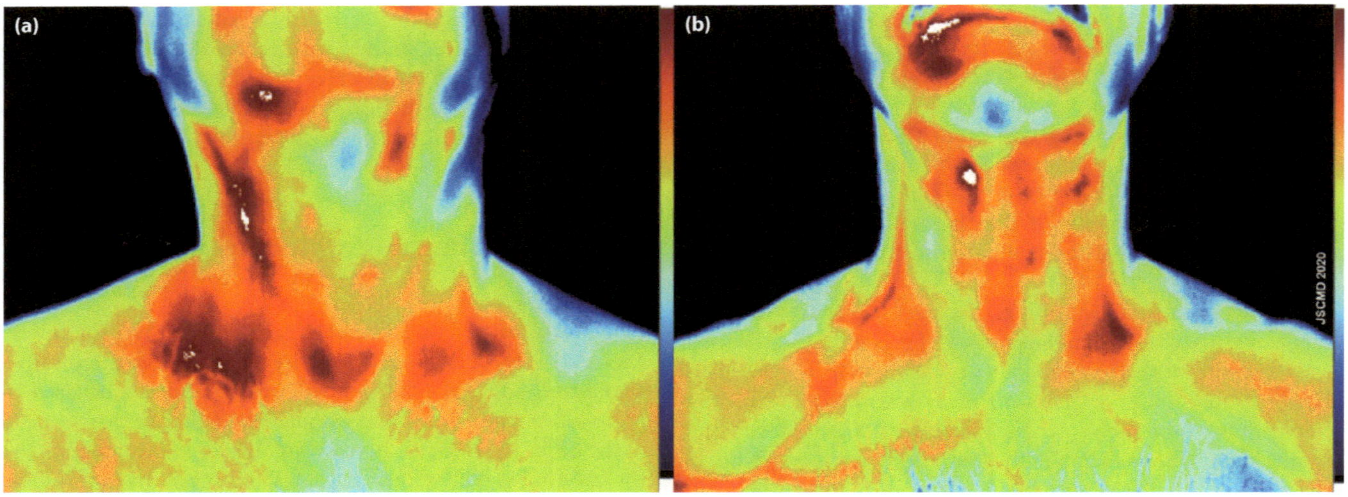

FIGURE 10.48 Thermal patterns of lymph node inflammation in the anterior neck: (a) 66 yoM; (b) 59 yoM.

warmth over the involved areas (Figure 10.48). Static thermographic signs of unilateral lymph node metastases include a surface temperature difference greater than 1°C (1.8°F) over the nodal sites compared to the site on the normal contralateral neck. An area of elevated surface temperatures over and around the nodes may also be detected.[151] This local skin warming over involved lymph nodes may be due to locally increased metabolism and increased NO production.[152] Dynamic thermography similar to QUAINT using a cool pack on the skin and watching temperature recovery over time is effective at detecting malignant lymph node metastasis.[153]

Thermal patterns over the posterior neck

The back of the neck consists of the occiput, cerebral vertebrae, and several thick muscular layers. The area is normally devoid of thermographically visible arteries or veins, but subdermal lymph nodes may be present. As described in Chapter 5, when upright or sitting, the posterior neck muscles are under constant tension to counter the forward rotation of the cranium on the cervical vertebrae. Chronic forward bending of the neck can put excessive strain on the posterior neck muscles, as can psychological tension and overuse of stimulants. If the subject has been properly cooled, with any long hair tied up off the neck area during the equilibration, thermography of the neck can detect this strain pattern as excess warmth over the upper portions of the trapezius muscles (Figure 10.49). Enthesiopathy of the trapezius insertion on the occipital bone can also be detected, in which case the inflammatory pattern may be limited to the junction where muscle attaches to bone.

Thermal patterns over the upper portion of the neck just below the occiput may also be augmented by the circulation of warm cerebrospinal fluid (CSF) surrounding the cerebellum, brainstem, and upper cervical spinal cord. Circulation of CSF is a physiologic mechanism that helps remove the heat of brain metabolism.[154] The heat from the brain may warm the upper posterior neck by conduction. Studies of normal subjects cooled in a prone position, as shown in Chapter 6 may help determine the contribution of CSF heat dissipation to the skin temperature of the occipital region.

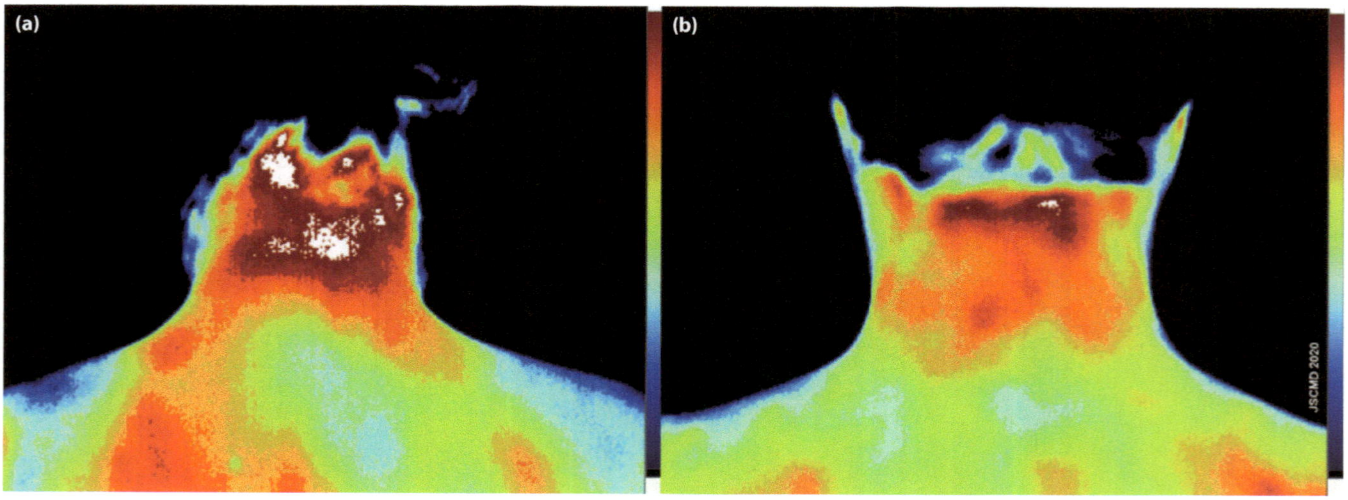

FIGURE 10.49 Thermal patterns of strain in the occipital muscle groups. (a) 49 yoF; (b) 44 yoM.

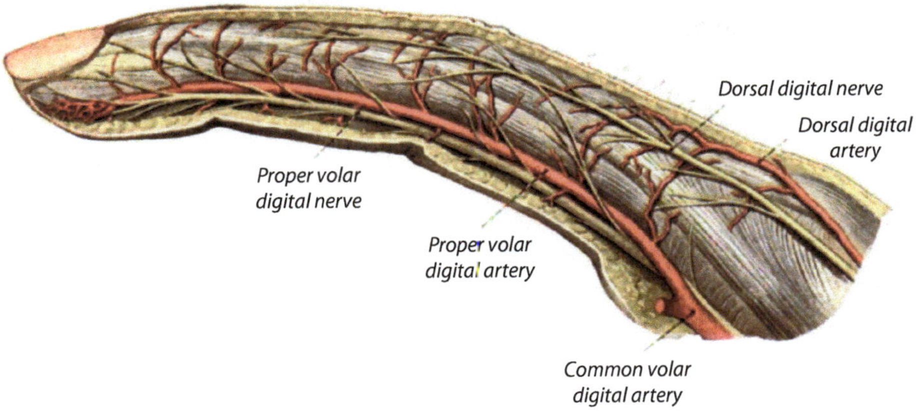

FIGURE 10.50 The arteries of the right forefinger, lateral (thumb) side. The two major arteries are on the palmar (volar) side, one lateral and one medial. The smaller dorsal digital artery extends only as far as the first phalanx.[155]

Thermography of the upper extremity and hand

Thermography of the arms is generally quite uniform when normal. The antecubital fossa is usually the warmest location in a normal arm, due to the venous and arterial vessels located close to the skin surface there. The skin over the volar radial head may also appear warm due to the radial artery coursing under the dermis in that location. The ulnar artery is sometimes visible at the wrist, but this is less common. Diffuse warmth is often seen over the hand extensor and flexor muscles located in the forearm. In the upper arm region, the main warm areas are seen over the deltoid muscles; the cephalic vein is sometimes visible coursing up the anterior upper arm. See the images of the arms in Chapter 13 for more details.

The digital arteries supplying the fingers are one of the few sites where arteries are located directly under the dermis. Though they are not detectable in normal cases, when inflamed, these small arteries can be visualized via thermography in the properly cooled individual. Warmth over the digital arteries cannot be due to an accompanying venous warmth, as the digital veins progress up the dorsal surface of the fingers, separate and away from the arteries. Anatomically, the digital arteries are found more to the palmar side of the phalanges (Figure 10.50). Thus, when inflamed, they are thermally visible, mainly on palmar hand views when the fingers are spread apart; in certain cases, oblique volar hand views may be needed to better demonstrate these small arteries (Figure 10.51). Thermal signs of digital artery inflammation may be due to vasculitis, autoimmune disease, and certain medications. More research into this thermal finding is needed.

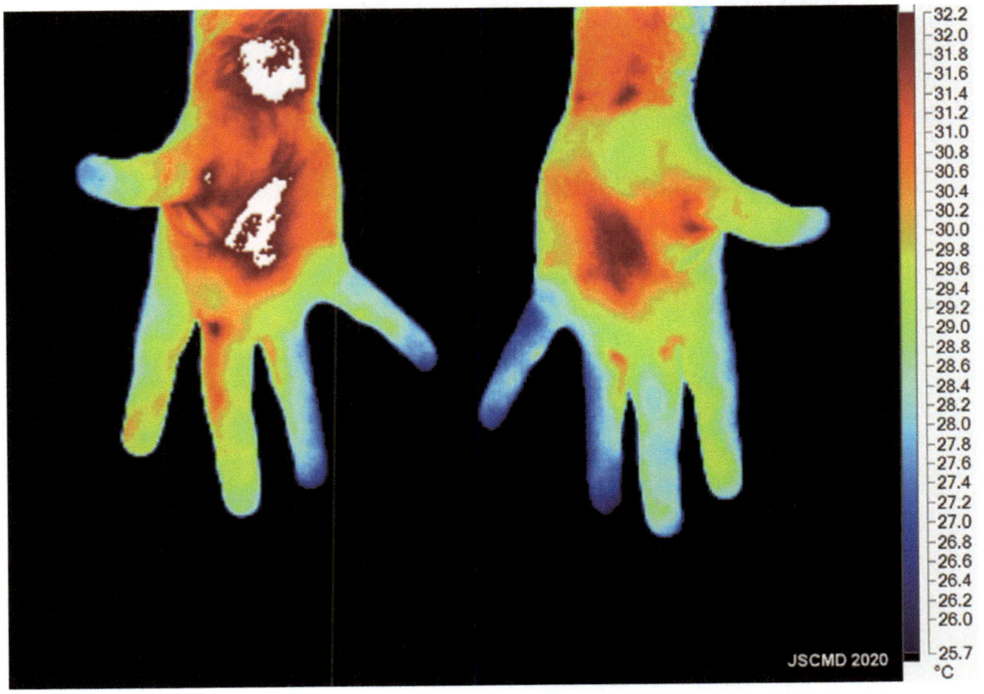

FIGURE 10.51 A thermographic image showing the pattern of digital arterial inflammation, most pronounced over lateral digit III right – 72-year-old male.

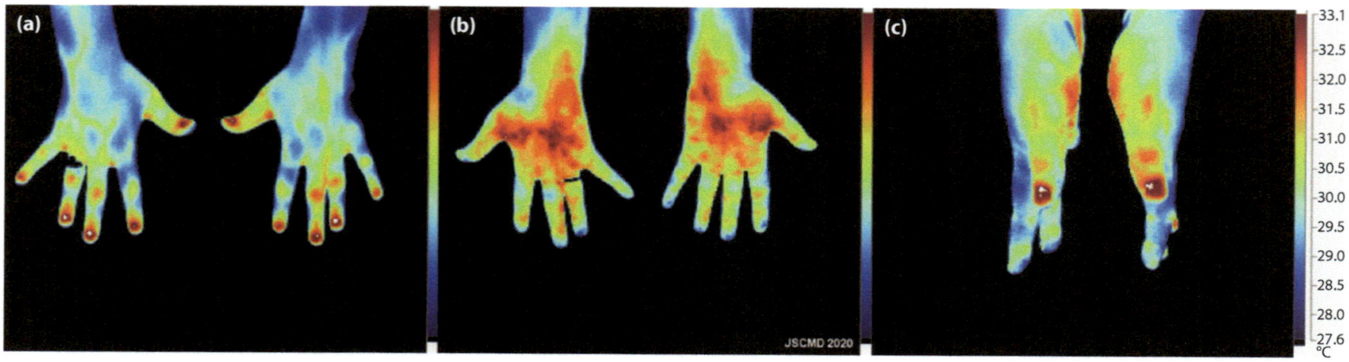

FIGURE 10.52 Isothermal images showing the appearance of paradoxical glomus AVA dilation in a cooled subject. The interphalangeal joints also appear warm. Note the warm veins over the dorsum of the hands draining the arterial blood flowing through the AVAs. (a) Dorsal view; (b) Palmar view; (c) Radial (thumb) view. Etiology unknown. – 32-year-old female.

At the termination of the digital arteries are located a large number of glomus bodies (AVAs), mostly concentrated under the fingernail and toenails (Figure 10.52). Blood flow through these AVAs is reduced by an increase in adrenergic sympathetic neural tone. If sympathetic enervation is disrupted, the AVAs remain open. AVAs are normally open after exercise at room temperature (Figure 10.53). Below equilibration temperatures of 20°C (68°F), properly enervated AVAs should remain closed unless affected by other factors such as increased circulating NO from autoimmune disease, active infection, or other pathology (Figure 10.54). Certain medications for blood pressure may also cause the AVAs to remain open at low ambient

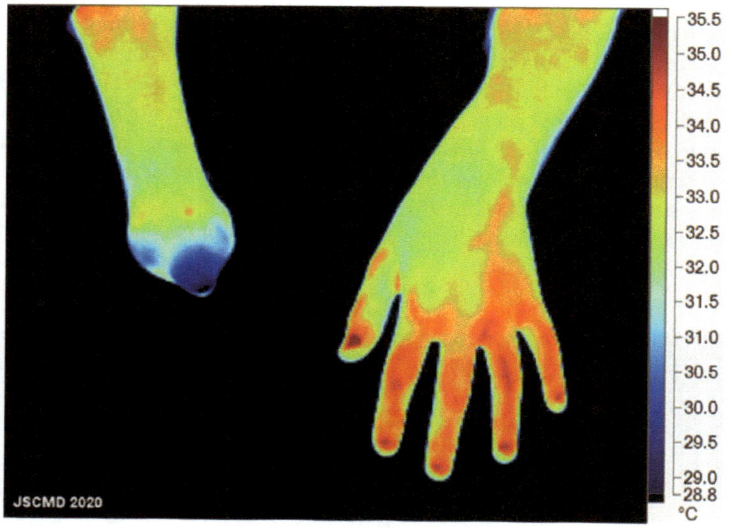

FIGURE 10.53 Congenital absence of right hand (ICD Q71.31) in a 13-year old male. This image was taken in a room-temperature environment after the subject exercised. The glomus AVAs of the left hand are dilated as is normal after exercise. The distal right limb is cool, indicating that glomus AVAs are not present.

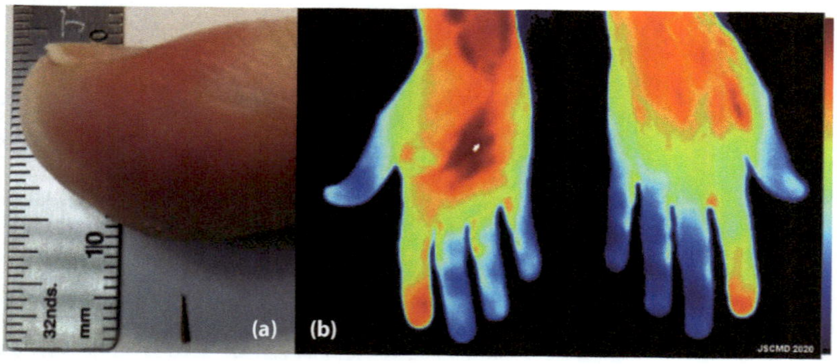

FIGURE 10.54 Infection caused by a 5 mm splinter retained 7 days in the pad of the right index finger. (a) Visual photograph of the swollen finger showing the removed splinter. (b) Thermogram of the right hand taken 18 hours after removal of the splinter. The veins over the dorsum of the hand appear cool, and no lymphangitis pattern is seen. – 73-year-old male.

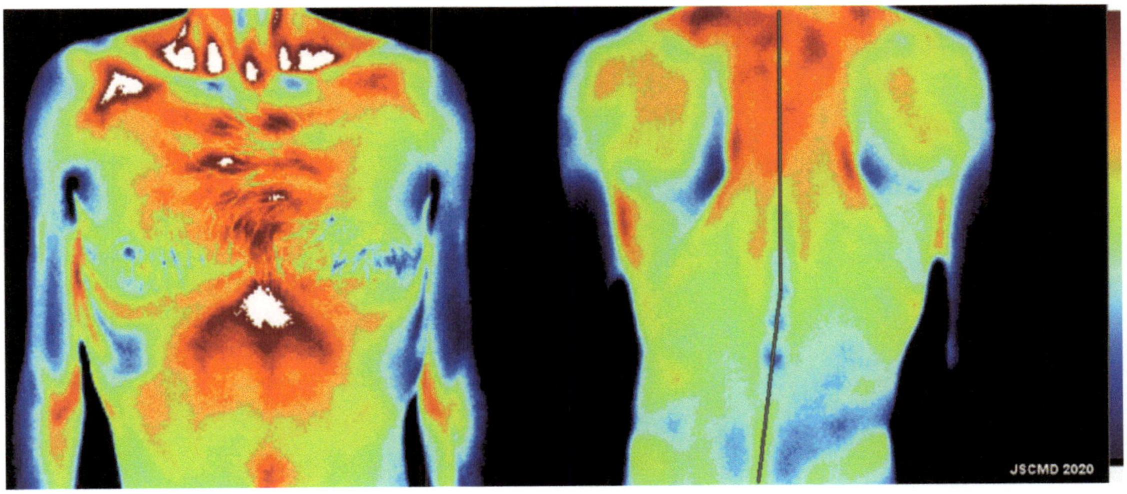

FIGURE 10.55 The appearance of the thorax of a 68-year-old male with mantle cell lymphoma. He recently lost 22.7 kg (50 lb.). Lower thoracic scoliosis is present. Following the course of the lower anterior ribs are warm stripes that may be heat conducted from the diaphragm muscle, or may be produced by the activity of the intercostal muscles.

temperatures. This phenomenon might be useful in detecting and following autoimmune diseases, but more study is needed to confirm the sensitivity and specificity of this Paradoxical Glomus Dilation (PGD).

Thermography of the chest and thorax

The thorax contains the lungs, heart, great vessels, and thymus gland surrounded by the ribs, rib cartilages, sternum, vertebral spine, and associated joints, ligaments, and muscles. Outside of the chest cavity are attached the scapulae, clavicles, and shoulder musculature. Because they are closer to the skin surface, the superficial structures block heat conduction from further inside the chest. The lungs, being constantly perfused with core blood, warm the chest wall by conduction. Pathology that reduces pulmonary blood flow reduces the temperatures detected over the outer chest wall. Increased chest wall temperatures may be seen over intrathoracic infections or tumors. Images of intrathoracic inflammation may show NO diffusing between the ribs. The ribs and their associated cartilages are seen thermographically in lean individuals where overlying structures are not present (Figure 10.55). The breasts in females may obscure findings over the anterior thoracic cage. Obesity in either sex may also hide thermographic details.

Fractures of the ribs, scapulae, or clavicles cause overlying warm patterns that appear acutely and may last for many months as the injury heals. Intercostal muscle strain or inflammation can be visualized thermographically where the anterior intercostal muscles are located close to the skin surface. Sites of costochondritis (inflammation of the junction of the rib and rib cartilage; Tietze's syndrome) are also detectable thermographically.[156] Even in the thermally uncontrolled environment of the emergency department, rib and lung injuries may be located quickly by thermography (Figure 10.56).[157] Traumatic chest wall injuries may affect the thermographic appearance for months (Figure 10.57).

The lungs are the largest organs in the thoracic cage and directly contact the internal chest wall over a wide area. Inflammatory diseases of the lungs or pleura may be detected thermographically over the external chest. Pleurisy appears as diffuse warmth over the affected lung.[159] Pneumonia appears as warmth over the area of infection, agreeing well with X-ray findings on disease location when thermography is positive. However, the positive predictive value of thermography

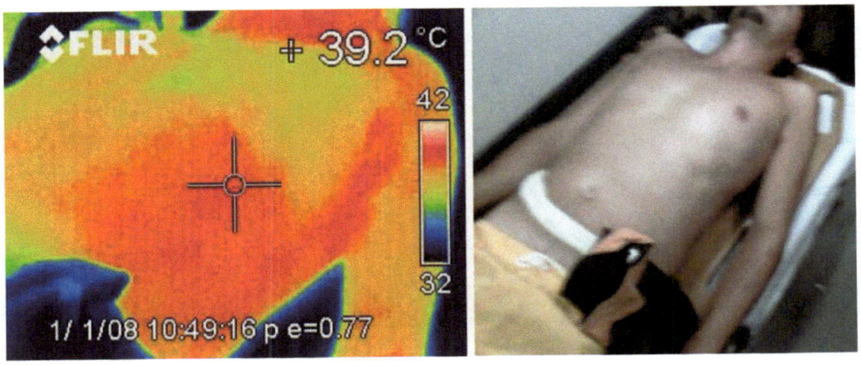

FIGURE 10.56 Pulmonary contusion caused by trauma at left thorax in an unconscious injured male. The red area indicates the troubled region and the spot meter points to the high temperature in the image coincident with a fracture of the ninth anterior left rib. (Images and caption from Brioschi 2008.)[158]

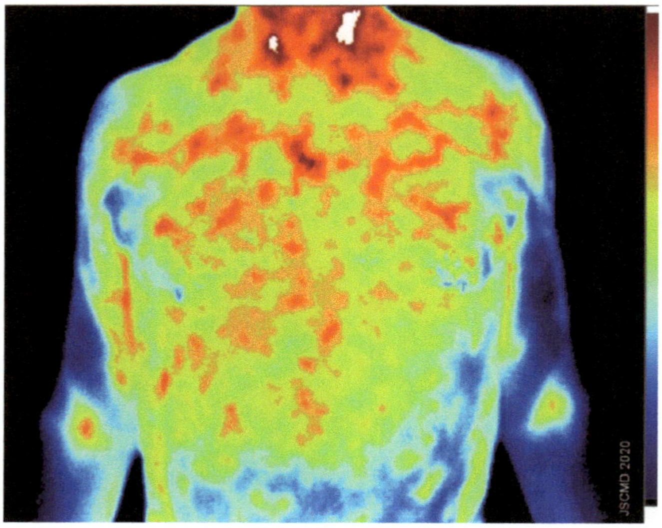

FIGURE 10.57 51-year-old man with unusual thermal markings over the anterior chest following an auto accident with forceful airbag deployment 3 months previously.

in pneumonia is less than 30%. The *negative* predictive value of thermography (pneumonia *not* present when thermography normal) approaches 94%, however, reducing the need for X-ray and CT scans in urgent care situations.[160] Another cause of an abnormal chest thermogram is malignancy of the lung or pleura, but thermal findings in chest malignancy are poorly correlated with X-ray diagnosis. Exceptions do occur, however, as shown in Figure 10.58. Thermographers should be aware of and report unusual chest findings, recommending further imaging to rule out significant disease states.

The heart is the second largest organ in the thoracic cavity. Most of the heart is surrounded by the lungs, which reduce the considerable heat generated by the heart from reaching the chest wall except at the precordial area. Unfortunately, thermography cannot estimate the functional state of a myocardium and pulmonary circulation due to the considerable ambiguity and variability in the interpretation of findings.[161] Other cardiopulmonary conditions can be detected thermographically, however. Inflammatory pericarditis may be detectable as a warm

TABLE 10.1 Thermographic Findings of Selected Cardiopulmonary Conditions

Condition	Temperature Difference	Location of Thermographic Findings
Acute angina	Cooler	Over area of pain in thorax and ipsilateral arm
Acute myocardial infarct	Cooler	Over area of pain and ipsilateral arm
Pericarditis, infectious	1.5–2.0°C Warmer	Precordial
Pericarditis, non-infectious	1.5–2.0°C Warmer	Precordial
Bacterial pneumonia	Warmer	Over the infected lobe
Active bronchitis	Warmer	T6 and cephalad paraspinal areas posteriorly
Active tuberculosis	Warmer	Over the infected lobe(s)
Lung carcinoma	Up to 2°C Warmer	Over the tumor area
Pleural Effusion, pleurisy	Warmer	Over chest wall on affected side
Pulmonary embolism	1.5°C Cooler	Over affected lobe(s)
Pulmonary fibrosis	1.5–2.0°C Cooler	Over affected area
Large lung abscess cavity	Cooler	Over location of cavity

Source: Adapted from Potanin (1970), Lobenko (1989), and Wang (2017).

zone over the precordial area near the sternal border.[162] Angina pectoris and acute myocardial infarct may produce cool areas over the zone of pain. This reduced temperature is likely due to a local sympathetic outburst which causes both sympathetic vasoconstriction and sympathetic cholinergic eccrine sweat production.

Other thermographic findings over the chest

A "vascular cape" pattern is often seen in subjects with active autoimmune disease or advanced malignancy, though it may be seen in patients unaware of any systemic disease (Figure 10.59). The cape pattern may be unilateral or bilateral. An occlusion of certain upper thoracic arteries or veins may theoretically cause a similar pattern. More research is needed into this unusual thermographic sign.

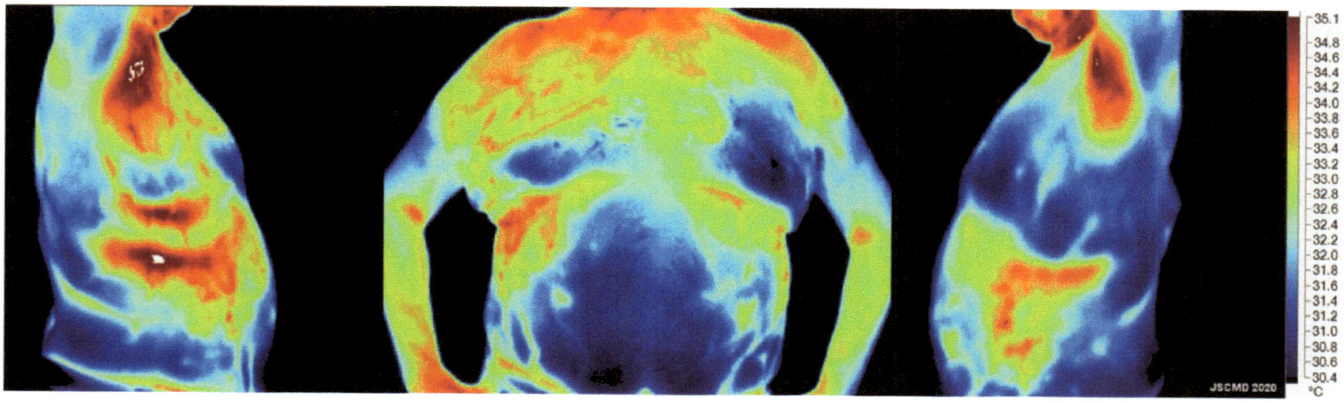

FIGURE 10.58 Thoracic thermogram of an afebrile subject with a 5 × 7 cm (2″ × 2.75″) mass in the lower right lobe of the lung recently found on CT scan. Note the very warm pattern over the right lateral chest, probably caused by nitric oxide diffusing from the mass; The areas of aberrant vessels over the lower right ribs and the right shoulder (a unilateral "vascular cape") are also unusual findings. Malignancy is strongly suspected.

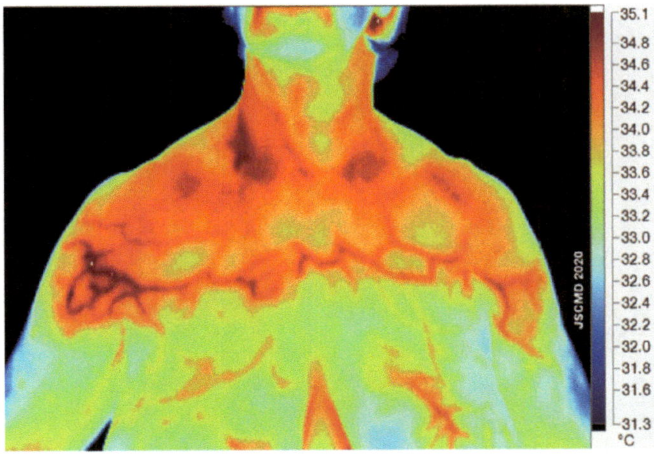

FIGURE 10.59 A bilateral vascular cape of idiopathic origin – 60-year-old female.

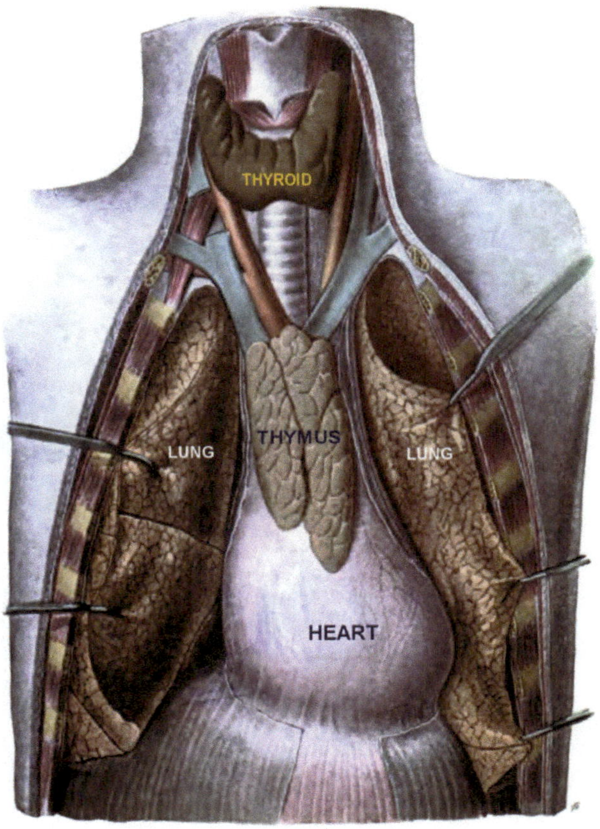

FIGURE 10.61 The organs of the anterior chest and neck in a young adult. The thymus gland shrinks considerably after puberty and weighs less than one ounce (30 gm) in older adults.[167]

Gynecomastia, or benign hypertrophy of the glandular breast tissue in males, may be detected thermographically as increased warmth over the affected site. The condition may be unilateral or bilateral. Pseudo-gynecomastia is caused by hypertrophy of breast fat and produces a cool thermal appearance (Figure 10.58). Though true gynecomastia is benign and usually resolves spontaneously in pubertal males, warm breast masses in adult men should be investigated further (Figure 10.60a).[163]

Supernumerary nipples are congenital growths that occur over the lower chest wall and abdomen, almost always caudal to the main breast nipple. They may occur singly or in multiples, extending in a line down the chest and abdomen. Unless inflamed, they appear as distinct cool spots on the thorax (Figure 10.60b). Males as well as females may have supernumerary nipples. These extra nipples may be surrounded by a visible areola. Supernumerary nipples are rarely cancerous, but they should be watched for inflammation, growth, or development of masses.[164]

The thymus gland is located in the anterior chest, in front of the upper portion of the heart and trachea (Figure 10.61). It is proportionally large in infancy but shrinks with age. At puberty, it weighs 30 to 50 grams, and by old age, it typically weighs 5 to 15 grams. The thymus rarely becomes neoplastic, developing into a lymphoma or thymoma. Lymphomas occupying superficial lymph nodes may appear warm on thermographic analysis, but this warmth is not associated with the thymus gland itself.[165] Thymomas, on the other hand, may become large enough to become detectable as a warm area in the upper anterior chest, but no studies confirming this have been published. Though some

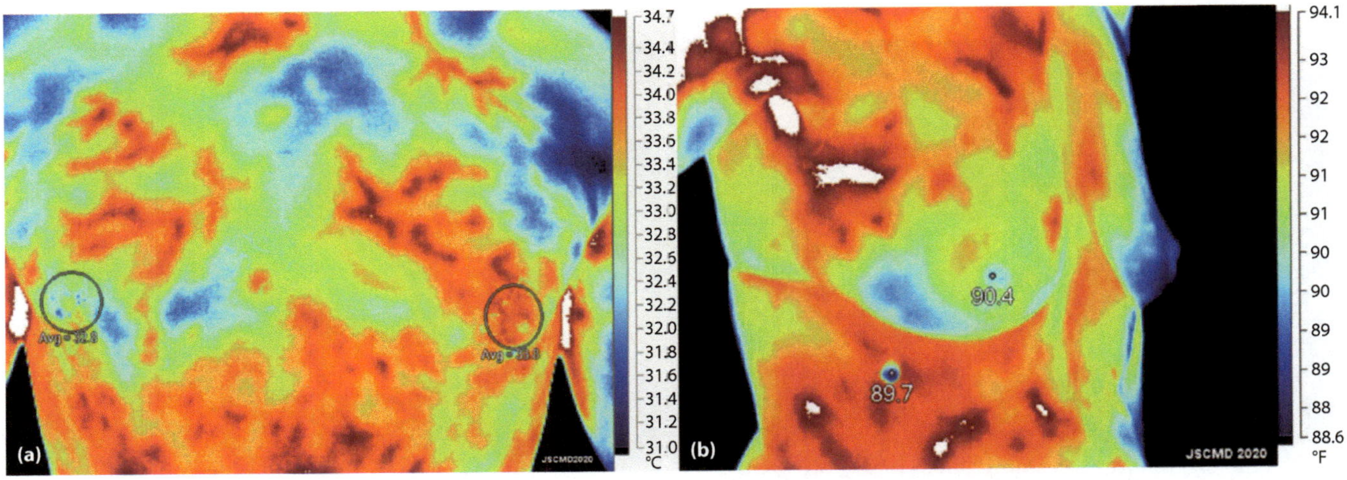

FIGURE 10.60 (a) 30-year old man with a mass in the left breast. This was later biopsied and found to be benign gynecomastia. An unusual vascular pattern is also present over the upper chest wall. (b) A supernumerary nipple is present over the lower right chest wall (site marked 89.7) – 37 yoF.

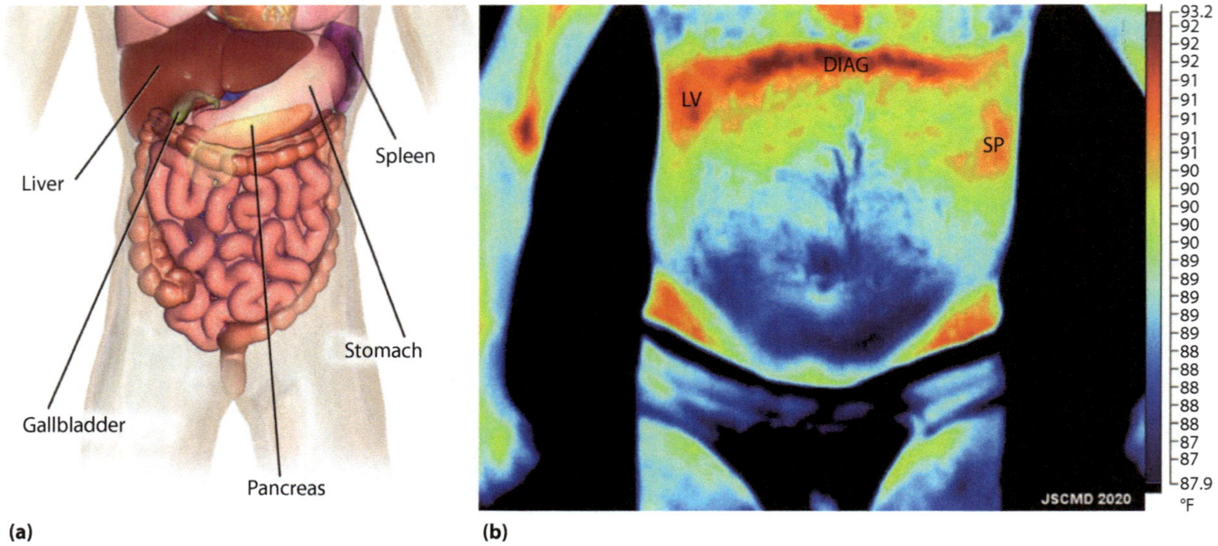

FIGURE 10.62 (a) The usual anatomical location of the abdominal organs. Thermographic findings may be expected directly over the organ involved. The gallbladder and pancreas are deep to other organs and may not affect the abdominal wall.[169] (b) Anterior abdominal thermograph of a 47-year-old male. Annotations: LV – liver area; SP – spleen area; DIAG – Warmth from diaphragm muscle. The normally warm umbilicus is cool in this case due to a small umbilical hernia.

thermographers claim that cool areas over the anterior or posterior upper chest are a sign of "underactive thymus," this is doubtful because of the small size and normally low metabolic activity of the gland in adulthood. A cool area over the upper sternum may instead be due to the presence of thymic cysts, which may become as large as 4 cm (1.6 in.) in diameter. No studies are available concerning cool areas over the thymus gland. MRI and CAT scans can determine anatomic thymus abnormalities, while hematology can monitor the physiologic and pathologic activity of the gland.[166]

Thermography of the abdomen

The anterior abdominal cavity contains the stomach, intestines, liver, spleen, and urinary bladder (Figure 10.62). The posterior abdomen contains the pancreas, kidneys, adrenal glands, and the great vessels (aorta, inferior vena cava, and cisterna chyli). Due to overlying structures, these posterior organs are rarely seen thermographically, though pyelonephritis may cause warmth near the costovertebral angle.[168] The anterior abdominal wall contains muscular and adipose layers that may obscure conducted heat or nitric oxide emitted from intestinal pathology, thus the stomach and intestines are rarely visible in thermal images unless markedly inflamed. Usually, the umbilicus provides a "thermal window" in the anterior abdominal wall through which the internal abdominal temperature can be approximated, though obesity or an umbilical hernia may obstruct this view.

The abdominal wall may show thermological changes independent of the organs underneath. Large injuries or chronic small injuries such as insulin injections can affect the abdominal wall (Figure 10.63a). Veins of the abdominal wall above the umbilicus generally flow cranially; veins below the umbilicus flow caudally. Antero-lateral abdominal veins are rare thermographic findings, but may be seen if inferior vena cava obstruction is present.[170]

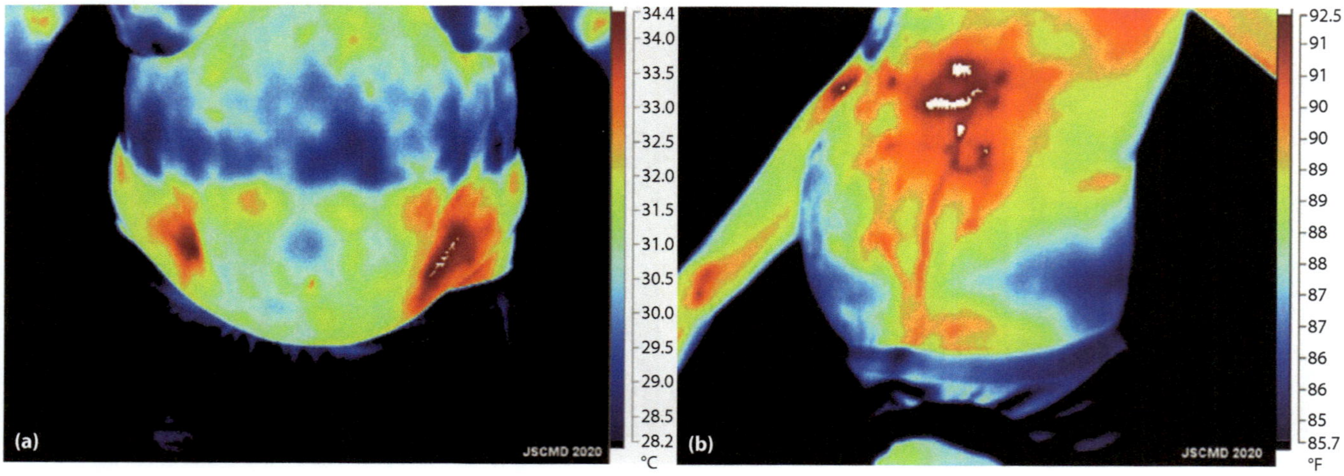

FIGURE 10.63 (a) Lipodystrophy of the abdominal wall from chronic insulin injections. The upper quadrants appear normal. – 63-year-old female. (b) Metastatic melanoma with possible spleen involvement. Left flank view. Antero-lateral abdominal vascular markings are present, representing either draining veins or inflamed lymphatics. – 61-year-old male.

The liver is the most metabolically active organ in the abdomen, and the heat generated can be detected thermographically in the upper portion of the right upper abdominal quadrant as an asymmetric warm area (Figure 10.62). This warm pattern persists in acute and chronic hepatitis, fatty infiltration of the liver, and early cardiac cirrhosis. Advanced cirrhosis with liver failure may appear cool, however.[171] The spleen is usually not detectable thermographically unless inflamed or enlarged (Figure 10.63b).

Acute infections of the abdomen, including appendicitis and biliary tract disease (cholecystitis) may be detected by thermography, but only in about 60% of cases.[172] Thermal differentiation of peritoneal infection from abdominal malignancy is not fully reliable because tumors can give the same thermal pattern as infection. Ascites (fluid accumulation in the abdominal cavity) has not been adequately studied with thermography. Detection of abdominal pathology in obese patients is poor, though thermography has application in the localizing of postoperative infections.[173]

Inflammatory bowel disease (IBD) and colorectal cancer can produce changes in the pattern of the abdominal thermogram. Colonic disease changes appear around the periphery of the abdomen, while small bowel inflammation tends to cause more central, periumbilical findings. Both IBD and colorectal cancer appear warm, however, making thermal differentiation between these conditions difficult. Thermography can, at best, be used as a screening tool for referrals for more definitive imaging or tests in these abdominal diseases.[174]

Thermography of the back and spine

Thermal images of the thoracic, lumbar, and sacral spine and musculature are useful for detection and follow-up of deformities, scoliosis, neural innervation, muscular strain, injuries, and inflammation. Though the vertebral bodies and spinal cord are generally too deep to be visible in the infrared, the general alignment of the spinal column is usually well visualized. The first layer of structures under the dermis – the trapezius muscles, latissimus dorsi, thoracolumbar fascia, iliac crests, and spinous processes of the vertebrae – can usually be assessed thermographically. Inflammation of the muscular layers under this layer may also be detected, though usually not as clearly and with less intensity (Figure 10.64). The kidneys, which are normally located on either side of the T12 to L2

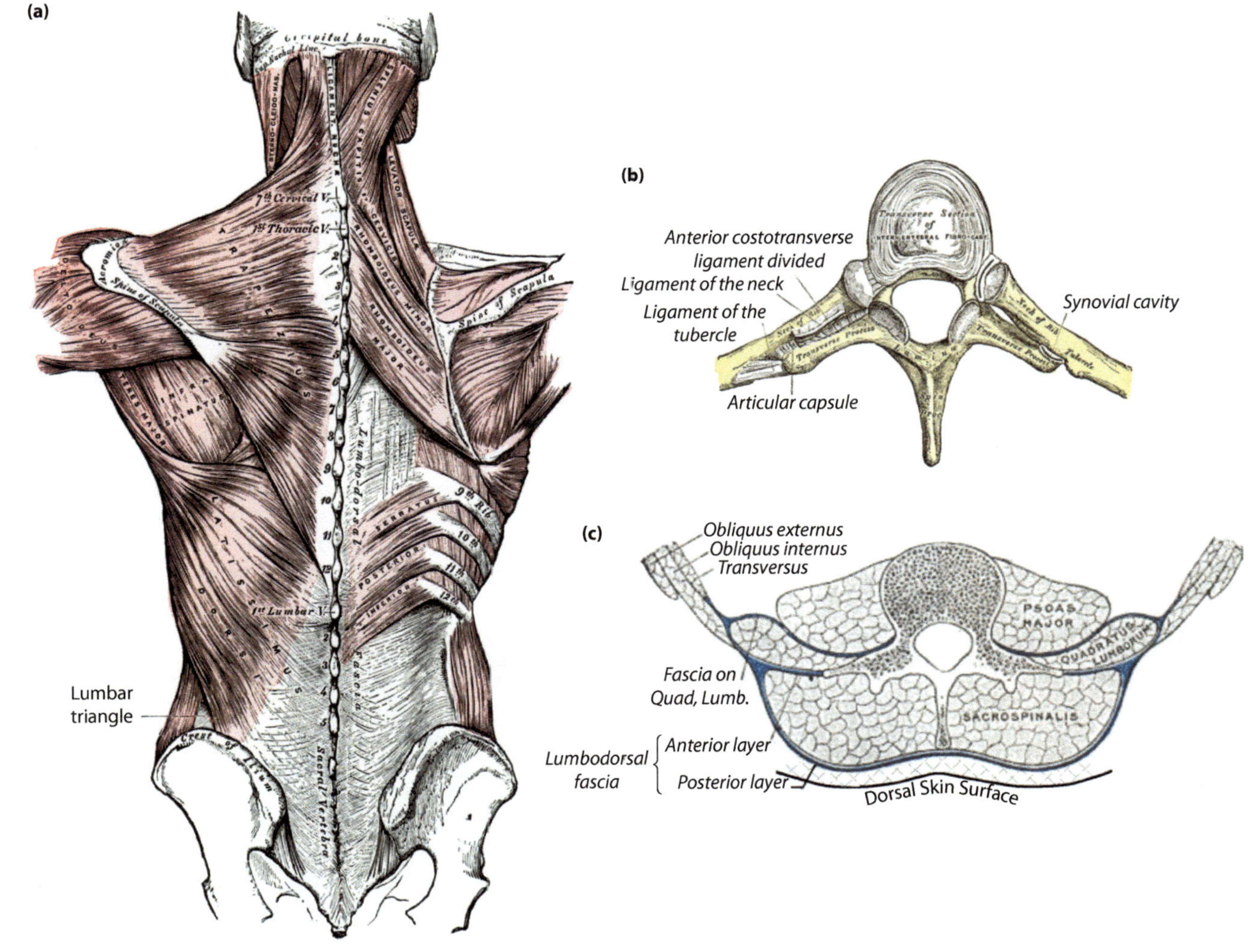

FIGURE 10.64 (a) Muscles of the back. The most superficial muscles are shown on the left. Intermediate layer structures are shown on the right. Muscles and ligaments in the deep layer are usually not visible thermographically.[175] (b) A thoracic vertebra with rib attachments, seen from above.[176] (c) cross-sectional view through a lumbar vertebral body. The erector spinae muscle group (formerly called the sacrospinalis) may be evaluated thermographically as it is only separated from the dermis by the lumbodorsal fascia. The psoas muscle lies deep to the transverse processes of the vertebral bodies and is too deep to affect the dorsal thermogram.[177]

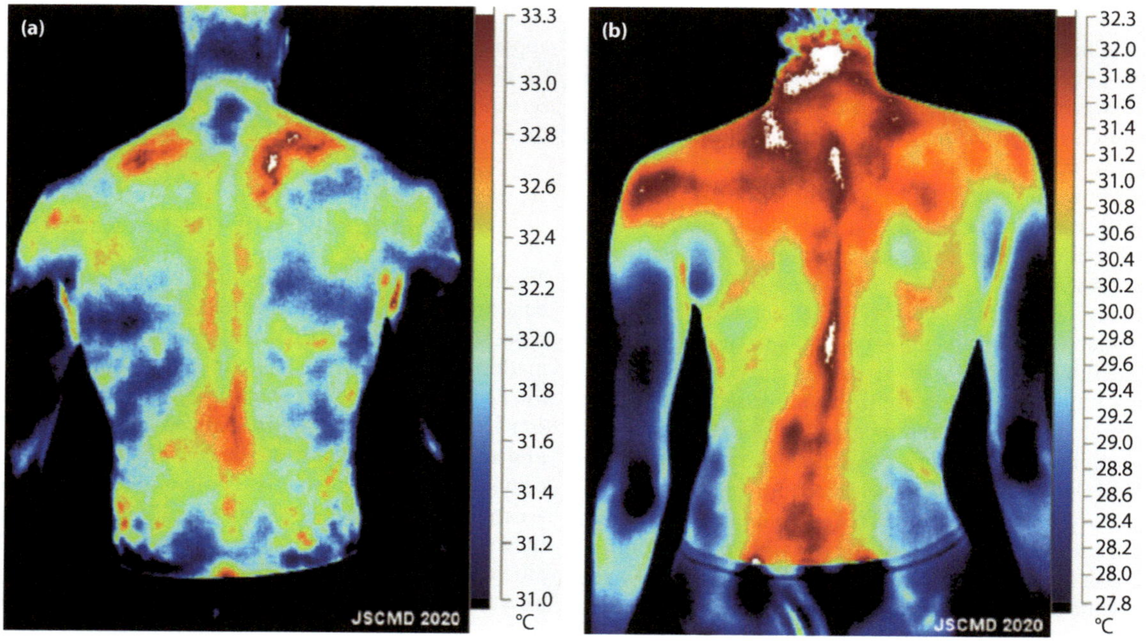

FIGURE 10.65 (a) This thoracic (T4–T12) paraspinal inflammatory pattern may be due to enthesiopathy of the origins of the trapezius muscles or inflammation of the deeper erector spinae groups. Also seen here are bilateral mid-Trapezius muscle and upper lumbar strain patterns. – 53 yoM. (b) complex scoliosis with a left lumbar strain pattern in a subject with foraminal stenosis. Trapezius and shoulder strain patterns are also present bilaterally. – 49 yoF.

vertebrae posteriorly, may develop thermally-detectable warmth at those spinal levels if infected. As with other imaging methods, spinal thermography may be less definitive if the subject is obese.

Thermographic images of the spine are usually taken with the subject standing. The subject may be temperature-equilibrated in a sitting position on a stool with no back, and then asked to stand for the images. If conducted heat from muscle tension due to gravity is not desired, the subject must be cooled in a prone position on a table with face and arm supports (Figure 6.4). The images may be taken while the subject remains prone, or the subject may be asked to stand up quickly for the images before any conducted heat from gravitational muscle contraction becomes apparent.

The lumbodorsal fascia provides a thermal "window" into several of the middle-layer muscles of the spine; especially the paravertebral muscles of the Erector Spinae group (see Figure 10.64). Difficulty may arise when trying to determine the origin of thermographic warmth over this area, however, because the inflammation may be due to either the lumbodorsal fascia itself, or the deeper underlying structures.

Scoliosis may be evaluated on spinal thermograms (Figure 10.65b). The midline of the back over the lumbar vertebrae is often warmer than the paraspinal areas; over the thoracic vertebrae, the midline may appear cooler (Figure 10.65a). The center of the nape of the neck serves as a landmark for determining scoliosis by drawing a straight line from there to the center of the sacrum and observing any spinal deviation from this line. Warmth may be seen over the interspinal muscles and ligaments, especially where those structures are under strain (Figure 10.66). Screening for spinal scoliosis in children may be done thermographically. Proper temperature equilibration is required, however.

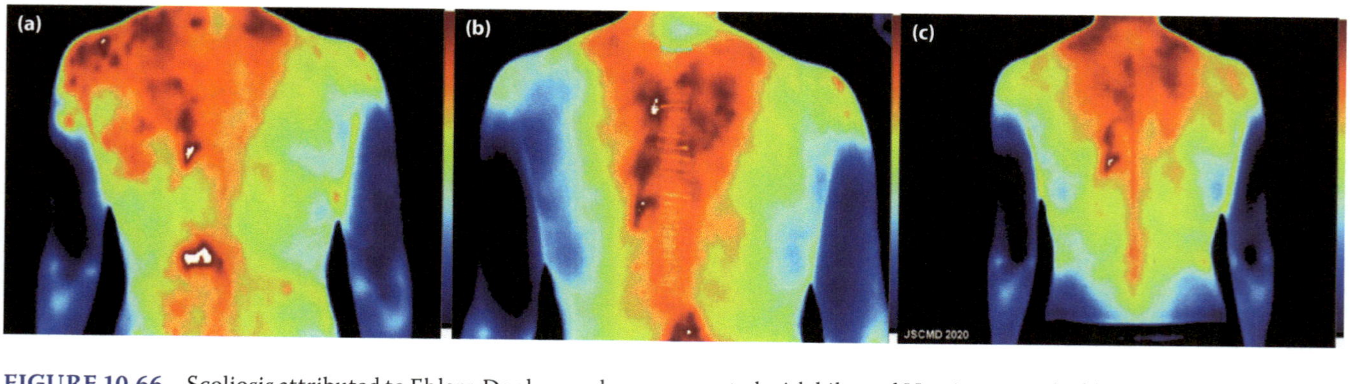

FIGURE 10.66 Scoliosis attributed to Ehlers-Danlos syndrome corrected with bilateral Harrington rods. (a) May 2011 – Harrington rods in place from T3 to L1. Marked strain pattern is present over left trapezius and shoulder. (b) August 2011 – rods removed 6 days previously. Shoulder inflammation much improved. (c) Apr 2014 – Scoliosis reported as stable. Moderate bilateral trapezius strain pattern is present. No scoliosis is seen thermographically. – 25–28 yoF.

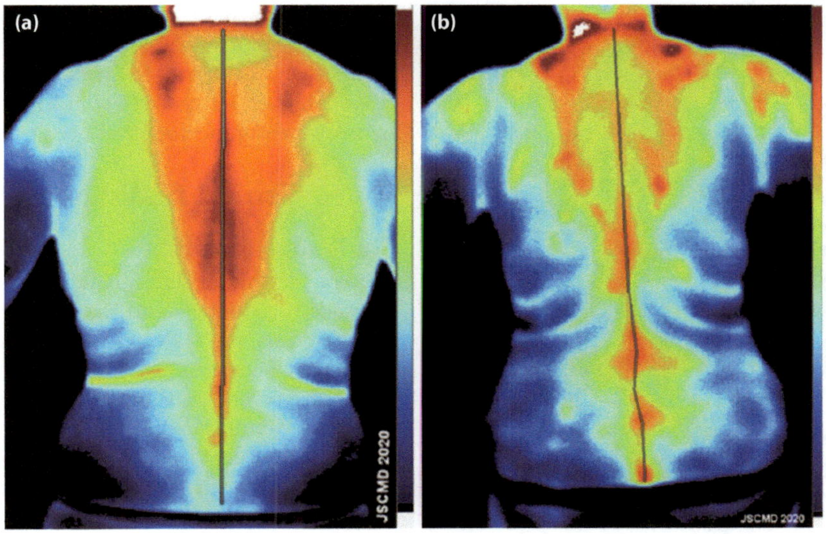

FIGURE 10.67 (a) Trapezius strain involving the tendinous vertebral attachments and muscle bellies bilaterally – 57 yoF (b) Trapezius muscle inflammation, bilateral, with the tendinous vertebral attachments mostly spared. A minor lumbar scoliosis pattern is also present. – 47 yoF.

Trapezius muscle strain and Trapezius tendinitis patterns are frequent findings (Figure 10.67). The Trapezius muscles are normally under tension to support the head and arms when in a standing or sitting position. As the Trapezii are large, flat muscles close to the skin surface, thermography can determine which parts of the muscle are inflamed. Muscle tissue or tendinous areas (or both) may be inflamed.

Lumbar strain

The skin over superficial lumbar muscles that are actively contracting will appear warm by conduction, a frequent finding on spinal thermograms. Inflammed ligaments, bursae, or muscles will appear warm due to the local production of NO (Figure 10.68). This may appear bilaterally or unilaterally, depending on the underlying condition. Except for the Erector Spinae group, the deeper muscles generally will not be visualized because of the overlying muscle layers.

Spinal nerve compression and laminectomy

Spinal nerve impingement from intervertebral disc protrusion or single-level foraminal stenosis does not cause dermatomal thermographically visible areas. The thermal finding of increased local warmth due to loss of sympathetic tone comes from the sympathetic trunks, not the spinal cord. The sympathetic trunks communicate both upward and downward across the dermatomes, thus compensating for and obscuring any sympathetic deficit caused by a single spinal nerve root compression. Paraspinal heat conducted from local muscle spasm caused by the pain of

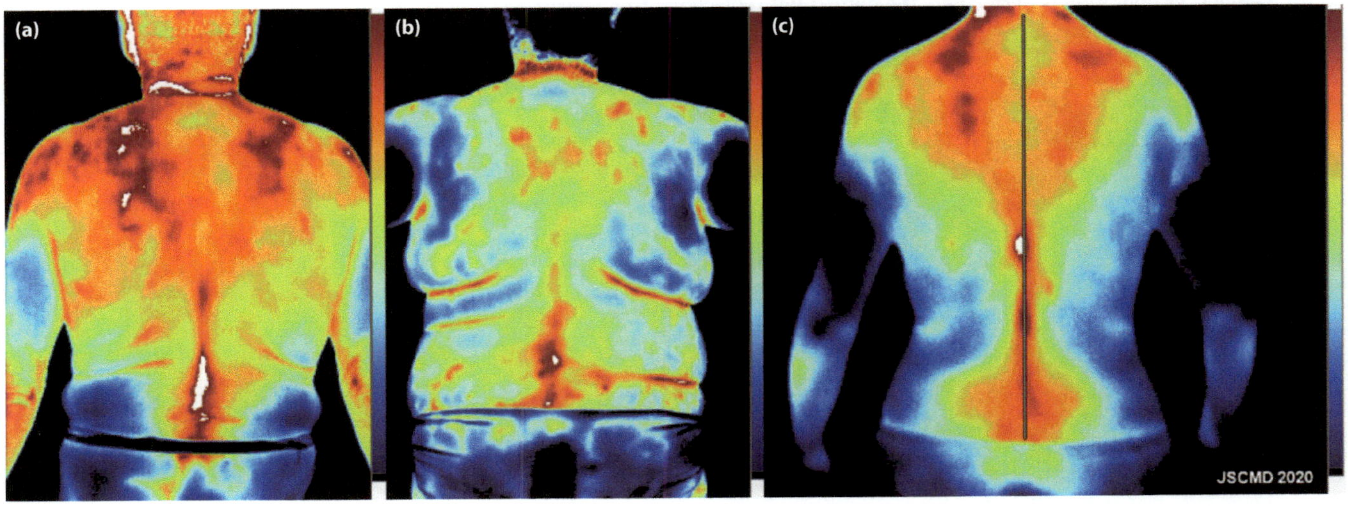

FIGURE 10.68 Lumbar inflammatory and strain patterns: (a) Tire salesman with midline lumbar and trapezius strain patterns. – 70 yoM. (b) Lumbar pain of unknown etiology in a subject with leukemia in remission. – 58yoF. (c) Diffuse bilateral lower lumbar strain pattern possibly due to fasciitis of the lower lumbodorsal fascia. Also seen are midline thoraco-lumbar and trapezius muscle strain patterns. – 38yoF.

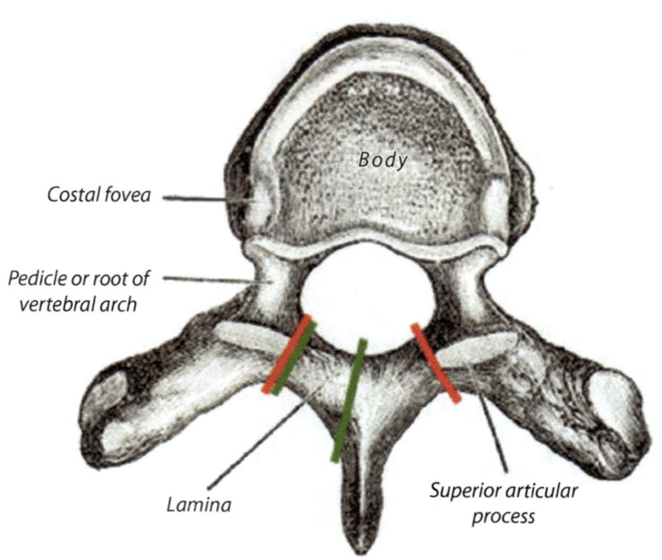

FIGURE 10.69 Unilateral vs. bilateral laminectomy. A unilateral procedure (left shown) removes the bone between the green lines, sparing the spinous process; a bilateral laminectomy removes the bone between the red lines, including the spinous process.[179]

spinal nerve impingement may be present, however. Skin warmth along a strictly dermatomal pattern should suggest nerve damage at or distal to the sympathetic trunks and proximal to the brachial or lumbar nerve plexuses. Due to stimulation of the corresponding sympathetic segment by the compressed nerve root causing increased vasoconstriction, the involved limb may have a *cool* area that corresponds roughly to the distribution of that nerve root.[178]

Laminectomy is a procedure necessary to gain surgical access to the spinal canal. Whether just one lamina is removed or both lamina and the spinous process are to be excised depends on the location and nature of the spinous pathology (Figure 10.69). Spinal tumor removal or correction of spinal stenosis generally require a bilateral laminectomy. Decompression of a herniated disk pressing on a nerve root may require only a unilateral procedure. Whichever operation is performed, the bone is not replaced afterward, leaving a "window" of thermal conduction from the circulating cerebrospinal fluid to the skin above. This postoperative increased warmth over the spine will appear in the midline in the case of bilateral laminectomy, and just lateral to the midline when a unilateral laminectomy has been performed (Figure 10.70).

Genital findings in thermography

Male subjects

Except for the prostate gland and seminal vesicles, which are too deep in the pelvis to significantly affect the overlying skin temperature, the male genitalia are easily observed with thermography. In normal subjects, the testicles should be about the same size on each side of the scrotum and of almost equal temperature. Scrotal temperature should be less than the inguinal skin temperature. The left testicle usually hangs lower when the cremasteric muscles are relaxed because the left spermatic cord is longer.[180] Thermographic cooling protocols may cause testicular retraction via the cremasteric muscle reflex. The glans penis is generally cooler than the penile shaft, though this may be partially obscured by a warm foreskin (Figure 10.71). The skin over the penis and scrotum is normally quite thin and has almost no subdermal fat, so it readily shows thermal anomalies.

Herpes simplex infections of the skin of the penis can be expected to create warm areas visible to thermography when prodromal or active. During the healing stage, any remaining crusts appear cooler.[181] Latent herpes generally cannot be detected thermographically over the perioral area, and the same lack of findings can be extended to genital herpes. Though no studies are available showing the penile changes with active gonorrhea or chlamydia, an inflammatory pattern over the glans or urinary meatus might be expected in these diseases.

Testicular or epididymal infections (orchitis or epididymitis) both cause painful inflammation and swelling within the ipsilateral scrotal sac, which should be visible to thermography. Varicocele is essentially a varicose vein within the scrotum. These usually painless varicosities appear warmer than the surrounding tissue in a serpentine pattern, similar to varicosities over other body locations (Figure 10.72).[182] Non-painful, chronic scrotal swelling that appears cool thermographically may be due to a hydrocele.

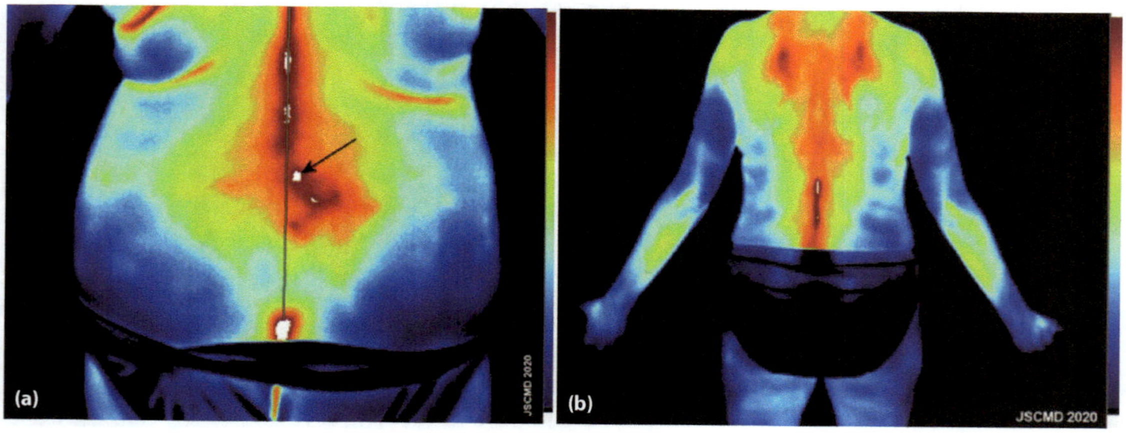

FIGURE 10.70 (a) Sciatica pain on right after unilateral right lumbar laminectomy. The midline warm areas over the upper lumbar vertebrae are likely due to tension or inflammation of the interspinalis lumborum muscles. Local lumbosacral warmth on the right is most likely due to the unilateral laminectomy (arrow) and local muscle spasm. No dermatomal pattern is seen. – 59yoF. (b) Bilateral laminectomy of the L1–L2 vertebrae for excision of a meningioma 4yrs previously – 70yoF.

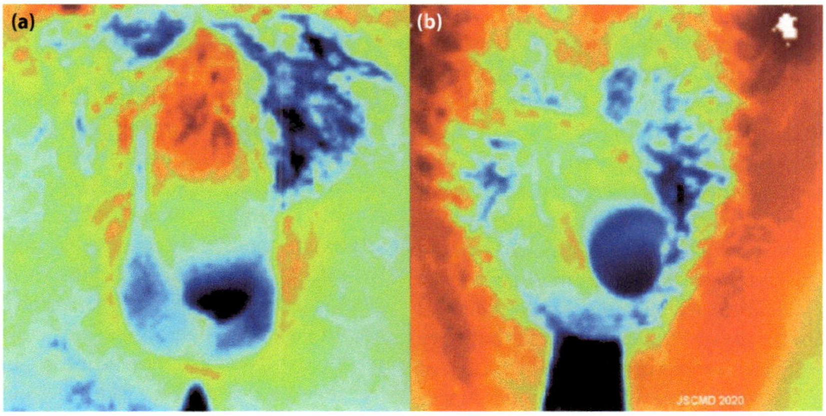

FIGURE 10.71 Normal external male genitalia. Note how the two sides of the scrotum appear about the same temperature. The glans penis is normally cooler than the penile shaft. (a) Uncircumcised 44-year-old male; (b) circumcised 68-year-old male.

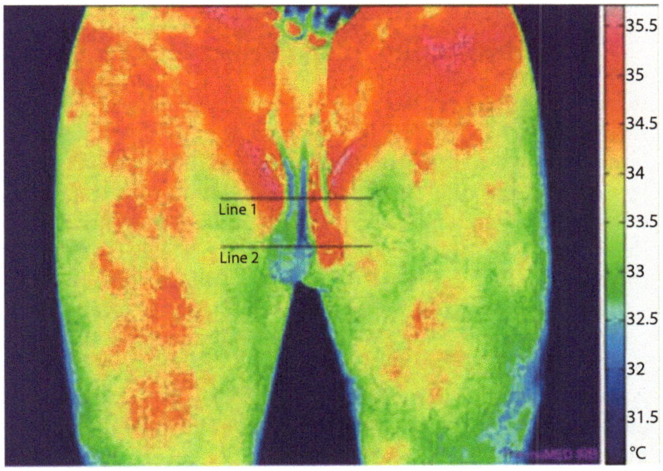

FIGURE 10.72 A varicocele in the left hemiscrotum appears much warmer than the normal, cooler right side. Incidental glomus dilation of the fingernails is also present.[183]

Testicular torsion is an emergency condition where one testicle rotates in the scrotal sac, occluding the testicular artery. The resulting testicular ischemia produces extreme pain of rapid onset on the affected side. Swelling may also be present, making the diagnosis of acute epididymitis a possible diagnosis. Since the arterial occlusion stops warm blood from entering the scrotum, the involved testicle should appear cool to thermography, as opposed to the warm appearance of epididymitis. Experimental torsion of the testicular artery in animals has confirmed this, testicular torsion results in significant testicular cooling as measured by thermography; rewarming occurs quickly upon reduction of the experimental torsion.[184] Thermography utilized in the emergency department may be extremely useful in the diagnosis of testicular torsion as well as in confirmation of its correction.

Female subjects

The external genitalia of females may be studied with thermography, though pubic hair and anatomical location may obscure the genital area as seen with normal thermographic views (Figure 10.73). In the standard lithotomy position with the labia majora parted, the labia minora, urethral meatus, and clitoral areas may be visualized. Proper thermographic cooling of the

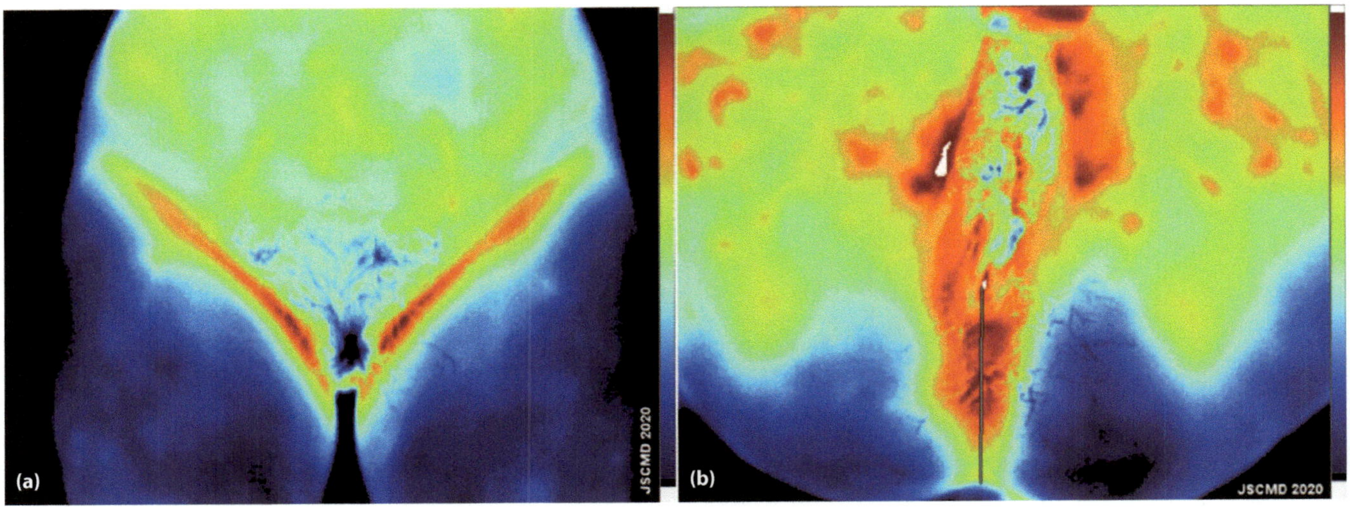

FIGURE 10.73 (a) Normal female pubic area, subject standing. – 64yoF. (b) Perineal and anal region in a normal female. The subject is supine with knees brought up and apart. The line indicates the anatomical midline. – 58yoF.

area may be difficult, however. Dynamic thermographic techniques might be required to provide suitable thermal contrast.

Infection of the Bartholin gland located in the female labia majora should, like other abscesses, appear unilaterally warmer, and may be detectable even in the standing position. A noninfected Bartholin cyst should appear relatively cool. Vulvar varicosities should appear warm, similar to varicose veins at other sites. Herpes simplex of the vulvar skin will, like oral herpes, be undetectable while latent, but show localized warmth while in the prodromal or active stages. Extensive hyperthermia may occur during an initial herpes attack. The thermal appearance of genital warts (condyloma accuminata) has not been reported, but they should appear cool as do other viral skin growths. More study of the external female genitalia is warranted using improved imager technology under proper thermographic conditions.

Culposcopic thermography of the cervix and vaginal walls is possible using a plastic speculum, though a temperature equilibration protocol for the internal vaginal surfaces has not been described. A high-resolution imager coupled with a telephoto infrared lens will be needed to provide an infrared view of the uterine cervix. Special cooling protocols may need to be developed. Whether the female ovaries and fallopian tubes can be evaluated by culpo-thermography has not been reported.

The peri-anal area can also be observed by thermography, but special positioning is required to expose the perineum during the equilibration period. A supine position with the knees pulled back and separated may be used, as can a face-down knee-chest position. Very little research has been done in perineal thermography. The extent of any external hemorrhoids, which are perianal varicose veins, should become apparent; whether thrombosis of a hemorrhoid can be detected is not clear. Proctitis may also be visible; though as the anal area is intrinsically warm due to a rich arterial supply, any inflammation of the area may be qualitatively less apparent. Recurrent rectal carcinoma may be detected as a significant rise in perianal temperature.[185] Postpartum infrared evaluation of the pelvic floor has also begun to be studied, though no conclusive results have yet been posted.[186]

Thermal findings in the human sexual response

As infrared thermography may be used at a distance, does not require visible light, and is totally noninvasive, it has become a research tool for observing the genital responses to visual sexual stimulation in both males and females. Such studies have demonstrated that genital temperature is strongly correlated with subjective ratings of sexual arousal; both men and women have significant genital temperature rises with sexual arousal (about 1.8°C/3.3°F rise in genital temperatures over controls); and men and women reach peak genital temperature in about the same time.[187] Most thermological research into the human sexual response has focused on the genitals, though other thermal responses may occur elsewhere on the body. Masters and Johnson reported a maculopapular flush over the anterior torso of both sexes during arousal; this subsides quickly following orgasm.[188] Whether this reaction is detectable thermographically remains to be studied.

Thermography of the lower extremity

Infrared imaging can assess tendon, ligament, bone, and joint injuries in the leg. Much of the clinical research in this area has focused on the knee joint. Ligaments within the knee are readily damaged by various forms of external trauma, including athletic activities, traffic accidents, industrial injuries, and falls. Although most of the thermography research has focused on osteoarthritis of the knee, some studies have addressed the issue of traumatic knee injury.[189]

A common form of knee injury involves damage to the medial collateral ligament (MCL), which connects the medial condyle of the femur to the medial side of the upper tibia (Figure 10.74).[190] An acute MCL tear is usually accompanied by pain, muscular guarding, swelling, and blood in the joint fluid. Careful evaluation and follow-up is needed when an MCL injury occurs because

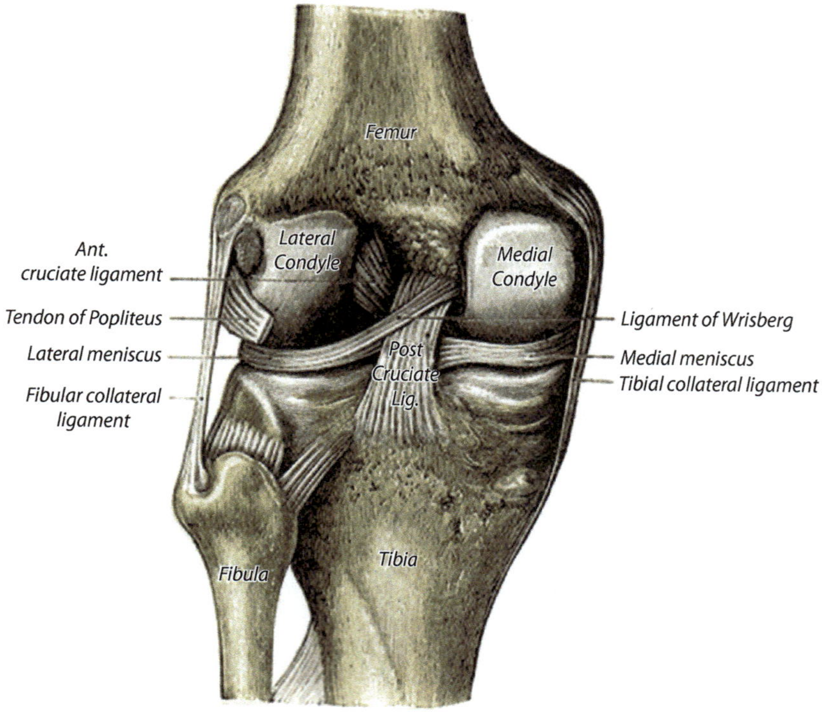

FIGURE 10.74 A posterior view of the left knee joint showing the bones, connecting ligaments, and menisci. The tibial collateral ligament is now called the medial collateral ligament (MCL).[192]

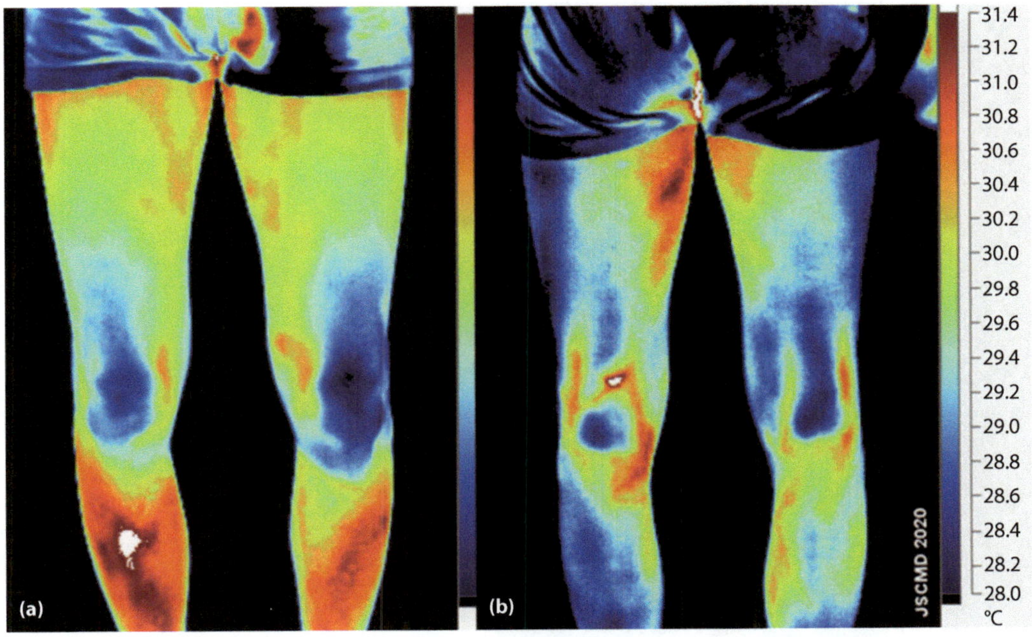

FIGURE 10.75 Continued pain in the left knee 1 year after surgical repair of a torn medial meniscus. (a) The anterior view shows warmth over the medial knees, greater on the left. (b) The posterior view has abnormal warm patterns over the left semimembranosus, semitendinosus, and biceps femoris tendons, possibly due to chronic muscular guarding of the left knee. – 53 yoM.

recurrence is possible if healing is not complete. Thermography provides an easy and noncontact assessment of joint morbidity.[191]

Infrared imaging of normal knee joints shows thermal symmetry between both knees, each of which is cooler than adjacent areas with the patella being coolest (see Figure 13.19). Temperature changes and asymmetries become significant when the knee ligaments are injured. Temperatures of the damaged knee show a significant increase over the unaffected knee. The temperature increase is due to inflammation from the ligament injury.[193] Thermography also helps in the assessment of physiotherapy for Anterior Cruciate Ligament (ACL) injuries.[194]

Other bony, ligamentous, and soft-tissue injuries can also be detected in the legs using static thermography (Figure 10.75). Enthesiopathies (inflammation or injury of the tendon-to-bone attachments) usually show distinct patterns. Bursitis and tendinitis also create areas of local warmth due to the emission of NO from the inflamed or healing tissues (Figure 10.76). The location of thermal signs from these various pathologies is strongly

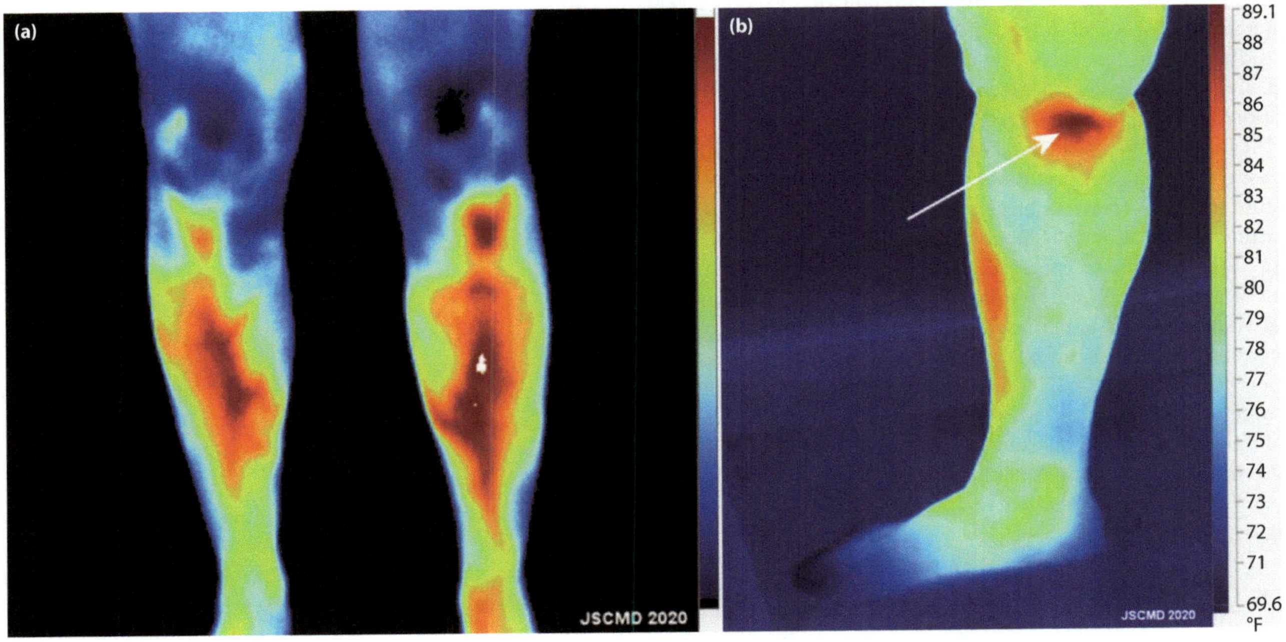

FIGURE 10.76 (a) Patellar tendon and tibialis anterior muscle enthesiopathy patterns, bilateral, greater on the left. Note the blurred thermal appearance due to NO diffusion. The knee joints both appear fairly normal. – 69 yoF. (b) Inflammation over the pes anserinus tendons of the medial right leg (arrow). This appearance may be due to tendinitis, enthesiopathy, or an overlying bursitis. – 68 yoF.

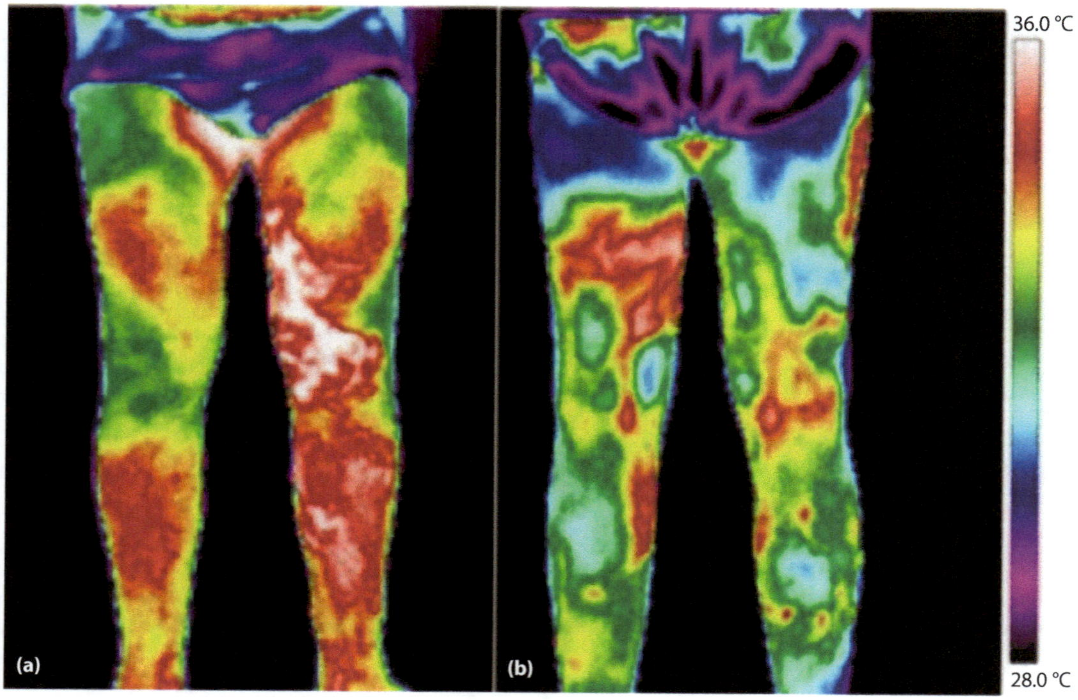

FIGURE 10.77 Thermograms of the legs of a patient with venous insufficiency primarily on the left. No venous ulceration is present. (a) Anterior view, (b) posterior view.[196]

dependent on the anatomy involved. Infection of the knee joint or surrounding structures can cause local temperature elevation. Active arthritis may be visible also, see Chapter 11 for more details.

Venous leg ulcers

A venous leg ulcer is a dermal wound on the leg or ankle caused by abnormally functioning veins. Major risk factors include varicosities, venous reflux, venous clotting, and obesity; hereditary factors may also play a role. Thermographically, venous ulcers generally appear 0.5°C to 1°C (0.9°F to 1.8°F) *cooler* than the surrounding dermis, probably due to the evaporative cooling of the wet surface, lack of dermal arterioles in the ulcer bed, and inflammation of the periwound skin.[195]

Thermography can assess venous ulcer healing potential by measuring temperature differences in the wound and the periwound skin.[197] A clean venous wound area larger than one square centimeter has about the same temperature as the peri-wound skin. The presence of bacteria in the wound produces a significant 0.4°C (0.72°F) differential temperature increases in the peri-wound skin; an increased number of bacterial species in the wound is associated with a highly significant temperature difference of 0.95°C (1.7°F). A lower temperature difference between these two areas is a reliable predictor of wound healing. Unfortunately, the correlation of infrared results in differentiating venous ulcer healing is confounded by the warmth of underlying varicose veins frequently associated with venous ulcers (Figure 10.77).[198]

Thermography of the feet

The feet, like the hands, have only a thin, albeit tough, layer of subdermal fat, allowing heat generated by muscle tension and NO produced by local inflammation or infection to be readily visible thermographically. Thermal images provide a convenient way to anatomically localize the underlying pathology, though identifying which layer is involved (fascia, muscle, ligaments, or bone) requires other clinical tests or imaging (Figure 10.78). A generally warm foot may be due to sympathetic denervation fromdiabetic nerve damage or other neuropathy, especially if the warmth is greater toward the toes. A cool foot may be seen in cases of arterial occlusion in the ipsilateral leg in subjects that have been equilibrated in a warmer environment. Massive sympathetic neural stimulation may also produce a cool foot, as can occur in acute compartment syndrome.

A thermal imprint made by standing on a room-temperature insulated pad provides qualitative information on the plantar surface of a subject.[199] This procedure is usually done on a warm patient just after they remove their shoes and socks. It may also be performed on a cooled subject to detect distal vasodilation or inflammation, or after "dry" cold immersion to detect diabetic neuropathy. The subject steps carefully onto the thermal pad, stands still for 5 seconds, and then steps off the pad. A thermal image is quickly taken of the pad, revealing the thermal footprints, which can be qualitatively analyzed (Figure 10.79). This technique can also be used for gait analysis by having the patient walk or run down a longer pad, then imaging and analyzing the thermal patterns retained on the pad. As this technique is dependent on heat conduction, both absolute and differential quantitative measurements will be affected by the temperature of the pad, making them unreliable.

To obtain both qualitative and quantitative plantar views of both feet, the supine or prone positions are preferred during equilibration. An image showing both soles will best visualize temperature patterns of the feet, as shown in Figure 10.78. To prevent thermal artifacts from affecting the ankles and Achilles tendons, the distal 7.6 cm (3 in.) of the tibia should be suspended off the exam table during the equilibration period. After the plantar view is obtained, the patient may sit or stand

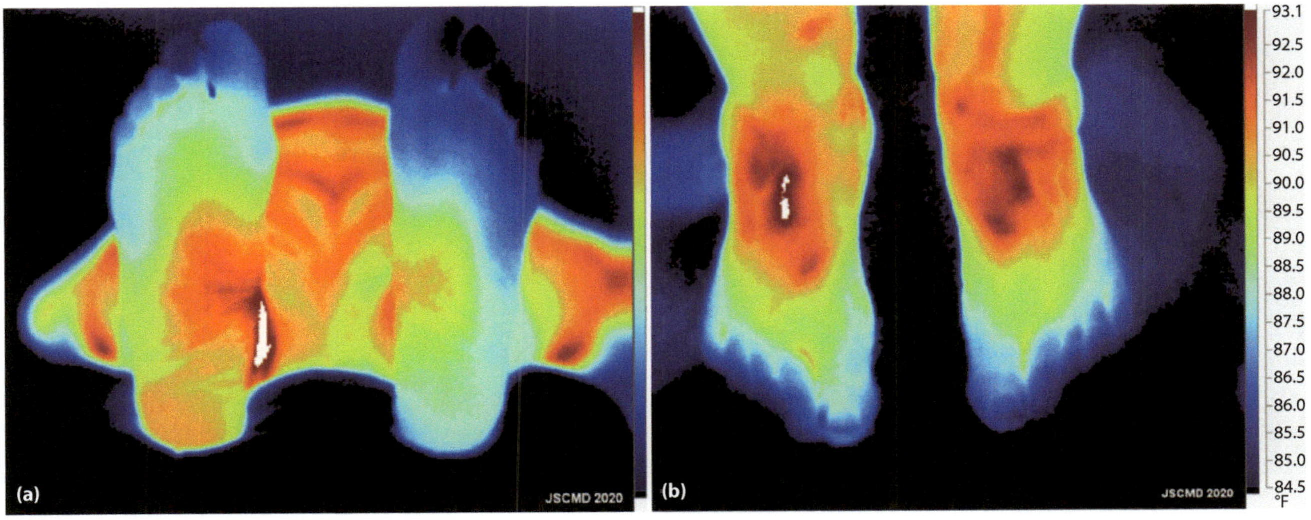

FIGURE 10.78 (a) Plantar view showing non-traumatic inflammation of the right foot involving the calcaneal area and the medial mid-foot. Inflammation of the plantar aponeurosis or strain of the flexor digitorum brevis muscle may be present. – 75 yoF. (b) Thermographic pattern of inflammation over the tarsal bones bilaterally. Inflammation or tension of the extensor digitorum brevis muscles may produce a similar image as can bilateral Charcot neuroarthropathy. – 65 yoF.

while the other images of the feet are taken to complete the series (Figures 10.80 and 10.81). As discussed in Chapter 6, five images are needed to fully evaluate a foot.

Foot ulcers and diabetic neuropathy

Diabetes mellitus adversely affects the peripheral nerves of the body. As the nerves to the foot are the longest in the human body, they are most likely to display diabetic neuropathy. Symptoms of diabetic neuropathy are numbness and paresthesias, accompanied by autonomic dysfunction. Loss of sympathetic vasoconstrictive control leads to skin warmth over the affected areas even in a cooled individual.[200] Because the neuropathic areas are numb, injuries such as blisters or small abrasions may go unnoticed. With repeated injury or infection, skin ulcers, sometimes deep enough to expose bone, may be seen thermographically.

Diabetic foot ulcers and related complications are debilitating and costly sequelae of diabetes.[201] Infection, neuropathy, and peripheral artery disease are key contributors to amputation risk in these patients.[202] When compared to normal subjects, diabetic patients tend to have warmer feet and exhibit significantly greater temperature differences between feet. Additionally, the presence of neuropathy raises foot temperature; both ischemic and neuro-ischemic feet are warmer than healthy feet.[203]

Increased skin temperature in the foot has high sensitivity but low specificity.[204] Charcot neuroarthropathy can mimic an injury

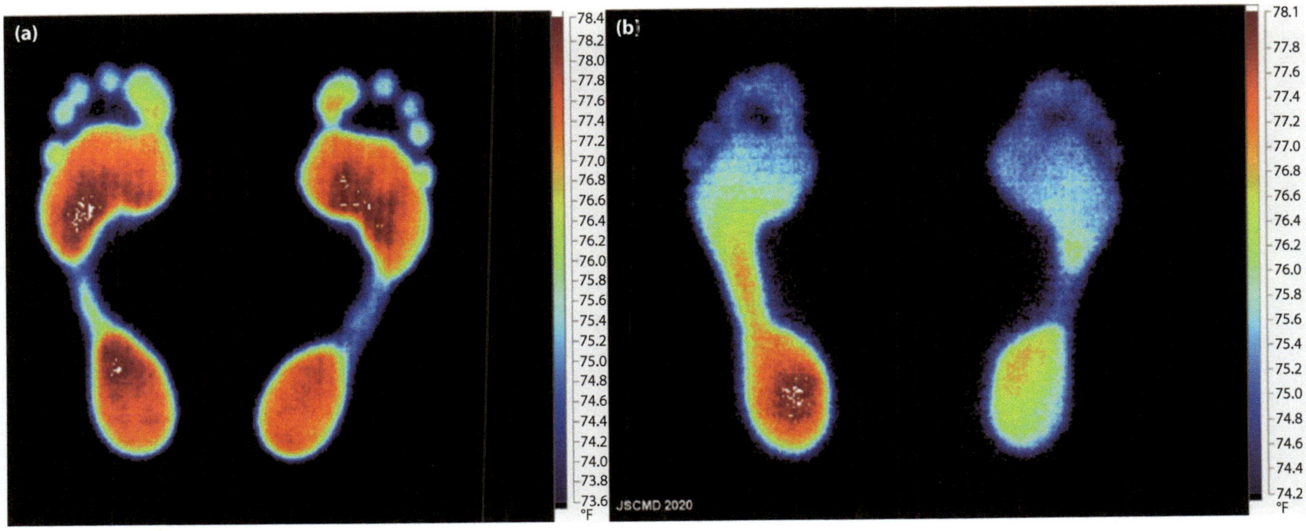

FIGURE 10.79 Stationary standing thermal prints. (a) 77-year old male with non-traumatic inflammation of the first metatarsal-phalangeal joint on the left. The entire left plantar surface is affected. (b) Same subject nine days later. The joint inflammation is clinically much improved, and the left plantar surface now appears slightly cooler than the right.

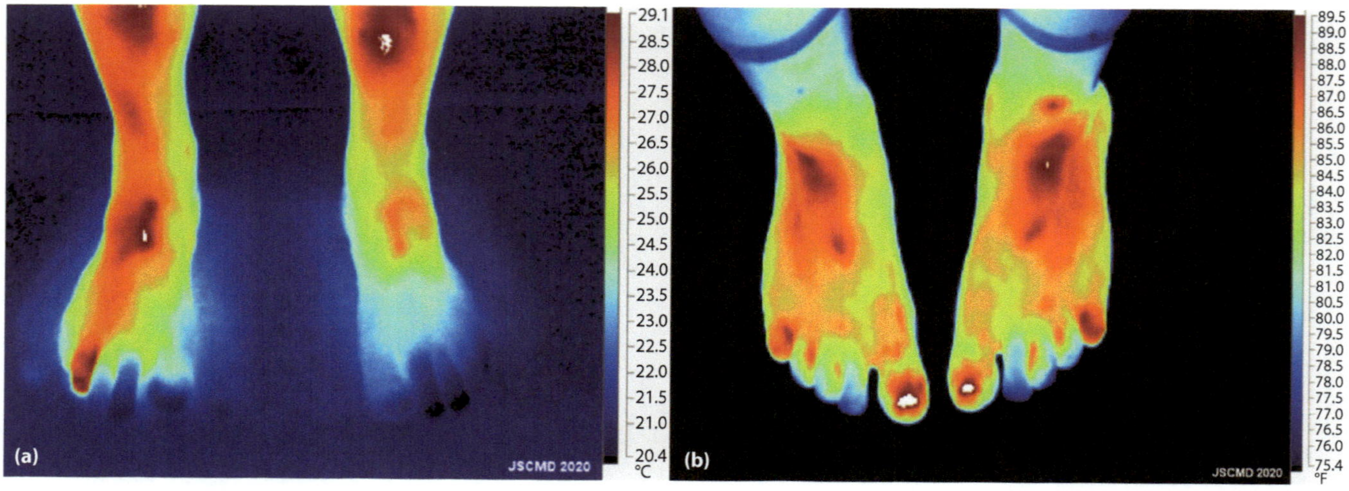

FIGURE 10.80 (a) Toe surgery on right digit IV seven days previously; clinically healing well. – 58 yoF. (b) Glomus AVA dilation of the toes mainly affecting the first and fifth digits bilaterally. The metatarsal and tarsal areas are also unusually warm bilaterally. Etiology unknown. – 47 yoF.

or infection of the mid-foot, with increased warmth (2°C/3.6°F) being an early sign.[205] Differences in skin temperature between the affected foot and the contralateral (non-affected) foot among patients with Charcot's neuroarthropathy can be detected well before other clinical signs emerge.[206]

In clinical settings, thermography offers non-contact visualization of the temperature distribution over the entire foot. Infrared imaging is useful as a method for risk screening diabetic feet at an early stage, particularly for patients with neuropathy, vasculopathy, and neurovascular disease.[207] Thermography-based diagnostic methods for diabetic feet emphasize asymmetric temperature analysis.[208] Though static thermal images can detect diabetic foot problems, dynamic thermography offers more information at an earlier stage (Figure 10.82). Serial thermograms or videothermography used to monitor the rewarming pattern of the plantar foot after "dry" cold water immersion in a thin plastic bag have shown good sensitivity but poor specificity.[209] An improved method of cooling the feet with cold packs and then imaging the plantar rewarming pattern is presently under study.[210]

Thermography is a useful method for following diabetic patients with neuropathy, plantar ulcer, peripheral arterial disease, and previous lower limb revascularization.[211] Monitoring diabetic patients via telemedicine is also a possibility; three randomized controlled trials have demonstrated that thermography is an effective home-monitoring tool for reducing the risk of recurrent diabetic foot ulcers.[212] Monthly thermographic examination of the feet has not reduced the occurrence of diabetic foot ulcers in high-risk patients, however.[213] Wearable thermometry devices may help improve the prevention of diabetic foot ulcers by detecting potential problems and enabling timely intervention.[214]

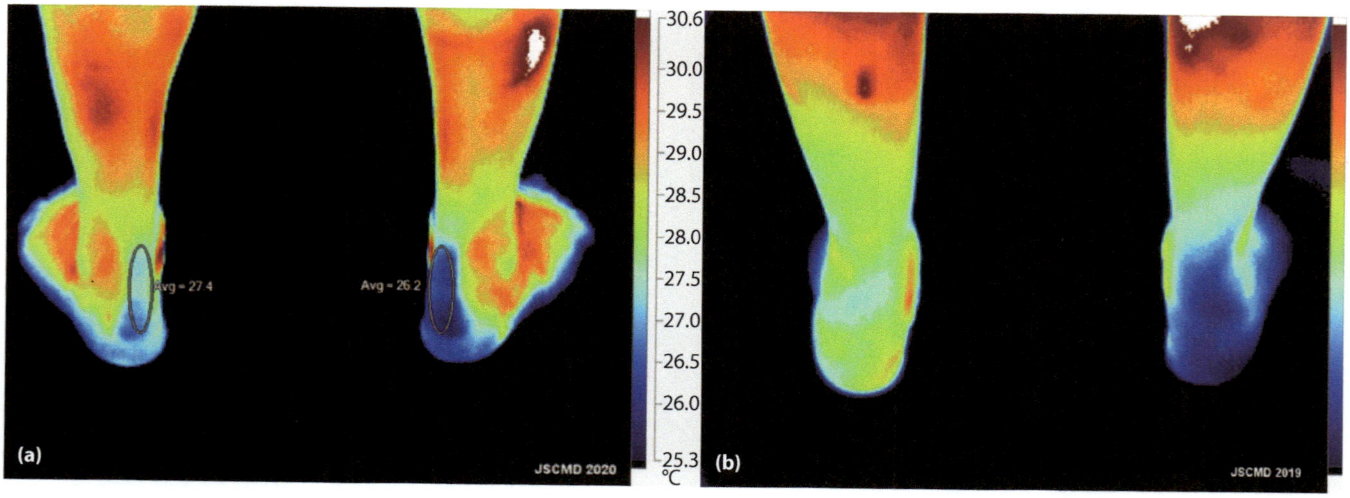

FIGURE 10.81 (a) Mild inflammation over the Achilles tendon on the left. – 70 yoM. (b) Asymmetric warmth over entire posterior left ankle. Etiology unknown, but ankle strain or sprain must be considered. – 37 yoF.

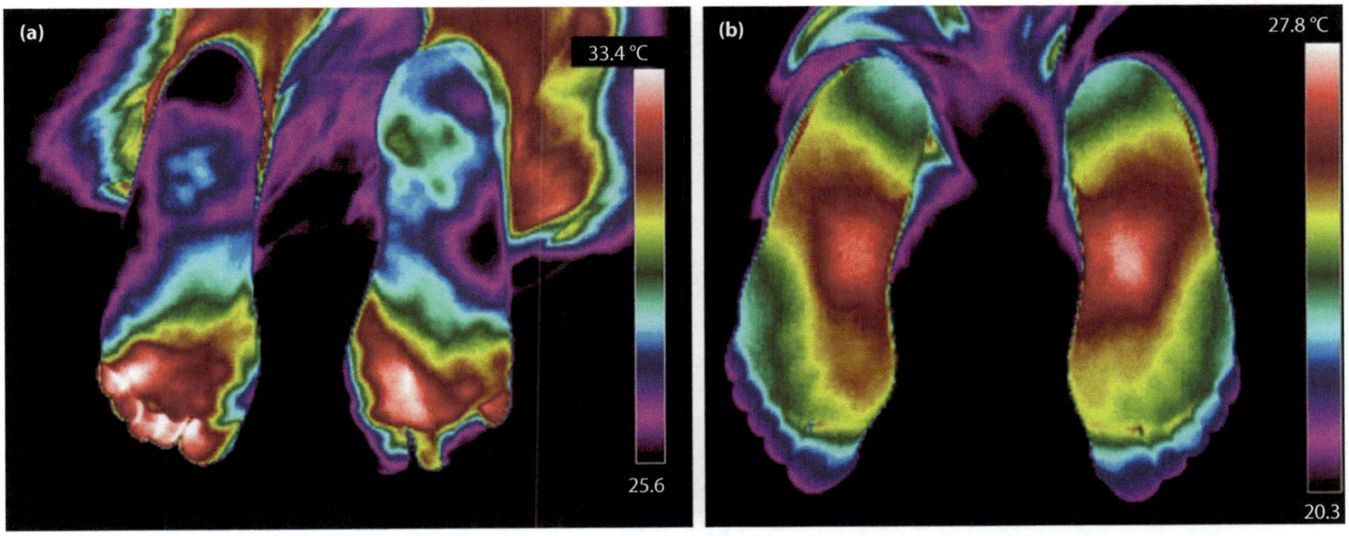

FIGURE 10.82 Plantar thermal rewarming patterns after "dry" foot immersion at 15°C (59°F) for 60 seconds. (a) Diabetic peripheral neuropathy (DPN) (b) normal subject. The qualitative thermal pattern is markedly different in DPN, with the distal portion of the foot warmest. Quantitatively the feet with DPN are also markedly warmer than normal (see scales), indicating poor sympathetic vasoconstriction. (Images courtesy of Dr. Luciane Balbinot, reprinted with permission.)

Thermal artifacts

Thermal artifacts are important for the thermographer to recognize and prevent (see figures 10.83-10.89). Artifacts may be caused by the subject's actions, the equilibration position, the thermal environment during imaging (rapid airflow, radiant heaters, sunlight, etc.), items used in the imaging protocol, and other factors such as medications. Microwave sources, especially cell phones, should be kept well away from the body during cool-down. For critical thermographic exams, video or direct monitoring of the subject during temperature equilibration may be necessary to assure that no artifacts have been introduced.

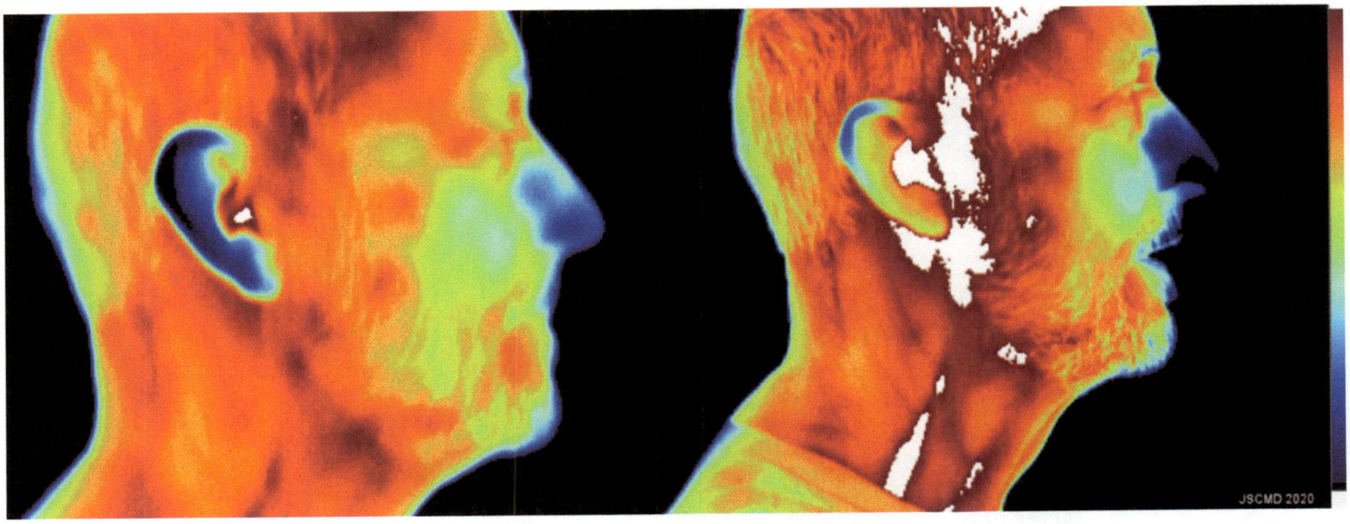

FIGURE 10.83 Cell phone artifact – isothermal images showing facial temperatures before (*left*) and after 5 minutes of cell phone use (*right*) with the phone held up to the right ear. Local tissue and venous blood warming can be detected. Microwaves are warming to body tissues up to 2.5 cm (1 in.) deep to the dermis. For this reason, a subject should not use, or even be very near, cellular telephones during a thermographic exam.

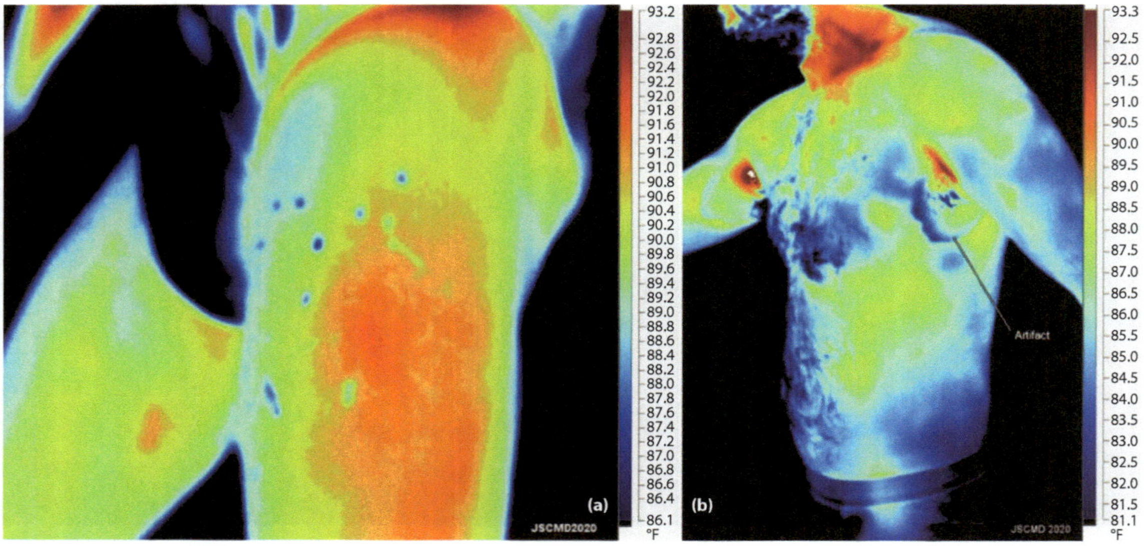

FIGURE 10.84 (a) Artifact: Water droplets on leg appear cool, similar to skin polyps or moles. – 55yoM. (b) Artifact from antiperspirant in both axillae. – 41 yoM, the artifacts appear cooler than the surrounding tissue due to the reduction in skin emissivity from the applied material.

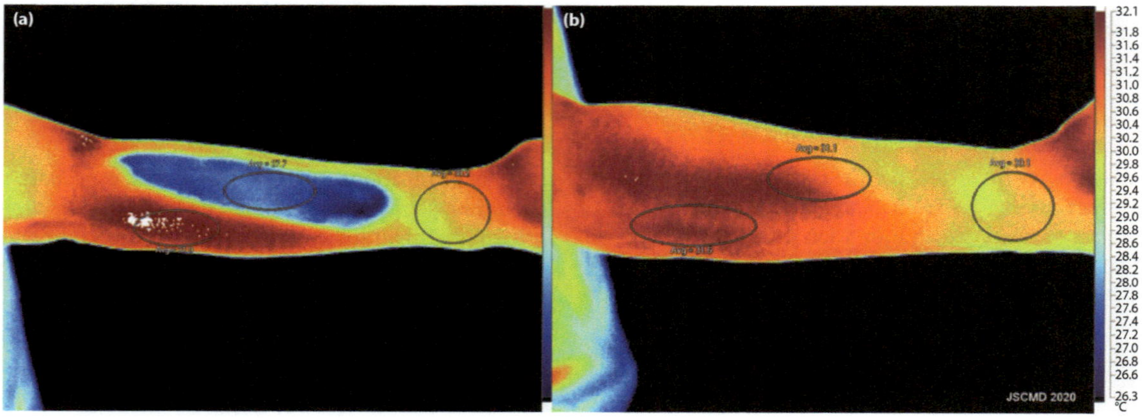

FIGURE 10.85 Isothermal images showing artifact from gel application to forearm (a) after 5 minutes and (b) after 15 minutes. The gel markedly lowers the apparent skin surface temperature, but the effect is short-lived. – 69 yoM.

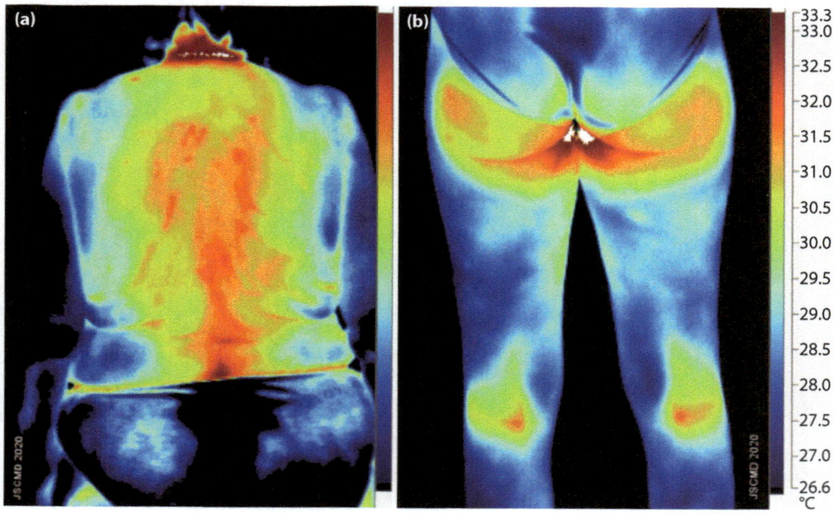

FIGURE 10.86 (a) Artifact: Subject cooled supine on a paper-covered exam table. The patient's skin did not appear scratched or excoriated. – 76 yoF. (b) Artifact: Buttocks warm from sitting on a round padded stool during equilibration. – 27 yoF.

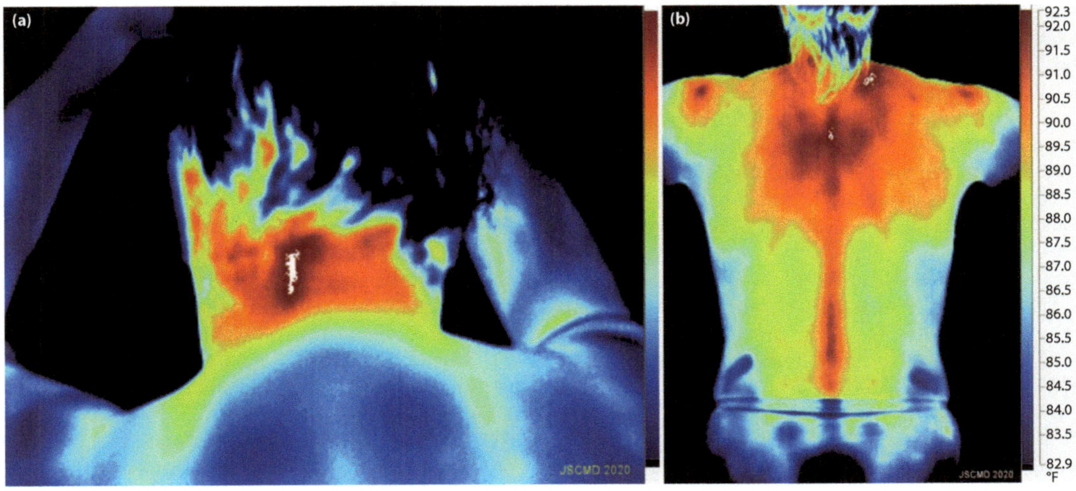

FIGURE 10.87 (a) Warm neck artifact – the subject just pulled her hair up off the neck. – 59 yoF. (b) Cool artifacts on both flanks from the subject placing her cold hands on her hips. – 46 yoF.

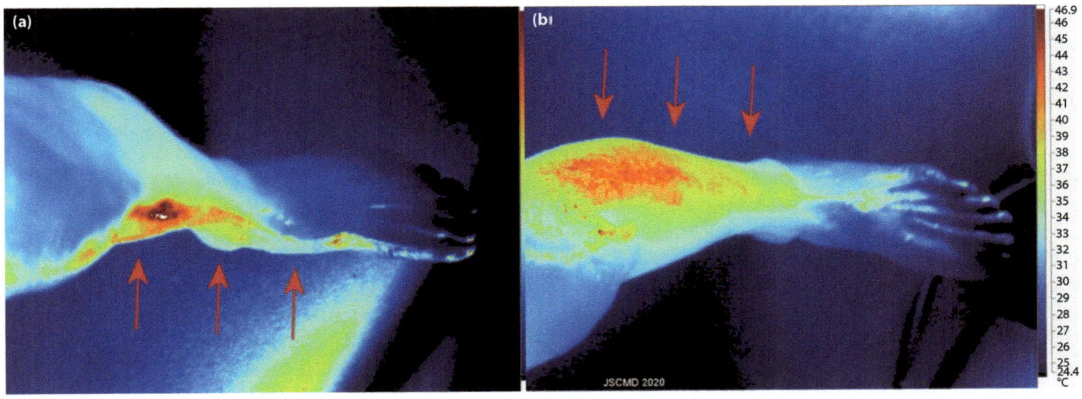

FIGURE 10.88 Thermal reflection artifacts in a 76-year-old male. Images of thermal radiation from a fanless infrared heater (red arrows) reflected off a normal leg. Note the uneven, speckled appearance. (a) Medial leg toward heater. (b) Lateral leg toward heater. Sunlight or incandescent lamps in a thermography room may create a similar appearance.

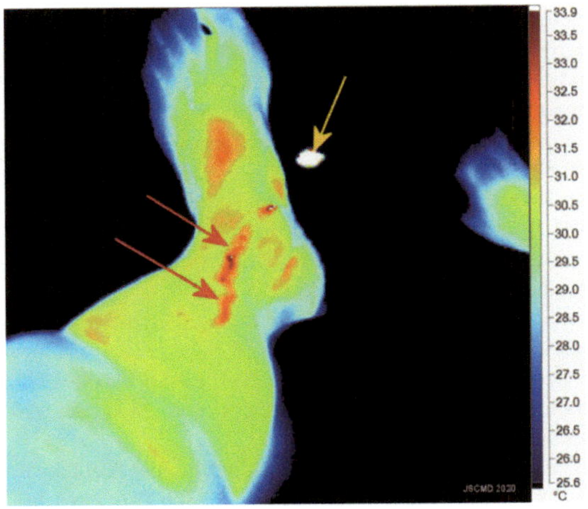

FIGURE 10.89 Thermal reflection artifact in a 76-year-old male. The heat from a 4 mm glowing tip of rope incense (yellow arrow) is reflected off the skin of the ankle and lower leg (red arrows). This thermographic appearance can be construed to represent stimulation of an acupuncture meridian, but is actually due to the 2% infrared reflectivity of human skin.[215]

Notes

1. Medina-Preciado JD et al., J Biomed Opt. 2013; Doi: 10.1117/1.JBO.18.6.061204
2. Romero-Méndez R et al., Math Med Biol. 2010; PMID: 19617302.
3. Pape SA et al., Burns. 2012; PMID: 22115981. See also: Jeng JC et al., Burns. 2003; PMID: 14556723. See also: Pape SA et al., Burns. 2001; PMID: 11311516.
4. Prindeze NJ et al., J Burn Care Res. 2016; PMID: 26284633. See also: Prindeze NJ et al., J Burn Care Res. 2015; PMID: 25412050.
5. Martı´nez-Jime´nez MA et al., PLoS ONE 2018; Doi: 10.1371/journal.pone.0206477
6. Images from: Martı´nez-Jime´nez MA et al., PLoS ONE 2018 CC-BY-4.0.
7. Simmons JD et al., J Am Coll Surg. 2018; PMCID: PMC5880281. See also: Jaspers MEH et al., Burns. 2017; PMID: 28536040. See also: Prindeze NJ et al., J Burn Care Res. 2015; PMID: 25412050. See also: Liddington MI et al., Burns. 1996; PMID: 8719312. See also: Burke-Smith A et al., Burns. 2015; PMID: 26421694. See also: Medina-Preciado JD et al., Noninvasive determination of burn depth in children by digital infrared thermal imaging. J Biomed Opt. 2013; PMID: 23111601. See also: Wearn C et al., Burns. 2018; PMID: 29032974. See also: Hardwicke J et al., Burns. 2013; PMID: 22652476.
8. Carrière ME et al., Wound Repair Regen. 2020; PMCID: PMC7217024.
9. Xue EY et al., Ann Plast Surg. 2018; PMID: 29489530.

10. Burmeister DM et al., J Burn Care Res. 2017; PMID: 27355653.
11. Personal experience of author jscmd glacier climbing near Zermatt, Switzerland, 1965.
12. Benrath J et al., Eur J Pain. 2001; PMID: 11465981.
13. Sunburn in Infrared by iRed Admin, 21 May 2015; https://ired.co.uk/news/sunburn-in-infrared/
14. Pandolf KB et al., Am J Physiol. 1992; PMID: 1566926.
15. Anbar M. Quantitative Dynamic Telethermometry in Medical Diagnosis and Management, 1st Ed, CRC Press, Boca Raton FL USA, 1994, p. 35.
16. Bobak Zonnoor MD, Medscape Drugs & Diseases, Emergency Medicine – Frostbite. https://emedicine.medscape.com/article/926249-overview
17. Norheim AJ et. al. Intl J Circumpolar Health2017; 76:1. Doi: 10.1080/22423982.2016.1273677
18. Department of the Army (USA), Technical bulletin TB MED 508, April 2005, p. 61.
19. Riquet D et al., J Med Eng Technol. 2016; PMID: 27270169.
20. Wang Zheng-Cai et al., Front Immunol. 2020; PMCID: PMC7746641.
21. Dini V et al., Wounds. 2015; PMID: 26479211. See also: Keenan E et al., Physiol Meas. 2017; PMID: 28430667.
22. Urakov AL et al., Thermol Int. 2015; 25(4):209–215.
23. Anderson JE, Mol Biol Cell 2000; PMCID: PMC14889.
24. Maria Conforti, Chapter 7 in Muscle Injuries in Sport Medicine, IntechOpen Ltd, London 2013; ISBN: 978-953-51-1198-6.
25. Ohtsuka E et al., Jpn J Pharmacol. 2001; PMID: 11430478.
26. De Medeiros CR et al., Rev Soc Bras Med Trop (RSBMT) 2017; doi: 10.1590/0037-8682-0390-2016, fig 2. Open-Source
27. De Medeiros CR et al., Rev Soc Bras Med Trop (RSBMT) 2017; doi: 10.1590/0037-8682-0390-2016, fig 3. Open-Source
28. De Medeiros CR et al., Rev Soc Bras Med Trop (RSBMT) 2017; doi: 10.1590/0037-8682-0390-2016, fig 1. Open-Source
29. Edwards G et al., BMJ. 2020; PMID: 32051117.
30. "Pseudocellulitis" is an inflammation of the dermis and hypodermis from a noninfectious etiology. See Korniyenko A et al., Am J Ther. July 2012; PMID: 22772033.
31. Ko LN et al., J Invest Dermatol. 2018; PMID: 28951240.
32. The FLIR One-Gen1 imager Toffset is not listed by the manufacturer; Toffset of the replacement version (FLIR Model 435-0006-03) is ±3°C (±5.4°F).
33. Ko LN et al., J Invest Dermatol. 2018; PMID: 28951240.
34. Park-Lee E et al., NCHS Data Brief No. 14, 2009; https://www.cdc.gov/nchs/products/databriefs/db14.htm
35. Gaskell P et al., Circ Res. 1958; PMID: 13547404.
36. Bhattacharya S et al., Indian J Plast Surg. 2015; PMCID: PMC4413488.
37. Haesler E, ed. Prevention and Treatment of Pressure Ulcers: Clinical Practice Guideline. Cambridge Media Perth, Australia, 2014; ISBN-13: 978-0-9579343-6-8.
38. Scafide KN et al., J Wound Ostomy Continence Nurs. 2020; PMID: 32068647.
39. Langemo DK et al., Adv Skin Wound Care. 2017;30(3):109–119. See also: Black J, Nursing September 2018;48(9):60–61.
40. Dini V et al., Wounds. 2015; PMID: 26479211.
41. Nakagami G et al., J Wound Care. 2010; PMID: 21135794.
42. Koerner S et al., Adv Skin Wound Care 2019; PMCID: PMC6716560.
43. Lee MHM & Cohen JM (eds.), Rehabilitation Medicine and Thermography, Impress Publications, Wilsonville OR, 2007. P. 92. ISBN: 978-0-6151-8721-1.
44. Mohammed JA et al., JAMA Dermatol. 2014; PMID: 25073587.
45. Shada AL et al., J Surg Res. 2013; PMCID: PMC4426199.
46. Ibid 15, p. 95.
47. Godoy SE et al., Biomed Opt Express 2017; PMCID: PMC5516826.
48. Gladfelter P et al., Melanoma Res. 2017; PMID: 28800028.
49. Shellenberger R et al., Ann Med. 2016; PMID: 26911192.
50. Tadiparthi S et al., Ann R Coll Surg Engl. 2008; PMCID: PMC2647196.
51. McClain SE et al., Int J Dermatol. 2012; PMCID: PMC4465919.
52. Menge TD et al., Semin Cutan Med Surg. 2016; PMID: 26963113.
53. Shada AL et al., J Surg Res. 2013; PMCID: PMC4426199.
54. Herman C et al., J Vis Exp. 2011; PMCID: PMC3197108.
55. The gel pack temperature can be anywhere from 15 to 25°C (59 to 77°F).
56. Shada AL et al., J Surg Res. 2013; PMCID: PMC4426199.
57. Images from: Shada AL et al., J Surg Res. 2013; PMCID: PMC4426199. Reprinted with permission from the Copyright Clearance Center.
58. Saxena, AK et al., Eur J Pediatr. 2008; PMID: 17762940.
59. Source: Hiroshi Shimizu, Shimizu's Textbook of Dermatology, Hokkaido University Press, 2007, ISBN-13 : 978-4521679211, p. 70.
60. Image from: Tanda G, J. Phys. 2015: Conf. Ser. 655 012062, Doi: 10.1088/1742-6596/655/1/012062. CC-BY-3.0
61. Alvarez-Prats D et al., Evidence-Based Complementary and Alternative Medicine 2019; Doi: 10.1155/2019/7126439
62. Pérez Atamoros FM et al., J Cosmet Dermatol. 2018; PMID: 29707877.
63. Bauer, J et al., EPMA J. 2020; PMCID: PMC7028894.
64. Images from Bauer, J et al., EPMA J. 2020; PMCID: PMC7028894, CC-BY-4.0.
65. Watts ME et al., Front Mol Neurosci. 2018; PMCID: PMC6023993.
66. Burhan H et al., Cerebrovascular Diseases, IntechOpen Ltd, London, 2020; Doi: 10.5772/intechopen.90484
67. Campbell JS et al., The American Academy of Thermology Annual Meeting, Greenville, SC, USA, 2019.
68. Crozier WR, De Jong PJ (eds.), The Psychological Significance of the Blush. Cambridge University Press, Cambridge, UK, 2012, pp. 16–19.
69. Valladolid, S et al., J Investig Dermatol. 2018; Doi: 10.1016/j.jid.2018.03.495
70. Gray's Anatomy of the Human Body – 27th Ed, Goss CM, ed., Leas & Febiger, Philadelphia, 1959, p. 733.
71. Nasal sinus locations added in color by JSCMD over open-source clip-art.
72. Fried MP, The MERCK Manual of Diagnosis and Therapy, 20th Ed, Porter RS, ed., Merck Sharpe & Dohme Pub, Kenilworth NJ, USA, 2018, p. 837.
73. Diaz I et al., Semin Respir Infect. 1995; PMID: 7761709.
74. Jung A et al., Chap 11 in Infrared Imaging – a Casebook in Clinical Medicine, Ring F et al. (eds.), IOP Publishing Ltd, London, 2015; ASIN : B01MXPQ2K4.
75. Godley FA, Am Fam Physician. 1992; PMID: 1575114.
76. Kalaiarasi R et al., Cureus. 2018; Doi: 10.7759/cureus.2298
77. Niedzielska I et al., Dentomaxillofac Radiol. 2017; PMCID: PMC5606276.
78. Ishimaru T et al., Int Arch Otorhinolaryngol. 2020; PMCID: PMC6986953.
79. Maciążek-Chyra B et al., Reumatologia. 2019; PMCID: PMC6409832.
80. Valladolid, S et al., J. Investig Dermatol. 2018; Doi: 10.1016/j.jid.2018.03.495
81. Andreychyn MA et al., Wiad Lek. 2020; PMID: 32285805.
82. Andreychyn M et al., Georgian Med News. 2018; PMID: 30358537.
83. Source: Wikipedia entry for Carotid triangle. Image author: Olek Remesz (wiki-pl: Orem, commons: Orem) Modified by user: madhero88, 2014.
84. Harshavardhan T et al., J Mahatma Gandhi Inst Med Sci. 2017; Doi: 10.4103/jmgims.jmgims_79_15 Also see: Mostovoy A, EAT2012 Book of Proceedings – Appendix 1 2012 http://uhlen.at/thermology-international/data/pdf/22A159.pdf
85. Snekhalatha U et al., Intl J Engr & Tech. 2018; Doi: 10.14419/ijet.v7i2.8.10353
86. Biagioni PA et al., Acta Derm Venereol. 1998; PMID: 9498027.
87. Chandra Mouli PE, IOSR J. Dent and Med Sci. 2012; Doi: 10.9790/0853-0113943
88. Dowling RH et al., Am I Dead Yet ... or Do I Just Feel Like It. Hobbies for Health, 2007; ASIN: B000QFWFV6. See also: Levy TE, MedFox Pub, 2017; ISBN-13 : 978-0983772873.
89. Campbell JS et al., The American Academy of Thermology Annual Meeting, Greenville, SC, USA, 2019.
90. Cordero OJ et al., Heliyon. 2018; PMCID: PMC6218413.
91. Söder B et al., Breast Cancer Res Treat. 2011; PMID: 20960226.
92. Baek SW et al., Evid Based Complement Alternat Med. 2018;PMCID: PMC5994269.

93. N = 1 study of 6 tongue thermograms taken in quick succession under varying respiratory conditions by author JSCMD, 26 January 2021.
94. Images from: Thirunavukkarasu, U, Evidence-Based Complementary and Alternative Medicine 2020; Doi: 10.1155/2020/3186208, Open access, CC-BY.
95. Ibi M, Biol Pharm Bull. 2019;42(4):538–542. PMID: 30930413.
96. Wang XD et al., J Dent Res. 2015; PMID: 25744069.
97. Temporal muscle. Deep dissection. Mummification process by Anatomist90, 2013. In Wikipedia, File:Slide8por.JPG. Annotations in yellow by jscmd.
98. Gratt BM et al., J Orofac Pain. 1994; PMID: 7812225. See also: McBeth SB et al., Am J Orthod Dentofacial Orthop. 1996; PMID: 8638592. See also: Canavan D et al., Oral Surg Oral Med Oral Pathol Oral Radiol Endod. 1995; PMID: 7621039.
99. Rodrigues-Bigaton D et al., J Bodyw Mov Ther. 2014; PMID: 24411149. See also: Barão VA et al., J Prosthodont Res. 2011; PMID: 20591761.
100. Rodrigues-Bigaton D et al., J Manipulative Physiol Ther. 2013; PMID: 23719519. See also: Dibai-Filho AV, et al., Saudi Dent J. 2015; PMCID: PMC4273257.
101. McBeth SB et al., Am J Orthod Dentofacial Orthop. 1996; PMID: 8638592. See also: Gratt BM et al., J Orofac Pain. 1993; PMID: 8467300. See also: Gratt BM et al., Dentomaxillofac Radiol. 1998; PMID: 9656869. See also: Johansson A et al., Acta Odontol Scand. 1985; PMID: 3866482. See also: Dibai-Filho AV et al., J Bodyw Mov Ther. 2014; PMID: 25042314.
102. Fikackova H et al., Oral Surg Oral Med Oral Pathol Oral Radiol Endod. 2004; PMID: 15583534. See also: Woźniak K et al., Med Sci Monit. 2015; PMCID: PMC4451701.
103. de Melo DP et al., Oral Surg Oral Med Oral Pathol Oral Radiol. 2019; PMID: 30482738.
104. Rodrigues-Bigaton D et al., J Manipulative Physiol Ther. 2013; PMID: 23719519.
105. Degowin, Bedside Diagnostic Examination, 2nd Ed., Macmillan Company, NY, 1969, p. 430.
106. Litmanovich DE et al., Insights Imaging. 2012; PMCID: PMC3505571.
107. Borkowski et al., Am J Pathol 2002;. PMCID: PMC1850706.
108. Lin, Peter H et al., J Vasc Surg Cases Innov Tech. 2017; PMCID: PMC5764859.
109. Nishiura H et al., BMC Infect Dis. 2011;. PMCID: PMC3096599.
110. Ng EY et al., Microvasc. Res. 2004; PMID: 15313119. See also: Chiang MF et al., J Formos Med Assoc. 2008; Doi: 10.1016/S0929-6646(09)60017-6. See also: Sun G et al., Ng E.Y.K., et al. (eds.), Application of Infrared to Biomedical Sciences, Springer, Singapore, 2017. Doi: 10.1007/978-981-10-3147-2_19 pp. 347–358
111. Ghassemi P et al., PLoS One. 2018; PMCID: PMC6145558.
112. Chan LS et al., Hong Kong Med J. 2013; PMID: 23535669. See also: Cheung BMY et al., Hong Kong Med J. 2012; PMID: 22865221.
113. Ring EFJ et al., J Mech Med Biol. 2013; Doi: 10.1142/S0219519413500450. See also: Ring FJ et al., Diakides M, Bronzino JD, Peterson DR (eds.), Medical Infrared Imaging: Principles and Practices, CRC Press, 2013. p. 23. See also: IEC 80601-2-59:2017 IEC / ISO, Geneva, Switzerland Pub, 2017.
114. Teunissen LP et al., J Med Eng Technol. 2011; PMID: 21329484.
115. Selent MU et al., Pediatr Emerg Care. 2013; PMID: 23426254.
116. Ng EYK et al., Microvasc Res. 2004; PMID: 15313119.
117. Ng EYK et al., Chapter 24 in The Biomedical Engineering Handbook, 3rd Ed, Medical Devices and Systems, Bronzino JD (ed.), CRC Press, Boca Raton, FL, USA, 2006.
118. Selent MU et al., Pediatr Emerg Care. 2013; PMID: 23426254.
119. Bitar D et al., Eurosurveillance. 2009; PMID: 19215720.
120. Negishi T et al., Conf Proc IEEE Eng Med Biol Soc. 2019; PMID: 31946564.
121. Negishi T et al., Sensors (Basel). 2020; PMCID: PMC7218727.
122. Image courtesy of US Food and Drug Administration 2020.
123. Mercer JB, Ring EFJ, Thermology Intl. 2009;19(3):67–69. See also: IEC 80601-2-59:2017 IEC / ISO, Geneva, Switzerland Pub. 2017.
124. IEC 80601-2-59:2017 IEC / ISO, Geneva, Switzerland Pub. 2017.
125. Recommendations from the US FDA 2021.
126. Heat generation of normal thyroid tissue averages 87.1 Watts per kg. See: Ammer K & Ring F, The Thermal Human Body – A Practical Guide to Thermal Imaging, 2019. Jenny Stanford, Singapore, 2019, p. 92.
127. Lumachi F et al., Cytokine. 2010; PMID: 20381375. See also: Łacheta D et al., Biomed Res Int. 2019; PMCID: PMC6875285.
128. Bindra A et al., Am Fam Physician. 2006; PMID: 16734054.
129. Sweeney LB et al., Am Fam Physician. 2014; PMID: 25251231.
130. Guarino V et al., Mol Cell Endocrinol. 2010; PMID: 19835928. See also: Pagano L et al., Front Biosci (Landmark Ed). 2018; PMID: 29772561. See also: Cunha LL et al., Endocr Relat Cancer. 2014; PMID: 24302667.
131. Bozec A et al., Curr Med Chem. 2010; PMID: 20738253.
132. Provatopoulou X et al., Inflamm Res. 2014; PMID: 24794392. See also: Yahyapour R et al., Mil Med Res. 2018; PMCID: PMC5859747. See also: Muzza M et al., Clin Endocrinol (Oxf). 2010; PMID: 20447069.
133. Samuels BI, Radiology. 1972; PMID: 5008156.
134. Helmy A et al., IEEE Trans Biomed Eng. 2008; PMID: 18334410.
135. Alves ML et al., Radiol Bras. 2016; PMCID: PMC5094820.
136. González JR et al., Stud Health Technol Inform. 2017; PMID: 29295121.
137. Rossato M et al., Endocrine. 2015; PMID: 24898902.
138. Jin C et al., Med Eng Phys. 2014; PMID: 23999383.
139. Di Maria C et al., J Clin Endocrinol Metab. 2014; PMID: 25238202.
140. Minatel Riguetto C et al., Int J Endocrinol. 2019; PMCID: PMC6532296.
141. Shaked Y et al., Postgrad Med J. 1988; PMCID: PMC2428841.
142. González JR et al., Ng E, Etehadtavakol M (eds.), Application of Infrared to Biomedical Sciences, Springer, Singapore, 2017. Doi: 10.1007/978-981-10-3147-2_26
143. Bahramian R et al., Infrared Phys. Technol. 2020; Doi: 10.1016/j.infrared.2019.103126
144. Bahramian F et al., Int J Numer Method Biomed Eng. 2019; PMID: 30801998.
145. F. Bahramian et al., 24th National and 2nd International Iranian Conference on Biomedical Engineering 2017; Doi: 10.1109/ICBME.2017.8430276
146. Han MA et al., Thyroid. 2018; PMID: 29160170. See also: De Santis M et al., Reprod Toxicol. 2005; PMID: 15925481.
147. Shatsova EN et al., Probl Endokrinol (Mosk). 1989; PMID: 2740312.
148. Korevaar TIM et al., Nat Rev Endocrinol. 2017; PMID: 28776582. See also: Preston-Martin S et al., Br J Cancer. 1987; PMCID: PMC2002082.
149. Goss CM (ed.), Gray H, Anatomy of the Human Body, 27th Ed, Lea and Febiger, Philadelphia, 1965, Fig. 616, p. 737.
150. Goss CM (ed.), Gray H, Anatomy of the Human Body, 27th Ed, Lea & Febiger, 1959, pp 735–739.
151. Dong, F et al., Sci Rep. 2018; Doi: 10.1038/s41598-018-24195-4
152. Guida G et al., Int J Immunopathol Pharmacol. 2009; PMID: 20074466.
153. Sarigoz T et al., Infrared Phys Technol. 2020, 10.1016/j.infrared.2020.103336
154. Burhan H et al., Cerebrovascular Diseases, IntechOpen Ltd, London, 2020; Doi: 10.5772/intechopen.90484
155. Drawing from Sobotta's Atlas and Text-book of Human Anatomy 1909. Public Domain, File:Sobo 1909 723.png. See Wikipedia file: "Proper palmar digital arteries."
156. Kalicki, B et al., Przegląd Elektrotechniczny 2012; R88, nr12b, pp. 135–138.
157. Brioschi, ML et al., InfraMation 2008 Proceedings, ITC 126 A 2008-05-14.
158. Image from Brioschi, ML et. al, InfraMation 2008 Proceedings, ITC 126 A 2008-05-14. Permission to reprint granted by author MLB.
159. Kuropka P et al., Acta Bioeng Biomech. 2019; PMID: 31798019.
160. Wang, L et al., BMJ Open 2018; Doi: 10.1136/bmjopen-2017-017964

161. Lazyuk DG et al., J Eng Phys Thermophys. 1996; Doi: 10.1007/BF02606967 UDC616.1-073.65
162. Potanin C, Ann Intern Med. 1 May 1970; Doi: 10.7326/0003-4819-72-5-785_4
163. Hirsch IH, Ch. 251 in MERCK Manual of Diagnosis and Therapy 20th Ed, Porter RS, ed., Merck Sharpe & Dohme, Kenilworth NJ, USA, 2018, p. 2132.
164. Cadman B et al., Medical News Today 2018; https://www.medicalnewstoday.com/articles/320710
165. Bianchi S, Radiol Med. 1976; PMID: 802918.
166. See Guyton and Hall, Textbook of Medical Physiology, 12th Ed, Ch.34. https://doctorlib.info/physiology/textbook-medical-physiology/34.html
167. Illustration by Sobotta and McMurrich 1906. File:Sobotta_1906_452, Wikimedia Commons. Public Domain. Annotations by JSCMD.
168. Panikratov KD et al., Urol Nefrol (Mosk). 1972; PMID: 5052357.
169. Abdominal Organs Anatomy.png by Bruce Blaus, 2016, Wikimedia Commons File CC-BY-SA-4.0. Cropped to exclude thorax by jscmd.
170. Degowin, Bedside Diagnostic Examination, 2nd Ed, Macmillan Company, NY, NY, USA 1969, p. 454.
171. Ibid 162
172. Ramirez-GarciaLuna JL et.al., Infrared Phys Technol. 2020; Doi/10.1016/j.infrared.2019.103165
173. Peltokallio P et al., Am J Roentgenol Radium Ther Nucl Med. 1975; PMID: 1200209.
174. Banic M et al., Period Biol. 2011; 113(4):439–444.
175. Illustration from Anatomy of the Human Body by Henry Gray 1918, Wikimedia Commons File: Gray409.png. In the public domain.
176. Illustration from Anatomy of the Human Body by Henry Gray 1918, Wikimedia Commons File: Gray313.png. In the public domain.
177. Illustration from Anatomy of the Human Body by Henry Gray 1918, Wikimedia Commons File:Gray388.png In the public domain. Graphic and labeling of the dorsal dermis added by jscmd 2020.
178. Uematsu S, J Neurosurg 1985; PMID: 2985769.
179. Illustration from Anatomy of the Human Body by Henry Gray 1918, Wikimedia Commons File: laminectomy.jpg Colored incision lines added by jscmd 2020.
180. Ibid 170, p. 568. Also see: Wikipedia entry for "testicle," edited 23 July 2020.
181. Biagioni P et al., Acta Derm Venereol (Stockh) 1995; PMID: 8578944.
182. Kulis T et al., Period Biol. 2011; Corpus ID: 5285414
183. Image from: Kulis T et al., Period Biol. 2011; 113(4), Fig. 1, Open-Access.
184. Capraro GA et al., J Urology 2008; PMID: 18951560.
185. Lenskaia OP et al., Med Radiol (Mosk). 1985; PMID: 4068939.
186. Oliveira M et al., ICS 2019 Programme S31 ePoster Station 7 Abstract 621. Sept 2019.
187. Kukkonen TM et al., J Sex Med. 2007; PMID: 17233778.
188. Masters WH & Johnson VE, Human Sexual Response, Little, Brown Co, Boston, 1966, p. 275.
189. Hildebrandt C et al., Sensors (Basel). 2010; PMCID: PMC3292141.
190. The medial collateral ligament was previously named the tibial collateral ligament. See Figure 10-74.
191. Keyl W et al., Fortschr Med. 1975; PMID: 1173237. See also: Shilo R et al., Handchirurgie. 1976; PMID: 992484.
192. Image Source: Gray's Anatomy 1918 edition, in the public domain. Wikimedia Commons File:Gray348.png.
193. Yang H et al., J Pharmacopuncture. 2014; PMCID: PMC4332010.
194. Litscher G et al., Medicines (Basel). 2014; Doi: 10.3390/medicines1010012
195. Cholewka A et al., J. Therm Anal Calorim. 2012; Doi: 10.1007/s10973-011-1934-6
196. Images from: Cholewka, A et al., J Therm Anal Calorim. 2017; Doi: 10.1007/s10973-017-6141-7 CC BY 4.0
197. Cwajda-Białasik J et al., Wound Repair Regen. 2020; PMID: 31705776.
198. Cholewka, A et al., J Therm Anal Calorim. 2017; Doi: 10.1007/s10973-017-6141-7
199. A suitably large piece of standard packing cardboard can be used as the thermal pad for this procedure.
200. de Sá Guimarães CMD et al., Surg Cosmet Dermatol. Rio de Janeiro 2018. Doi: 10.5935/scd1984-8773.20181021154
201. Brownrigg, JR et al., Diabetologia. 2012; PMID: 22890823. See also; Holman, N et al., Diabetologia. 2012; PMID: 22398645. See also: Vamos, EP et al., Diabetes Care. 2010; PMCID: PMC2992196.
202. Boyko, EJ et al., 2018; PMID: 29439130.
203. Ilo A et al., J Diabetes Sci Technol. 2020; PMCID: PMC7189167.
204. Vanore J. The Podiatry Institute Update, 2003, Ch. 28. http://www.podiatryinstitute.com/pdfs/Update_2003/2003_28.pdf
205. Vopat ML et al., Kans J Med. 2018; PMCID: PMC6276967.
206. Armstrong DG et al., Phys Ther. 1997; PMID: 9037217.
207. van Doremalen RFM et al., J Diabetes Sci Technol. 2020; PMCID: PMC7189170. See also: Astasio-Picado Á et al., Curr Diabetes Rev. 2019; PMID: 30727903. See also: Quinn S et al., Conf Proc IEEE Eng Med Biol Soc. 2019; Doi: 10.1109/EMBC.2019.8856900
208. Adam M et al., Comput Biol Med. 2017; PMID: 29121540.
209. Balbinot LF et al., Clinics (Sao Paulo) 2012; PMCID: PMC3521805.
210. Peter Soliz, US Patent # 8868157, 2014.
211. Ilo A et al., J Diabetes Sci Technol. 2020; PMCID: PMC8258513.
212. Hazenberg CEVB et al., Diabetes Metab Res Rev. 2020; PMCID: PMC7079242.
213. Petrova NL et al., Diabet. Med. 2020; Doi: 10.1111/dme.14152
214. Najafi B et al., Diabetes Metab Res Rev. 2020; PMID: 31909547.
215. See Chen et al., Biomed Eng OnLine 2011; 10:80. Doi: 10.1186/1475-925X-10-80

11

THERMOGRAPHY BY SPECIALTY

Orthopedic and sports thermography

Bone fractures

Musculoskeletal injuries are typically accompanied by local inflammation. Skin temperature around the injury site increases in response to trauma-induced release of NO. Injury usually produces thermal asymmetry, with the damaged region of interest (ROI) being warmer than contralateral unless the damage occurs in both limbs. The temperatures can be affected by other factors, such as reduction in skin blood flow due to the injury. Skin temperatures will tend to decrease in tissues that have poor perfusion.[1] This may lead to reduction in the thermographic visualization of musculoskeletal injuries in elderly individuals or those with accelerated aging of the microvasculature due to stress and illness.[2]

Infrared imaging can detect temperature changes associated with increased blood flow around a healing fracture due to the production of nitric oxide (NO) at the fracture site (Figure 11.1).[3] These surface temperature changes correlate well with the different stages of bone healing and follow the NO production curve with only a slight lag.[4] During the initial inflammatory phase, there is increased temperature of the surrounding tissue; thermography can indicate bone injury very soon after it has occurred.[5] In the repair phase, as the bone undergoes healing, the temperature over the fracture decreases. In the remodeling phase following the injury, there should be no significant temperature difference because the bone has fully mended (Figure 11.2).[6] The hyperthermia seen thermographically over a healing fracture may spread widely both proximally and distally, most likely due to tissue diffusion of the copious amounts of NO generated at the fracture site (Figure 11.3).

Thermography can detect stress fractures in the tibia and fibula, reducing the need for radioactive scans.[7] Thermography is an accurate way to differentiate between stress fracture and other causes of shin-splint syndromes in runners (see Figure 10.76a).[8] Infrared imaging offers only moderate accuracy for detecting stress fractures, however, unless performed with modern imaging technology.[9]

Modern infrared imaging is useful to rule out fractures, having a sensitivity of 91% and a negative predictive value of 95% (Figure 11.4).[10] Thermography can identify a professional soccer player's risk of having an injury, reducing the injury severity and days lost following the injury.[11] In pediatric trauma, wrist strains and fractures increase the average skin temperature significantly compared with the uninjured wrist.[12]

Thermography of osteogenesis

In the pediatric population up to the age when the epiphyses of the long bones fuse (about 12–18 years for girls and 14–19 years for boys), the metabolism of the epiphyseal growth plates creates heat as well as NO that is conducted to the surrounding skin surface (Figure 11.5). NO is also generated along the shafts of the long bones as osteoblasts increase the bony diameter during growth.[13] The thermographic pattern of this warmth will evolve and change due to epiphyseal fusion as the subject ages. When thermographically assessing only one limb for fracture in the pediatric age group, normal NO production due to osteogenesis may be mistaken for the warmth seen over a fracture or sprain. As normal bone growth and NO production are generally a symmetrical process, comparing the injured limb to the contralateral limb should differentiate between osteogenesis and injury. A thermographic atlas of normal osteogenic heat patterns with age would be a useful addition to the practice of pediatrics.

Sometimes thermographically mistaken for the warmth of osteogenesis, chronic nonbacterial osteomyelitis (CNO) is an auto-inflammatory bone disease seen in children characterized by multiple foci of painful swelling of bones mainly in the metaphyses of the long bones, pelvis, spine, and shoulder girdle. Children with active CNO lesions in the distal tibia/fibula exhibited higher regional temperatures when compared to healthy extremities.[14] Thermography may be useful for detecting active bone lesions in these children. Unfortunately, the thermographic appearance of children, both normal and abnormal, has not been well researched and more thermal studies of younger age groups are needed.

Muscle, joint, and ligament injuries

Soft-tissue injuries and inflammation are of three main types: (1) Involving muscle, including traumatic myopathy or myositis; (2) Involving tendons, i.e., tendinopathy or tendinitis; and (3) Involving the junction where a tendon or ligament attaches to bone (enthesiopathy or enthesitis). To these conditions may be added injury or inflammation of bursal sacs (bursitis) as well as extravasation of whole blood into or around soft tissues (hematoma). These conditions have various findings in common. They result in subjective pain. They cause at least a minimum loss of function. And they increase the local production of NO as well as other cytokines.[15]

NO increases local blood flow to the damaged area. This increased NO surrounding the damaged tissue diffuses in all directions, causing capillary vasodilation. If the injured tissues are close to the skin surface, that vasodilation will be detected as localized warmth over the injured tissues (Figure 11.6). Injuries to the deeper muscle layers or joints may not be as thermographically visible due to attenuation of NO diffusion by more superficial structures. When the injury has fully healed, NO production slows and eventually returns to baseline levels with a concomitant return of normal thermographic appearance.

Whether the increased NO helps or harms the underlying injury is a matter of considerable debate. Therapeutic NO delivery systems such as nitroglycerine transdermal patches are being used to treat enthesiopathy or tendinitis.[16] The thermographer must be made aware of the use of these patches because they may cause artefactual local skin vasodilation.

Exercise-induced muscle and ligament damage are common problems in the sports world. Elevations in skin temperature correlate with inflammation from these conditions. An infrared image of recently injured areas will typically show local skin temperature increases when compared to the temperature of

DOI: 10.1201/9781003281764-12

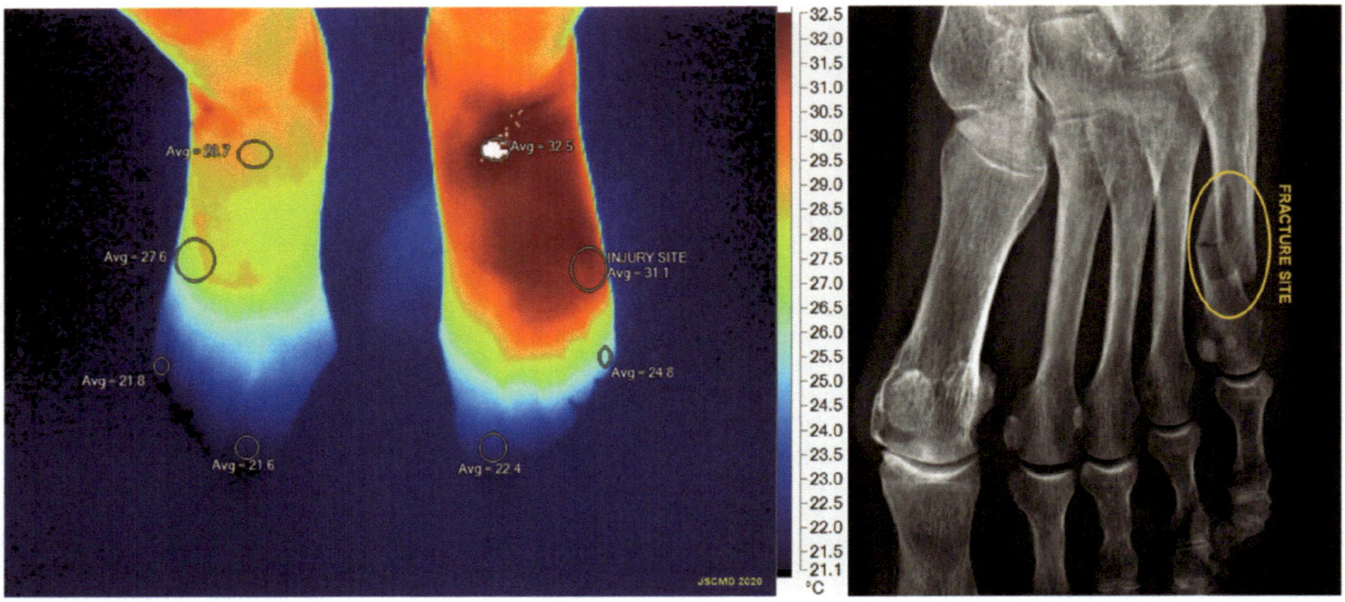

FIGURE 11.1 Thermographic appearance of a fracture of metatarsal V imaged 3 days post-injury. The increase in skin temperature extends from the toes to the level of the ankle – 79-year-old female.

otherwise healthy skin. Thermal monitoring of the patient over the course of weeks or months can provide a quantitative and qualitative assessment of the extent of damage as well as the healing progress of the injury.

Muscle damage due to intensive exercise creates local inflammation and delayed-onset muscle soreness, one of the most common forms of recurrent sports injury.[17] This problem is commonly experienced in individuals who have been physically inactive for long periods of time and then begin to exercise intensively; however, it can also occur in athletes who exert themselves beyond their usual training limits. Symptoms can range from slight muscle tenderness to severe debilitating pain. Lasting anywhere from 24 hours to seven days, muscle damage is a concern for athletes because it can markedly impair performance.

Thermography has been used twice a week to detect major temperature differences in professional soccer players' leg muscles. If a temperature difference higher than 0.4°C (0.72°F) initiates a prevention protocol, a 63% reduction in muscle injuries can be expected.[18] Thermography may help prevent injuries by identifying players potentially at risk, thus enabling adjustments to reduce the severity and frequency of injury.[19] Thermography may be less effective, however, when used to predict exercise-induced muscle damage in untrained soccer players, for reasons that are not entirely clear.[20] Sports

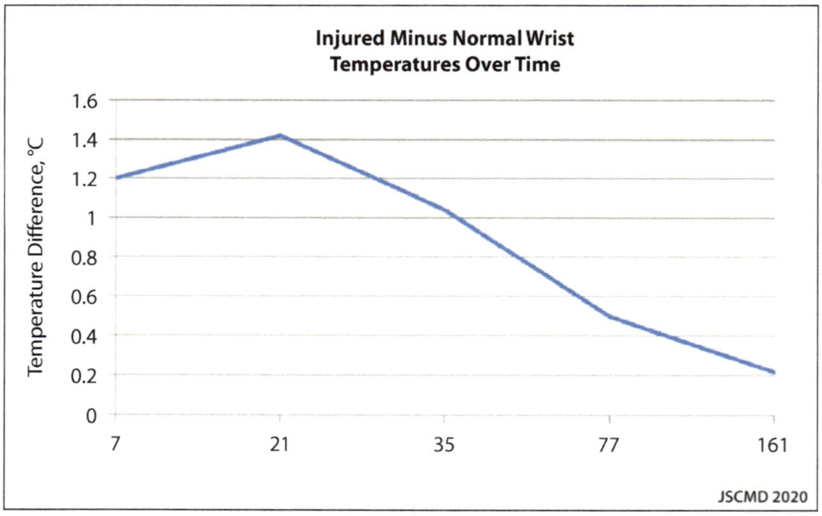

FIGURE 11.2 Average temperature differences over time between arm with Colles' fracture and uninjured arm. (Graph of data from Haluzan, 2015.)

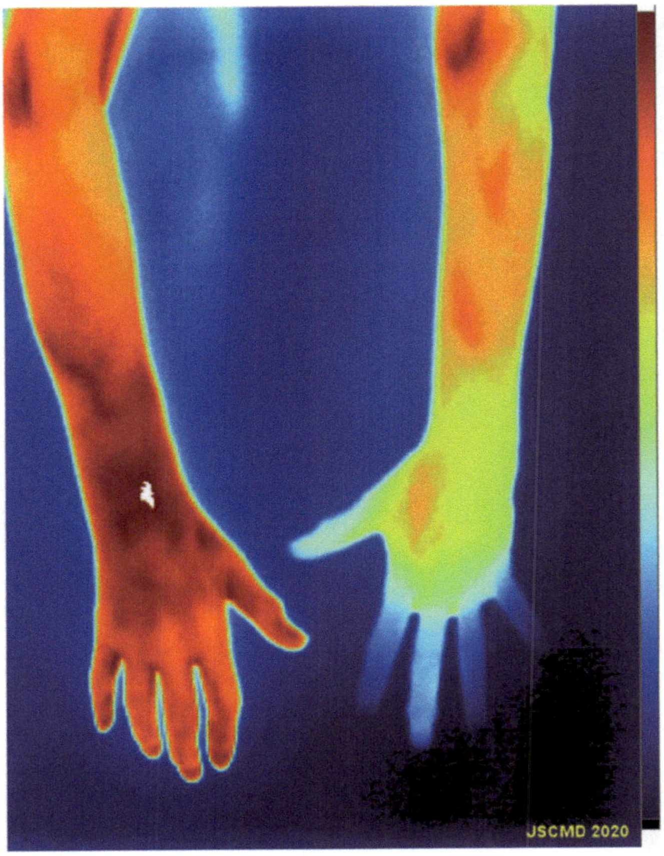

FIGURE 11.3 Thermal appearance of a healing right Colles' fracture 80 days post-injury. The fracture was treated by casting without fixation. The patient went on to heal fully by X-ray, without residual pain. Incidental osteoarthritic changes in the digits are present bilaterally – 64 yoF.

thermographers are encouraged to learn more by reading recent publications on the subject.[21]

Muscle paralysis, disuse, and fibrosis

Any skeletal muscle under active contraction produces heat as a byproduct; this in turn directly warms the muscle and any surrounding tissues via heat conduction. Thus the skin over active, enervated muscles appears warmer than skin over non-metabolizing tissues. A muscle at rest or with flaccid paralysis can be expected to be cooler than active muscle. (Figure 11.7)[22] A completely fibrosed muscle is cooler than active muscle because it has become a low-metabolizing tissue similar to tendons or ligaments. Increased muscle tone due to CNS disruption from brain stroke or cerebral palsy may appear paradoxically cool due to reduced blood flow to the overlying dermis (see the section on Neurology for more details). The thermal appearance of abnormal muscle contraction due to recent tendon rupture requires further study, though an acute increase in local skin temperature is expected from possible inflammation, with later decrease in local temperature due to muscle atrophy if the tendon is not repaired.[23] Muscles acting across a chronically painful or "frozen" joint may also appear relatively cool due to reduced contractions caused by the pain and resultant inactivity.[24]

Compartment syndrome

Severe crush injuries or comminuted fractures of the limbs may be complicated by the development of Compartment Syndrome (CS), where hematoma or edema increase the tissue pressure inside a closed fascial space, cutting off the arterial blood supply to the muscles within that space. Even milder injuries or a cast that is applied too tightly may cause CS. Arterial pulses distal to the injury usually remain full. Severe pain occurs and muscle necrosis may result unless emergency fasciotomy is performed to relieve the compartment pressure. Forearm fractures involving both radius and ulna, as well as tibial fractures of the leg, are most prone to CS complications.[25] A study using thermography to aid in the detection of CS showed a highly significant "thigh-foot index" (TFI), or difference between thigh and ankle temperatures, of over 8°C

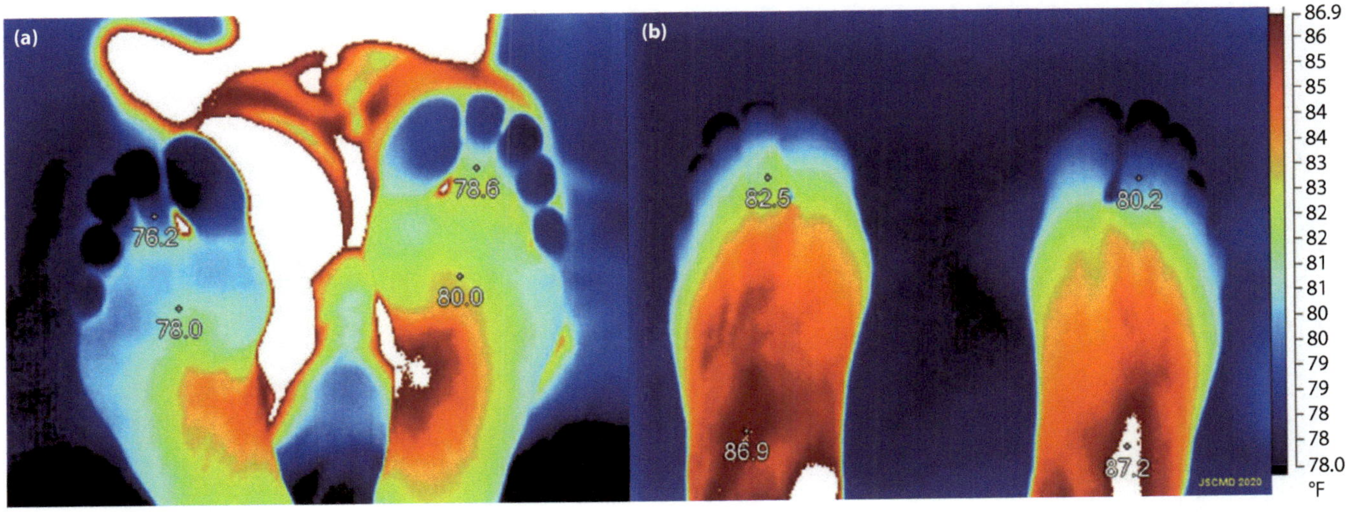

FIGURE 11.4 Fracture of the distal portion of the proximal phalanx, digit II of the left foot at 42 days post-injury. (a) Plantar view; (b) Dorsal view. – 70-year-old male.

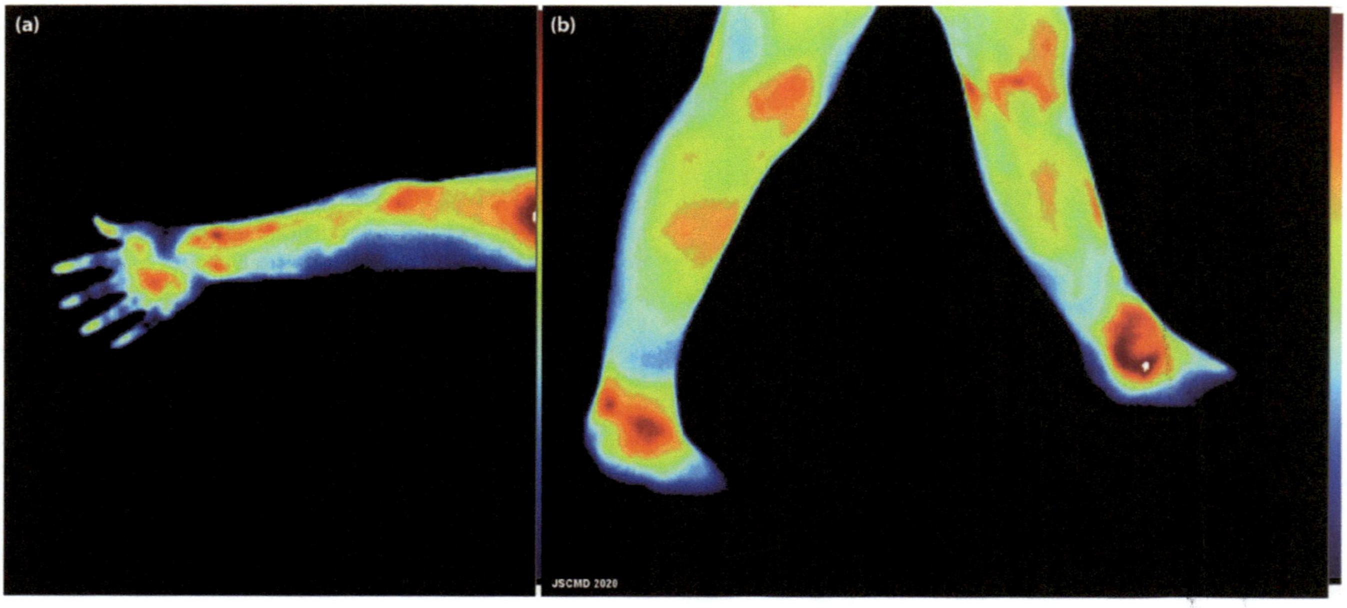

FIGURE 11.5 The skin surface warmth due to osteogenesis is visible over both the ends and shafts of the long bones in pediatric subjects. (a) Right volar forearm view; (b) Right lateral view of the lower legs – Normal 8 yoM.

(15°F) in the involved leg as compared to about 2°C (3.6°F) in the uninvolved normal leg (Figure 11.8).[26]

As all limbs in the study had intact distal leg pulses, reduced arterial blood pressure is not the cause of the reduced foot temperature seen in CS (arterial occlusion causing a pulseless foot *could* cause an abnormal TFI). Venous or lymphatic congestion in the foot due to proximal pressure on returning vessels is also an unlikely cause, as 80 mm Hg pressure-cuff occlusion of the calf has little, if any, effect on dorsal foot temperatures despite causing visible venous engorgement.[27] This leaves distal vasoconstriction of the foot due to adrenergic sympathetic hyper-stimulation as the most likely cause of the increase in TFI, similar to the local drop-in skin temperature seen with myocardial ischemia. For centers without access to a thermal imager, these temperature differences should be easily measurable with a noncontact infrared thermometer to determine relative skin temperatures over the quadriceps and the dorsum of the foot. Whether these data apply to CS of the forearm is not known. With further research, thermography could become an invaluable tool in the emergency detection of Compartment Syndrome.

Osteoarthritis

Osteoarthritis (OA), the most common form of arthritis, is a degenerative disease in which the cartilage between the bones

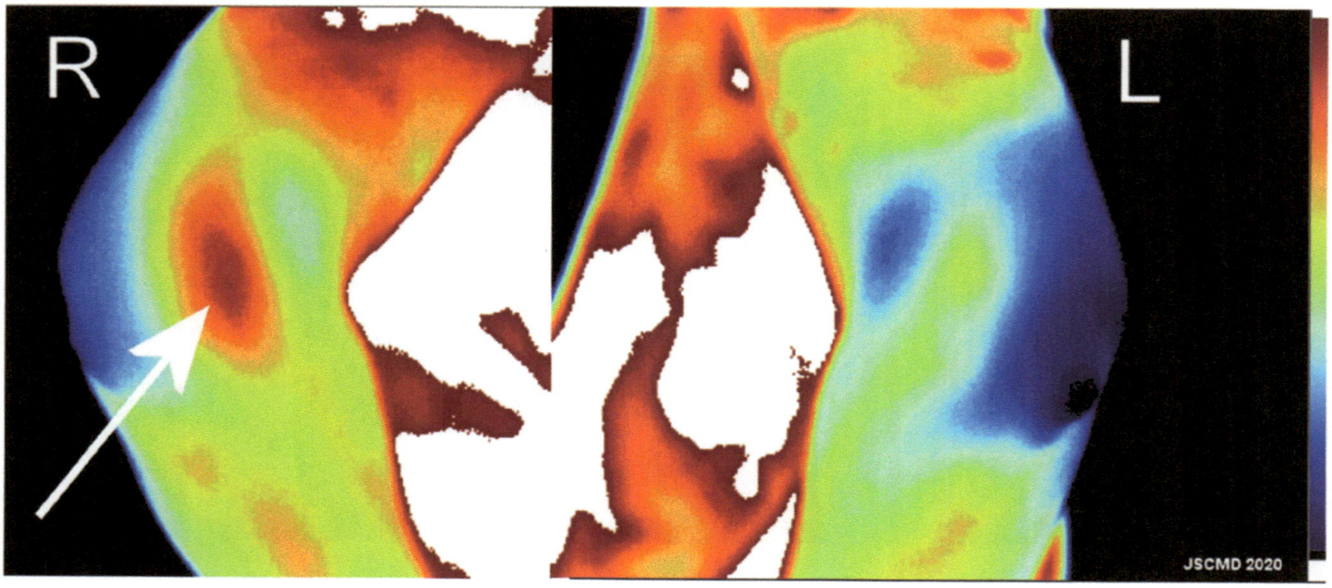

FIGURE 11.6 Lateral epicondylitis of the right elbow ("tennis elbow") – arrow. This enthesiopathy is close to the skin surface, so thermography detects it easily. The left elbow is shown for comparison – 46 yoF.

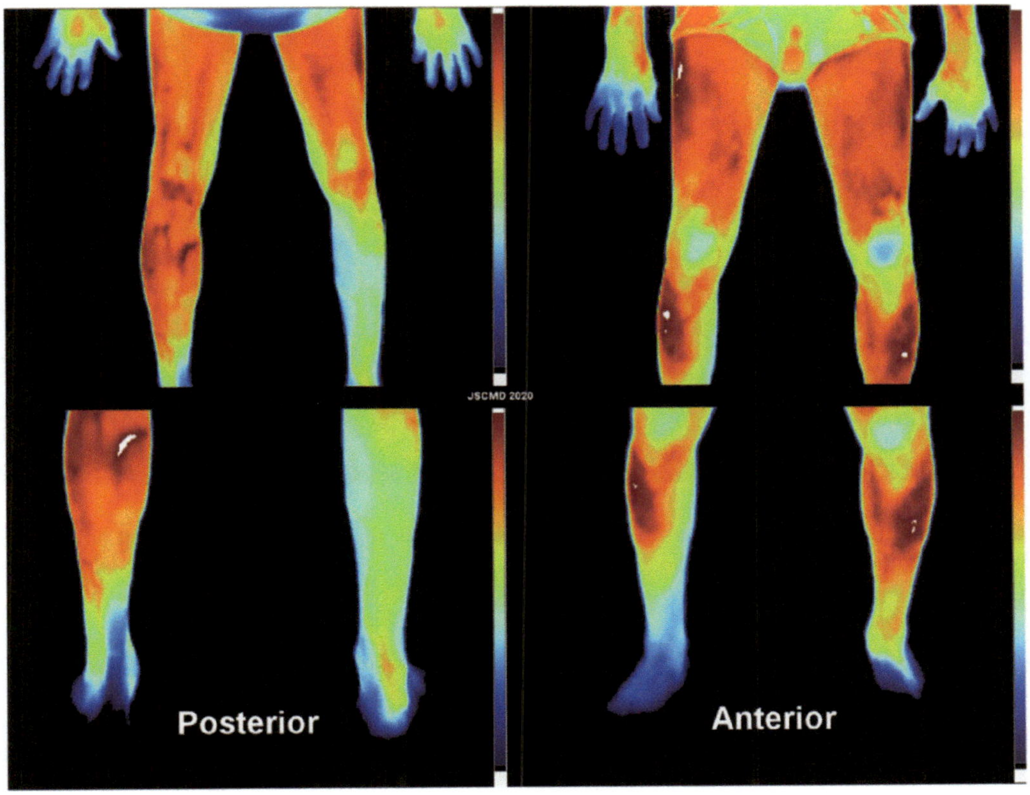

FIGURE 11.7 An 81-year-old man with chronic painless right calf weakness after a severe illness in childhood during which he could not walk and had to be carried around. No edema is present. Pulses are full in both feet by palpation. Note the cool and atrophied appearance of the lower right leg. Presumed diagnosis: Post-polio muscle atrophy and fibrosis in the pattern of the right tibial nerve.

is progressively degraded, causing pain, swelling, stiffness, and limited motion in the affected joints. Chronic low-level inflammation is involved in the pathogenesis of OA.[28] Traumatic joint injury triggers a chronic inflammatory process that may cause OA-related joint tissue degradation and remodeling.[29] OA is more common in the elderly; aging has been linked with elevated levels of cytokines that increase the risk of OA.[30]

The inflammatory picture of osteoarthritis may change significantly over time, as shown in Figures 11.9 and 11.10. Active inflammation seems to have little to do with the underlying bony deformities produced by the disease. Marked bony deformities may show little active inflammation, though one can infer from these deformities that inflammation has been present. In other subjects, osteoarthritic inflammation indicated by periarticular warmth may be variable, showing little anatomic correlation to the bony changes. This variability is confirmed by studies of NO concentrations in and around the affected joints in OA patients.[31]

Inflammatory signs over osteoarthritic joints are associated with disease progression and clinical severity. Although this inflammation can be detected by thermography, it tends to be thermally subtle compared with the changes seen in rheumatoid arthritis and other types of arthritis.[32] There is a significant

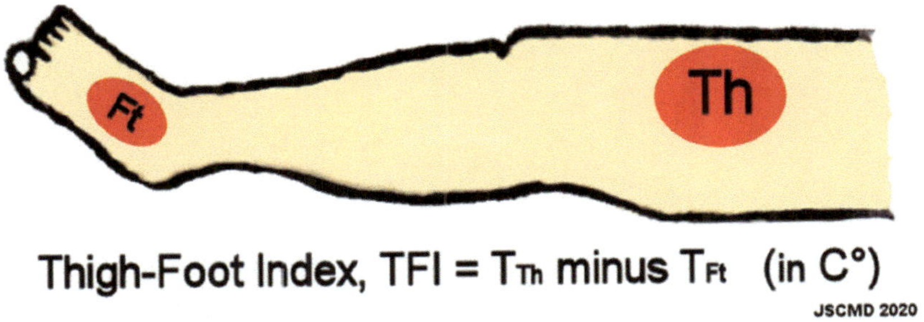

FIGURE 11.8 Diagram showing the skin surface temperatures measured to determine the thigh-foot index (TFI) in diagnosing compartment syndrome. (See Katz LM, 2008.)

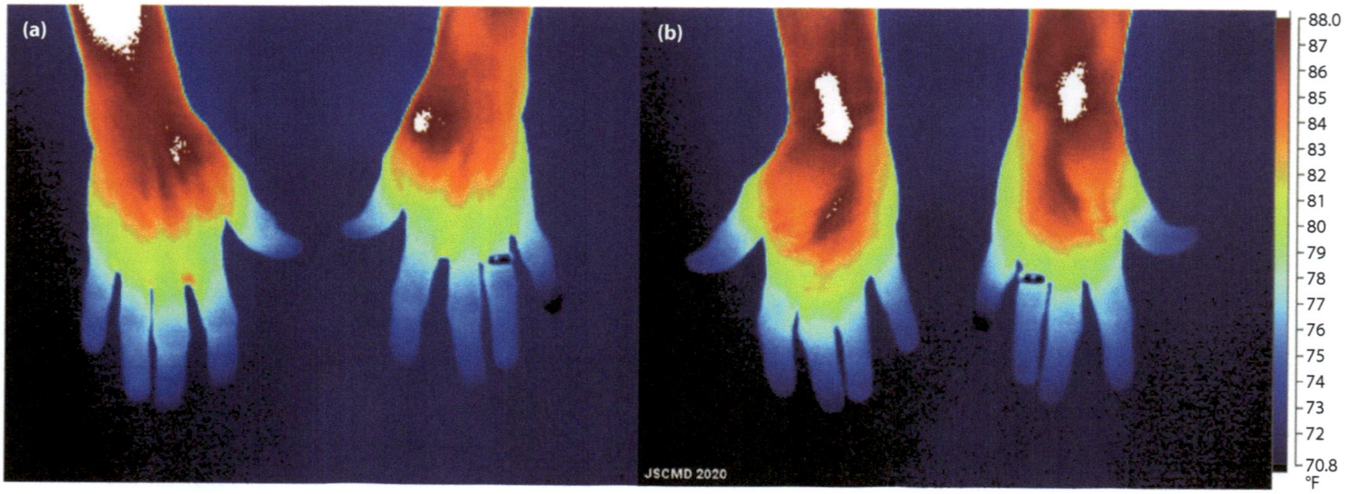

FIGURE 11.9 Osteoarthritis of hands, quiescent. Though bony deformities are present, there is almost no sign of active inflammation. (a) Dorsal view; (b) Palmar view – 64-year-old female.

correlation between local skin temperature and the severity of knee pain in OA, though the data are more robust for rheumatoid arthritis.[33] Skin temperature of the patellar region is significantly correlated with X-ray-confirmed severity of knee OA (Figure 11.11).[34]

Paget disease of bone (*Osteitis deformans*)

Paget's disease of bone interferes with the normal remodeling process so that the bones eventually become fragile and deformed. As its scientific name *Osteitis deformans* suggests, Paget Disease is an inflammatory process.[35] Often affecting the skull, Paget Disease may involve any bone, especially the pelvis, femur, tibia, humerus, clavicle, and vertebrae. Bone metabolism and turnover are accelerated locally, and affected bone is metabolically hyperactive and highly vascular, unlike healthy bone. Thermography over a site of Paget Disease shows distinct and significant warmth patterns.[36] This warmth has three sources: core heat from increased blood flow within the affected bone, the increased metabolic activity of bone turnover, and NO diffusing from the inflamed bone. Osteoclasts express both iNOS and eNOS.[37] Thermography is useful for identifying the location of Paget Disease and following the response to treatment.[38]

Thermography in rheumatology

Gout and crystal-induced arthritis

An attack of gout entails acute inflammation due to crystallization of uric acid within a joint, bursa, or tendon sheath. The distal joints of the feet are most affected because the needle-like urate crystals form where the tissues are coolest. Though gout is commonly regarded as an affliction of the feet, it can also affect any joint or other tissue. Inflammation during an acute attack produces skin redness and palpable warmth, a prominent

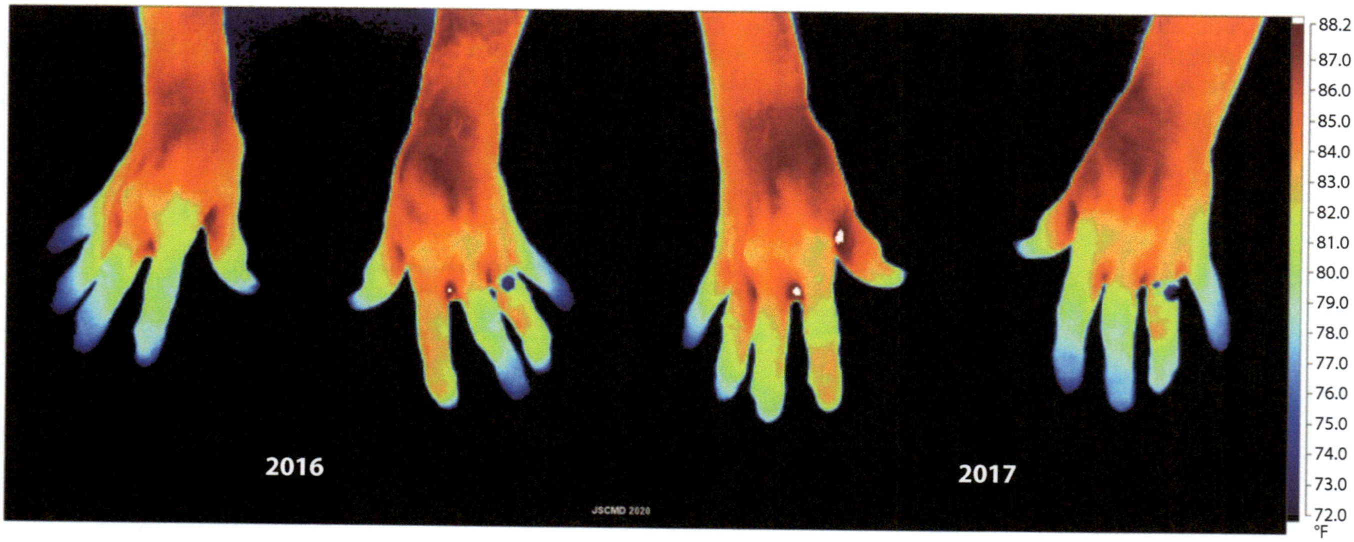

FIGURE 11.10 Osteoarthritis of hands showing changes in the active inflammatory pattern over 1 year. The bony anatomy has remained stable. – 62-year-old female.

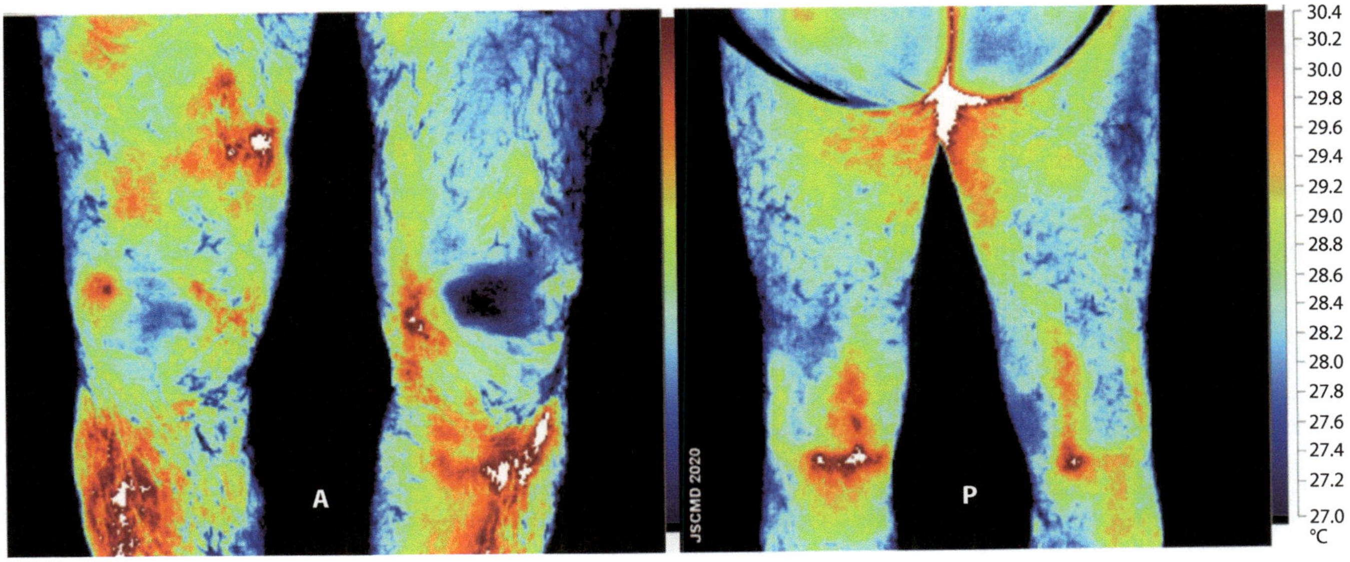

FIGURE 11.11 Bilateral knee osteoarthritis in a 70-year-old man two years after left knee replacement.

feature that can be readily detected, quantized, and followed by thermography. The affected joints are marked by an area of intense hyperthermia with clear contours, an area larger than the visible extent of hyperemia.[39] Thermal findings become less defined and may persist for several days as clinical remission occurs.[40]

Besides gout, there are other crystal-induced arthropathies caused by calcium phosphate or calcium oxalate deposits. All the crystal-induced arthritides present the same thermographic picture of inflammation. "Pseudo-gout" arthropathies tend to involve the larger peripheral joints, unlike true gout, which usually attacks the distal foot. Crystalline deposits that remain in tissues between acute gout attacks, also known as gouty "tophi," may cause chronic subclinical inflammation. A 1°C (1.8°F) temperature rise compared to the contralateral side can be detected over an olecranon bursa containing tophaceous deposits. This difference can be easily documented by thermography.[41]

Thermography in autoimmune arthropathy and myopathy

The four major autoimmune diseases that fall under the specialty of rheumatology are: rheumatoid arthritis (RA), systemic lupus erythematosus (SLE), giant cell arteritis (GCA), and psoriatic arthritis (PsA). All four disorders generate copious NO at locations of active disease.[42] The excess NO is visible thermographically due to increased local skin blood flow over the active areas. The hands, feet, elbows, and knees where the joints are close to the skin surface best display the thermal effects of local NO (Figure 11.12). Deeply located joints such as the hip may not affect the surface thermogram. The NO also diffuses into the circulating blood. During autoimmune attacks, plasma NO levels increase significantly along with the exhaled NO concentration. Increased circulating serum NO levels occur in active autoimmune arthropathy, increasing with the severity of the inflammation.[43] Further research is needed to determine whether these

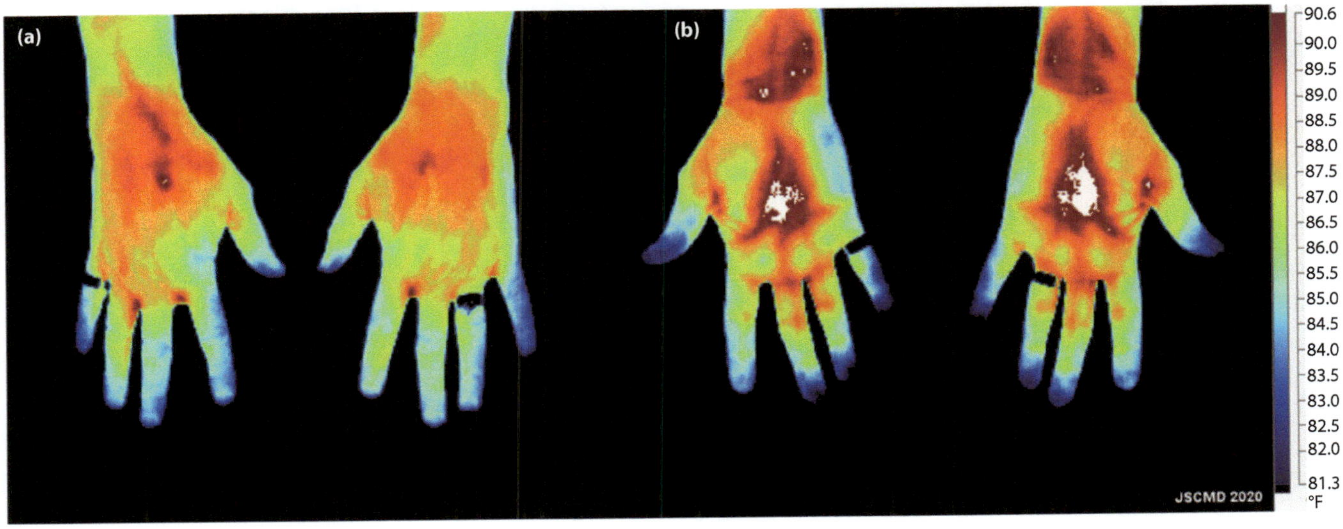

FIGURE 11.12 Inflammatory arthritis of hands, active. The interphalangeal, metacarpal, and carpal joints appear warm. Note the lack of bony deformity indicating an early stage of the disease. (a) Dorsal view; (b) Palmar view – 58 yoF.

increased blood levels of NO cause systemic signs such as the "vascular cape" or dilation of glomus AVAs.

Joint inflammation from active RA produces copious NO, which then increases the concentration of other cytokines. The NO is produced by the upregulation of iNOS in the rheumatic joint.[44] On the other hand, certain autoimmune diseases are linked to an eNOS genetic variant or a *decrease* in NO production. These pathologies, such as Behçet's disease, Wegener's granulomatosis, Polymyalgia rheumatica, and others may not generate the inflamed thermological appearance of the four major autoimmune diseases.[45] More study is needed to delineate the thermal findings in various arthritic conditions.

Psoriasis and psoriatic arthritis (PsA)

Psoriasis involves immune stimulation of the skin keratinocytes. Psoriatic skin lesions involve hyperkeratosis, dermal inflammation, and increased angiogenesis.[46] In 90% of cases, psoriatic dermatitis (PsD) creates well-demarcated inflamed skin plaques. Involved areas may be minimal; the cleft of the buttocks, the umbilicus, elbows, and knees are preferred sites. In more generalized disease, PsD plaques form groups, sometimes disseminating over the entire skin surface including the nails. Initially, the plaques are inflamed and thermally detectable well beyond the edges of the visible plaque. Mature psoriasis plaques become covered with silvery scales, which might lower surface emissivity and increase the thermal insulation over the plaque. As the lesions age, the surrounding skin becomes less inflamed, with warmth limited to the visible plaques.[47] Thermographic monitoring of PsD during certain therapies shows initial warming of the lesions before they become less inflamed. The role of thermography in PsD staging is well established.

PsD is associated with psoriatic arthritis (PsA), with up to 30% of dermal cases developing PsA. Though any joint may be involved, the distal interphalangeal joints of the hands and feet are most often affected. PsA generally appears asymmetrically in the limbs, sacroiliac joints, or spine. Often it follows the same course as the skin lesions. Active PsA can often be detected by static thermography. Mild isometric exercise increases the thermal contrast over inflamed joints.[48] More investigations of the thermal findings of PsA are needed, including studies of the acute and chronic effects of therapy.

Rheumatoid arthritis (RA)

Rheumatoid arthritis is a debilitating autoimmune inflammatory disease that results in the destruction of joints. Patients develop warm, swollen, and painful joints in a symmetrical pattern involving the wrists and hands, though any joint may be involved. Severe inflammation is relatively easy to detect by visual examination of the joints. Assessment of an RA patient with mild to moderate inflammation is more challenging, however. Thermography becomes important in these mild cases. It is important to recognize even mild active disease to prevent chronic joint deterioration and loss of functioning.

The standard imaging tools for assessing disease activity in RA patients include magnetic resonance imaging (MRI), ultrasonography, and X-rays.[49] Ultrasound can detect synovitis in the wrist and finger joints of RA patients, though performing a multi-joint survey is tedious.[50] Thermography can observe skin temperature changes over the inflamed joints, visualizing many at a time. As RA is often a migratory disease, with inflammation and involved joints varying over time, thermography becomes useful in following these changing patterns as well as documenting changes in overall inflammation.[51]

The presence of inflammation in the knee is an early indication of both RA and osteoarthritis (Figure 11.13). The combination of thermography and ultrasound imaging may offer improved detection of early-stage RA of the knee.[52] New segmentation techniques improve the classification of arthritis-affected knee thermograms as well as superior diagnostic accuracy compared to other thermography methods.[53] With automated segmentation techniques, infrared imaging may enable the evaluation of RA at an earlier stage compared to radiography.[54]

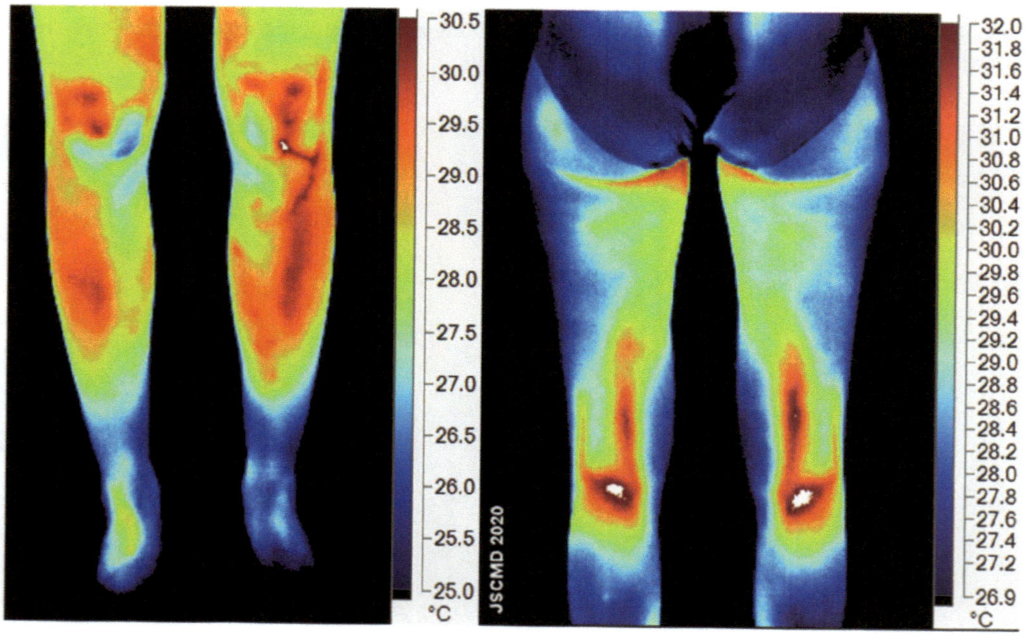

FIGURE 11.13 Arthritis of the knees with anterior inflammation bilaterally in a 50-year-old woman. The "J-L" sign over the posterior knees is also more pronounced than usual.

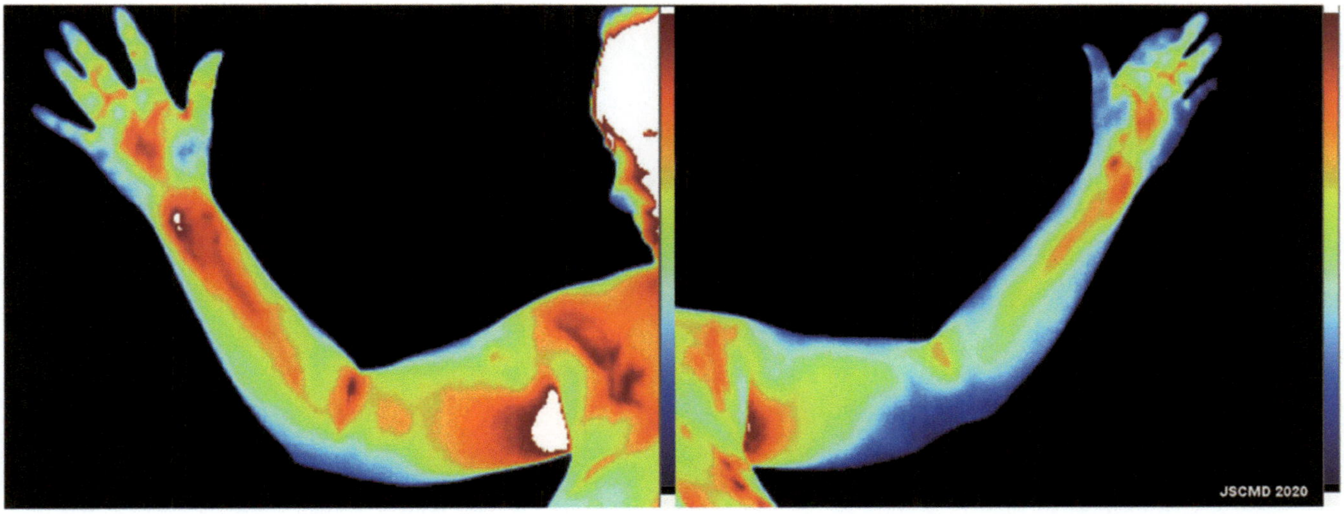

FIGURE 11.14 A 59-year-old female with bilateral wrist flexor muscle inflammation, greater on the right. The etiology is unknown. The interphalangeal joints also appear inflamed.

The distribution of temperatures in the hand and knee joints of RA patients is significantly different from that of non-RA individuals.[55] Thermography is effective for evaluating larger joints, but it may be less reliable for assessing the small joints of the hand.[56] Diagnostic accuracy in the hands improves with the help of a cold provocation test, which increases thermal contrast along the RA patient's fingers.[57] Computer-aided diagnostic software performing thermal image segmentation and feature extraction enhances thermography's reliability in detecting arthritis in hand thermograms.[58] Elbows, wrists, and ankles of RA patients have also shown significant temperature differences compared to contralateral sites. Thermographic findings are correlated with pain scores, grip strength, morning stiffness, inflammatory blood markers, and the Ritchie articular index.[59]

Thermal images have been compared to clinical evaluations of the knee and ankle in juvenile patients with inflammatory arthritis.[60] Skin temperatures are significantly higher over inflamed ankle joints, but not for inflamed knee joints. This difference may be due to the normal warmth from bone growth in children; osteogenesis must be taken into account when performing thermographic studies of juvenile arthritis.

Ankylosing spondylitis (AS)

Ankylosing Spondylitis is a systemic disease that causes inflammatory arthritis, eye inflammation (uveitis), and cardiac problems. Sacroiliitis is often the major symptom, but other joints may be involved, especially the hips, spine, and joints of the hand. Achilles and patellar tendinitis may also occur in AS.[61] Many of these sites of inflammation can be detected thermographically, thus aiding in the detection, staging, and treatment of AS.[62] As the sacroiliac joints are fairly deep anatomically, thermographic signs over the lumbosacral spine are rarely seen in early cases. Thermographic signs over the sacroiliac area are more likely in advanced cases.[63]

Myopathy and myositis

Myopathy refers to disorders with muscle weakness due to dysfunction of muscle fiber. Muscle cramps, stiffness, and muscle spasms can also occur. Pain is not a typical symptom of myopathy. Upon thermal imaging, flaccid myopathies with weakness and muscle disuse appear cool over the involved muscles, while muscular cramps or "tight" myopathies will appear warm due to the heat produced by prolonged, intense muscular contraction. This heat is conducted to overlying skin where it can be viewed thermographically (Figure 11.14). White blood cells and macrophages are generally absent in non-inflammatory myopathy, thus production of NO is not a major feature. The muscular dystrophies, mitochondrial myopathies, and glycogen storage diseases are non-inflammatory myopathies.[64]

Although technically a myopathy, *myositis* is a condition causing inflammation in muscles. Infection, trauma (acute or chronic), autoimmune conditions, and drug effects may cause myositis (Table 11.1). Weakness, local swelling, and pain are the most common symptoms, generally occurring in central muscles in younger individuals, and in peripheral muscles in older subjects. The onset of myositis may herald an occult malignancy. Myositis involves local invasion of mast cells releasing histamine and macrophages generating NO.

Inducible nitric oxide synthetase (iNOS) is upregulated in skeletal muscle under severe inflammatory conditions, such as autoimmune inflammatory myopathy and acute muscular injury.[65] This iNOS produces an excess of NO, which diffuses away from the affected muscles and causes vasodilation of overlying skin visible to thermography. The thermal effect of rhabdomyolysis

TABLE 11.1 Some Features of the Inflammatory Myopathies (Myositis) as Described in Current Medical Literature. Necrotizing Myopathy May Not Cause Thermographically-Visible Signs Over Affected Muscles

Main Idiopathic Inflammatory Myopathies

Myositis Type	Age Affected	Notes
Dermatomyositis	5–15 and 40–60	Facial rash, joint pain, muscle wasting
Polymyositis	31–60	In proximal muscles at first, then distal
Inclusion body myositis	>50, M > F	Thigh and arm weakness and atrophy
Necrotizing myopathy	~40	proximal, little inflammation, high CK

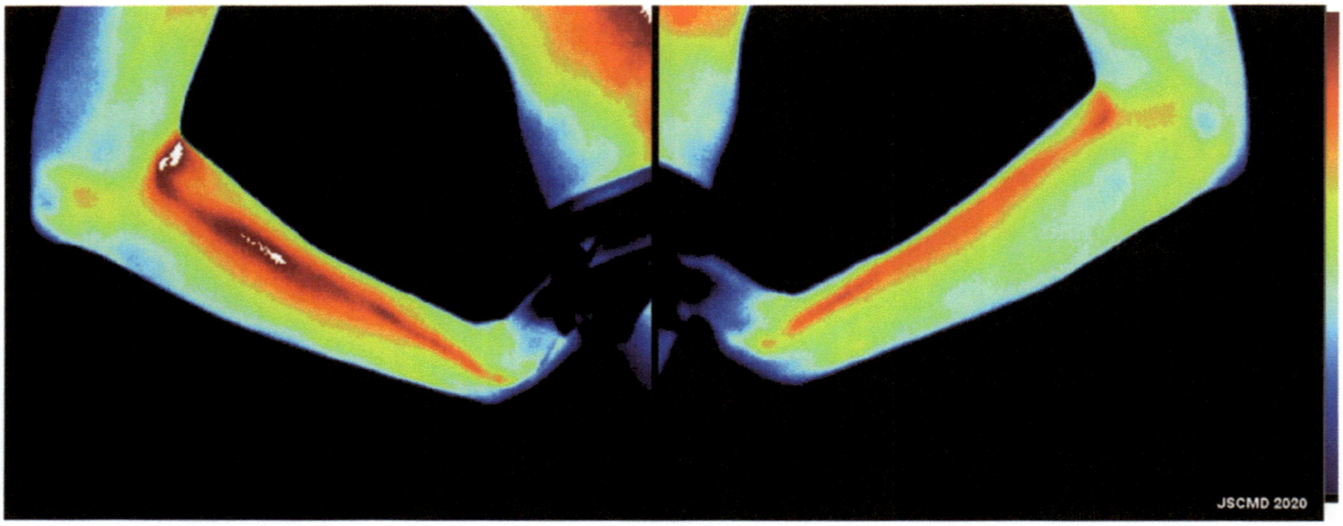

FIGURE 11.15 A 49-year-old female with a bilateral brachioradialis inflammation pattern, etiology unknown. Posterior standing views with hands-on hips.

from 'statin-induced necrotizing myopathy merits further investigation. Thermography may provide the rheumatologist with important information about the location, extent, and type of weakness-causing myopathies (Figure 11.15).

Ophthalmic thermography

With the advent of high-resolution thermal imagers, thermography of the eye and orbit has become useful in the detection of certain eye diseases. Thermal imagers can take clinically-useful close-up views of the eyes and orbital structures. Thermographers are advised to examine eye temperatures closely, report any abnormal findings, and make referrals for ophthalmic examination if necessary.

The average temperature of the cornea is between 34.1°C (93.4°F) and 35.4°C (95.7°F) as measured by microbolometer imagers with no mention of the temperature offset of the devices.[66] These different results could be due to the ± 2°C (3.6°F) typical temperature offset of microbolometer imagers. In ophthalmic thermography it is better to rely on differential, not absolute, corneal temperatures. Still, in cases with bilateral pathology, it is important to detect whether the corneal temperatures are warmer or cooler than normal (Figure 11.16). Emissivity for the cornea is 0.98, thus the corneal surface has about the same infrared temperature as the surrounding conjunctiva and eyelids.[67] As the cornea is a moist surface, however, significant evaporative cooling takes place on the corneal surface when the eye is open. The rate of evaporation is inversely proportional to the Relative Humidity (RH) of the examination room. Comparing the corneal temperatures to the glabellar area of the frontal bone is often useful as long as the area of nasal vasoconstriction is avoided and no local inflammation is present.

The globe of the eye sits in the orbital cavity surrounded by a thick layer of thermally insulating fat. The muscles that control ocular

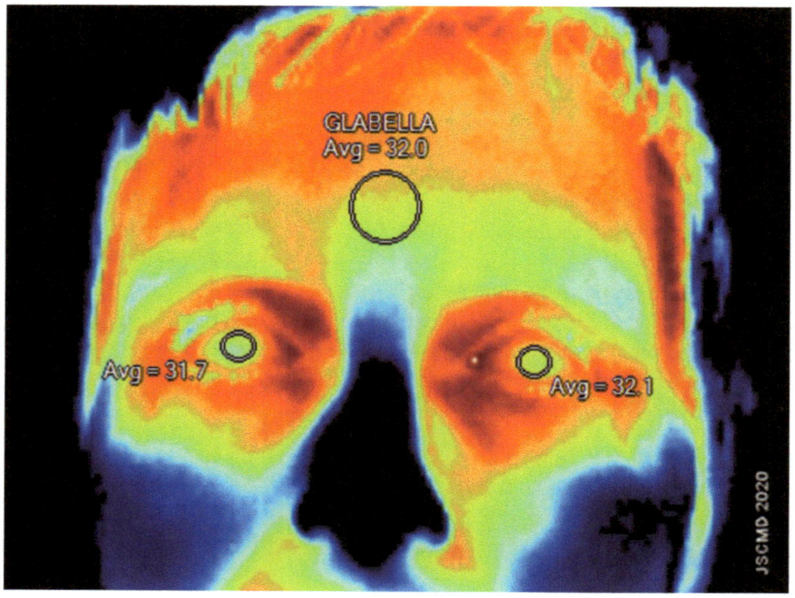

FIGURE 11.16 The glabella may often be used as a "normal" temperature reference to compare corneal temperatures.

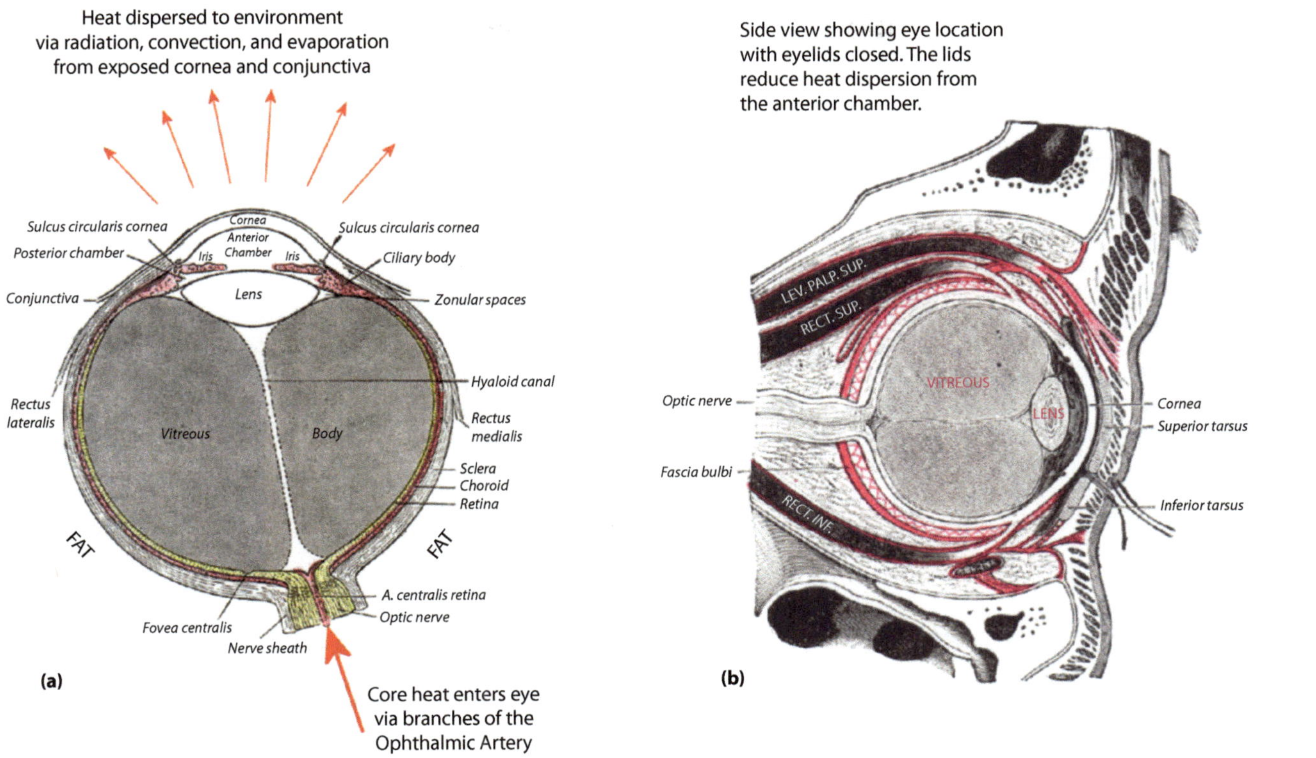

FIGURE 11.17 (a) Top view of the left eye showing the basic internal structures and the flow of heat through the globe.[68] (b) Side view showing the location of the eye in the orbit with the eyelids closed.[69]

The surface temperature of the central cornea comes from two sources: the aqueous humor and the inner surface of the upper eyelid. As the central cornea is essentially non-vascular, there is no close contact with the circulating blood except around the periphery of the cornea (the limbus). The eyelid is vascular and provides heat to the corneal surface when the lids are closed (Figure 11.17b). **On opening the eye, significant corneal cooling takes place within one second, providing a convenient method to observe dynamic thermal changes. In a normal individual in still air, this cooling should occur in both eyes equally. Radiometric video thermography at 9 fps or more can be useful in documenting the rate of corneal cooling on opening the eyes.**

motion lie outside the fat layer. The arterial supply to the eye comes from the ophthalmic artery, which enters the globe posteriorly, coursing forward towards the anterior chamber and cornea. This arterial supply brings core heat into the globe. The anterior portion of the eye is exposed to the environmental temperature; heat flows anteriorly out of the eye at room temperatures (Figure 11.17a). The temperature of the vitreous and aqueous humors depends on the balance between the incoming arterial heat and outgoing heat from the anterior eye surface. The non-vascular cornea provides a thermal window where the internal globe temperature may be evaluated.

A corneal temperature difference greater than 1.0°C (1.8°F) may be considered abnormal. Although some thermographers consider 0.55°C (1°F) significant, this may be too strict a criterion considering that the right eye is statistically 0.28°C (0.5°F) warmer than the left – see Figure 11.18. Significant corneal temperature differences may be due to unilateral contact lens wear, corneal inflammation, "dry eye," conjunctivitis, scleritis, eyelid inflammation, glaucoma, pterygium, eye blood supply differences, and other ophthalmic conditions (Figures 11.19 and 11.21). Paresis due to oculomotor cranial neuropathy has little effect on the corneal temperatures (Figure 11.22)

A contact lens in one eye appears cooler than the bare contralateral cornea (Figure 11.20a). This is due to the evaporative cooling of tear fluid on the surface of the lens as well as the thermal insulation of the lens material.[70] Patients should be asked to remove their contact lenses during cooldown to best detect any eye pathology. Eyeglasses should also be removed at the start of equilibration as they may cause localized orbital warming as well as pressure artifacts over the bridge of the nose (see Figure 10.30).

Occult **glaucoma** is a serious condition that may be detected during routine facial thermography. Glaucoma may be unilateral or bilateral. Central corneal temperatures in patients with clinically-diagnosed glaucoma are *cooler* than normal by 0.57°C (1.0°F) (Figure 11.20b). This decrease in temperature correlates with decreased flow velocity in the ophthalmic artery.[71] Though this temperature difference may be easily detected in unilateral glaucoma, it may go unnoticed in bilateral cases. Dynamic thermal testing may be required to thermally detect bilateral glaucoma. On opening the eyes after keeping them shut for 10 seconds, the corneal temperature in glaucoma decreases about 0.49°C (0.88°F) during the first second compared to 0.24°C (0.43°F) in normal subjects.[72] Certain therapeutic eye drops for glaucoma may alter the central corneal temperature. Brimonidine, but not latanoprost drops, significantly decreases corneal temperature 30 to 120 minutes after administration. Saline drops have no effect. This corneal cooling of brimonidine may be due to the reduction of blood circulation in the ciliary body and iris, thus affecting the temperature of the aqueous humor.[73]

The eyelids, being thin and sensitive, may become quite warm during infection or when traumatized. Thermography is good at detecting these conditions, sometimes appearing quite abnormal when the visible appearance of the lids is almost normal. A stye

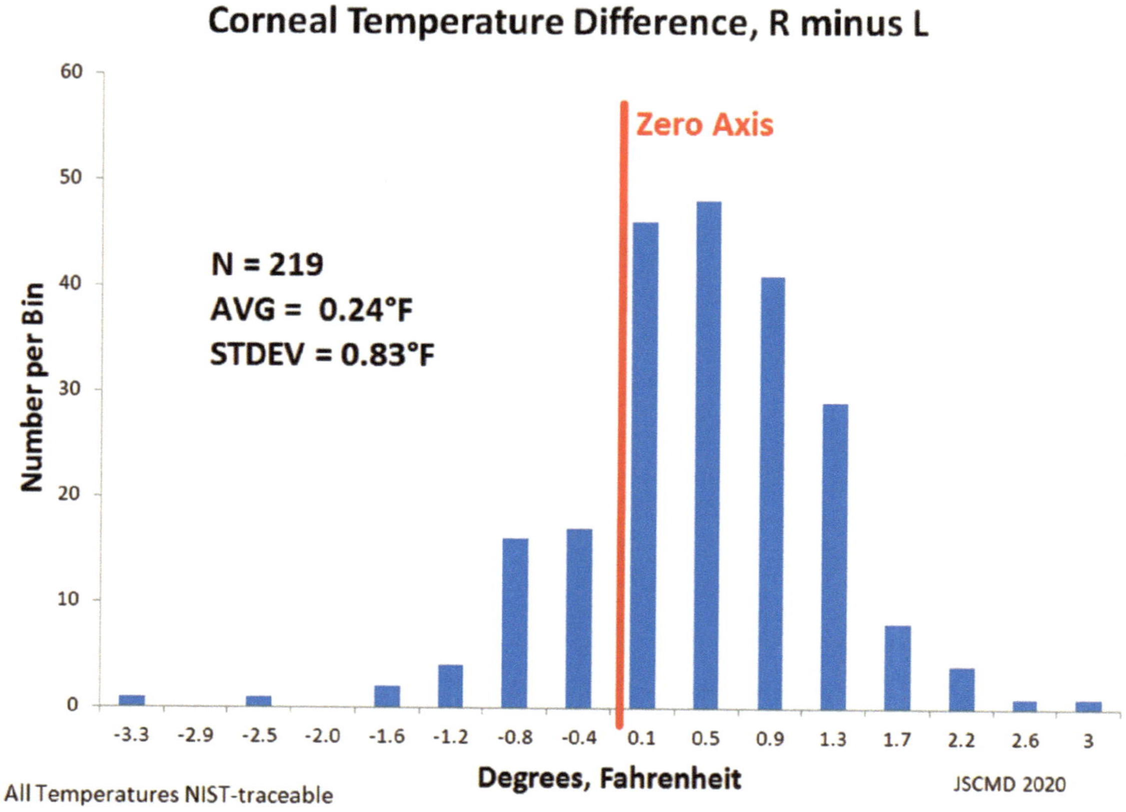

FIGURE 11.18 Histogram of corneal temperature differences in 219 subjects undergoing routine thermography, showing that the right cornea is usually warmer than the left.

(infection of a meibomian gland in the lids) shows up well in facial thermograms (Figure 11.21b).

Dry eye syndrome presents with significantly lower central corneal temperatures. Corneal temperatures in these conditions may range from 0.55°C (1°F) to 0.95°C (1.7°F) below normal.[74] This decrease may be due to increased evaporation by the more aqueous tears found in dry eye. Dry eye caused by meibomian gland dysfunction (MGD) may also be detected by thermography, but special measurements may be required for this analysis. Upper eyelid margin temperature as measured by thermography increases normally from the lateral lid to the medial lid (Figure 11.23). This increase in temperature is significantly higher in cases of MGD.

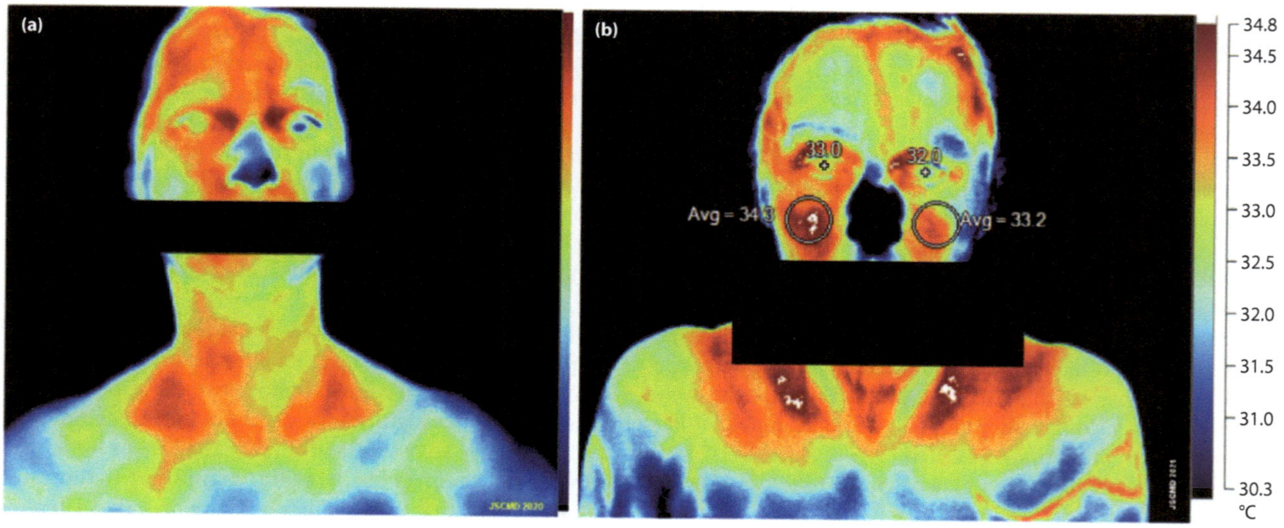

FIGURE 11.19 (a) Unequal corneal temperatures after neurosurgical removal of a benign tumor on the left optic nerve 12 years previously. Patient reports poor vision on the left. The left cornea is abnormally cool. An autonomic imbalance pattern is also present over the face, right side warmer. – 50 yoF. (b) Unequal corneal temperatures – Left cornea cooler by 1°C (1.8°F). Subject underwent a right craniotomy for carotid aneurism repair 6 years previously. Both the right eye and maxilla are significantly warmer than the left. – 66 yoF.

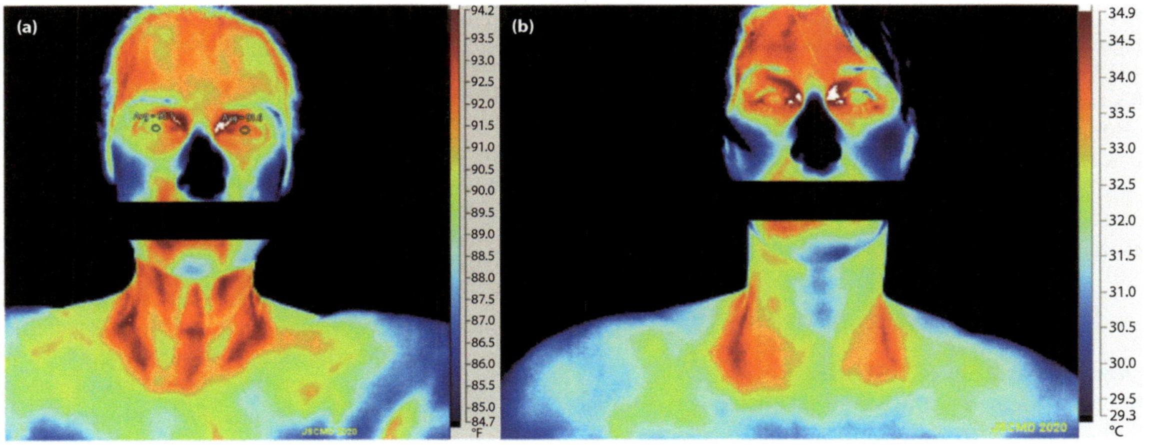

FIGURE 11.20 (a) Unequal corneal temperatures – contact Lens in right eye only. The Lens appears 0.83°C (1.5°F) cooler – 58 yoF. (b) Unequal corneal temperatures – Left cornea 1°C (1.8°F) cooler in a subject *not* wearing contact lenses. No eye symptoms or previous surgery reported. Differential diagnosis includes occult glaucoma on the left – 49 yoF.

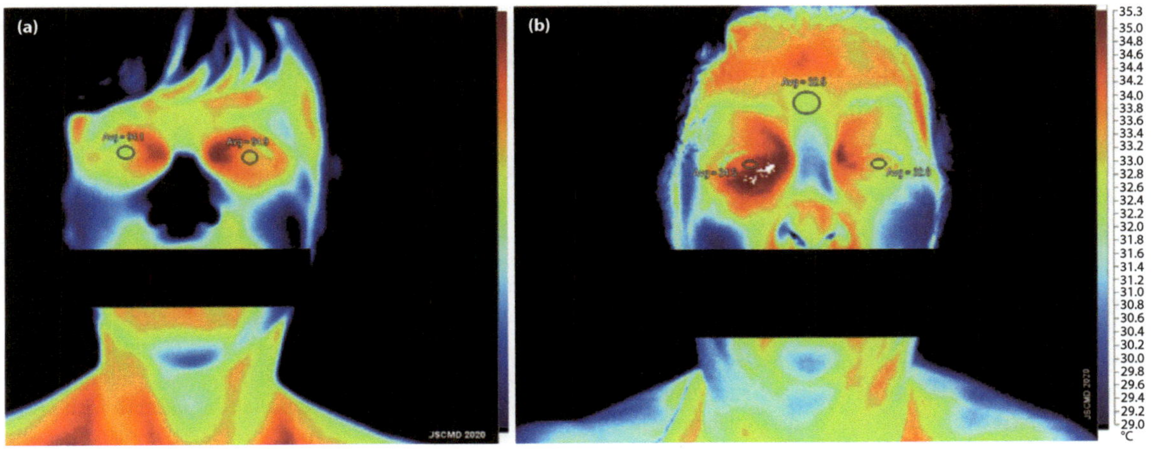

FIGURE 11.21 (a) Conjunctivitis (Pinkeye) on left. The entire eye appears warm, and the orbital skin is warmer than contralateral – 37 yoF. (b) Acute stye (Hordeolum internum) of right lower lid. Thermography of this condition can be much more striking than the visual image, which showed minimal lid inflammation in this case. Even the conjunctiva and corneal surface are warm, though they appeared visibly normal on examination – 78 yoF.

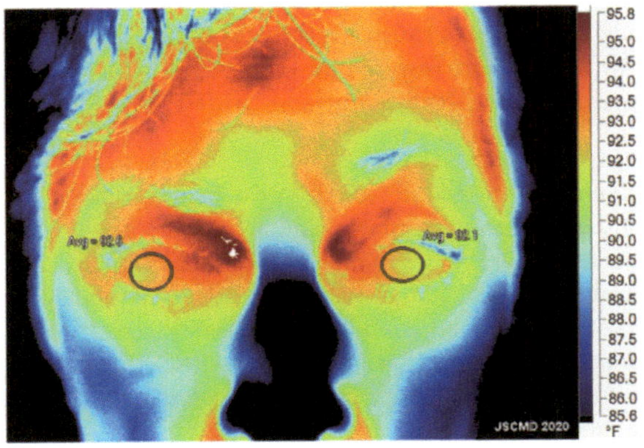

FIGURE 11.22 Post-viral oculomotor cranial neuropathy with marked exotropia on the right. Cranial MRI with contrast was essentially normal. The patient recovered full oculomotor function in 2 months. The thermogram looks unremarkable (except for the easily-missed exotropia) because the neuropathy is intracranial, invisible to thermography – 77 yoF.

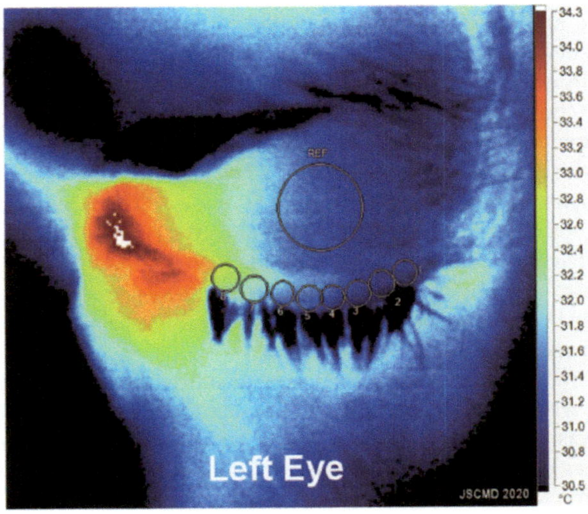

FIGURE 11.23 Measurement areas used to detect meibomian gland dysfunction. In this case, the area 8/REF ratio measured 1.035, within the normal range. (After Su TY, 2016.)

To normalize this difference to an individual's body temperature, the lid margin measurements can be divided by the reference temperature (REF) taken over the main portion of the upper lid. At Area 1, this ratio is less than 1.0 in both MGD and control subjects, becoming greater than 1.0 at Area 4 in MGD cases, and Area 6 in normals. In normal individuals, the ratio remains less than 1.2 at Area 8, while in MGD, that ratio is between 1.2 and 1.5, increasing with the severity of the condition.[75] Further investigations into these measurements should be undertaken.

Thermography in neurology

Central nervous system (CNS) effects

Though the primary temperature thermostat of the body is located in the hypothalamic region of the brainstem, the cerebral cortex also plays a role in peripheral temperature control as observed in patients following hemiplegic stroke. The cortical effect on the neural tone of the sympathetic trunks appears to be one of inhibition, with increased peripheral sympathetic vasoconstrictor tone when communications from the cortex have been disrupted, although this may take weeks or months to develop.[76] Subjects with hemiplegia have cooler feet bilaterally that normal controls, and the paralyzed side is cooler than the normal side. This difference is independent of the time since the stroke. The level of motor function in the paralyzed side is not a significant factor in the temperature difference between the limbs.[77] Reduction in local limb temperature may be a disturbing symptom in patients after hemiplegia. Patients show reduced finger skin temperatures and reduced blood flow at rest in the paralyzed hand.[78]

Spinal cord injury

The spinal cord (SC) is also part of the CNS and can produce local and systemic thermal effects when transected either partially or completely. These thermal changes may be seen in cord transection caused by mechanical disruption, ischemia, or infection. Partial SC injury may produce mixed or reduced thermal findings.[79] If the cervical cord is completely transected, the entire sympathetic and sacral parasympathetic systems may continue functioning, albeit without modulation from cerebral control. Patients with complete SC injuries in the mid-thoracic area maintain some cerebral control of the sympathetic trunks and peripheral vasomotor function, though pelvic parasympathetic control is lost.

In cases of complete spinal transection, sensory and motor functions are sharply reduced below the level of SC injury. Autonomic sympathetic regulation, however, is affected across several dermatome levels and does not create a distinct thermographic demarcation at the level of SC injury.[80] This is because the sympathetic trunks, which lie outside of and lateral to the central spinal canal, are not usually injured. These trunks communicate rostro-caudally, "smearing" the autonomic vasomotor effects as seen thermographically. Thermography cannot be used to detect the precise level of SC injury.

The thermographic effects seen distal to SC injury depend on whether the disruption is acute or chronic. Initially, there is vasodilation distal to the injury, with warmer skin temperatures and venous dilation consistent with decreased sympathetic stimulation. In chronic cervical cord injury, profound autonomic dysreflexia occurs; adrenergic sympathetic constriction of the skin vasculature increases, while cholinergic sympathetic sweating is inhibited. These two effects can cause hyperthermia in warm environments.[81] Thermographic or non-contact infrared monitoring of the patient's head and face may be useful to monitor body temperature non-invasively.

Lumbar spinal stenosis (LSS)

Lumbar spinal stenosis is technically known as Cauda Equina Compression Syndrome. The Cauda Equina (CE) is a bundle of peripheral nerves that exits the adult spinal cord at the conus medularis about the level of T12 and courses downwards, contained in and protected by the dura mater and bathed in cerebrospinal fluid. Individual CE nerves exit the bony spinal canal as they reach their corresponding lumbar and sacral dermatomal levels. Patients with LSS develop pain in the lower extremities on standing or walking due to increased pressure on the CE by venous congestion or bony impingement on the dura. As this pressure creates temporary partial nerve damage due to reduced local blood flow, sympathetic vasoconstrictor tone is increased over the lumbar and sacral skin areas, which become demonstrably cool. The areas over the buttocks (sacral nerves) and the quadriceps (lower lumbar nerves) best demonstrate this decrease in temperature.

The increase in lumbar and sacral sympathetic tone is due to reflex sympathetic stimulation in the conus medularis; nerves of the lower lumbar CE do not carry sympathetic fibers.[82] LSS patients without pain, and patients with non-LSS back pain, do not show this thermographic cooling.[83] Lumbar thermography is a sensitive tool for evaluating LSS patients.[84]

Cerebral palsy (CP)

Cerebral Palsy is not a distinct disease; symptoms and physical limitations of CP vary widely from patient to patient. CP is due to brain injury from anoxia, infection, or other brain insult occurring from the prenatal period up to two years of age. Muscle spasms and dystonia are frequent features. Although in normal subjects, muscle tension and spasm create local heat that may be visualized thermographically, the areas affected by CP appear cool. This is especially apparent in patients with hemiplegic-type CP, where the affected side appears cooler that the contralateral side; this temperature difference increases when the subject is exercised. This increased temperature difference is due to decreased temperature over the affected muscles on the hemiplegic side.[85] Thermography of horse-riding therapy provided to teenagers with CP shows that this skin-cooling effect occurs in both markedly affected legs as well as in the more normal contralateral leg, indicating a CNS or spinal cord etiology in some cases. Simulated horseback riding exacerbates this decreased temperature finding.[86] More research into this paradoxical thermal cooling may improve therapy for patients with CP.

Peripheral nerve injury

All human peripheral nerves from the first cervical to the fifth sacral contain sensory, motor, and autonomic nerve fibers once they course lateral to the sympathetic trunks. Damage to sympathetic fibers medial to the trunks may sometimes be detected as diffuse thermographic cooling. Nerve lesions lateral to the trunks produce more distinct thermal changes with better-defined edges as there are no significant sympathetic connections between the distal peripheral nerves.

With complete mechanical or anesthetic interruption of a peripheral nerve, adrenergic sympathetic vasoconstrictive fibers are blocked, resulting in a warm area over the skin supplied by that nerve. This finding may be useful to detect nerves damaged by trauma. Initially, the totally denervated skin area appears warm but may later appear cool as the nerve heals and recovers over several months. Confirmation of successful anesthetic nerve block may also be made thermographically.[87] With complete block, the anesthetized skin appears thermographically warm, with the surface temperature returning to normal as the block wears off over several hours.

Incomplete or diffuse damage to a peripheral nerve, such as found in partial nerve injuries or compression neuropathies, produces a different thermographic picture. In partial nerve damage, there is sympathetic over-activity due to neural irritation. This produces dermal vasoconstriction distally, with the enervated skin appearing cool. Sensory impairment (numbness) is usually only partial in these cases. If the partial nerve damage is healed or pressure relieved, the enervated skin will return to normal temperatures and normal sensation. A mixed thermographic picture may occur where intact nerve bundles are mixed with damaged bundles, causing a "scattered" neuropathic dermal appearance. In this condition, the thermogram may show cooler areas mixed with areas of increased temperature, or a cooler area surrounded by a warmer zone.[88]

Entrapment and pressure neuropathies

"The sympathetic nerve can also develop a pathologically overactive state ... due to irritative lesions, as in partial nerve injury or compression neuropathy." – Sumio Uematsu MD, 1985

All clinical entrapment neuropathies and most pressure neuropathies have the same thermographic appearance as a partial nerve injury: cool areas caused by overactive sympathetic vasoconstriction. Severe pressure neuropathies may progress to total neuropathy, however, appearing warm from vasodilation of the supplied skin areas. A complicated thermal picture may appear if the damaged nerve also causes significant muscle paresis. The paresis decreases the warmth from affected muscles, enhancing the cool appearance of a partial neuropathy, but reducing any vasodilatory warmth from a complete nerve injury. When evaluating the appearance of peripheral neuropathies, thermographers must keep these basic pathological mechanisms in mind.

Carpal tunnel syndrome (CTS)

Carpal tunnel syndrome, a common form of peripheral nerve entrapment, is caused by compression of the median nerve as it traverses under the flexor retinaculum at the wrist, accompanied by the flexor tendons of the fingers and thumb. Irritation of the flexor tendons or their synovial sheaths can result in swelling that narrows the carpal tunnel, placing pressure on the nerve. Bony deformities at the wrist due to injury or arthritis can also compress the median nerve. The neural distribution of the median nerve includes the volar thumb, index, and middle fingers, and the radial half of the ring finger (see Figure 11.48). Classically, CTS patients experience numbness, weakness, tingling, burning, and pain affecting at least two of the digits supplied by the median nerve.[89]

Using older infrared scanning technology, thermal irregularities of wrists and digits were found in many patients with CTS, but no clear diagnostic pattern was found.[90] Today, using microbolometer imagers, thermographic assessments are performed in both hands, from fingertips to the wrist on the dorsal and palmar sides. Blood flow regulation in CTS as monitored by finger temperatures appears to be abnormal, possibly due to disturbances in sympathetic vasomotor regulation.[91]

Temperatures of the median nerve distribution area in the hands are *decreased* in subjects with CTS, because CTS is a partial nerve injury. Partial neural irritation produces sympathetic over-activity with resulting dermal vasoconstriction, thus the enervated skin appears cool. Thermography can differentiate CTS from other peripheral compressive neuropathies.[92] Most patients with CTS have thermographic abnormalities over the dorsal hand; specificity ranges from 98 to 100%.[93] The early expectation that entrapment neuropathies caused warming of the skin has caused much confusion in older studies. Adding to the confusion, normal fingers and fingernails are not all the same temperature. The thumb, forefinger, and middle finger are, on average, warmer than the ring and little finger (Figure 11.24).

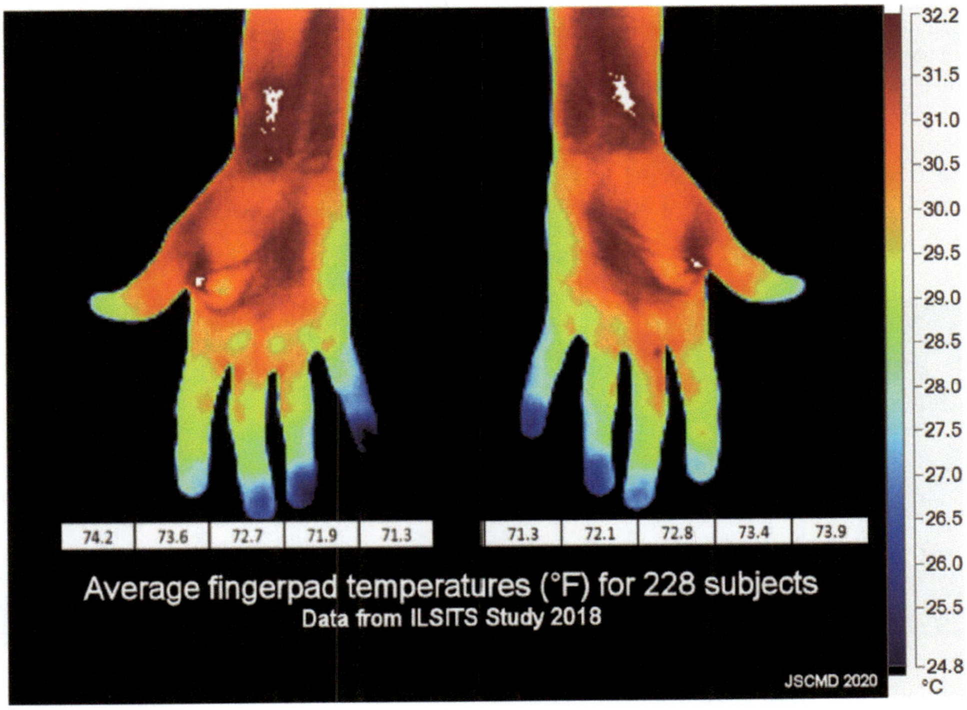

FIGURE 11.24 Qualitative view of the palms of a normal 69-year-old female; shown with the average temperatures of the finger pads of 288 cooled subjects. The pad temperatures normally decrease gradually from thumb to little finger by about 1.5°C (2.7°F).

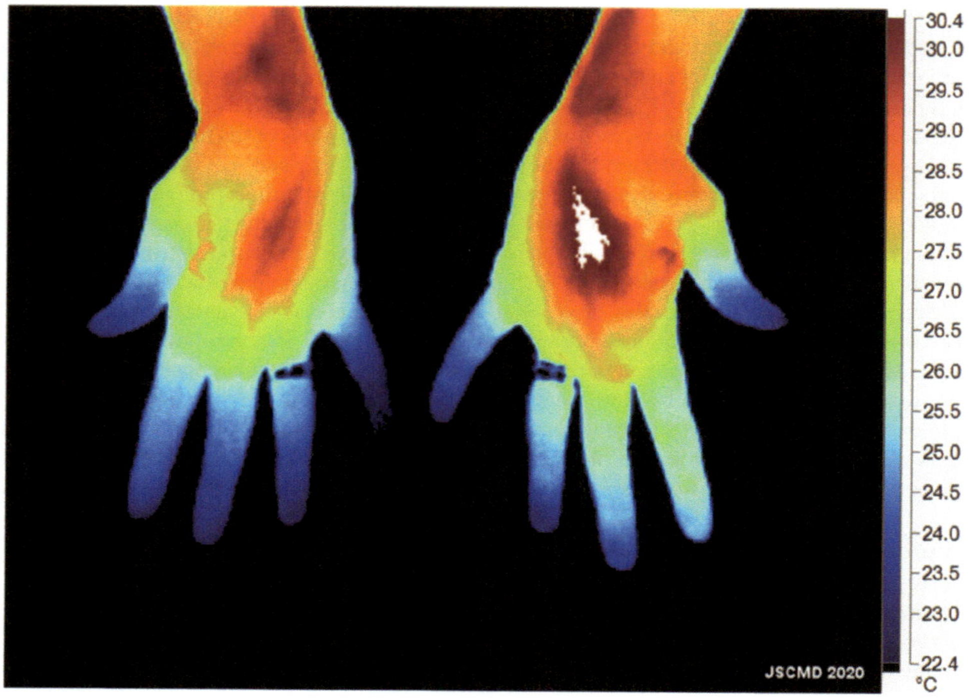

FIGURE 11.25 A 55-year-old woman with possible CTS symptoms in the *right* hand.

Patients with advanced CTS show normalization of the temperature distribution in the hands following decompression surgery.[94] CTS may make digits I through III cooler than normal, bringing them into the same temperature range as digits IV and V (Figure 11.25). In one study, all fingertips of the CTS-afflicted hand, including those innervated by the ulnar nerve, were cooler before but warmer after decompression surgery; CTS is a partial nerve injury.[95]

Dynamic thermography may detect CTS. In a recent study, control subjects and patients with CTS were equilibrated at 22°C, and then placed their palms on a block of ice (0°C, 32°F) for 60 seconds.[96] After cooling, thermograms of the palms were taken every 30 seconds for up to 11 minutes (Figure 11.26). Distinctly different qualitative thermograms were observed in the CTS patients versus controls. CTS patients showed faster reheating over the areas supplied by the median nerve, with the ulnar areas remaining the coolest; the controls showed normal warming of the palms with the ulnar areas warming the most.[97]

Thermography may play a role as a tool for monitoring CTS. Thermography can be used as a screening tool for severe CTS cases in populations with high ergonomic risk factors. If surgical decompression is planned, thermography may be helpful as a tool for assessing CTS pre- and post-operatively. Computer-based systems employing artificial neural networks to analyze thermograms should further improve the tool's accuracy and may lessen the need for other costly and painful tests.[99]

Fibular neuropathy (peroneal neuropathy)

The common peroneal nerve, now called the common fibular nerve, is subject to chronic pressure or acute trauma where it

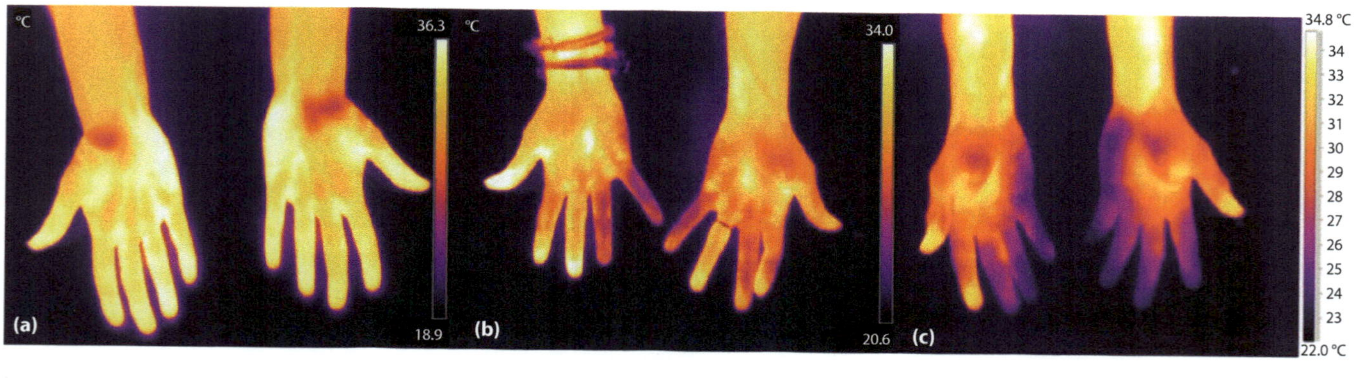

FIGURE 11.26 Proposed dynamic testing protocol for CTS. (a) Thermogram of a normal, healthy patient 180 sec after contact with ice block. (b) Thermogram of a subject diagnosed with carpal tunnel syndrome in three fingers of the right hand, at 90 sec after contact with ice. (c) Thermogram of a subject diagnosed with carpal tunnel syndrome on the two first fingers of the right hand 240 sec after contact with ice.[98]

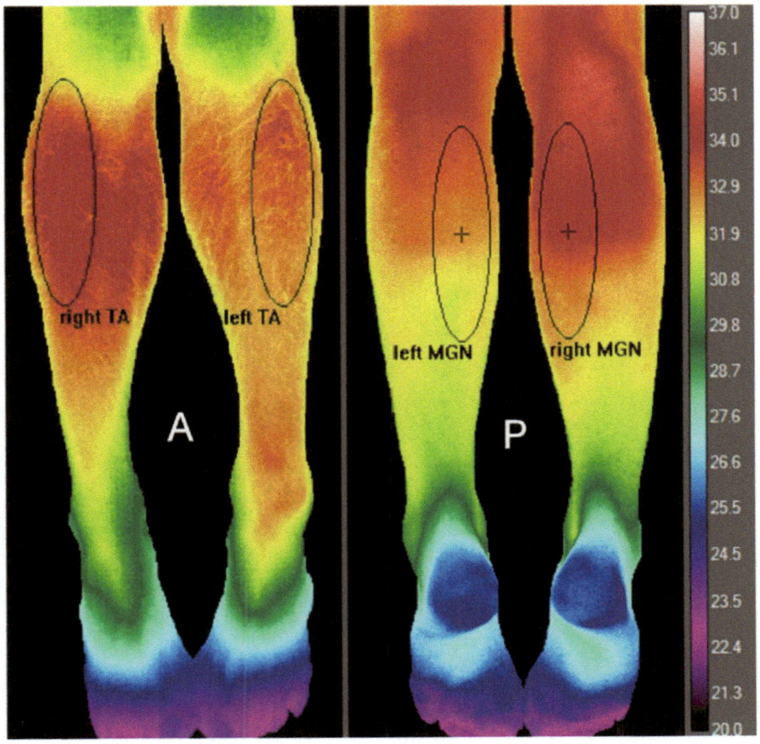

FIGURE 11.27 Static thermal images showing decreased temperatures over the left lower leg. This appearance may be due to left fibular neuropathy or a left L5 nerve root compression. (a) Anterior view. (p) Posterior view. TA = tibialis anterior muscle; MGN = medial gastrocnemius muscle.[101]

courses laterally over the fibula at the knee.[100] This nerve supplies sensory and sympathetic enervation to the lateral skin of the lower leg and dorsum of the foot as well as enervating several muscles of the lateral lower leg (Figure 11.27). Being both a sensory and motor nerve, the thermal picture may vary, with partial neuropathy always appearing cool, and complete neuropathy showing coolness over the paretic muscles and warmth from vasodilation down the lateral leg and dorsum of the foot.

Thoracic outlet syndrome (TOS)

Thoracic Outlet Syndrome encompasses three basic compression pathologies: neural, venous, and arterial (Figure 11.28). One or more of these pathologies can be involved in an individual case. These TOS-related problems stem from compression of the large neurovascular bundle to the arm at the exit point between the structures of the upper thorax. Trauma, skeletal deformities, poor posture, or tumors are possible causes of the syndrome. The thermographic appearance of TOS may vary depending on which structures are involved. TOS may be dangerous by damaging the subclavian artery or vein, producing intravascular clotting.

- **Neural TOS** may cause wasting in the thenar muscles at the base of the thumb from compression of the brachial plexus, creating an area of coolness over those muscles visible to thermography. A picture of partial nerve injury can also be expected in the areas of the brachial plexus being compressed, with cool areas appearing over the arm and hand. These areas can vary from patient to patient.
- **Venous TOS** entails compression of the subclavian vein, thereby restricting blood flow returning from the arm. This causes arm swelling, cyanosis, and enlarged arm veins. The enlarged veins, which can be visualized thermographically, may not drain normally when the arm is raised.
- **Arterial TOS** features pallor and coolness in the hands and fingers, often made worse by raising and dorsiflexing the involved arm, acutely compressing the subclavian artery, and obliterating the pulse in the ipsilateral wrist. Because arterial flow is blocked by this maneuver, thermography can detect a drop in hand temperature. Subjects who use their folded arm as a pillow may awake with the entire arm numb and cold "like a corpse" from compressing the subclavian artery at the thoracic outlet for several hours. This should be discouraged as major arterial damage may result.

Lateral femoral cutaneous nerve (LFCN) syndrome

The lateral femoral cutaneous nerve of the thigh is a purely sensory nerve that supplies sensation to the upper lateral leg, extending as far as the knee (Figure 11.29). It exits the pelvis just lateral to the psoas tendon, where it can be compressed or damaged, causing numbness and possibly burning pain (meralgia paresthetica) over the lateral upper leg. The compression syndrome may be caused by chronic use of weight-bearing belts, heavy body armor, tight clothing ("skinny jeans syndrome"), or pressure from body positions such as leaning over the hood of a car for long periods. If numbness is the only symptom, many people will be unaware that the condition exists.

LFCN neuropathy produces a scattered appearance of warmth over the lateral upper legs. If thermal anomalies should progress below the knee, other pathology should be considered. A good

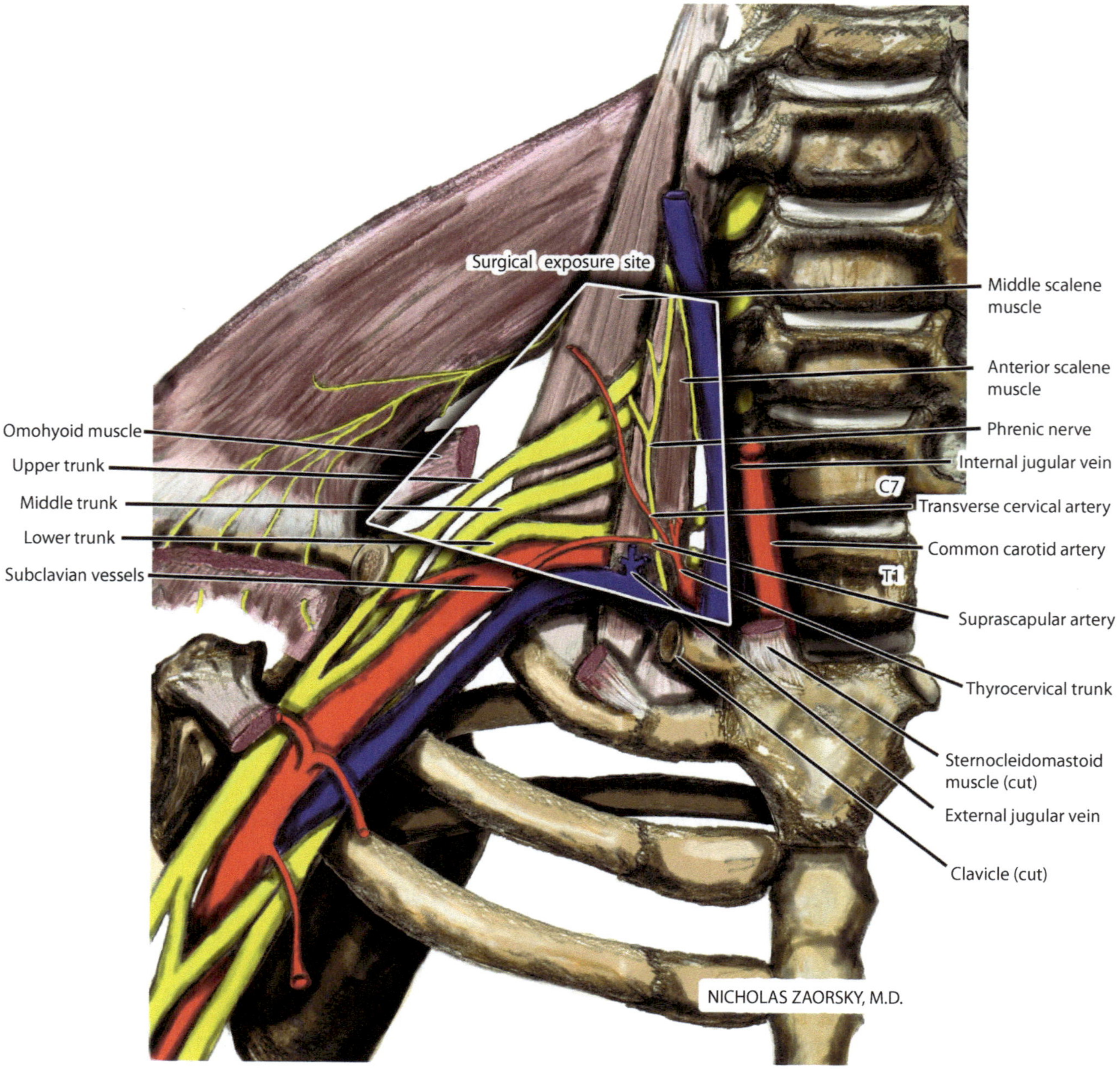

FIGURE 11.28 Anatomy of the right thoracic outlet showing the relationship of the brachial nerve plexus and subclavian artery and vein.[102]

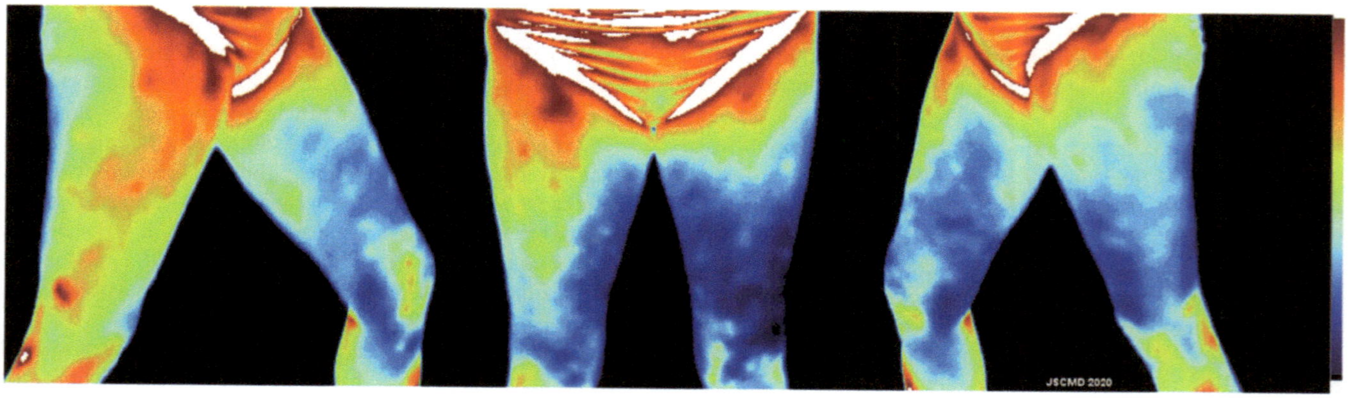

FIGURE 11.29 Isothermal views showing a pattern of lateral femoral cutaneous nerve compression on the right – 64 yoF.

diagram of the peripheral nervous system is useful when encountering thermal signs of possible neural origin (Figure 11.30).

Thermographic findings in headache

Although thermography has been used in headache research for over 50 years, few definite signs have been found to detect headache or distinguish headache types. Acute migraine has received the most attention; migraine headache has no clear thermographic features to separate it from tension headache.[104] Here is presented a partial synopsis of headache features that have been studied thermographically.

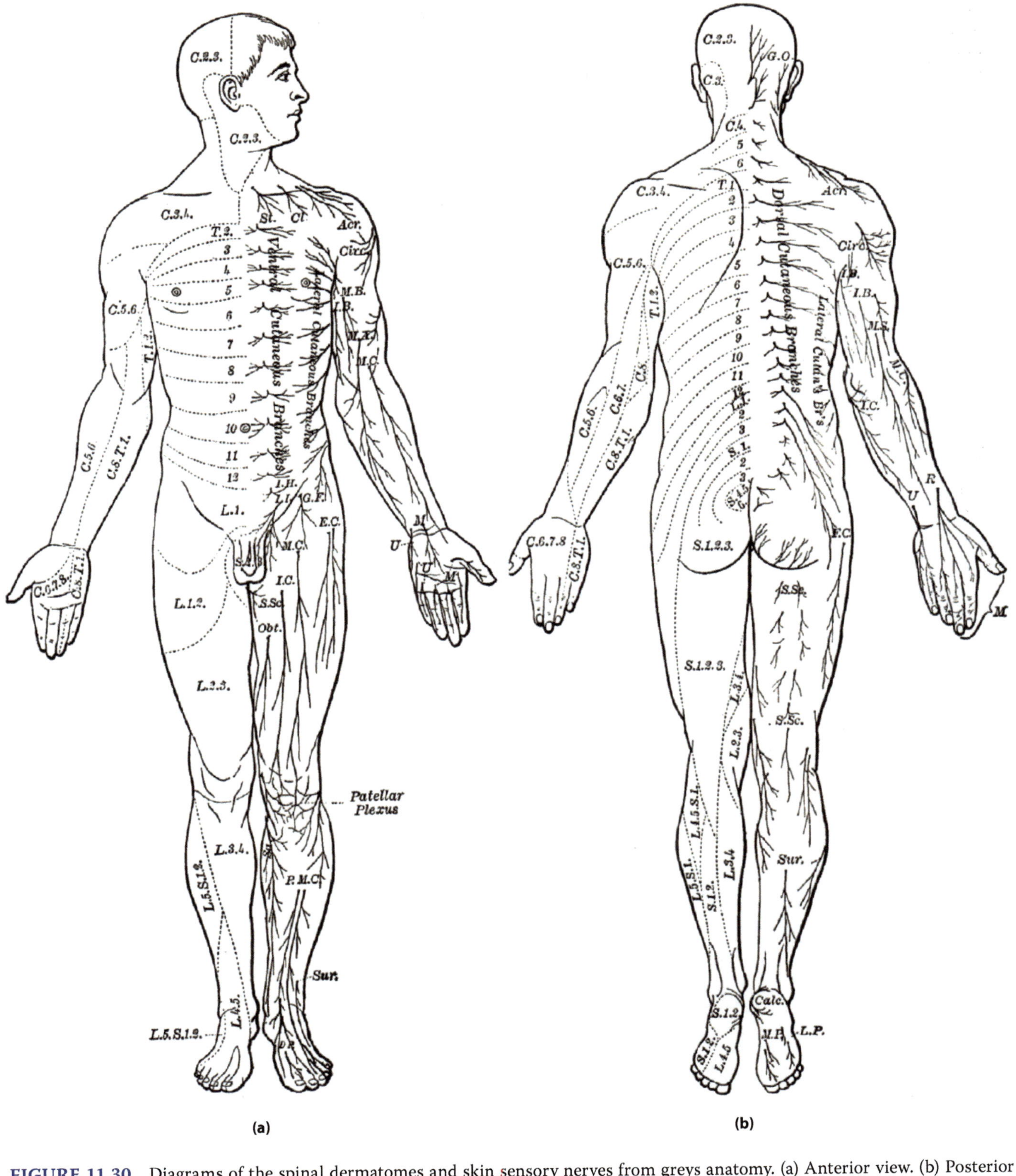

(a) (b)

FIGURE 11.30 Diagrams of the spinal dermatomes and skin sensory nerves from greys anatomy. (a) Anterior view. (b) Posterior view.[103] Anatomical diagrams depicting dermatomal and peripheral nerve enervations can help to correctly identify abnormal areas seen in thermographic images.

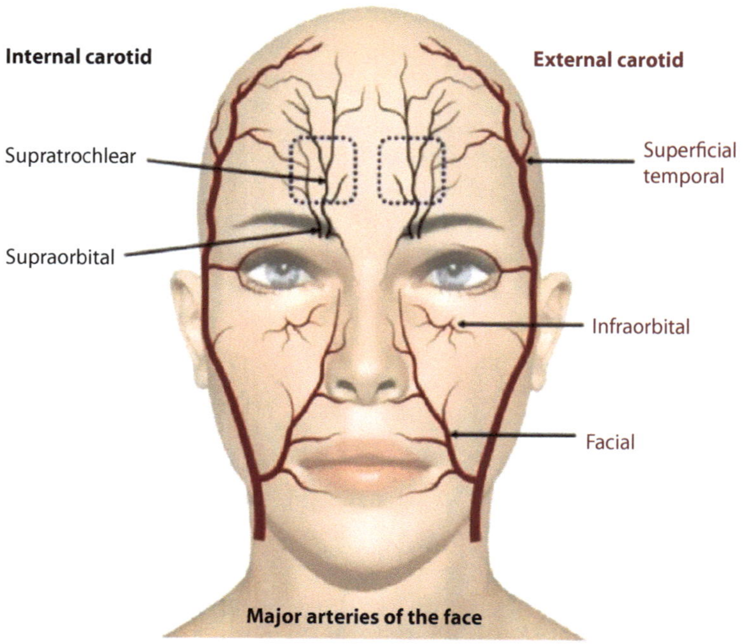

FIGURE 11.31 Anatomy of the blood supply to the skin of the face. Red color indicates the arteries from the external carotid artery system. Black color shows the branches of the arteries of the internal carotid system. The dotted areas indicate areas where thermography can examine the state of cerebral blood flow. See also **Figure 11.38** in this chapter.[105]

Thermal patterns of the arteries supplying the face and forehead have been studied qualitatively (Figure 11.31). One such pattern, similar to the Hebrew "Chai" (חַי) depicts warmth over the anastomotic pattern of the facial arteries (Figure 11.32). This sign may be seen in 25% of cluster headache patients, and 14% of subjects with classical migraine or hemiplegic migraine attacks, but not in the more frequently encountered "common migraine." Quantitative measurements of active migraine show a decreased supraorbital temperature over the side of the headache in 67–75% of patients; this becomes more prominent with the more severe headache.[106] Measurements over the dotted areas shown in Figure 11.31 confirm a distinct decrease in temperature over the headache side as compared to the contralateral side, most likely due to increased unilateral sympathetic tone from the pain. The magnitude of this temperature difference could determine active headache patients from the control group.[107] Both supraorbital and periorbital temperatures decrease in cases of active migraine compared to "control" periods of no migraine. Home thermal monitoring may be useful to confirm migraine occurrence.[108]

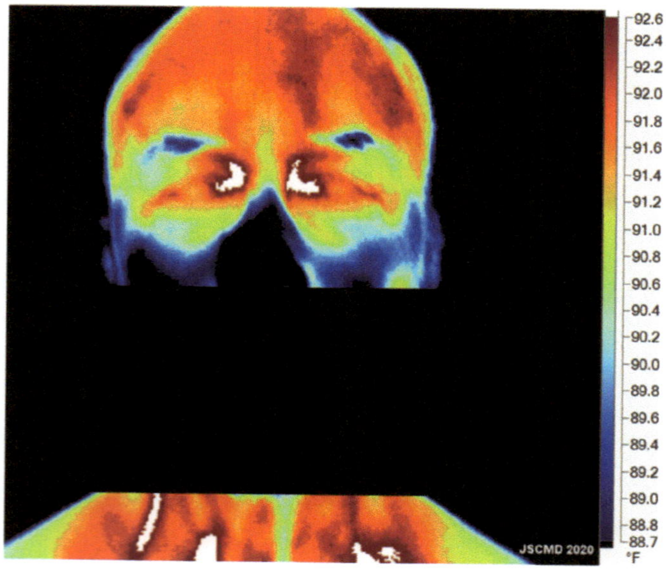

FIGURE 11.32 "Chai" sign over left forehead – 72-year-old male with known migraine headaches imaged while symptom-free.

When evaluating a subject for headache, it is important to obtain seven views of the head and neck: frontal craniocervical, left and right craniocervical laterals, apex cranial, posterior craniocervical, posterior upper chest, and anterior neck – chin up. The frontal view should be taken with eyelids open to observe the corneal temperatures. Posterior views of the neck and upper trunk may reveal muscle tension as the cause of a headache. Sinusitis and tooth abscess pain can be causes of headache. On the lateral views, it is important to comb back any hair to observe the temporal arteries. Temporal arteritis (Giant Cell Arteritis, GCA) is a potentially dangerous headache that should be treated promptly (Figure 11.33).

Cervicogenic vertigo (Barre-Lieou syndrome)

An unusual headache pattern that may cause thermographic abnormalities is the *Barre-Lieou Syndrome,* now called Cervicogenic Vertigo (CV). The occipital headache of this syndrome is due to pressure on the cervical spinal cord from spinal stenosis that is often position-dependent. Involuntary tension of the neck muscles occurs to hold the head steady, augmenting the headache and possibly increasing stenosis. The warmth from this muscle tension can be visualized thermographically.

The vestibulospinal tract in the cervical spinal cord, when compromised by cervical stenosis, creates a feeling of unsteadiness, often interpreted as vertigo.[109] Horner's Syndrome is not part of CV. Pressure on the cervical cord may stimulate cerebral sympathetic inhibition, making the enervated skin of the ipsilateral neck warm to thermographic imaging.[110]

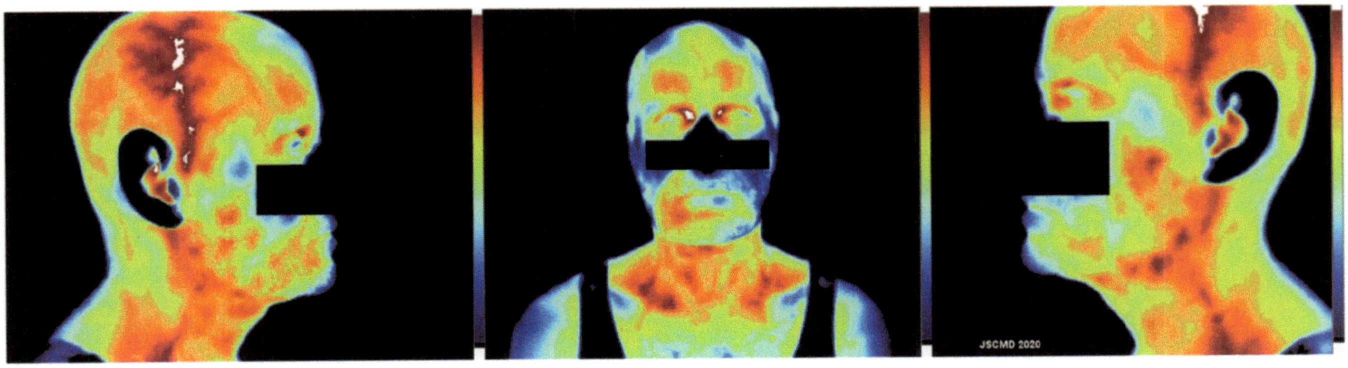

FIGURE 11.33 Isothermal views of a 50-year-old man showing warm, temporal artery patterns bilaterally. Note how the frontal facial view misses this important finding. Though the specificity of these arterial markings in detecting GCA is not known at present, referral of a patient showing signs of this arterial inflammation is advised, especially those over 55.

Trigeminal neuralgia

Patients with trigeminal neuralgia generally have normal thermographic findings, but subjects severe enough to undergo radiofrequency ablation of the trigeminal nerve may show significant hypothermia over the affected area preoperatively. Those cool areas return to normal after the procedure.[111] Normal subjects and those with trigeminal neuralgia, pre-trigeminal neuralgia, and tooth pain without abscess show no thermal difference over the painful site when compared to the contralateral side. Subjects with sympathetically-maintained post-traumatic trigeminal neuralgia show locally warm thermograms. Approximately half of those patients with sympathetically independent traumatic trigeminal neuralgia present with warm thermograms; the other half display cool thermograms in the area of pain.[112]

Parkinson's disease (PD)

Parkinson's disease is a chronic neurodegenerative condition. PD is primarily a disease of aging, but genetic variations can initiate symptoms as early as age 20. Though regarded as a disease of the central nervous system, PD also affects the neurons of the autonomic nervous system. The majority of patients with PD develop sympathetic denervation of the heart. PD also causes autonomic dysfunction of the bowels and urinary bladder.[113] Patients with PD are known to have problems with decreased skin blood flow and their limbs are usually cooler than normal individuals. Thermography has been studied as a clinical tool to detect the autonomic effects of PD.

Static thermographic methods to detect PD have not yielded significant results. Dynamic thermography, however, shows distinct differences compared to control groups (Figure 11.34). To

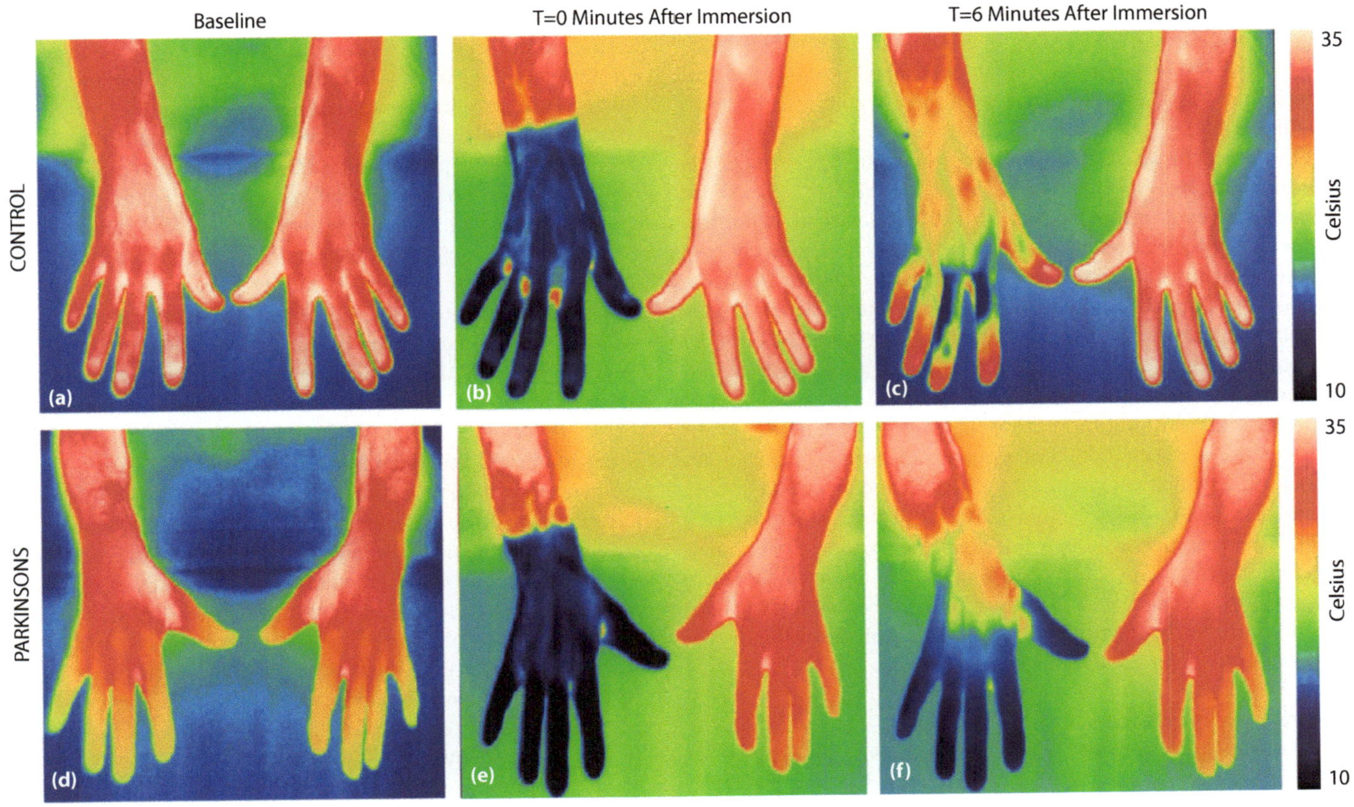

FIGURE 11.34 Dynamic cold challenge in Parkinson's disease.[115] See text for explanation.

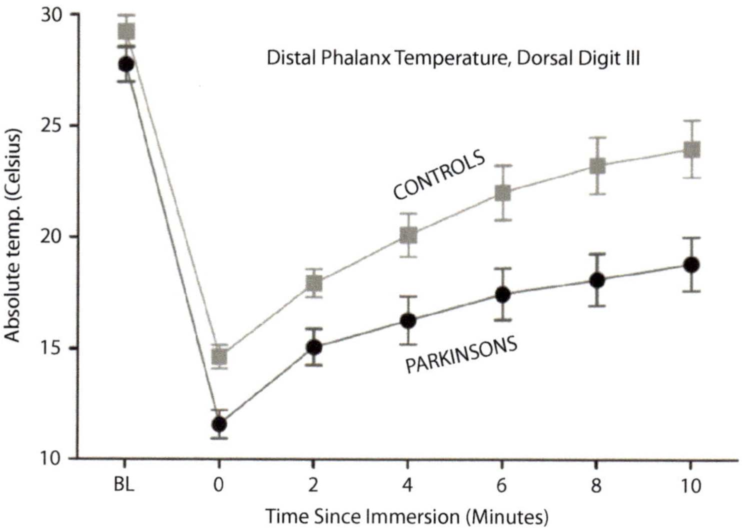

FIGURE 11.35 Quantitative data during dynamic cold challenge in Parkinson's disease. A cutoff temperature of 20°C (68°F) at 6 minutes would separate these two groups.[116]

observe the thermal effects of PD, baseline (BL) images are taken after equilibration in a thermographic environment at 23°C (73.4°F) (Figure 11.34a&d). The subjects immerse one hand in 3°C (37.4°F) water up to the wrist for 2 minutes, creating a large thermal contrast for analysis (Figure 11.34b&e). The immersion technique is "dry" – the hand is encased in a plastic bag during immersion. The contralateral hand serves as control. Subsequent images are taken at 0, 2, 4, 6, 8, and 10 minutes after immersion.

Qualitative and quantitative differences between PD and normals become significant by 6 minutes post-immersion. Hands in normal subjects show a pattern of glomus AVA dilation; the fingernails and distal phalanges of all fingers display rapid rewarming (Figure 11.34c). The PD patients display almost no distal arterial flow as the digits remain uniformly cold at 6 minutes (Figure 11.34f).[114]

Observing the quantitative data as graphed in Figure 11.35, the dorsal distal phalangeal temperatures of the subjects with PD are consistently cooler than normal. This difference at BL is not significant, but by 6 minutes after cold immersion, the two curves diverge to achieve statistical significance. Assuming the temperature offset of the imager is corrected to zero and the thermal gain is unity, a dorsal distal phalangeal temperature below 20°C (68°F) at 6 minutes post-immersion would support a diagnosis of PD. The sensitivity and specificity of this cutoff temperature cannot be determined without further studies.

The effect of PD on peripheral sympathetic tone is one of excess stimulation, which closes the glomus AVAs and arteriolar shunts in the distal extremities.[117] This is similar to the distal effect of a partial nerve injury, although the effect may be due to unknown CNS mechanisms.[118] These results may only apply to the early stages of PD. Nonetheless, dynamic thermographic findings are useful in the early diagnosis of PD as well as in the evaluation of new treatments for the disease.

Dementia syndromes

The mental deterioration syndromes known collectively as "dementia" encompass a number of different diseases, including Alzheimer's dementia (AD), "vascular" dementia stemming from multiple small brain infarcts, and a variety of less common disorders. Though often considered a non-threatening problem of advancing age, dementia can be a terminal disease in many cases. Early diagnosis and staging of dementia is therefore important.

Thermography may help in the diagnosis of dementia; patients with the disease often show autonomic system alterations, which can affect thermoregulatory activity. By applying cognitive and mnemonic tests as a stressor, then using functional infrared imaging and sample entropy analysis techniques, patients with AD are found to have stronger sympathetic activity compared to healthy controls. No differences in the groups are seen during rest periods. Frequency-based analysis of the subjects' thermal responses shows no significant differences.[119] More research into these autonomic phenomena associated with AD is needed.

Thermography can help in the nursing care of demented individuals. Patients with dementia may not be aware of, or be able to communicate, their thermal comfort level in institutional care settings. Patients with dementia tend to rate the temperature of their environment as cold or cool compared to residents without dementia. Thermography, by observing the hand temperatures of residents, can objectively determine the autonomic temperature balance of the subject. A patient showing strong sympathetic vasoconstriction will display room-temperature fingers and hands. Warm hands may detect an overheated patient before sweat appears. By using thermal imaging, a patient's thermal comfort may be detected and documented.[120]

Complex regional pain syndrome (CRPS)

Complex regional pain syndrome is a chronic, debilitating pain condition that most often affects one limb (arm, leg, hand, foot), usually after a traumatic injury or surgery. CRPS is produced by a complicated neurological dysfunction, with many of the symptoms stemming from an autoimmune attack on self-antigens found in the peripheral and central nervous systems.[121] The severe prolonged pain occurs without dermatomal distribution and typically is accompanied by changes in skin color and temperature, as well as disuse atrophy and bone loss in the affected limb.[122] There are two types of CRPS: CRPS1 occurs following trauma or surgery without significant nerve injury, and CRPS2, which involves partial or complete damage to a peripheral nerve. "Phantom" limb pain after amputation is similar to the CRPS1 category.[123] The specific diagnosis is based on medical history and clinical examination, along with tests to confirm CRPS and exclude other diagnoses.

Thermographic studies have focused on CRPS1, *algodystrophy*. The neuropathic pain of CRPS1 is characterized by significant autonomic and inflammatory features.[124] In general, CRPS patients initially exhibit the classic signs of inflammation, i.e., heat, pain, redness, and swelling.[125]

Other mechanisms involved in CRPS include autoimmunity, altered cutaneous innervation, and excessive sympathetic nervous system activity.[126]

In the acute stage of CRPS, sudomotor (sweat gland) function in the affected limb is increased, whereas vasomotor control is decreased.[127] As CRPS progresses, the skin temperature of the affected limb changes from warm to cold due to sympathetic vasoconstriction, with the affected area appearing bluish, blotchy, or pale.[128] Secondary peripheral mechanisms involving vasomotor and sudomotor function affect autonomic responses at all stages of CRPS.[129]

Thermography is clinically recommended as a test for CRPS.[130] Infrared imaging is an effective way to detect CRPS by observing static or dynamic temperature asymmetry between the limbs.[131] Skin temperature asymmetry with a minimum difference of 1°C (1.8°F) is among the diagnostic criteria for CRPS.[132] A substantial temperature discrepancy between limbs supports the diagnosis of CRPS (Figure 11.36).[133] Thermography has shown high sensitivity and specificity compared to bone scans and magnetic resonance imaging of CRPS patients.[134] During cold and warm temperature challenges, the temperature asymmetries markedly increase, resulting in improved sensitivity and specificity in detecting CRPS1.[135]

The protocol for dynamic CRPS testing should be explained fully to the patient before the examination to assure compliance. The protocol as performed should be documented in the examination report, including any deviations from the standard protocol. For medical-legal reasons, both the temperature equilibration period and the actual thermographic examination may need to be performed under direct surveillance or video monitoring to document that the patient did not create any artifacts.[136]

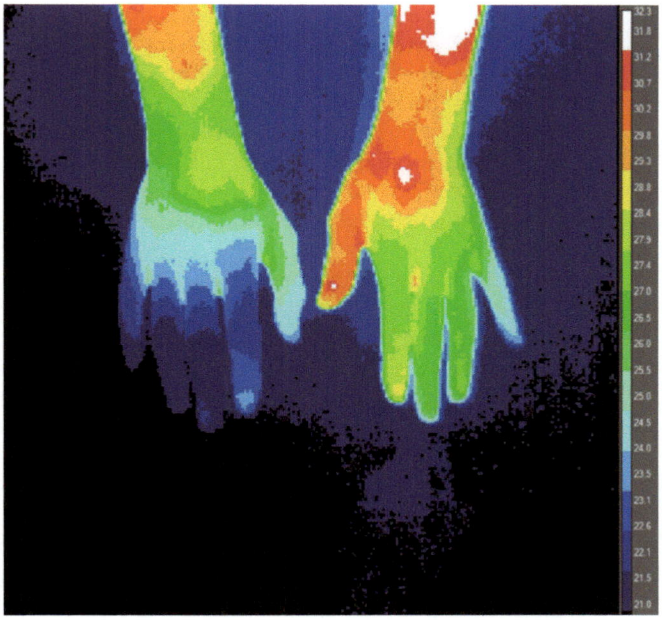

FIGURE 11.36 Static image of CRPS in a 31-year-old man after his right hand was crushed in a door. (Image courtesy of George Schakaraschwili, MD, used by permission.)

Precautions must be taken to ensure patient privacy and confidentiality if video monitoring is used.

When subjects are in the resting state, thermography has been shown to be a reliable tool for detecting early-stage CRPS1; temperature asymmetries usually correlate with pain severity and disease duration.[137] Thermography may become a useful tool for monitoring therapeutic interventions for CRPS1. Temporary yet immediate thermal changes may be observed with diagnostic nerve blocks.[138] Any injections or surgery in cases of CRPS must be used conservatively if at all, however, as they may exacerbate the pain.

Static thermography detects a patterned difference in skin temperature (Figure 11.37).[139] These patterns can vary

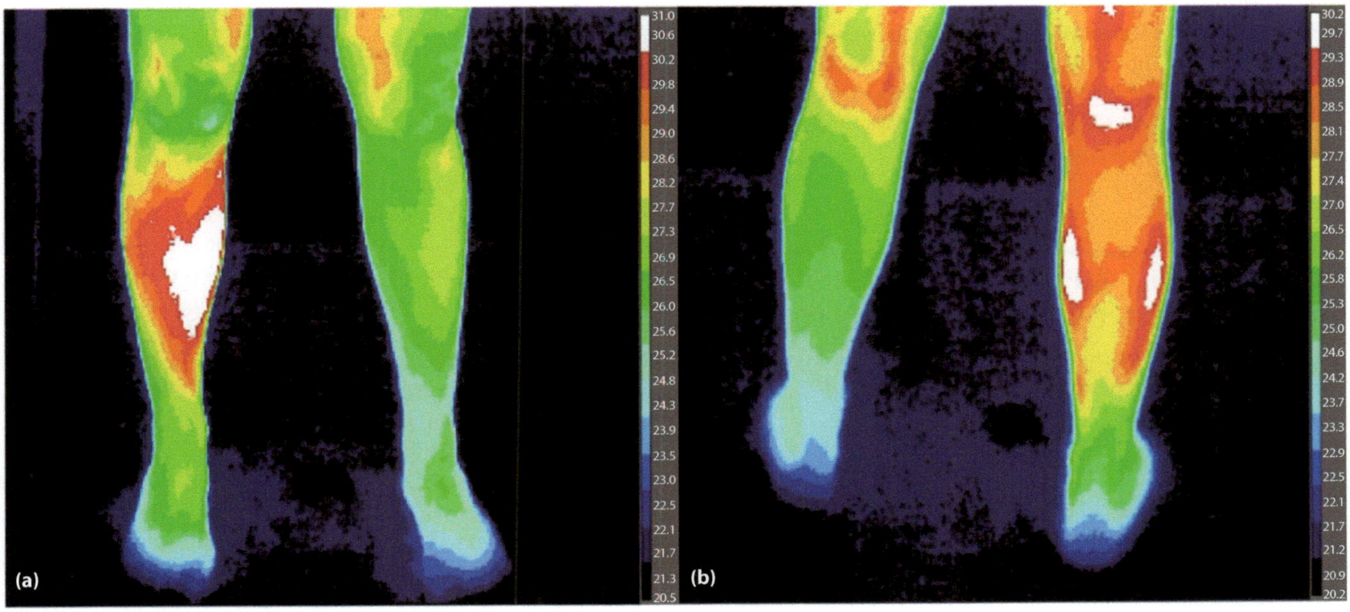

FIGURE 11.37 Static images of CRPS in a 44-year-old man who sustained multiple ligament tears around the left ankle. (a) Anterior view; (b) Posterior view. (Images courtesy of George Schakaraschwili, MD, used by permission.)

considerably, and the accepted thermal criteria may not always apply. Fourty-four percent of patients exhibit a static skin temperature difference between bilateral limbs of 1°C (1.8°F) or less, and 30% of patients may not have cool skin temperatures.[140] There is only poor correlation between skin temperature difference and duration or severity of CPRS symptoms.[141] Sensitivity and specificity vary considerably depending on the method used to calculate the temperature difference between extremities.[142]

To increase the accuracy of thermography in detecting CRPS, consideration of the patient history and symptoms should be included.[143] Infrared imaging offers a more reliable way to evaluate CRPS when the thermographer is supplied with basic clinical data; the thermographer can better plan the examination depending on the location of symptoms. Incorporation of thermography into clinical practice provides additional information, aiding the diagnosis of CRPS and other diseases of neurological origin.[144]

In severe cases of CRPS, the decreased temperatures over the affected limb are virtually pathognomonic of CRPS as long as the distal pulses of the limbs are normal and the affected limb is not grossly edematous. Full distal pulses in the affected limb rule out significant arterial occlusion, which is the major pathological condition that could also cause a cold, painful limb.

Not all cases of genuine CRPS are as thermally clear-cut as seen in Figures 11.36 and 11.37. Even in patients who have developed trophic skin changes and osteoporosis, static thermal images may not show the 1°C (1.8°F) thermal asymmetry cutoff for presumed CRPS. In patients where CRPS is suspected, but local skin temperatures are not significantly different, dynamic thermography utilizing temperature challenge testing may confirm the disease. Dynamic testing should be done with the patient equilibrated for medium vasoconstriction (22.2–23.9°C/72–75°F) in order to detect skin temperature changes in both directions.[145]

In studies using a thermally-controlled body jacket, CRPS asymmetries occur within 20 minutes of temperature challenge, decreasing to zero at 40 minutes. Cold challenge at 15°C (59°F) and warm challenge at 40°C (104°F) are appropriate.[146] A variable-temperature, water-filled body jacket, however, is not practical for routine clinical use. Whether deep cool-warm immersion of one or two uninvolved limbs (hand and forearm for leg CRPS, foot, and calf for arm CRPS) will have the same results as a body jacket remains to be studied.

SIDEBAR 11.1 A PRACTICAL PROTOCOL FOR DYNAMIC CRPS THERMOGRAPHY

Purpose: To augment the autonomic response by thermally challenging the patient as an adjunct test for the detection of CRPS.

Equipment:

Calibrated thermal imager with time-stamped images
Standard thermography room with temperature set at 22.2–23.9°C (72–75°F)
Special support furniture for the water vessels if needed
For limb immersion: Two vessels approximately 12 in. (30.5 cm) diameter by 18 in. (46 cm) deep
A source of water at 15°C (59°F) [and one at 40°C (104°F), if warming is to be included]

Procedure:

The patient is thermally equilibrated with minimal clothing for 15–20 minutes.
Baseline thermograms are taken of the symmetrical Regions of Interest.
Cold Immersion begins on one or both unaffected arms or legs.
An immediate image documents the start of immersion.
Thermograms of all ROIs are taken at 2–5 minute intervals.
The cool immersion imaging session lasts for 25 minutes.
Warm immersion (if needed) begins, using the same image timing as for cool immersion.
The patient may dry off and get dressed.

Interpretation:

Sagittal asymmetry of symptomatic area temperatures is of primary importance.
Significant asymmetry may mean >1°F to > 1°C, depending on the study.
Qualitatively, unequivocal visible asymmetry over the comparable ROIs in full-span, isothermal images is significant.
For dynamic exams, significance may not be met for 15–20 minutes.
The affected ROI is usually cooler but can be warmer than contralateral.
The magnitude of the thermal changes may not correlate with the duration and severity of the subjective pain.
A spreadsheet program helps calculate and graph quantitative thermal data.

Thermography of the arterial system

Arteritis

As discussed in Chapter 5 (Physiology), the arteries generally run deep in the body, avoiding injury and heat loss. Arteries can only be seen thermographically, where they run close to the skin surface. An exception is seen in arteritis – arterial inflammation occurring in various autoimmune diseases. Arteritis may be detected thermographically not because the arteries involved are warmer than the surrounding tissues, but because the inflammatory process emits NO, which diffuses through to the local skin surface, preventing it from vasoconstricting. Thus arteritis affecting the more superficial arteries may appear in thermograms of properly cooled and vasoconstricted subjects. The thermographic signs of arteritis should prompt a search for underlying disease. As arteritis may cause intraluminal blood clotting and embolism, thermal signs of arteritis are important to disclose to the patient and emphasize in exam reports.

Peripheral artery disease (PAD)

Thermography has been used to non-invasively detect peripheral artery disease. Though thermography offers a non-contact method to detect PAD, it is not as accurate as the ankle-brachial index (ABI).[147] The ABI test often fails in diabetic subjects, however, due to calcified arterial walls preventing occlusion at reasonable cuff pressures. Though non-invasive blood pressure (NIBP) devices may avoid this problem, they have not been evaluated in large-scale studies.[148] Sudden surgical cross-clamping of the aortoiliac arteries slowly decreases the skin temperature at the toes, foot, and calf levels, with a rise in temperatures 30–60 minutes after the restoration of blood flow. This delay in thermal response to arterial occlusion reduces the clinical usefulness of thermography in arterial surgery.[149] Static thermographic methods have shown poor ability to detect PAD unless the disease is advanced, in which case static ankle and toe temperatures are negatively correlated with disease severity.[150] Complicating this observation, the mean toe and forefoot temperatures in diabetic patients with PAD is higher than in those with diabetes only, a finding that might hide PAD severity.[151]

To increase the sensitivity of thermography in the detection of PAD, dynamic challenge tests have been evaluated. Post-occlusion Reactive Hyperemia (PORH) does not show a correlation with PAD severity. On the other hand, exercising the subject with a 6-minute treadmill walk shows promise. Thermograms are taken of the lower legs and soles of the feet before, immediately after, and 1-minute after the exercise. The soles of normal subjects get warmer with exercise by about 0.3°C (0.54°F), while the soles of PAD patients get significantly cooler by an average of 1.3°C (2.3°F).[152] The level of the arterial occlusion can be roughly estimated by the location of the decreased temperature change post-exercise along the affected limb. Thermal imaging can be a useful addition to the diagnostic capabilities of noninvasive vascular laboratories.

Cerebral artery thermography

Atherosclerosis of the carotid arteries is a common finding in PAD, with much of the problem occurring at the bifurcation of the common carotid artery, where it divides into the internal and external branches. The internal branch supplies the brain, while the external branch supplies most of the facial structures except for the lower forehead. Small branches of the ophthalmic arteries (the supraorbital and supratrochlear arteries) supply this forehead area via the internal carotid system.[153] The terminal arterioles of the supraorbital and supratrochlear arteries anastomose with the ipsilateral superficial temporal artery (see Figure 11.31). There are only minor arteriolar anastomoses across the midline of the forehead. Normally, blood flow in these forehead vessels is directed out of the cranium, bringing warm intracranial blood to the periorbital skin located just above the eyes (see Figure 11.38).[154] If obstruction occurs anywhere in the internal carotid system, flow reversal will occur, and the usually warm areas above the eyes become cool on thermographic images. If the flow in the ophthalmic artery is compromised, the cornea may also appear cool. Other vascular pathology, such as a meningioma or intracranial arterio-venous malformation (AVM), may lower the blood pressure of the internal carotid system, reversing flow in the supraorbital and supratrochlear arteries and producing similar cool areas over the forehead. A micro-embolic blockage of the ophthalmic artery, which later cleared, has been observed to cause a temporary appearance of forehead coolness. Fibromuscular hyperplasia of the internal carotid artery may also cause flow reversal.[155]

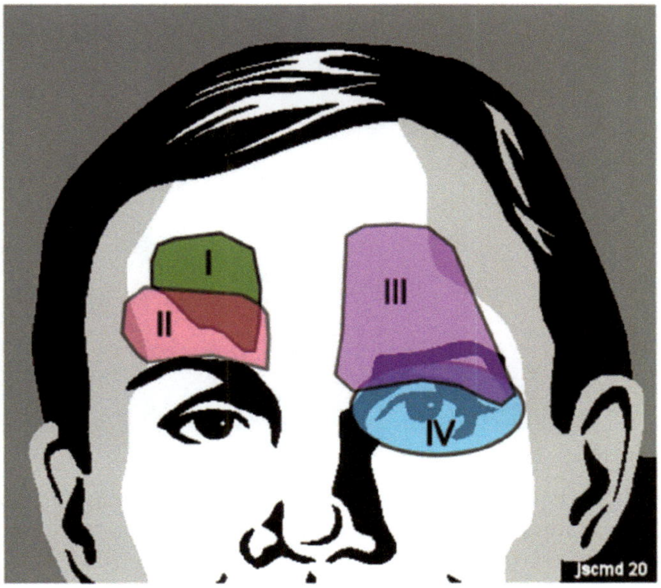

FIGURE 11.38 The four basic patterns of thermal asymmetry recognized in patients with flow reversal in the supratrochlear, supraorbital, and ophthalmic arteries. These areas may appear cool in cases of internal carotid occlusion or other pathology. (After Capistrant, 1973.[156])

Arterio-venous shunts

"Short-circuits" from the high-pressure arteries to the low-pressure veins are known as arterio-venous (AV) shunts. Glomus bodies (AV anastomoses) are normal physiologic, controllable AV shunts that gently lower the pressure as blood flows through convoluted vessels to empty into the low-pressure veins. Abnormal AV shunts have uncontrolled high flow rates that may be detected by palpation or auscultation. The cause of abnormal shunts is usually congenital, traumatic, or surgical. Examples include infantile hemangiomas and artificial AV shunts for chronic hemodialysis. If close to the skin surface, AV shunts may be detected thermally as they carry warm arterial blood. Compared to the contralateral side, the dermal temperature over a patent hemodialysis shunt increases in a linear fashion with the blood flow through the shunt. A temperature difference of 2.5°C (4.5°F) may be reached at high flow rates (~2000 ml/min). A rough estimate of the blood flow through a hemangioma may be made by observing the temperature of the overlying skin. If a shunt is surgically corrected or becomes obstructed, the skin temperature over the shunt drops to the temperature of nearby uninvolved skin.[157] In addition, large AV shunts may "steal" blood supplied by the involved artery, reducing the downstream arterial pressure, which may be detected thermally as cool skin distal to the shunt.[158]

Raynaud's disease

Vasoconstriction in response to cold is a normal thermoregulatory response; the cooled area restricts blood flow via adrenergic sympathetic vasoconstriction to prevent further loss of heat. In the case of Raynaud's phenomenon (RP), this response becomes exaggerated and can even be triggered by emotional distress.[159] RP patients exhibit a dramatic discoloration of the fingers and/or toes, often recurring in episodes.[160] Anatomically,

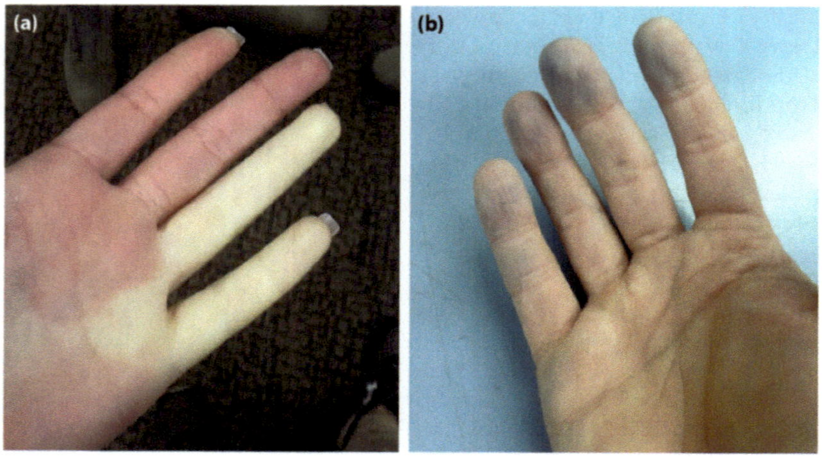

FIGURE 11.39 Raynaud's disease during a vasospasm episode: (a) The fingers initially become white. (b) With prolonged vasospasm, the fingers may become cyanotic.[166]

total restriction of blood flow to a finger or toe requires closure of both arteries supplying that digit (Figure 11.39). The disorder may range from relatively benign temporary vasospasm to severe progressive microangiopathy brought on by systemic sclerosis or other autoimmune diseases.[161]

A similar vasospastic disease of the fingers, typically brought on by working with machine tools, is known as Hand-Arm Vibration Syndrome (also called Vibration-Induced White Finger Syndrome, VWF). This condition can be assessed in the same manner as RP using cold challenge protocols. Workers exposed to chronic hand vibration may complain of a cold sensation in their fingers and hands even when not working, and the occurrence of VWF is more likely at low ambient temperatures.[162]

There are two types of RP, primary and secondary. Primary RP may encompass several entities, including functional vasospastic disorder, subclinical atherosclerosis, and cold intolerance.[163] Primary RP is generally self-limiting and runs a benign course without producing ischemic damage. Secondary RP has an identifiable underlying disease. Secondary RP may progress to severe digital vasculopathy, with patients developing ischemic complications such as digital ulceration, sometimes leading to the loss of digits.[164] Regardless of whether RP is primary or secondary, the symptomology involves spasm of the small muscular arteries and arterioles of the fingers and toes.[165]

Following exposure to sudden cold, the hands or feet of RP patients show a triphasic color change: first blanching, then cyanosis if the vasospasm lasts long enough, and finally redness during recovery.[167] Medical observation of these three phases can be challenging, however, because the vasospasm often will disappear once the patient spends a few minutes in a warm waiting room, and the classic tricolor phenomenon only occurs in only a small portion of patients with RP.[168]

Attempting to induce RP by equilibrating a patient at 20°C (68°F) or below will normally vasoconstrict *all* the digits to the point where their surface temperatures equal the room temperature. If RP does occur under these conditions, the thermal phenomenon is hidden as the RP digits cannot cool further. However, infrared imaging of the hands as they *recover* from a cold challenge offers a practical way to evaluate and monitor RP.[169] The different temperature recovery between fingers is a useful parameter for evaluating RP patients.[170] RP may be suspected when differences between mean temperatures of the metacarpals and digits are at least 3°C (5.4°F) at a room temperature of approximately 25°C (77°F).[171] Research has shown that thermography overcomes the limitations of self-reporting in RP.[172]

Most thermography studies of RP have focused on the fingers, presumably because they are easier to examine than the toes. Patients also tend to complain more frequently about RP symptoms in their hands than in their feet. In the summertime, the dominant hand of RP patients has been found to be cooler than the dominant hand of non-RP patients.[173] The thumb and little finger are least affected by RP, thus the three middle fingers (digits II, III, & IV) of the dominant hand are best for RP assessments.[174] The coolest fingertip temperature can be identified in a hand thermogram, and this finger can serve as the reference for future monitoring. In women with RP, the ring finger (digit IV) displays a linear behavior in both hands and is the coldest one and slowest to reheat after cold challenge testing. Thermographic focus on this finger can serve as a helpful reference for thermography studies.[175]

Infrared assessment of the hands alone may be insufficient, especially in women with RP. Comparing RP patients to controls, temperature differences are significantly higher between the center of the palm and the coolest finger, and also between the center of the dorsal foot and the first toe. Thermographic assessment of the coolest finger has greater sensitivity and specificity in men than in women. This gender difference does not apply to the toes; however, temperature differences between the foot dorsum and first toe consistently distinguish RP patients from normal controls in both sexes. Thermographic assessments of the feet are recommended in cases of RP, even in the absence of any pedal symptoms.[176] For proper classification of RP, a combined approach is recommended using thermography in conjunction with autoantibody testing and nailfold capillaroscopy, which is normal in primary RP but abnormal in most patients with systemic sclerosis.[177]

Static thermographic images of patients who are between attacks of RP or VWF may provide a hint to the diagnosis. At ambient temperatures of 30°C (86°F), a fingertip temperature 1°C (1.8°F) less than the dorsum of the ipsilateral hand is specific for secondary RP. Also, under static conditions, the temperature change along a finger from the radial carpal-metacarpal joint to the fingertip is the best way to detect secondary RP.[178] See Figure 7.21 for details on this technique. Dynamic cooling protocols, however, yield greater diagnostic accuracy for both RP and VWF.

A practical dynamic procedure for detecting Raynaud's/VWF

- The subject must abstain from nicotine, alcohol, and hot food or drinks for 3 hours before the procedure.
- Equilibration temperature is set between 23°C and 25°C (73.4°F and 77°F) to observe the rewarming time of the digits.
- Only light clothing is worn (e.g. shorts and T-shirt) during a 15-min equilibration.
- Baseline close-up thermograms of both the hands and feet (toes) are taken after cool-down.
- The hands and feet are enclosed in loose-fitting plastic bags 1–2 mil (25–50 µm) thick. Fingers should be kept spread apart before and during immersion
- The limbs are immersed in 12°C (53.6°F) water for 5 minutes[179]
  - Hands immersed to the wrist
  - Feet immersed to the ankle
- The limbs are removed from the water and uncovered; any water on the skin is removed gently with paper towels.
- Thermograms of the palmar and dorsal hands and the toes are taken at 1-minute intervals for up to 20 minutes.
- Interpretation criteria:[180]
  - Asymmetry between the hands and differences between the fingers are seen in VFW and secondary RP.
  - In VFW, the fingers rewarm from the tip to the base.
  - Rewarming in Secondary RP appears "blotchy" or uneven.
  - Symmetrical temperature distribution indicates Primary RP
  - Rewarming is delayed compared to normal subjects.
  - A specificity of 100% and a sensitivity of 60% can be expected from this type of dynamic test.

Thermography can serve as an objective tool for documenting RP. With the ongoing development of smartphone thermography, infrared monitoring of RP episodes could become standard practice, especially in young children and adolescents.[181] Laser Speckle Contrast Imaging (LSCI) offers a reliable method to visualize blood perfusion within the microcirculation. The combination of LSCI with thermography after cold challenge has shown validity in patients with RP related to systemic sclerosis.[182]

Thermography of the venous system

As with other anatomic locations where arteries and veins run close together, the head and neck veins are larger in diameter, have less of a muscular wall, and are almost the same temperature as the arteries, so they show up well on thermograms. Engorged supratrochlear veins (previously the frontal veins) which appear over the medial forehead are often seen in thermograms and photographs of normal subjects (Figure 11.40). As these veins drain the diploic veins that run within the frontal cranial bone, they may become visibly warm with increased neural activity in the frontal lobes. Local increased venous pressure from bending forward, neck occlusion, or increased intrathoracic pressure from forced vocalization or the Valsalva maneuver may cause enlargement of the supratrochlear veins but not the arteries. The supraorbital vein is much smaller than the supratrochlear and tends to run laterally above the orbit to meet the ipsilateral superficial temporal vein. It is seen only rarely on thermograms.

The venous system holds most of the blood in the circulatory system. A large reservoir of blood is stored in the veins of the legs, abdomen, and chest. In a resting subject at a room temperature of 20°C (68°F), the temperature of returning venous blood at the elbow is about 33°C (91.4°F).[184] The subdermal veins may show up in thermographic images especially if they are carrying warm blood via AVA dilation, muscular activity, or inflammation. Veins that run through deeper tissues may not be detectable due to overlying structures. The walls of a vein contain smooth muscle which contracts via neural and local stimuli, most notably in response to cold. Because venous blood pressure is quite low (5–10 mmHg), gravity and body position must be considered

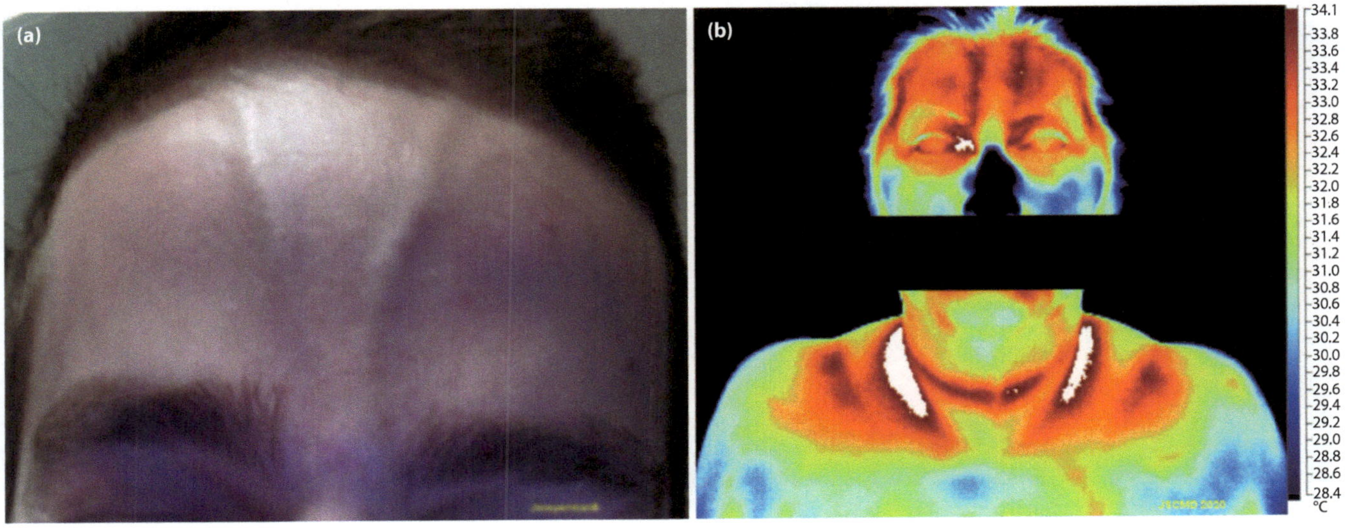

FIGURE 11.40 The supratrochlear veins: (a) visual appearance when engorged.[183] (b) Thermographic appearance in a different subject. These venous markings are often mislabeled as arterial markings. The vessels should not be pulsatile to palpation.

when evaluating venous thermograms. Larger veins normally contain valves at intervals that restrict backflow. The function of these valves can be assessed thermographically by first raising the leg of a cooled supine subject to drain the venous blood from that limb, then having the subject stand up.

Video thermography of the leg may show the superficial veins rapidly rewarming due to blood flowing "backwards" through incompetent venous valves (venous "insufficiency"). Likewise, the veins of the forearm may appear engorged when the arm is down, but they should drain quickly if the arm is raised (if not, venous *thoracic outlet syndrome* might be considered along with other possible diagnoses). The superficial veins of the neck including the external jugular vein, may appear engorged thermographically in cases of congestive heart failure. This is best seen with the subject reclined at a 45-degree angle. Similar to arteritis (arterial wall inflammation), the veins may develop phlebitis (venous wall inflammation), usually from infection or autoimmune disease. Arteritis and phlebitis may appear concurrently. *Thrombophlebitis* refers to clots forming in an inflamed vein. Even with the old infrared scanners of the 1970s, thermography was found useful in the detection of phlebitis.[185]

Deep venous thrombosis (DVT)

The thermally invisible deep veins of the legs and pelvis can hold the large, dangerous clots, which sometimes result in life-threatening pulmonary emboli. These clots may damage the delicate venous valves, leading to increased venous reflux and the generation of varicosities. Using older scanning technology, thermography studies of limbs having symptoms of DVT (aching leg pain with swelling, vein tenderness, distal pitting edema, and erythema) have shown a combined sensitivity of 93% but a specificity of only 74% when compared with venograms. Typical thermographic findings in significant DVT are a 1°C (1.8°F) surface temperature increase of the involved leg versus the contralateral limb, and dilation of the superficial veins of the affected limb. The low specificity of thermography in DVT is because many other conditions of the leg – i.e., edema, dermatitis, infection, sprains, and stress fractures – can lead to unilateral increased skin temperatures, and the presence of varicose veins can mimic flow-induced venous dilation.[186]

Since those early years of investigation, thermography has been found to be less reliable for detecting DVT than ultrasound imaging combined with a blood test to detect fibrinolysis.[187] More recent studies show that venous thrombosis may occur as a complication of *arterial* vasculitis because the damage to the endothelial lining of the vessels with subsequent clot formation occurs in veins as well as arteries. In large-vessel arteritis, there is a 2.5-fold increased risk of both deep vein thrombosis and pulmonary embolism compared to the normal population.[188] Similar complications may occur in polymyalgia rheumatica, systemic lupus, rheumatoid arthritis, systemic sclerosis, and other vasculitides.[189] Migratory SVT, an inflammation that may come and go in otherwise normal veins of the limbs and trunk, is associated with pancreatic cancer and other adenocarcinomas.[190] To non-invasively detect thrombophlebitis, a combination of thermography and Doppler ultrasound imaging has proven very effective. While ultrasound imaging is excellent for detecting deep thromboses, thermography can readily visualize superficial phlebitis due to the NO produced by venous inflammation. In the absence of visible varicose veins, a vein that appears significantly warmer than the surrounding tissue should arouse suspicion for active phlebitis.[191] The "vascular cape" seen thermographically at times across the upper chest wall may be a migrant phlebitis similar to Mondor's disease.[192]

Phlebitis

A clinical picture of active phlebitis (erythema, tenderness) is a common finding in patients with indwelling intravenous catheters or lines. The etiology of the inflammation may be infectious in nature or caused by endothelial irritation from the substance being injected. The incidence of phlebitis increases with the time the catheter has been in place (the catheter "dwell time"). Superficial venous thrombophlebitis (SVT) in the arms most likely results from intravenous infusion causing localized redness, tenderness, and heat visible to thermography. By thermographically monitoring the temperature of the catheter insertion site and subtracting it from a distal reference skin site, a "delta-T" (ΔT) value can be computed (Figure 11.41). Negative ΔT values indicate no phlebitis, while a positive ΔT is associated with clinical signs of phlebitis. Even in the uncontrolled environment of an Intensive Care Unit, the ΔT is highly correlated with the clinical

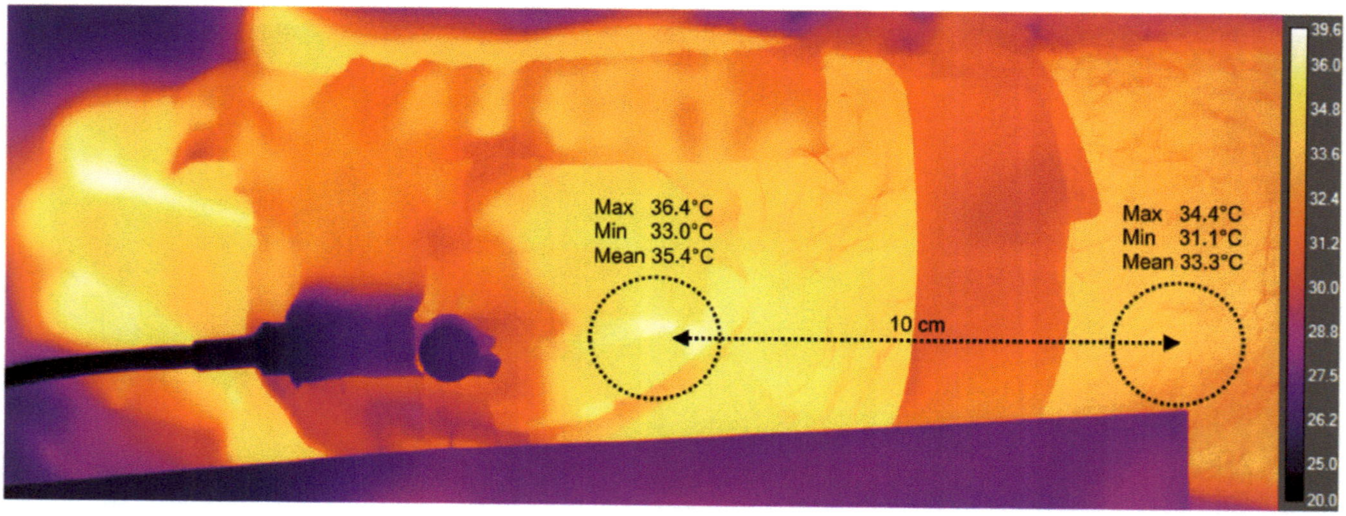

FIGURE 11.41 A qualitatively unscaled thermogram showing a possibly infected indwelling intravenous catheter. The catheter site temperature is compared with a site 10 cm proximal to the catheter site. The *maximum* temperature at the insertion site (left circle) is 36.4°C and that of the proximal reference point (right circle) is 34.4°C. The ΔT in this case is 2.0°C, indicating clinical phlebitis.[194]

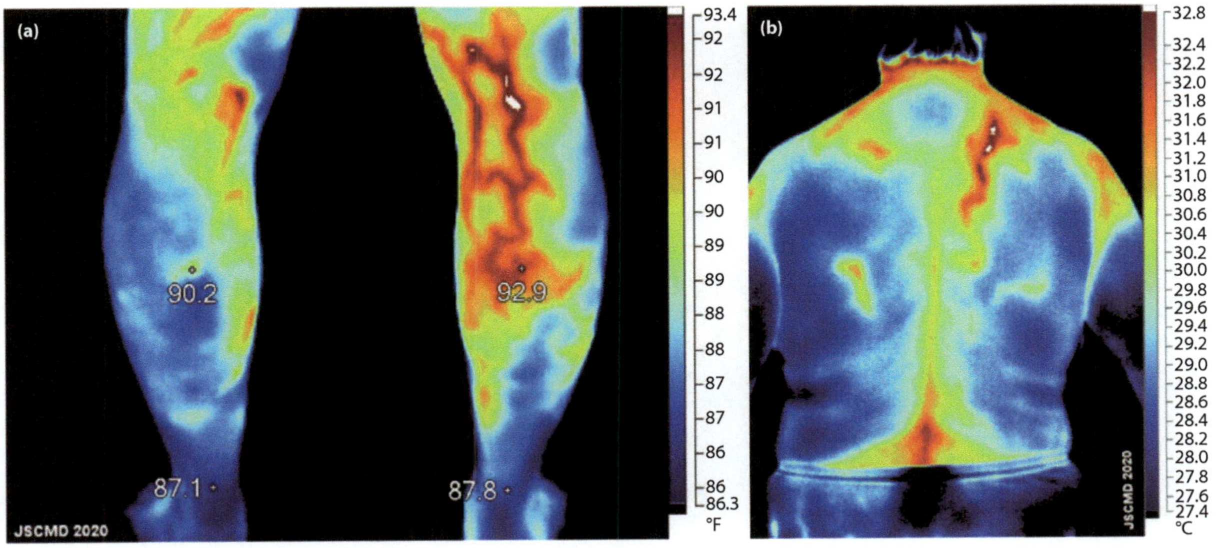

FIGURE 11.42 (a) Varicose veins over the posterior knee and calf, worse on the right – 53 yoM. (b) A varicose vein over the right trapezius. Superficial varicose veins can occur anywhere on the body surface – 58 yoF.

diagnosis of local phlebitis ($p = 0.001$).[193] Thermography is useful in the early detection of phlebitis associated with indwelling intravascular catheters and other conditions.

Varicose veins

"Varicose" veins are superficial veins that have enlarged and elongated, producing ropy, convoluted venous masses in the subdermal fat layer just under the skin surface, usually in the lower extremities. The saphenous veins are often implicated in forming complex varicosities. Hemorrhoids, scrotal varicoceles, and venous masses forming in the female labia can also be considered varicosities; varicosities may occasionally form over any part of the body. Insufficiency (reverse leakage) of venous valves is a frequent cause of leg varicosities. Varicose veins are usually patent, with blood flow bringing deep body warmth to the skin surface. Leg varicosities without thrombophlebitis may appear warm when engorged, but should flatten and have a reduced thermal appearance if the limb is raised above heart level. If clots form in a varicose vein, the resulting thrombophlebitis releases NO, causing the skin over the affected vein to appear warmer. Clotting in varicose veins may be induced therapeutically by intravenous injection of sclerosing agents; if successful, the vein no longer carries warm venous blood, becoming cooler. Because of their superficial location, thermography provides an excellent way to find, evaluate, map, and monitor treatment of varicose veins.

Thermographic mapping of superficial varicose leg veins is best performed with the subject standing and properly equilibrated at 20°C (68°F) (Figure 11.42). This position increases the static pressure within the leg veins, causing them to fill with warm blood. Venous reflux speeds up this venous engorgement. The enlarged veins located just under the skin surface are easily detected with thermal imaging, and their course and extent can be readily visualized, aiding in the preoperative mapping and marking of the offending veins.[195]

Thermography of the lymphatic system

Though the vascular system is often thought to be confined to the arteries and veins, the lymphatics or "third vascular system" must also be considered. The lymphatic system is generally invisible or overlooked by thermographers except when disrupted by trauma or surgery, obstructed by parasites such as filariasis, inflamed by infection, or invaded by malignant metastases. A prominent thermal finding is "blood poisoning" – lymphatic inflammation from ascending lymphangitis, usually due to streptococcal bacteria (Figure 11.43). The thermographic appearance

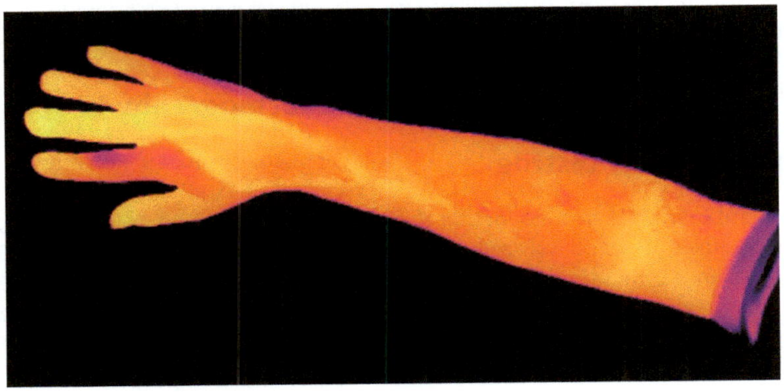

FIGURE 11.43 Infection in the distal portion of digit III of the right hand showing the warm pattern over the vessels draining the finger in this thermogram. This pattern may be due to warm venous blood or ascending lymphangitis.[197]

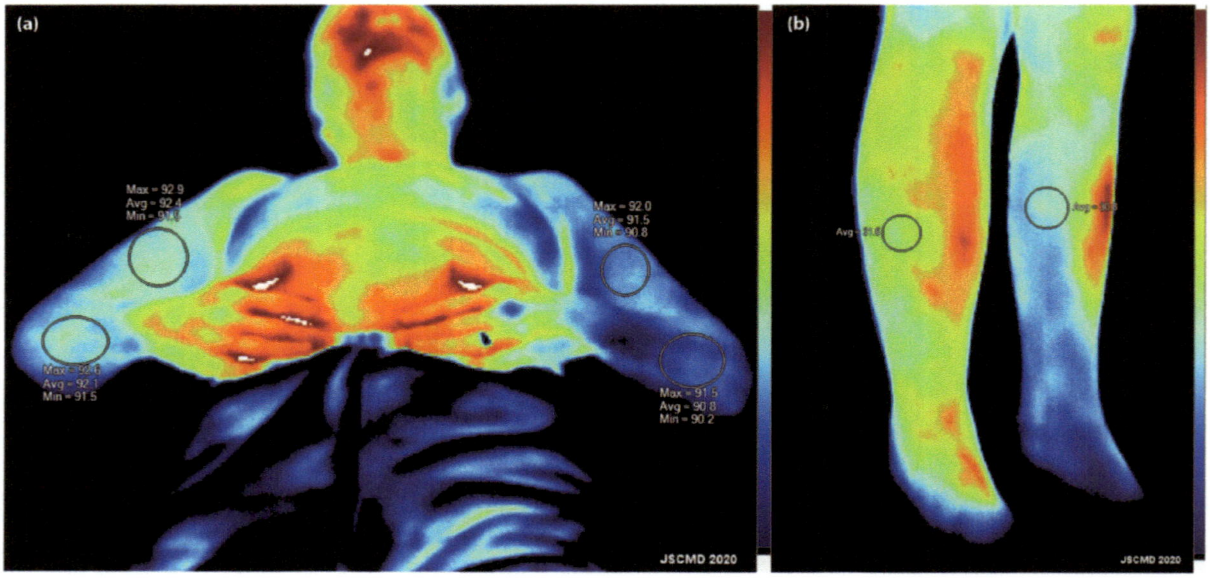

FIGURE 11.44 (a) Mild lymphedema of the right arm 5 years after lymph node dissection for breast cancer. The skin of the right arm and hand is diffusely warmer than the left – 64 yoF. (b) Moderate edema of the right lower leg secondary to lymphatic obstruction by a pelvic sarcoma – 77 yoF.

of inflamed lymphatics tends to be "wispy," like cirrus clouds, due to the interweaving network of small lymph vessels, as opposed to the well-defined thermal borders of a warm vein.[196] The lymph vessels become more linear and less branched as they progress up the limbs toward the trunk. The presence of visible and warm red streaks extending up a limb indicate possible lymphangitis. Acting as waystations along the lymphatic flow, groups of superficially-located lymph nodes appear thermographically as warm spotty or blotchy areas when reacting to an infection or other invasion. Lymph nodes deep in the body cannot be detected by thermal imaging.

Obstruction or destruction of the lymphatic channels may lead to the condition of *lymphedema*, an accumulation of normal, non-infected lymph fluid within the tissues distal to the lymph blockage creating a swollen limb. Surgical disruption of lymph vessels or removal of lymph nodes is the major cause of lymphedema in developed countries (Figure 11.44). Lymphedema can be classified as mild (10%–20%), moderate (20%–40%), or severe (>40%), referring to the percentage of increase in limb volume. In mild and moderate cases, the involved limb is diffusely warmer than contralateral by up to 2°C (3.6°F), though this increase may not be present in the case of decreased arterial inflow. Also, as lymphedema becomes severe, skin warming may not be present due to decreased muscular activity, soft tissue degeneration, skin fibrosis, and deposition of dysfunctional subdermal fat in the affected limb.[198]

Thermography in allergy testing

Thermography can provide useful information in evaluating the skin reaction to allergen patch testing by objectively measuring the rise in temperature of the skin surrounding active allergic reactions. This reaction can be measured even with a low-resolution cell phone infrared imager.

When equilibrated at 21°C (70°F), subjects who demonstrate erythematous reactions to standard 48-hour allergen patch testing show allergic patch test reactions with temperature increases of 0.72°C ± 0.67°C (1.3°F ± 1.2°F) compared to surrounding skin. Non-allergic irritant reactions result in only 0.17°C ± 0.31°C (0.31°F ± 0.56°F) temperature increases.[199] Although these results overlap, the mean temperature difference between the two groups is highly significant ($p < 0.0001$). On removal of the offending substance, allergic reactions become worse (warmer) at 24 hours; irritant reactions partially fade by 24 hours.[200]

Prick testing may also be evaluated by thermography, though the micro-injury to the dermis might affect the results. A 15-minute time period to reduce this reaction seems sufficient as long as the skin pricks are not too traumatic. Digital subtraction techniques can be used to compare pre-prick versus post-prick temperatures, which increase up to +3.5°C (6.3°F) (Figure 11.45).[202] Precision digital subtraction of serial images is difficult, however, due to subject motion and misalignment. Considering the magnitude of these temperature changes, allergic reactions may be evaluated qualitatively by using a full-span color scale without the need to perform image subtraction.

Image registration to determine which prick-test allergen in a matrix of challenge sites produces a reaction has been a problem in both visible and infrared allergen studies. Small (1 mm) pieces of aluminum tape "fiducials" placed on the skin at intervals around the testing area should help this problem in that they can be seen in both visual and infrared images.

Thermography in acupuncture and TENS

Acupuncture involves inserting thin, solid needles into the skin to various depths at defined locations (acupuncture points) to treat disease. Twisting, vibrating, heating, or electrically stimulating the needles is said to induce certain effects. Transcutaneous electrical nerve stimulation (TENS), which uses flat dermal electrodes, is a western therapeutic system based on the acupuncture points. In TENS, specific effects are purportedly produced by varying the stimulation current levels and frequencies applied to the electrodes. Thermography has been studied as an objective way to assess the point locations and effects of acupuncture-type therapies, with some thermographers claiming that the acupuncture meridians

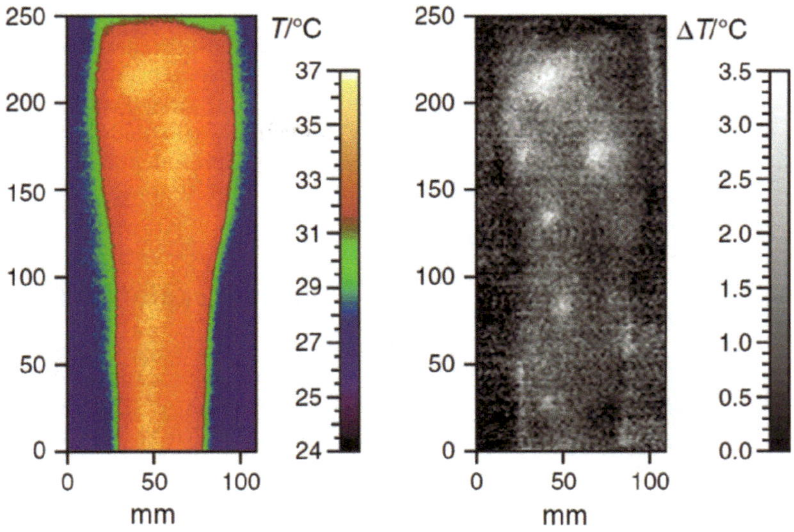

FIGURE 11.45 Prick testing for allergy sensitivity: Left image: Volar forearm after injection of the allergens. Right image: Greyscale image showing post-injection skin temperature change compared to a pre-injection image of the same anatomical site (image subtraction).[201]

(lines connecting families of points) are visible to thermal analysis, especially if the points on that meridian are stimulated. However, well-designed studies have shown this to be artefactual, not an actual property of meridians (see Figure 10.88).[203]

Acupuncture of the Hoku point

The effect of acupuncture on sympathetic vasoconstrictive tone has been studied using quantitative thermography as the measurement device. In 1985, researchers using a calibrated thermal scanner under controlled conditions studied the sympatholytic effect of manually or electrically stimulating the hand acupuncture point, Hoku (L.I. 4).[204] Only the left hand was given acupuncture, but a resultant temperature increase occurred equally in both hands and both feet. No local reaction was seen at the needling site. Manual stimulation proved more effective than electrical. The face showed the most consistent warming of 1.5°C (2.7°F) above that of the control group. The next most consistent warming appeared in the hands, while the feet showed the least reaction. The authors concluded that the Hoku acupuncture sympatholytic effect was a cranio-caudal phenomenon under central nervous system control, not a peripheral effect.[205]

A more recent study also examined the effect of Hoku-point needling of the left hand in subjects under controlled equilibration conditions at 23.5°C (74.3°F). No manual or electrical stimulation was given to the needle once in place. A warming of all fingers of the left hand over 1.5°C (2.7°F) was seen almost immediately with deep needling into the muscle under Hoku but not with cutaneous Hoku needling, non-Hoku muscular needling, or no needling (controls). A matrix of qualitative color images printed in the study clearly shows these temperature differences.[206] This thermographic finding should be repeated in other laboratories for validation and clarification as it could not be replicated by the authors (Figure 11.46).[207]

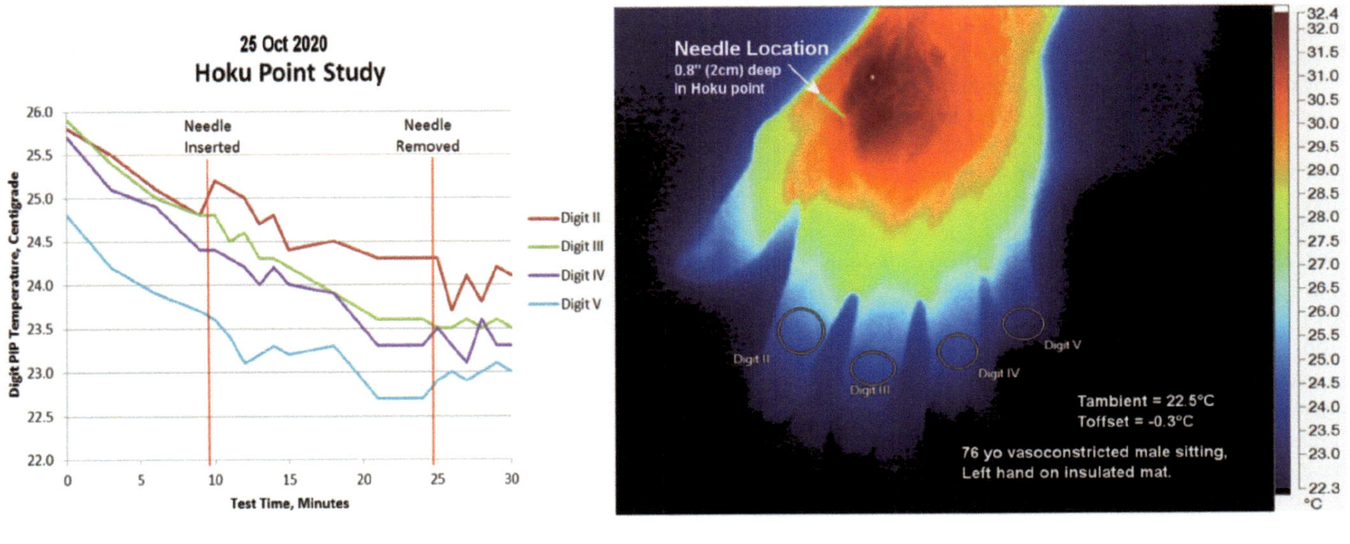

FIGURE 11.46 An N = 1 study by author JSCMD attempted to reproduce the warming of the hands from Hoku acupuncture reported in previous studies. No peripheral warming was detected thermographically in the hand. More study on the Hoku sympatholytic effect is needed.

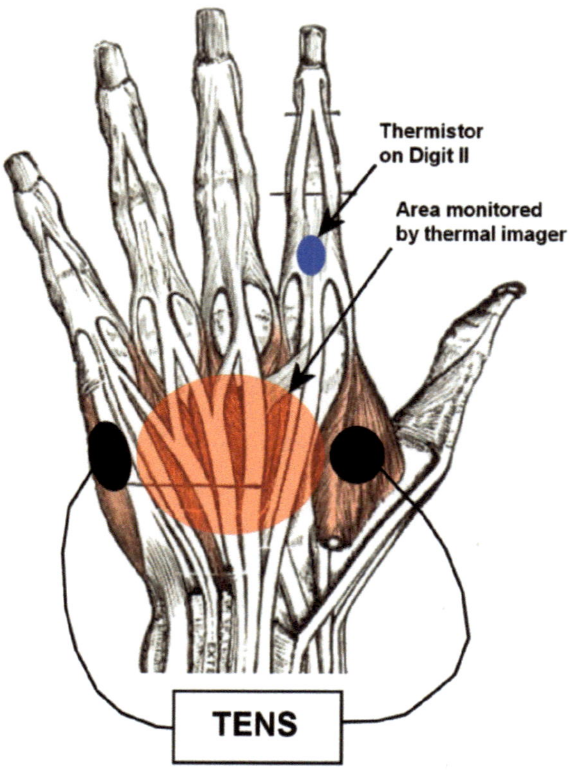

FIGURE 11.47 Image of the dorsum of the left hand showing the experimental setup to test TENS effects as described in RJ Scudds, 1995.[208]

TENS

Thermography also has been used to study the effects of transcutaneous electrical nerve stimulation (TENS) on local and regional skin temperatures. In a 1995 experiment involving temperature-equilibrated, healthy young subjects, TENS was applied to electrodes on either side of the back of the hand (Figure 11.47). 4-Hz TENS, 100-Hz TENS, or control (no TENS) was applied for 30 minutes. Stimulation at 4-Hz caused warming over the dorsum of the hand; 100-Hz stimulation and controls showed no warming. Any warming effect reversed quickly as soon as the stimulation was stopped. A thermistor on digit II, placed to determine any distal effects, showed no warming in any of the three groups. The authors concluded that "high-intensity, low-frequency TENS prevents cooling of the hand."[209] They postulated that low-frequency TENS might have an effect on reflex sympathetic dystrophy (now called CRPS).

On closer inspection of the study, however, the current of the pulsed 4-Hz stimulation was turned up to be unpleasant, causing the muscles between the electrodes (the dorsal interossei) to rhythmically contract, presumably four times a second. The 100-Hz stimulating current was adjusted to be "comfortable," and muscle contractions did not occur. The control group likewise showed no muscle contractions. The authors dismissed these muscle contractions as a heat source. It is well known, however, that muscular contractions create waste heat, and also increase regional blood flow. The heat from rapidly contracting interosseous muscles and increased local blood flow will diffusely warm the dorsal hand skin by conduction, where the reported 1.6°C (2.9°F) rise in temperature is easily detected by thermography. The thermistor located on Digit II did not sense any warming because there are no skeletal muscles in the fingers to contract and generate heat.[210] The warming effects of TENS stimulation seen in this experiment do not appear to be due to axonal, sympathetic, or central nervous system mechanisms, but are instead due to strong TENS stimulation causing local muscle contractions. Further experimental study into the thermographic appearance and effects of TENS is needed.

Thermography in the practice of surgery

In the context of surgery, infrared imaging can serve a variety of purposes, such as locating tumors or infection, documenting revascularization, monitoring anesthesia, and evaluating wounds. In the early history of thermography, infrared scanners were large devices without the agility to provide a good image of the surgical field. With the advent of miniature scanners such as the Agema devices in the 1980s, practical thermal evaluation within the surgical theatre became possible. Even with these smaller devices, however, a trained operator was required to arrange large cables connecting the scanner to the display and supply liquid nitrogen to cool the infrared detector, thus limiting their use in the operating room. Modern microbolometer imagers require no cooling, can be miniaturized, and may operate either wirelessly or with very small cables; these developments have made infrared monitoring of surgical procedures possible with little or no disturbance to the surgeons or to the sterile field. Standard silvered-glass mirrors can be placed above the patient to reflect the infrared findings to an imager away from the sterile field, thus lowering the possibility of post-surgical infection.[211] It is beyond the scope of this section to describe in depth all the ways in which thermography can be utilized in surgical practice, but several important topics will be covered.

Preoperative thermography

Thermograms can aid in surgical planning by documenting the status of arterial circulation to a limb or flap, or mapping varicose veins for removal. Preoperative thermal evaluation of burn depth and frostbite damage is possible. The preoperative status of an arterial occlusion should be imaged after exercise stress to be most effective and to provide a baseline for postoperative evaluation. The location of vascular perforating bundles prior to forming a flap for plastic surgery procedures can be assessed thermographically. The level, location, and extent of peripheral nerve damage can be visualized thermally. Denervated or fibrosed muscles may appear cooler than the background, allowing preoperative planning in orthopedic cases. And the presence and approximate location of superficially-located occult infections may be detected preoperatively.

Thermography in anesthesia monitoring

Thermography may be used in local anesthesia to determine the onset and extent of nerve blocks and spinal/epidural anesthesia procedures.[212] Perineural injections of local anesthetic agents such as lidocaine cause a total nerve block as the agent diffuses into the nearby neural tissue. This block affects the sympathetic fibers as well as the sensorimotor fibers, inhibiting the sympathetic vasoconstrictive action over the distribution of the blocked nerve. The warmer thermographic appearance of a successful nerve block in a vasoconstricted hand or foot will show a distinct and sharp-edged delineation (Figure 11.48). Areas supplied by other unaffected nerves will remain cool.[213] This thermographic

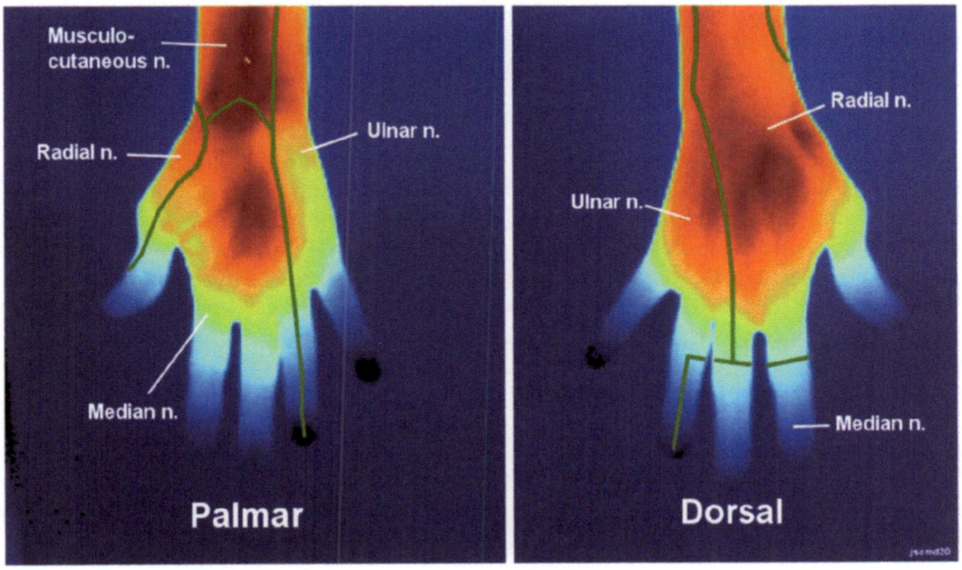

FIGURE 11.48 Approximate areas of innervation of the right hand. A successful anesthetic block (or complete transection) of any one of these nerves will cause the area supplied by that nerve to become significantly warmer than the surrounding areas.[214]

appearance may precede the sensory blockade by a few minutes. More proximal areas supplied by the blocked nerve may show less distinct and lower amplitude thermal changes. If epinephrine is added to the anesthetic to make the block last longer, the injection site may appear cool due to local adrenergic vasoconstriction.

Spinal and epidural anesthesia also entail perineural infiltration of local anesthetics. They interrupt the spinal nerves *before* they communicate with the sympathetic trunks, however, thus the skin temperature changes are less well defined (more diffuse and extended) compared to block of a peripheral nerve (Figure 11.49). Both spinal and epidural blocks act like an acute spinal transection, with warmer skin temperatures and venous dilation consistent with decreased sympathetic stimulation. When observing the spinal level of skin temperature rise compared to the level of numbness, the sympathetic block level is five to seven dermatomes *higher* than sensory block.[215] Also, because the sympathetic fibers are small and more susceptible to the local anesthetic, they are blocked at lower anesthetic concentrations more distal to the injection site.[216] When the temperature increase from a spinal or epidural block reaches the T-4 level, the blood pressure may decrease due to the considerable loss of sympathetic vasoconstrictive tone below that level. The skin temperature rise over the distal limb within the block area may provide a guide for when to start the surgical procedure as shown in Table 11.2.

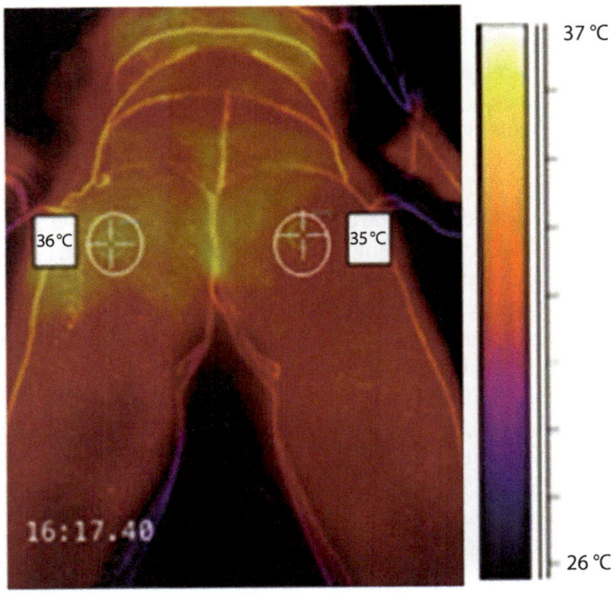

FIGURE 11.49 Thermogram of a supine patient 20 minutes after an epidural block taken with a cell-phone infrared camera attachment. The block did not "take" symmetrically, with the right side being more anesthetized (warmer).[218]

Open surgical procedures

In an open surgical procedure, a relatively large incision is made to expose the organ(s) to be worked on, allowing the relatively cool and dry air of the operating theatre to contact the exposed internal surfaces of the body. These exposed surfaces, which are normally at body temperature, cool down due to convective and evaporative heat losses, especially if blood flow to the exposed surfaces is restricted either by disease or the operative procedure. Modern thermographic equipment can detect perfused versus ischemic tissues, allowing the surgeon to evaluate whether an arterial anastomosis has been successful before the incision is closed.

TABLE 11.2 Elapsed Time to Reach 95 Percent of Skin Temperature Rise in the Distal Portions of an Extremity (Hand or Foot) after Injection of the Anesthetic. More Proximal Areas of a Limb Usually Show a Slower and Less Pronounced Skin Temperature Rise. Ambient Temperature May Affect These Measurements.[217]

Spinal	Epidural	Sciatic Block	Brachial Block
9 Min	17 Min	20 Min	23 Min

During coronary artery bypass grafting procedures (CABG), the vessels of the anterior heart are readily visualized. Posterior vessels may only be seen by carefully rotating the heart. Because the temperature of the circulating blood is almost equal to that of the myocardium, visualizing graft patency requires special techniques.[219] By using a thermal imager to observe the vessel as it is infused with either cold or warm saline, any blockage of the vessels may be easily visualized even with cardiac movement.[220] This procedure can replace intraoperative radiographic coronary arteriography, which requires injection of a contrast agent and X-ray equipment in the operating room.[221] Thermography is used in CABG procedures to visualize temperatures as the cardiac surface is cooled with a stream of cold CO_2. Adequate coronary blood flow can be confirmed by observing the surface temperatures of the heart.[222]

In order to temporarily paralyze the myocardium during heart bypass surgery, about one liter of cold (4°C, 39°F) Cardioplegic Solution is rapidly infused into the coronary arteries, causing myocardial ischemia and hypothermia, which induces asystole. This hypothermia must be maintained to preserve the myocardium until normal blood flow returns. Myocardial distribution of the Solution may be uneven, however, due to local arterial stenosis or blockage. Under-perfused warm myocardium may be damaged by myocardial metabolism during ischemia.[223] As the temperature difference is quite large between tissue adequately cooled to an estimated 10°C (50°F) and a (low) body temperature of 32°C (90°F), radiometric thermography can be an ideal way to accurately monitor the myocardium during hypothermic induction, maintenance, and recovery.[224]

Thermography in neurosurgery

Major neurosurgical procedures on the brain are often started by partially or totally removing the calvarium, exposing the brain tissue to the temperature and humidity of the operating theatre. Within the brain, an even outflow of heat is maintained by a 0.5°C (0.9°F) temperature difference between the deeper tissues and the cooler superficial layer.[225] With the brain exposed to room air, evaporative heat losses additionally cool the surface, providing thermal contrast between blood vessels and the brain tissue. During craniotomy procedures, the arteries and veins of the brain can be qualitatively visualized with properly-scaled images. In an operating theatre at an ambient temperature of 20°C (68°F), the surface of the brain can be expected to be up to 4°C (7.2°F) lower than the normal body core temperature (37°C).[226] In experiments on exposed primate brains, areas of reduced blood perfusion due to arterial occlusion cooled rapidly by 0.3 to 1.3°C (0.5–2.3°F) and then rewarmed equally rapidly upon the resumption of blood flow.[227] This cerebral rewarming can be seen in patients undergoing cerebral artery anastomosis for Moyamoya disease. An increase in brain surface temperature can be observed and graft patency monitored with thermography. Brain hyperperfusion can also be observed and treated accordingly.[228]

Neurosurgical thermology relies on determining the rate and variance of temperature change with time using both static images and radiometric video thermography. The static technique, also known as Spot-Averaging Analysis or SAA, entails averaging the pixel temperatures over a small area, thus reducing the thermal noise value. The first derivative of the SAA is called the Spot-Slope Analysis (SSA). Mathematically, $SSA = dT_{SAA}/dt$, usually determined over a 20-second time period. As with any derivative calculation based on an in-vivo measurement, motion artifact is a problem that must be strictly controlled by stabilization of both imager and patient; synchronization of image acquisition with the electrocardiogram may also be required. Videothermography is useful to observe cranial blood flow distribution by injection of a 10 cc bolus of 4°C (39°F) saline into the vena cava, causing a drop in cerebral temperature 11 seconds after the injection. Post-processing of the multiple images is required to visualize the subtle temperature changes, which decrease and then return to baseline rapidly. Subdural hematoma and middle cerebral artery ischemia are among those conditions revealed by this method.[229]

Brain tumors of glial origin are usually 0.5°C to 2.0°C (0.9°F to 3.6°F) cooler than the surrounding normal brain, while metastatic tumors may be up to 3.3°C (5.9°F) warmer. Increased vasculature of the metastatic neoplasms may be the cause of this surface heat, though nitric oxide effects may also be involved as the brain's immune system attempts to repel the "foreign" cellular invasion.[230] Although thermography can detect the basic tumor location, thermal conduction between the tumor and surrounding normal brain precludes observing margins distinctly enough to guide precise tumor resection.

Intraoperative neurosurgical thermography may be useful in determining the focal site of seizures. Seizure foci are usually cooler than the adjacent cortex, but warm foci may be encountered. A mean 3.40°C (6.1°F) temperature decrease compared to normal brain tissue can be expected.[231] In some patients, there was more than a 90% reduction in seizure burden after focal resection of the thermally abnormal cortex seen on infrared imaging.[232]

Thermographic monitoring of arterio-venous malformation (AVM) excision provides important information. AVMs show significantly increased temperatures compared to adjacent normal brain tissue, and this warmth pattern corresponds well with the anatomical edges of the AVM. On correction of the AVM, the bed of the lesion becomes cooler while the adjacent brain becomes warmer due to increased blood flow; the AVM is no longer "stealing" circulation from the surrounding brain.[233]

Sensory-motor mapping of the cortex is aided by thermal imaging of the exposed brain. These mapping studies require sensitive, low-noise thermal imagers because heat fluctuations caused by the metabolism of somatosensory stimulation are minuscule (0.06–0.09°C/0.11–0.16°F) compared with cortical temperature changes caused by arterial occlusion (0.3–1.3/0.54–2.3°F).[234] Using SAA averaging, however, speech motor functions can be convincingly mapped using thermography.[235]

Neurosurgical procedures on the spinal cord must often be performed through a small-diameter deep dissection requiring removal of vertebral bone to expose the cord. When correcting a spinal A-V fistula, 7–14 µm imagers are best to delineate blood flow without the use of cold saline applications. However, as the surgical exposure is quite limited and the air of the operating room does not fully cool the deeper portions, the intermittent use of an air blower (presumably sterile air) helps in obtaining images with adequate temperature contrast.[236]

Thermography of limb revascularization procedures

Vascular surgeons are frequently called upon to restore arterial blood supply to a limb made ischemic from atherosclerosis, trauma, or other problem. As arterial blood flow is the major physiologic mechanism for bringing core body warmth to an extremity, successful return of blood flow can be detected and monitored thermographically. Thermography has an advantage over other blood flow-monitoring techniques in that it is non-contact. In cases of lower leg ischemia treated by endovascular techniques, pre- and post-operative thermographic comparisons reliably detect successful recanalization by monitoring the metatarsal, heel, and shin areas. Comparison with normal hand temperatures also shows significant improvement. Toe temperatures are less useful in cooled patients due to sympathetic vasoconstriction reducing toe temperatures. Unsuccessful procedures show no change in limb temperatures compared to pre-operative values.[237]

Infrared imagers that can plug in to a cellphone have proven useful for the evaluation of ischemic limbs before and after revascularization. This highly mobile technology has proven useful, though smartphone imagers presently have low spatial thermal resolution, large thermal offsets, and the images acquired are often not properly scaled for optimum qualitative analysis.[238] As the resolution, accuracy, and image scaling of these devices improve, they will become more useful in the diagnosis and documentation of limb blood flow.

Thermography in plastic surgery

As the specialty of Plastic Surgery includes the correction of problems of the skin and soft tissues just underneath the skin, thermography can provide useful information in both clinical practice and research settings. Postoperative thermograms of facial plastics procedures, such as blepharoplasty, often reveal extensive subdermal bruising (Figure 11.50). This extravasated blood attracts inflammatory cells that emit NO, and the area of warmth seen on thermograms may appear larger than the visible bruising.

Skin flap perfusion

Thermography is useful in the pre-op planning, surgery, and post-op monitoring of full-thickness skin flaps. Skin flaps come in two main types – pedicle flaps and free flaps. In both types, it is important for the surgeon to locate the arterio-venous bundles ("perforators") supplying the dermis in order to plan the surgery and prevent damage to the blood supply of the flap.

Pedicle flaps consist of dermis that is elevated along with at least one of its normal arteries and veins intact to supply the pedicle with blood. If this supply is interrupted by twisting, sharp bends, or other occlusion, the flap temperature will drop as the warm arterial blood supply is no longer flowing. Occlusion of the draining vein(s) will have the same thermographic effect, though the cooling may be delayed, and the flap may turn violaceous in color due to venous congestion.

Free flaps are technically more difficult because the arterio-venous perforators must be located and preserved so that they can be microsurgically re-anastomosed to vessels in the placement site.[239] Problems arising with arterial or venous flow in a free flap will appear similar to those appearing in a pedicle flap.

The location of arterial perforators may be visualized thermographically in a cooled subject (see Figure 10.20); additional local skin cooling may help locate the perforating bundles.[240] Even with local cooling, whole-body cooling is important to close the glomus AVAs that can mimic the perforators (see Figure 10.19). Any additional local cooling over the flap donor site should be diffuse and evenly distributed. Alcohol spray, local cooling air currents, or room-temperature thick metal plates applied to the skin have been utilized successfully (Figure 11.51). A hand-held Doppler can confirm that a "hot spot" seen on rewarming after cold challenge is due to a vascular bundle.[241]

Once fully dissected from the underlying tissues, a free, non-vascular flap will cool toward room temperature as it has no arterial input. When the vessels are attached and flow reestablished,

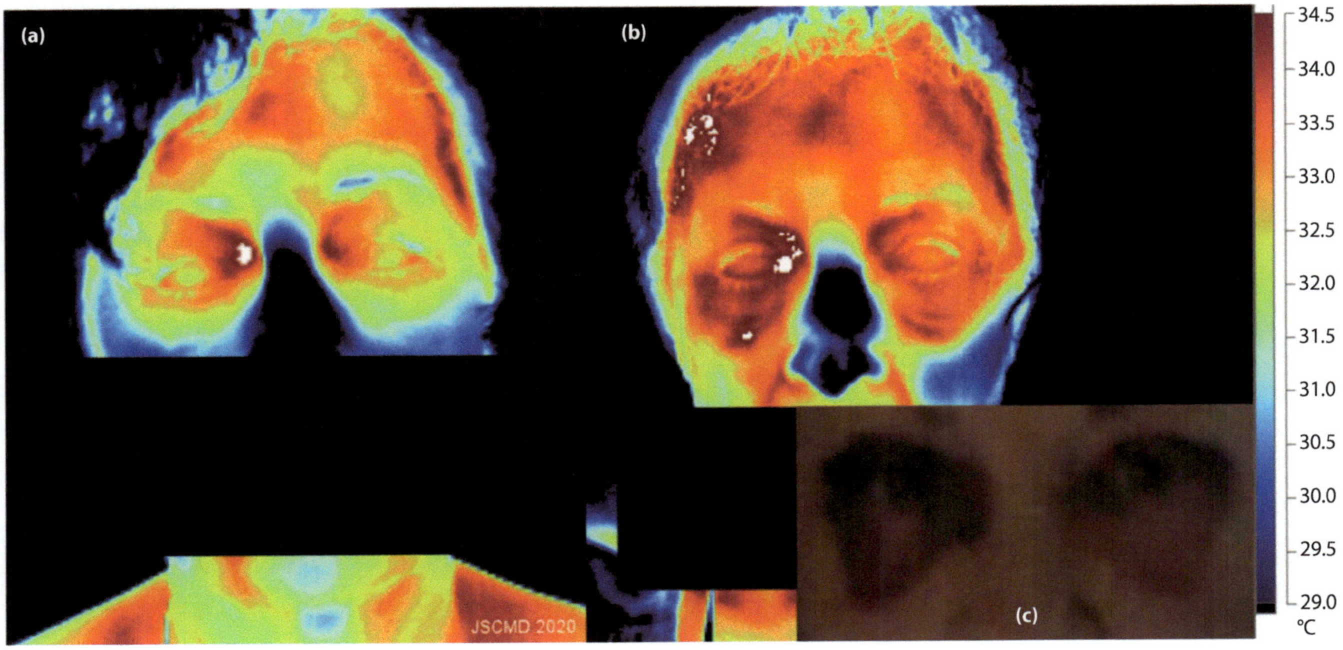

FIGURE 11.50 Bilateral upper lid blepharoplasty – 78 yoF. (a) Pre-op view. (b) 6 hours post-op thermal image. (c) 6 hours post-op visual appearance.

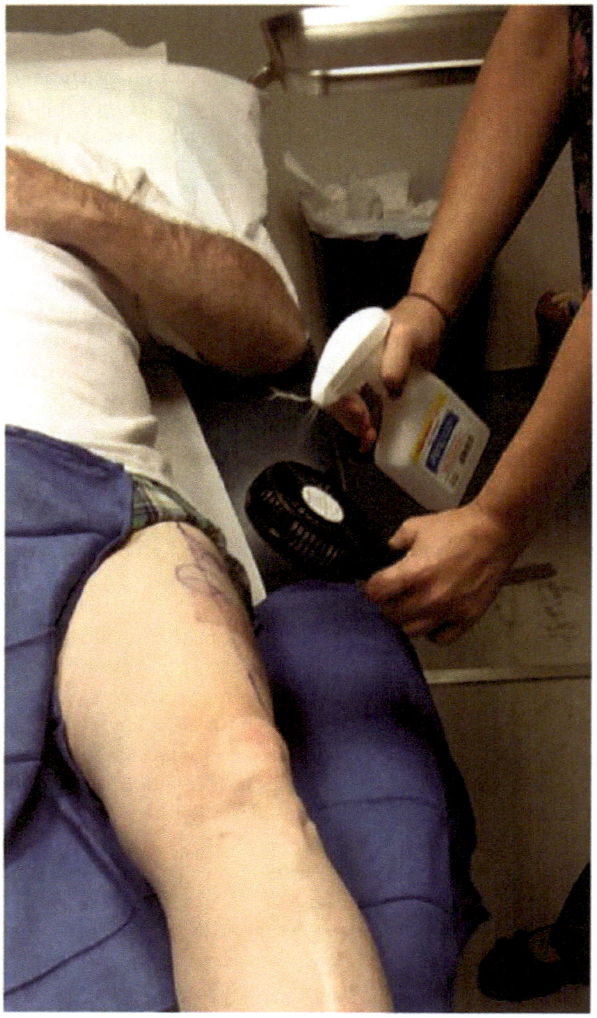

FIGURE 11.51 Dynamic cooling of a donor flap site to better locate perforator vessels. An alcohol spray is additionally cooled using a small electric fan.[242]

the flap will increase in temperature, indicating a successful anastomosis (Figure 11.52). Real-time quantitative thermography can provide the surgeon with information on the state of the graft before the surgery is concluded.

Continued thermographic monitoring in the postoperative period is an effective method to visualize flap viability. Pedicle flaps may maintain their neural input including sympathetic vasoconstrictive enervation, making the flap appear cool; patient warming may be necessary. If a flap has no neural input, it should appear warm due to lack of sympathetic vasoconstriction(Figure 11.53). By their nature, free flaps have no neural connections and thus no neural vasoconstriction. If well supplied with arterial blood and venous drainage, they will often appear warmer than the surrounding vasoconstricted skin in a properly cooled individual. In neither type of flap, however, will the flap temperature approach room temperature as long as flap blood flow is maintained.

Thermology in endoscopic procedures

Endoscopic surgeries use insufflation of an inert gas into the body space where the surgery is to be performed – generally the abdomen – thus creating a non-flammable gas-filled cavity allowing visualization of the procedure by an endoscopic visual camera. Gasses used for endoscopic surgery include carbon dioxide, nitrous oxide, helium, argon, nitrogen, and room air.[245] Though CO_2 and argon are known thermal insulators, the close quarters within a body cavity prevent gaseous attenuation of infrared radiation to any appreciable extent. Because a cavity insufflated for endoscopic surgery quickly takes on the core temperature, thermography cannot visualize infected or inflamed areas within the cavity as warmer than other tissues. Continuous insufflation of a cooled moist gas might theoretically allow endoscopic thermography to detect ischemic or inflamed tissues, but this has not been reported in studies.

Thermographic monitoring of laser ablation temperature during endoscopic surgery is now possible with the advent of miniature calibrated radiometric thermal imagers (Figure 11.54a). An intra-cavity imager can observe the thermal ablation procedure, assuring and documenting the proper location and extent of tissue destruction (Figure 11.54b).[246]

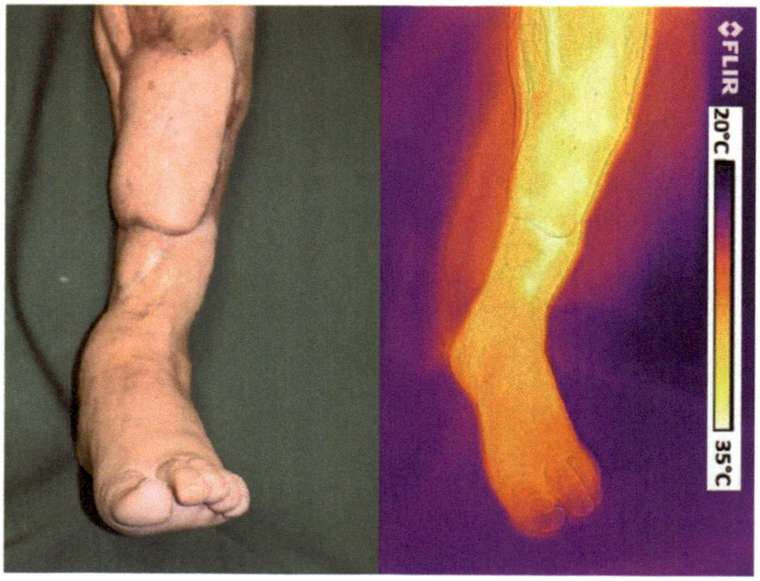

FIGURE 11.52 Photograph and thermogram of a successful free flap graft over the anterior left shin 40 days post-op. The flap shows good color and the flap surface temperature is warm. Because the flap skin has no sympathetic innervation to cause vasoconstriction, it appears warmer than the adjacent normal skin.[243]

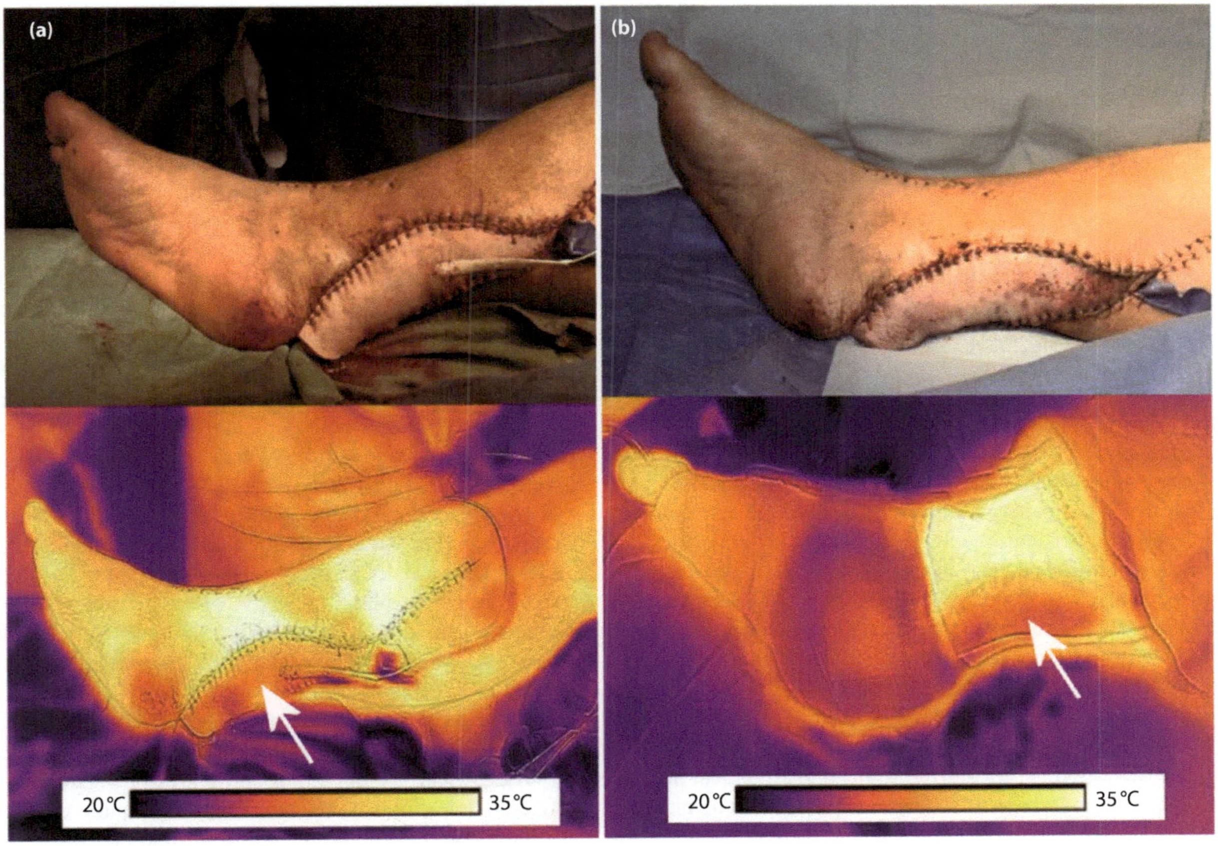

FIGURE 11.53 Failure of a free-flap graft. (a) Immediate postoperative view taken on the operative table shows good flap color and acceptable warmth of the flap (arrow). (b) Postop day one: The graft (arrow) shows a violaceous hue and is significantly cooler than the anterior leg. The flap subsequently failed due to thrombosis in the flap veins.[244]

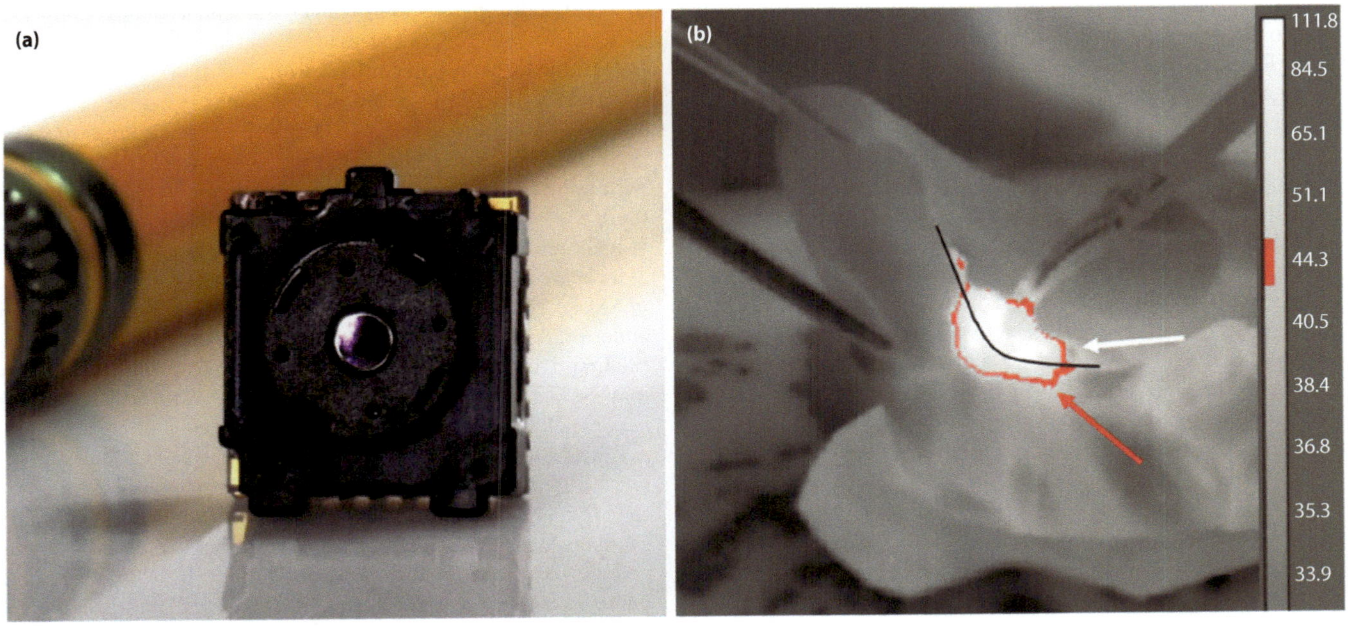

FIGURE 11.54 (a) A "Lepton" calibrated radiometric thermographic imager small enough to fit through a surgical endoscope to visualize and document internal tissue temperatures during thermal ablation.[247] (b) A greyscale thermogram of the cecum (to the left of the black line) during mesoappendix dissection (to the right of the black line). Inside the red zone, the temperature is over 45°C; outside the red zone, it is below 42°C.[248]

In both endoscopic and open surgical procedures, electrosurgical dissection and hemostasis are commonly employed techniques. Care must be taken, however, not to apply too much current to the surrounding tissues, as the stray heat produced may cause necrosis and even bowel perforation. Also, "shorting" of an electrosurgical instrument may damage tissues away from the actual surgical site. Experimental surgery on rabbits has shown that thermographic monitoring of electrosurgical procedures can monitor the current flow and any unwanted shorting by observing the tissue temperature. The current application time (seconds) is found to be more significant in predicting bowel damage than is the electrical power (watts) applied.[249]

Flexible optical fibers made of amorphous arsenic triselenide (As_2Se_3) could be used in endoscopes to visualize thermal events within the body. When purified, As_2Se_3 transmits infrared with wavelengths between 0.7 and 19 µm.[250] Infrared transmitting fibers have been used to cauterize and bond tissues using high-power infrared laser energy, however, more research is needed to develop thermal fiber endoscopes.[251] Concomitant fiber optic or intra-cavity thermography may be useful in evaluating tissue temperatures during cautery by fiber-directed infrared laser energy.

Endoscopic surgery of the urinary bladder is a common procedure. In this case, however, the bladder is filled with a clear liquid (saline), not a gas. As thermal imaging cannot detect infrared radiation through saline, it has not been used in this type of procedure. However, infrared cautery from holmium:yttrium-aluminum-garnet (Ho:YAG) lasers delivered through an optical fiber is common in urology and can be strong enough to break up bladder or kidney stones.[252] Orthopedic endoscopic procedures are also performed within joint spaces distended with clear saline, thus they share the same thermal characteristics and limitations as cystoscopic procedures. Laryngoscopic thermography is useful in determining pathology of the vocal cords; however, as the cords are exposed to cool air (thereby providing more thermal contrast, at least during inspiration), this is a different physical situation than true endoscopic closed-cavity thermography.[253]

Surgical bonding using a 2-watt, 10-µm laser to heat a "tissue solder" of aqueous albumin has been found effective in bonding external tissues and could work through a standard endoscopic port. Researchers have developed a laser tissue soldering system using a silver halide ($AgCl_{0.3}Br_{0.7}$) 0.9 mm fiber. With this system, the laser beam is optically interrupted ("chopped") at an 8 Hz rate. When the laser is switched on, 10 µm infrared heat is transmitted down the fiber to the tissue target. When the laser is switched off, the infrared generated by the temperature of the tissue target is transmitted up the same fiber to a calibrated infrared detector. Electronic circuitry then provides feedback to automatically adjust the laser power, keeping the tissue temperature within 2°C (3.6°F) of the 60°C (140°F) required to activate the albumin solder while minimizing any tissue damage. Delicate tissues such as the cornea can be repaired using this instrument.[254] As this method uses 10-µm radiation, standard thermographic imagers should be useful to monitor the suturing procedure in real time.

Surgical wound healing and post-operative complications

Following surgery, infections in the surgical wound area can greatly prolong or disrupt the healing process. Traditionally, clinicians have gauged the presence and severity of a wound infection by visual inspection and palpation, confirming the diagnosis through wound culture and laboratory markers. Thermography provides an imaging modality for better observing, locating, and quantifying these postoperative wound infections.

Because the white cell response to infection generates nitric oxide, which dilates nearby skin vasculature, many perioperative and postoperative infections can be detected by utilizing thermography. Thermography can detect prosthetic joint infections, thus supporting the perioperative care of patients after arthroplasty of the knee and hip joints.[255] The technology can also be used to screen for reinfections following successful surgery.

Sternal wound infections after midline sternotomy for cardiac repair can be detected by thermography, even when using the older infrared scanners.[256] If images taken at three to four weeks postoperatively show local elevation of skin temperatures over the presternal skin, deep wound infection, possibly osteomyelitis, is likely. As patients recovering from major surgery may "normally" have low-grade fevers and elevated white blood counts, the use of thermographic monitoring of wound temperature provides additional indication of a developing local infection three to six weeks postoperatively.[257]

Thermography has been found useful in evaluating the postpartum infection after caesarean section (C-section). Large healing wounds normally form a "healing ridge" of collagen about 2 cm (0.79 in.) wide along the length of the incision.[259] Due to tissue metabolism and NO production, skin over this healing ridge is normally 1.5°C (2.7°F) warmer than surrounding undisturbed skin for up to 30 days after surgery; qualitative and quantitative thermal criteria that differ from this normal healing temperature can detect wound infection. Paradoxical cold spots along the surgical scar are potential biomarkers of infection.[260] Areas of arterial compromise, hematomas, seromas, and collections of purulent exudate show up on infrared imaging as discrete cool spots over the incision. Surgical disruption of arterial inflow to an area of the wound shows up by the second day postoperatively, predicting slow wound healing or local infection. These cool spots tend to be small compared to the total wound size, thus a quantitative average of wound ROI temperatures may miss them. To predict problems in wound healing, qualitative thermographic surveillance must begin early, prior to the appearance of purulent exudate or dehiscence.[261]

In clinically obese women (BMI ≥ 30) who undergo emergency or elective C-section, the average postpartum wound site temperature minus abdominal temperature difference (WATD) is greater in patients who develop wound infection (see Figure 11.55). On day two, the quantitative WATD cut-off for predicting infection is >1.7°C (3°F). A 1.0°C (1.8°F) increase in WATD is associated with approximately a 2-fold increase in surgical site infections (SSI). On postoperative day seven, the WATD cut-off is 2.40°C (4.3°F), and a 1°C (1.8°F) increase in temperature difference is associated with approximately a 2.5-fold increased incidence of SSI.[262] These findings extend to the healing pattern of other abdominal incisions; properly healing incisions appear warm for the first five days, and then become gradually cooler. 'Cold spots' may be detected qualitatively over incisions that subsequently become clinically infected.[263]

Injuries to the nerves in the vicinity of a surgical intervention are fairly common occurrences. The sensory nerves to the skin tend to be very small and have variable anatomic locations, making their identification and protection difficult, especially during endoscopic procedures or trauma repair. These unintentional nerve injuries may be either complete, causing distal vasodilation, or partial, causing vasoconstriction. As an example, the femoral branch of the genitofemoral nerve, which is located close to the site of inguinal hernia repair, may be damaged during herniorrhaphy. Injury to this nerve causes postoperative pain in the distribution of the nerve over the upper inner thigh (see Figure 11.56).[264]

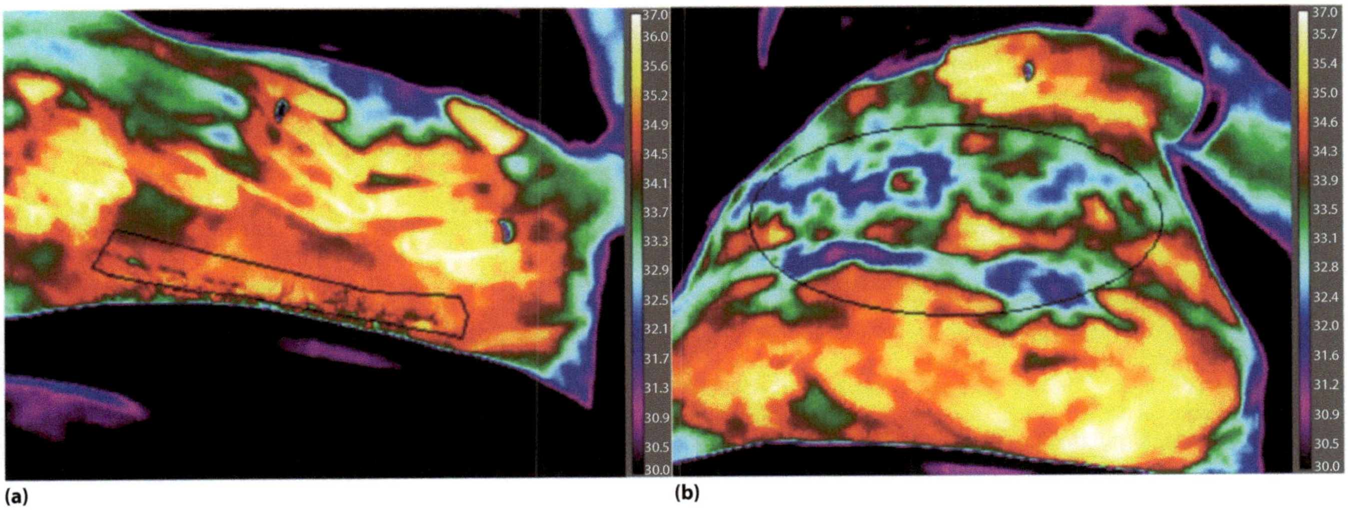

FIGURE 11.55 Postsurgical thermographic evaluation of a C-section wound in an obese subject. (a) the wound ROI (black rectangle) outlines the C-section Pfannenstiel "bikini" incision. The lower abdominal pannus is being manually retracted upwards by two hands. (b) the abdomen ROI (black oval) is taken over uninjured cool skin. Note the warm handprints over the lower abdomen from exposing the wound site as shown in image (a). Color scale range is 30–37°C.[258]

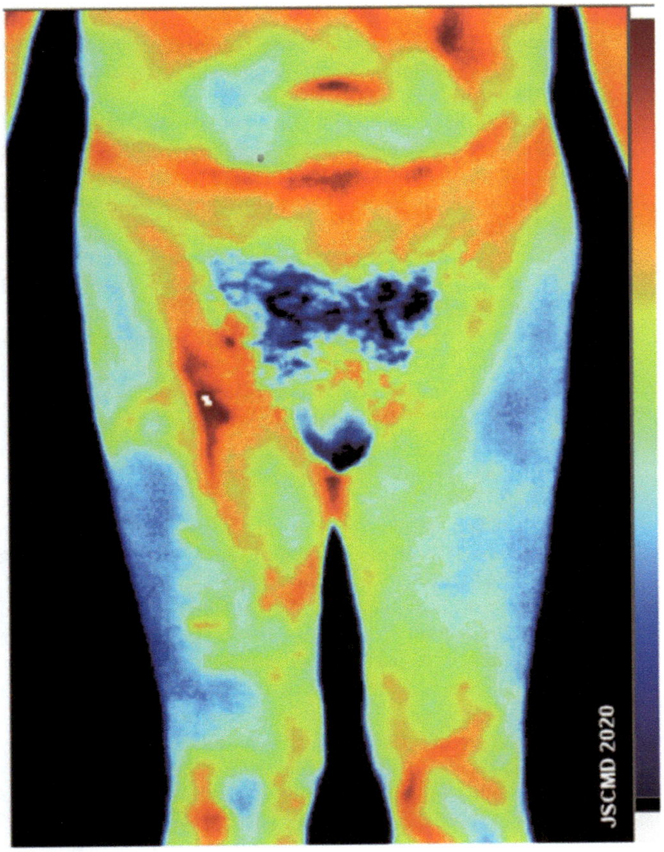

FIGURE 11.56 Thermal image of a 69-year-old male with right inguinal pain 1 year after right herniorrhaphy surgery. The thermal pattern is asymmetrically warm over the distribution of the femoral branch of the right genitofemoral nerve, indicating complete transection of the nerve. He also has a history of bilateral knee arthritis, and a right proximal saphenous varicosity pattern is present.

The pain of a chronic nerve injury is difficult to treat, but it generally does not have the debilitating effects of postoperative CRPS, a neurological disease of autonomic and central origins discussed earlier in this chapter. Because the vasomotor effects of these two conditions may be quite different, thermography can help establish the correct diagnosis.

Notes

1. Bentov I et al., Microvasc Res. 2015; PMCID: PMC4461519. See also: LeBlanc AJ et al., Microcirculation 2016; Doi: 10.1111/micc.12264
2. Houben AJHM et al., J Am Soc Nephrol. 2017; PMCID: PMC5698072.
3. Diwan AD et al., J Bone Miner Res. 2010; Doi:10.1359/jbmr.2000.15.2.342; See also: ZHU W et al., J Bone Miner Res. 2002; Doi:10.1359/jbmr.2002.17.8.1470
4. Haluzan D et al., Injury 2015; Doi: 10.1016/j.injury.2015.10.046
5. Silva CT et al., Emerg Radiol. 2012; Doi: 10.1007/s10140-012-1027-2
6. Haluzan D et al., Injury 2015; Doi: 10.1016/j.injury.2015.10.046
7. Devereaux MD et al., JAMA 1984; Doi:10.1001/jama.1984.03350040061027
8. Goodman PH et al., Phys Sportsmed. 1985; Doi: 10.1080/00913847.1985.11708772
9. Sanchis-Sánchez E et al., Am J Roentgenol. 2014; Doi: 10.2214/AJR.13.11716
10. Sanchis-Sánchez E et al., Eur J Pediatr. 2015; Doi: 10.1007/s00431-014-2425-0
11. Gómez-Carmona P et al., J Sport Rehabil. 2020; Doi:10.1123/jsr.2019-0056
12. Reed C et al., Med Biol Eng Comput. 2020; Doi: 10.1007/s11517-020-02167-z. See also: Ćurković S et al., Injury 2015; Doi: 10.1016/j.injury.2015.10.044. See also: Silva CT et al., 2012; Doi: 10.1007/s10140-012-1027-2
13. Saura M et al., Sci World J. 2010; Doi 10.1100/tsw.2010.58
14. Zhao Y et al., Arthritis Care Res (Hoboken). 2019; Doi: 10.1002/acr.23804
15. Sudoł-Szopińska, I et al., J Ultrason. 2015; Doi:10.15557/JoU.2015.0006. See also: Liu, Xing Hui et al., Int J Biol Sci. 2015; doi:10.7150/ijbs.10283. See also: Szomor ZL et al., BMJ Ann Rheum Dis. 2001; PMCID: PMC1753611.

16. Murrell GAC, Br J Sports Med. 2007; Doi: 10.1136/bjsm.2006.034447
17. Al-Nakhli HH et al., J Vis Exp. 2012; Doi:10.3791/3551. See also: Lewis PB et al., Clin Sports Med. 2012; Doi: 10.1016/j.csm.2011.09.009
18. Côrte AC et al., BMJ Open Sport Exerc Med. 2019; Doi:10.1136/bmjsem-2018-000431
19. Gómez-Carmona P et al., J Sport Rehabil. 2020; Doi:10.1123/jsr.2019-0056
20. da Silva W et al., Physiol Meas. 2018; Doi:10.1088/1361-6579/aae6df
21. see Application of Infrared Thermography in Sports Science, J, Quesada (ed.), Springer International Publishing, 2017. Doi: 10.1007/978-3-319-47410-6
22. Zurlo F et al., J Clin Invest. 1990; Doi: 10.1172/JCI114857
23. Heikkinen, J et al., Paper #189, ISAKOS ABSTRACTS 2017 https://www.arthroscopyjournal.org/article/S0749-8063(17)30957-X/pdf
24. Ring FE et al., Ch 25 – Thermal Imaging in Diseases of the Skeletal and Neuromuscular Systems, in Diakides M, Bronzino JD & Peterson DR (eds.), Medical Infrared Imaging: Principles and Practices, CRC Press, Boca Raton FL USA, 2013. Section 25.4.1.
25. Campagne D, Ch. 359. Fractures, Dislocations, and Sprains, in Section 23 of the MERCK Manual of Diagnosis and Therapy, 20th Ed, Porter RS (ed.), Merck Sharpe & Dohme, Kenilworth NJ, USA, 2018.
26. Katz LM et al., Crit Care Med. 2008; Doi: 10.1097/CCM.0b013e318174d800
27. N = 1 Personal Experiments by author jscmd 2020.
28. Robinson WH et al., Nat Rev Rheumatol. 2016; Doi:10.1038/nrrheum.2016.136
29. Scanzello CR, J Orthop Res. 2017; Doi: 10.1002/jor.23471
30. Greene MA et al., Osteoarthr Cartil. 2015; Doi:10.1016/j.joca.2015.01.008
31. Abramson SB, Arthritis Res Ther. 2008; Doi:10.1186/ar2463
32. Scanzello CR, Curr Opin Rheumatol. 2017; Doi:10.1097/BOR.0000000000000353
33. Fokam D et al., J Basic Clin Physiol Pharmacol. 2018; Doi:10.1515/jbcpp-2017-0218
34. Denoble AE et al., Clin Med Insights Arthritis Musculoskelet Disord. 2010; PMCID: PMC2998980.
35. Altman RD, Ch. 43. Paget Disease of Bone, in Section 4 of the MERCK Manual of Diagnosis and Therapy, 20th Ed, Porter RS (ed.), Merck Sharpe & Dohme, Kenilworth NJ, USA, 2018.
36. Cosh JA et al., Rheumatology 1970; Doi: 10.1093/rheumatology/10.7.342
37. Osdoby PA, Nitric Oxide, Osteoclasts and Metabolic Bone Disease. Abstract for NIH Grant Request 6534426, 2002.
38. FJ Ring et al., Proceedings of 17th International Conference of the Engineering in Medicine and Biology Society 1995; Doi: 10.1109/IEMBS.1995.579904
39. Mudra U et al., Georgian Med News. 2020; PMID: 32841189.
40. JA Cosh et al., Rheumatology 1970; Doi: 10.1093/rheumatology/10.7.342
41. Schiavenato, M et al., J Rheumatology 2012; Doi: 10.3899/jrheum.110581
42. Husni, ME et al., Rheumatology & Immunology / Research 2018 – Cleveland Clinic, USA. https://acrabstracts.org #2677.
43. Weinberg, et al., Arthritis Res Ther. 2006; Doi: 10.1186/ar2030
44. Nagy, G et al., Arthritis Res Ther. 2010; Doi: 10.1186/ar3045
45. Löffers, C et al., Clin Exp Rheumatol. 2015; PMID: 26314610 Also See: Orem, A et al., Dermatology 1999; Doi: 10.1159/000018061
46. Zalewska, A et al., Conf Proc IEEE Eng Med Biol Soc. 2005; Doi: 10.1109/IEMBS.2005.1616491. PMID: 17282260.
47. Zalewska, A et al., Conf Proc IEEE Eng Med Biol Soc. 2004; doi: 10.1109/IEMBS.2004.1403381. PMID: 17271900.
48. A Capo et al., Microvasc Res. 2015; Doi: 10.1016/j.mvr.2015.08.008
49. Mathew, AJ et al., Curr Opin Rheumatol. 2016; Doi: 10.1097/BOR.0000000000000282
50. Takase-Minegishi, K et al., Rheumatology (Oxford). 2018; Doi: 10.1093/rheumatology/kex036. See also: Haavardsholm, EA et al., BMJ 2016; Doi: 10.1136/bmj.i4205
51. Collins, AJ et al., Ann Rheum Dis. 1974; Doi: 10.1136/ard.33.2.113
52. Umapathy, S et al., Biomed Tech (Berl). 2020; PMID: 31821162. See also: Pauk, J et al., Sensors (Basel). 2019; Doi: 10.3390/s19163444
53. Bardhan, S et al., Australas Phys Eng Sci Med. 2019; PMID: 30706334.
54. Snekhalatha, U et al., Proc Inst Mech Eng H. 2017; PMID: 29076764.
55. Frize, M et al., Stud Health Technol Inform. 2012; PMID: 22874260.
56. Jones, B et al., Clin Rheumatol. 2018; PMID: 29679167.
57. Pauk, J et al., Med Biol Eng Comput. 2019; Doi: 10.1007/s11517-019-02055-1
58. Snekhalatha, U et al., Proc Inst Mech Eng H. 2015; PMID: 25934260.
59. Devereaux, MD et al., Ann Rheum Dis. 1985; PMCID: PMC1001672 See also: Lerkvaleekul, B et al., Physiol Meas. 2017; PMID: 28248195.
60. Lasanen, R et al., Physiol Meas. 2015; PMID: 25582734.
61. Kontzias, A, Ch. 39. Joint Disorders, in Section 4 of the MERCK Manual of Diagnosis and Therapy 20th Ed, Porter RS (ed.), Merck Sharpe & Dohme, Kenilworth NJ, USA, 2018, pp. 311 & 313.
62. Ring, EF, Bibliotheca Radiologica 1974; PMID: 170907.
63. Grennan, DM et al., Rheumatol Rehabil. 1982; Doi:10.1093/rheumatology/21.2.81
64. Source: https://www.ninds.nih.gov/Disorders/All-Disorders/Myopathy-Information-Page, downloaded 31 August 2020.
65. Liu, X et al., Int J Biol Sci 2015; Doi:10.7150/ijbs.10283
66. Tkáčová, M et al., MEASUREMENT 2011; https://www.measurement.sk/M2011/doc/proceedings/406_Tkacova-2.pdf. See also: Tan, JH et al., J Med Syst. 2011; PMID: 20703645.
67. Konieczka, K et al., TVST 2018; Doi: 10.1167/tvst.7.3.14
68. Image: Gray869 by Henry Vandyke Carter from Wikimedia Commons in the public domain, annotated to add heat flow by author JSCMD.
69. Image: Gray891 by Henry Vandyke Carter from Wikimedia Commons in the public domain, annotated with explanation by author JSCMD.
70. Nishimura, S, The investigation of the thermal effect of contact lens wear. Master's thesis for the School of Optometry & Vision Sciences, Cardiff University, UK, 2014.
71. Galassi, F et al., Br J Ophthalmol. 2007; PMCID: PMC1955655.
72. García-Porta, N et al., J Opt Soc Am A Opt Image Sci Vis. 2019; Doi: 10.1364/JOSAA.36.001015. PMID: 31158132.
73. Konieczka, K et al; Trans. Vis. Sci. Tech. 2019; Doi: https://doi.org/10.1167/tvst.8.3.47
74. Abreau, K et al., Ocul Surf. 2016; Doi: 10.1016/j.jtos.2015.09.001
75. Su, TY et al., J Formos Med Assoc. 2017; Doi: 10.1016/j.jfma.2016.09.012. PMID: 27817990.
76. Wanklyn, P et al., The Cold Hemiplegic Arm. Stroke 1994; pp. 1760–1770.
77. Alfieri FM, et al., NeuroRehabilitation 2016; PMID: 27935558.
78. Wanklyn, P et al., The Cold Hemiplegic Arm. Stroke September 1994; 25(9):1760–1770.
79. Song, Y-G et al., Ann Rehabil Med. 2015; Doi: 10.5535/arm.2015.39.5.696
80. Roehl, K et al. Spinal Cord. 2009; https://doi.org/10.1038/sc.2008.128
81. Mathias, CJ et al., Ch. 66 in Autonomic Failure, 5th Ed, Mathias CJ & Bannister R (ed.), 2013, Oxford University Press, Oxford, UK, p. 812.
82. Netter FH, Nervous System. Plate 54, p. 81 in The CIBA Collection of Medical Illustrations, Volume I. Case-Hoyt Corp, Rochester, NY USA, 1972. ISBN 0-914168-01-0; See also: Figure 5.9.
83. Kim, TS et al., Asian J Pain 2018; Doi: 10.35353/ajp.4.2.25
84. Chafetz, N et al., Spine (Phila Pa 1976) 1988; PMID: 2973135.
85. Volovik, MG et al., 15th Quantitative InfraRed Thermography Conference, Porto, Portugal, July 2020; https://easychair.org/publications/preprint_open/mxxn
86. Zurek, G et al., J Physiol Pharmacol. 2008; PMID: 19218709.
87. Pascoe, D et al., Ch. 6 – Physiology of Thermal Signals in Diakides, M et al. (eds.), Medical Infrared Imaging: Principles and Practices, CRC Press, Boca Raton FL USA, 2013, Section 6.6.3.
88. Uematsu, S, J Neurosurg. 1985; Doi: 10.3171/jns.1985.62.5.0716
89. Wipperman, J et al., Am Fam Physician. 2016; https://www.aafp.org/afp/2016/1215/p993.html
90. Reilly, PA et al., Br J Rheumatol. 1989; PMID: 2590817.
91. Ming, Z et al., Clin Neurol Neurosurg. 2007; PMID: 17400369.

92. Herrick, RT et al., J Hand Surg Am. 1987; PMID: 3655269.
93. Tchou, S et al., J Hand Surg Am. 1992; PMID: 1629541.
94. Baic, A et al., Medicine (Baltimore). 2017; PMCID: PMC5626262.
95. Ming, Z et al., Clin Neurol Neurosurg. 2007; PMID: 17400369.
96. A thin sheet of food-grade plastic wrap over the ice could keep the moisture of ice melt away from the skin to prevent evaporation artifact.
97. Maxel, X et al., Mechanics & Industry 2014; Doi: 10.1051/meca/2014034
98. Images and caption from: Maxel, X et al., Mechanics & Industry 2014; Doi: 10.1051/meca/2014034. Used with permission.
99. Jesensek Papez, B et al., J Int Med Res. 2008; PMID: 19094447.
100. The term "peroneal" can be easily confused with "perineal" and "peritoneal." "Fibular" is more anatomically descriptive.
101. Thermal images courtesy of: Ali, SS et al., Cureus 2019; Doi: 10.7759/cureus.4087, CC-BY 3.0.
102. Image Credit: Nicholas Zaorsky, MD, File: Wikipedia medical illustration thoracic outlet syndrome brachial plexus anatomy with labels.jpg Created: 11 June 2010.
103. Anatomic diagrams from Grays Anatomy 1918. From Wikimedia Commons. Anterior view file: Gray 797. Posterior view file: Gray 798.
104. Drummond, P et al., Cephalalgia. 1984; Doi:10.1046/j.1468-2982.1984.0403149.x
105. Image from: Fedorovich, AA et al., Clin. Pract. 2018; 15(2):561–567. CC-BY-4.0.
106. Kudrow L, Headache 1985; Doi 10.1111/j.1526 4610.1985. hed2501033.x
107. Antonaci, F et al., Cephalalgia. 2019; Doi:10.1177/0333102418788341
108. Pavlidis, I et al., IEEE J Biomed Health Inform. 2019; PMID: 30004895.
109. Takahashi, S, J Rural Med. 2018; PMCID: PMC5981019.
110. Pearce, JMS, J Neurol Neurosurg Psychiatry 2004; PMCID: PMC1738935.
111. Hampf, G et al., Pain 1990; Doi: 10.1016/0304-3959(90)91121-X
112. Graff-Radford, SB et al., J Orofac Pain 1995; PMID: 7488983.
113. Gonzalez-Usigli, HA, Ch. 232. Movement and Cerebellar Disorders, in Section 17 of the MERCK Manual of Diagnosis and Therapy, 20th Ed, Porter RS (ed.), Merck Sharpe & Dohme Pub, Kenilworth, NJ, USA, 2018, p. 1936.
114. Purup, MM et al., Hindawi Parkinson's Disease, 2020; Doi: 10.1155/2020/2349469
115. Images © 2020 MM Purup et al., CC-BY-4.0 Graphic design edited and labels added by jscmd.
116. Graph © 2020 MM Purup et al., CC-BY-4.0 Text labels added and edited by jscmd.
117. Studies using peripheral nerve block may confirm that the lack of distal arterial circulation in PD is due to sympathetic hyper-stimulation and not humoral or local constriction.
118. Cortelli, P et al., A Textbook of Clinical Disorders of the Autonomic Nervous System, 5th Ed, Mathias & Bannister (eds.), Oxford University Press, Oxford UK, 2013, p. 556.
119. Perpetuini, D et al., Physiol Meas. 2019, Doi:10.1088/1361-6579/ab057d
120. Childs, C et al., Int J Environ Res Public Health 2020; PMCID: PMC7557728.
121. David Clark, J et al., Mol Pain. 2018; Doi:10.1177/1744806918799127. See also: Cooper, MS et al., J Neuroimmune Pharmacol. 2013; Doi:10.1007/s11481-012-9392-x
122. Marinus, J et al., Lancet Neurol. 2011; PMCID: PMC5511749.
123. Acerra, NE et al., J Rehabil Med. 2007; Doi: 10.2340/16501977-0027. PMID: 17351691.
124. Pagani, S et al., Pain Physician. 2017; PMID: 28934787.
125. Borchers, AT et al., Autoimmun Rev. 2014; PMID: 24161450.
126. Knudsen, LF et al., Clin Auton Res. 2019; PMID: 31104164.
127. Birklein, F et al., Clin Auton Res. 1998; PMID: 9613797.
128. Eldufani, J et al., Heliyon 2020; Doi:10.1016/j.heliyon.2020.e03329. See also: Goebel A. Rheumatology (Oxford). 2011; PMID: 21712368.
129. Birklein, F et al., Clin Auton Res. 1998; PMID: 9613797.
130. Markman, J et al., MERCK Manual of Diagnosis and Therapy 20th Ed, Porter RS (ed.), Merck Sharpe & Dohme, Kenilworth, NJ, USA, 2018, p. 1977.
131. Shah, A et al., Foot Ankle Clin. 2011; PMID: 21600455. See also: Kim, SH et al., Pain Physician. 2016; PMID: 27454281.
132. Dholakia, M et al., in Challenging Neuropathic Pain Syndromes, Elsevier, 2018; ISBN: 9780323485661, pp. 41–42.
133. Jeong, MY et al., J Invasive Cardiol. 2013; PMID: 23995728.
134. Schurmann, M et al., Clin J Pain 2007; PMID: 17515744. See also: Krumova, EK et al., Pain. 2008; PMID: 18723287.
135. Niehof, SP et al., Biomed Eng Online. 2006; Doi:10.1186/1475-925X-5-30
136. Patients who are lawsuit litigants, drug users in a time of drug prohibition, or who may otherwise gain from having a diagnosis of CRPS could possibly induce thermal artifacts. Cooling with alcohol spray or warming by holding a transmitting cell phone near the body are possible ways to create convincing artifacts.
137. Huygen, FJ et al., Eur J Appl Physiol. 2004; PMID: 14735366.
138. Dhatt, S et al., Am J Phys Med Rehabil. 2020; Doi:10.1097/PHM.0000000000001522
139. Veldman, PH et al., Lancet 1993; PMID: 8105263.
140. Cho, CW et al., Medicine (Baltimore). 2016; PMCID: PMC5207547.
141. Jeon, SG et al., Korean J Pain. 2014; PMCID: PMC4196499.
142. Niehof, SP et al., Anesth Analg. 2008; PMID: 18165590.
143. Choi, E et al., Skin Res Technol. 2013; PMID: 23331254.
144. Neves, EB et al., Open Neurol J. 2015; PMCID: PMC4503831.
145. Robertson D. (ed.), Primer on the Autonomic Nervous System, 3rd Ed, Academic Press, 2012. ISBN:978-0-12-386525-0. p. 583.
146. Niehof, SP et al., BioMedical Engineering OnLine 2006; Doi:10.1186/1475-925X-5-30
147. Ilo, A et al., Adv Skin Wound Care 2020; Doi: 10.1097/01.ASW.0000694156.62834.8b
148. Lee, BY et al., J Vasc Surg. 1996; PMID: 8558726.
149. Griffin, LH et al., Ann Surg. March 1971; 173(3):389–397.
150. Sowa, MG et al., Measurement 2009, Proceedings of the 7th International Conference, Smolenice, Slovakia. https://www.measurement.sk/M2009/proceedings/427_Sowa2.pdf
151. Gatt, A et al., Prim Care Diabetes 2018; Doi: 10.1016/j.pcd.2018.01.001
152. Chi-Lun Huang, et al., J Vasc Surg. 2011; Doi:10.1016/j.jvs.2011.03.287
153. The Supratroclear artery was previously called the Frontal artery.
154. Brockenbrough EC, in Vascular Diagnosis, 4th Ed, Bernstein EF (ed.), Mosby Publishing, St. Louis MO USA, 1993, p. 409.
155. Capistrant, TD et al., Stroke 1973; PMID: 4685809.
156. Open-source clipart annotated after Capistrant TD & Gumnit RJ, Stroke 1973; PMID: 4685809. p. 63.
157. Kalicki, B et al., in Infrared Imaging, Ring, F et al. (eds.), IOP Publishing Ltd, London, 2015.
158. Allen, J et al., Ch. 21 in Infrared Imaging, Ring, F et al. (eds.), IOP Publishing Ltd, London, 2015.
159. Freedman, RR et al., Br Med J (Clin Res Ed). 1983; PMCID: PMC1549944.
160. Coffman JD, Hypertension. 1991; Doi: 10.1161/01.HYP.17.5.593. See also: La Montagna, G et al., Semin Arthritis Rheum. 2002; PMID: 11836657.
161. Pauling, JD et al., Clin Rheumatol. 2019; PMID: 31420815.
162. Laskar, MD et al., Environ Health Prev Med. 2005; Doi: 10.1007/BF02898196
163. Hadler NM, J Rheumatol. 1998; PMID: 9858419. See also: Pauling, JD et al., Clin Rheumatol. 2019; PMID: 31420815.
164. Tiev, KP et al., J Rheumatol. 2009; PMID: 19487271. See also: Khimdas, S et al., Arthritis Care Res (Hoboken). 2011; PMID: 20740608.
165. Block, JA et al., Lancet. 2001; PMID: 11438158.
166. (A) File: Raynaud syndrome on female airman's hand.jpg Created: 25 January 2018 by User: Profpedia – Wikipedia. (B) File: Blue finger tips 2.jpg Created: 3 June 2013 by Walt Fletcher – Wikipedia. Both images CC BY-SA 4.0.

167. Lambova, S et al., J Clin Rheumatol. 2011; Doi: 10.1097/RHU.0b013e31822be4e8. See also: Sari-Kouzel, H et al., Rheumatology (Oxford). 2001; PMID: 11312379.
168. Edwards, JM et al., in Vascular Diagnosis, 4th Ed, Bernstein EF (ed.), Mosby Publishing, St. Louis MO USA, 1993, p. 603.
169. Hwang, Y et al., Conf Proc IEEE Eng Med Biol Soc. 2017: PMID: 29060127.
170. Horikoshi, M et al., Intern Med. 2016; PMID: 26935364.
171. Chlebicka, I et al., Acta Derm Venereol. 2013; Doi: 10.2340/00015555-1508
172. Pauling, JD et al., Clin Exp Rheumatol. 2012; PMID: 22691218. See also: Schlager, O et al., Microvasc Res. 2010; PMID: 20144625.
173. Gardner-Medwin, JM et al., Br J Clin Pharmacol. 2001; PMCID: PMC2014513.
174. Heslop, J et al., J R Coll Gen Pract. 1983; PMCID: PMC1972650.
175. Campos, MF et al., Conf Proc IEEE Eng Med Biol Soc. 2018; PMID: 30441211.
176. Lim, MJ et al., J Korean Med Sci. 2014; PMCID: PMC3991792.
177. Herrick, AL et al., Autoimmun Rev. 2018; PMID: 29526628.
178. Cohen, JM, in Rehabilitation Medicine and Thermography, Lee HM & Cohen JM (eds.), Impress Publications, Wilsonville OR USA, 2007, p. 78. See also Schuhfried, O et al., Arch Phys Med Rehabil. 2000; PMID: 10768542.
179. Laskar, Md et al., Different Conditions of Cold Water Immersion Test for Diagnosing Hand-Arm Vibration Syndrome. Environ Health Prev Med. 2005; PMCID: PMC2723502.
180. From: Lindsell, CJ, Environ Health Prev Med. 2005; Doi 10.1007/BF02898195
181. Martini, G et al., Pediatr Rheumatol Online J. 2019; Doi:10.1186/s12969-019-0371-0. See also: Mosdósi, B et al., Pediatr Rheumatol Online J. 2018; Doi: 10.1186/s12969-018-0237-x
182. Wilkinson, JD et al., A Multicenter Study of the Validity and Reliability of Responses to Hand Cold Challenge as Measured by Laser Speckle Contrast Imaging and Thermography: Outcome Measures for Systemic Sclerosis-Related Raynaud's Phenomenon. Arthritis Rheumatol. 2018; PMCID: PMC6001804.
183. (A) Photo Source: https://commons.wikimedia.org/wiki/File:Supratrochlear_artery_forehead.png, Date: 27 February 2012, Author: Jmeyerman8, CC BY-SA 3.0.
184. Bazett, HC et al., J Appl Physiol. 1948; PMID: 18887571.
185. Soulen, RL et al., Radiology 1972; PMID: 5057292.
186. Wheeler, HB et al., in Vascular Diagnosis, 4th Ed, Bernstein EF (ed.), Mosby Publishing, St. Louis MO USA, 1993, p. 867.
187. Douketis, JD, in MERCK Manual of Diagnosis and Therapy, 20th Ed, Porter RS (ed.), Merck Sharpe & Dohme, Kenilworth, NJ, USA, 2018, p. 757.
188. Novikov, P et al., Ann Rheum Dis. 2015; PMID: 25381230.
189. Emmi, G et al., Thrombosis J. 2015; PMCID: PMC4399148.
190. Douketis, JD, in MERCK Manual of Diagnosis and Therapy, 20th Ed, Porter RS (ed.), Merck Sharpe & Dohme, Kenilworth, NJ, USA, 2018, p. 764.
191. Vijayakumar C, IOSR J Dent Med Sci. 2018; Doi: 10.9790/0853-1706056469
192. Ben Hamida et al., J Med Case Reports 2021; doi. 10.1186/s13256-021-02708-6
193. Doesburg, F et al. PloS one 2019; PMCID: PMC6415825.
194. Image and caption from Doesburg F, et al., PloS One 2019; PMCID: PMC6415825 (CC-BY-4.0).
195. Martins, M et al., Conference: 12th European Congress of Thermology At: Porto, Portugal 2012; https://www.researchgate.net/publication/280111240
196. *See* plates of the lymphatic system in Spalteholz-Spanner Atlas of Human Anatomy 16th Ed, Spanner R (ed.), Sheltema & Holkema NV, Amsterdam, 1967. Lymph vessels in the forearm are about 1 mm (0.039 inch) diameter.
197. Image Credit: Thermal Vision Research. In the Wellcome Collection, Image N0037142 (CC BY 4.0).
198. Dębiec-Bąk, A et al., Lymphat Res Biol. 2019; Doi: 10.1089/lrb.2019.0002
199. Common irritants include: solvents, rubbing alcohol, bleach, detergents, shampoos, hair permanent applications, sawdust, wool dust, plants, fertilizers, and pesticides. Source: https://www.mayoclinic.org/diseases-conditions/contact-dermatitis/symptoms-causes/syc-20352742
200. Anzengruber, F et al., Allergol Int. 2019; PMID: 30598404.
201. Image from: Rok, T et al., J Therm Anal Calorim. 2017; Doi: 10.1007/s10973-016-5676-3 CC-BY-4.0
202. Rok, T et al., J Therm Anal Calorim. 2017; Doi: 10.1007/s10973-016-5676-3
203. Litscher, G, BioMed Eng. 2005; Doi: 10.1186/1475-925X-4-38
204. An Outline of Chinese Acupuncture by The Academy of Traditional Chinese Medicine, Foreign Language Press, Peking, China, 1975, p. 102; ISBN-13 : 978-1299232068.
205. Ernst, M et al., Pain 1985; PMID: 3982836.
206. Agarwal-Kozlowsk, K et al., Anesthesiology 2009; PMID: 19672170.
207. See Figure 11.46 illustrating N = 1 study by author JSCMD on 28 February 2021.
208. Image from Wikipedia: Extensor compartments of wrist (back of hand), File:Gray418.png, User: James Bedford, Public Domain. Image cropped. Additional graphics and text by JSCMD showing experimental conditions as described by RJ Scudds, 1995.
209. Rosenblum, J et al., *in* Rehabilitation Medicine and Thermography, Lee & Cohen (eds.), Impress Publications, 2007, p. 116.
210. Scudds, RJ et al., Phys Ther. 1995; PMID: 7604081.
211. Szabo, T et al., IEEE Eng Med Biol. 2000; PMID: 10834120.
212. Kim, J et al., J Clin Monit Comput. 2019; PMID: 30426322.
213. Pascoe, DD et al., in Diakides, M et al. (eds.), Medical Infrared Imaging: Principles and Practices, CRC Press, Boca Raton FL USA, 2013, Section 6.6.3.
214. Neural boundary outlines as described in Clemente CD, Anatomy – A Regional Atlas of the Human Body, 3rd Ed, Lea & Febiger Publishing, Malvern PA USA, 1987, Figures 38 & 39.
215. Chamberlain, DP et al., Anesthesiology 1986; PMID: 3740502.
216. Hermanns, H et al., Acta Anaesthesiol Scand. 2018; PMID: 29938773.
217. Data from Hermanns, H et al., Acta Anaesthesiol Scand. 2018; PMID: 29938773.
218. Image from: Bruins, AA et al., J Clin Monit Comput. 2018; Doi:10.1007/s10877-017-0026-y. CC-BY-4.0 Image modified for clarity by jscmd.
219. Szabo, T et al., IEEE Eng Med0 Biol. 2000; PMID: 10834120.
220. Fujimasa, I et al., In Ring &Phillips (eds.), Recent Advances in Medical Thermology, Springer, Boston, MA, 1984; ISBN: 978-1-4684-7697-2.
221. Sönmez, B et al., Eur J Cardio-Thorac Surg. 2003; PMID: 14643815.
222. Suma, H et al., Ann Thorac Surg. 2000; PMID: 11093537.
223. CARDIOPLEGIA SOLUTION A – Data Sheet, 2018, Baxter Healthcare Ltd, New Zealand.
224. Ekroth, R et al., Ann Thorac Surg. 1980; PMID: 7362327.
225. Ecker, RD et al., J Neurosurg. 2002; PMID: 12507150.
226. Kateb, B et al., Neuroimage. 2009; PMID: 19332140.
227. Watson, JC et al., J Neurosurg 2002; PMID: 12005400.
228. Nakagawa, A et al., J Neurosurg. 2009; PMID: 19425891.
229. Steiner, et al., J Biomed Opt. 2011; Doi: 10.1117/1.3528011
230. Kateb, B et al., Neuroimage. 2009; PMID: 19332140.
231. de Font-Réaulx, E et al., Surg Neurol Int. 2020; PMCID: PMC7110298.
232. Ecker, RD et al., J Neurosurg. 2002; PMID: 12507150.
233. Ecker, RD et al., J Neurosurg. 2002; PMID: 12507150.
234. Watson, JC et al., J Neurosurg. 2002; PMID: 12005400.
235. Ecker, RD et al., J Neurosurg. 2002; PMID: 12507150, Figure 8.
236. Nakagawa, A et al., Minim Invasive Neurosurg. 2004; PMID: 15343427.
237. Sturgeon, CD et al., J Angiol Circulat Sys. 2019; 1:104.
238. Lin, PH et al., J Vasc Surg Cases Innov Tech. 2017; PMCID: PMC5764914.

239. Mercer, JB et al., EAT2012 Book of Proceedings – Appendix 1 of Thermology international 22/3 (2012), pp. 9-15. http://www.uhlen.at/thermology-international/data/pdf/223A09.pdf
240. Hallock GG, Plast Aesthet Res 2019; Doi: 10.20517/2347-9264.2019.029
241. John, HE et al., Gland Surg. 2016; PMCID: PMC4791361.
242. Photo courtesy of Dr. G.G. Hallock 2019. CC-BY-4.0.
243. Photo courtesy of Dr. G.G. Hallock 2019. CC-BY-4.0.
244. Photos and images courtesy of Dr. G.G. Hallock 2019. CC-BY-4.0.
245. Yu, Tianwu et al., The Cochrane Database Syst Rev. 2017; PMCID: PMC6481852.
246. Kenneth Ogan, et al., Urology 2003; PMID: 12837456.
247. Photo courtesy of FLIR Corporation, Wilsonville, OR. Used with permission.
248. Image courtesy of TV Nechay 2020. Image and caption CC-BY-4.0.
249. Nechay, TV et al. BMC Surg. 2020; PMCID: PMC7251678.
250. Guillevic, E et al., J Non-Cryst Solids 2011; Doi : 10.1016/j.jnoncrysol.2011.03.030
251. Gabay I, J Biomed Opt. 2013; PMID: 24057125.
252. Sandhu, AS et al., Medical Journal, Armed Forces India 2007; PMCID: PMC4921716.
253. Jahan, A et al., J Voice. 2020; PMID: 31924431.
254. Gabay, I et al., J. Biomed Opt. 2013; PMID: 24057125.
255. Scheidt, S et al., Z Orthop Unfall. 2019; PMID: 31525794. See also: Yaghmour, KM et al., J Clin Med. 2019; PMCID: PMC6406500.
256. Robicsek, F et al., Thorac Cardiovasc Surg. 1984; Doi: 10.1055/s-2007-1023400
257. Abdelmaseeh, TA et al., In: StatPearls [Internet]. StatPearls Publishing, Treasure Island, FL, USA; 2020; https://www.ncbi.nlm.nih.gov/books/NBK482299/
258. Image credit: Childs, C et al., Antimicrob Resist Infect Control 2019; Doi: 10.1186/s13756-018-0461-7 CC-BY-4.0, image layout edited for clarity.
259. World Union of Wound Healing Societies Consensus Document. Surgical Wound Dehiscence: Improving Prevention and Outcomes. Wounds International, London UK, 2018.
260. Childs, C et al., J Wound Care 2016; PMID: 27608511.
261. Henrikson, NA et al., J Hosp Infection 2010; PMID: 20338667. See also: Siah, CJ et al., J Wound Care 2012; PMID: 22399080.
262. Childs, C et al., Antimicrob Resist Infect Control 2019; Doi: 10.1186/s13756-018-0461-7
263. Siah, CJR et al., J Wound Care 2015; PMID: 25764955.
264. Gupton, M et al., In StatPearls. Treasure Island (FL): StatPearls Publishing, Treasure Island FL USA, 2020, PMID: 28613484.

12

FUTURE DEVELOPMENTS IN HUMAN THERMOGRAPHY

Though no one can see through the quantum fog to accurately predict the future, there are certain trends in human medical thermography that can advance the technology if properly nurtured. This chapter will investigate these trends, and offer a "wish list" of hardware, software, and research developments that can make clinical thermography easier, more standardized, better understood, globally available, and compatible with modern medicine. Clinical thermography has become a reliable tool for the early detection and monitoring of a multitude of disease states and physiologic conditions. Improvements in imager technology and thermographic protocol design have played a major part in establishing thermography as a scientifically-based imaging method. Future developments, as discussed here, will qualify human thermography as a respected addition to the practice of medicine.

Hardware

Beyond the microbolometer – Solid crystal 10-µm detectors

The workhorse sensor of today's thermal imagers, the microbolometer, is delicate and difficult to produce in quantity in large arrays. It must be operated in a vacuum, and can be damaged by even moderate physical shock. A more rugged, solid-state planar 10-µm radiation sensor that can be placed in 20-µm arrays on a chip would be a big advance for thermography. At present, there are several metalloids – transition metal alloy possibilities that could replace the microbolometer, providing their operating temperature, sensitivity, and thermal noise level can match the present-day instruments. If an improved thermal array sensor is found to provide lower cost, higher resolution, lower noise, and smaller imager size, it will become the next generation in thermal imaging technology. Present candidates for practical thermal detectors include Silicon with Gallium (Si:Ga), Silver (Si:Ag), or Antimony (Si:Sb); Germanium with Cadmium (Ge:Cd), Copper (Ge:Cu), or Gold (Ge:Au); Mercury/Cadmium/Tellurium (HgCdTe); and Indium/Arsenic/Antimony (InAsSb).[1] Which one will the quantum bless?

Thermography suite design

When designing a thermography suite, patient privacy, technician convenience, and time efficiency must be addressed. In the design shown in Figure 12.1, the thermography room and the two equilibration rooms each have their own thermostat to accommodate different equilibration and examination temperatures. The suite can then accommodate both static and dynamic examinations. As the 15-minute temperature equilibration period is usually longer than the time it takes to acquire the thermal images, it makes sense to have two or more separate, adjacent equilibration areas to maximize the number of thermography examinations that can be done. If an observation window is used, it should have argon-filled double-pane glazing, and be located behind the camera.

Facilitating thermography worldwide

Motorized or easily transportable inexpensive thermal imaging modules should be designed and manufactured for use in areas where air conditioning is not commonly available (Figure 12.2). These could be built into standard international shipping containers, bringing state-of-the-art thermographic facilities to remote regions around the globe.

Software

An interpreting thermographer's wish list

- Easier side-to-side visual comparisons over time. Images may vary between sessions, even with positioning fixtures and software alignment algorithms. Imaging analysis displays must accommodate unavoidable patient movement and body habit changes.
- Auto full-span palette formatting where a user-defined area would automatically be made a full-span graded spectral image (Figure 12.3).
- A differential 0.5°C or 1.0°C temperature "contour line" overlay would include a Vernier control for up-down adjustment to compare the temperature of features in an image (Figure 12.4).

Ongoing Tasks

Education and regulation of thermography

Hypothesis: Better regulation, education, and certification of thermographers and technicians will improve the practice of human medical thermography.

Though technological advances have improved the ease of recording high-resolution thermal images, the process that follows is more complex because the level of information provided is so much more refined. Thermograms must be reliably interpreted, documented, and relayed to the patient and their medical provider, with proper follow-up care advised. Accordingly, interpretation of thermograms must be done by professionals who hold credentials as thermographers. Collaboration will help. The collection of accurately-interpreted, pathologically-confirmed, and standardized images accumulating from trained thermographers can provide a rich database for development of future C-A and AI systems (and humans).

Although originally promoted as easy to perform and simple to interpret, thermography has proven to be quite complex, requiring specialized training of both the technician and physician. Clinical thermal imaging should only be performed by one properly trained and certified. Such training is essential for analyzing infrared phenomena in relation to human pathologies and conditions. Qualified thermography organizations are helping to promote the scientific validity and quality of thermal imaging.

The standards and guidelines issued by qualified thermography organizations may form the basis for regulating the clinical application of thermographic imaging. These standards and guidelines take into account various criteria for thermal imaging and are updated on a regular schedule to keep abreast of advances in thermographic equipment and interpretation standards.[3]

The future regulation of thermography will be especially important for breast cancer screening, as illustrated by the

DOI: 10.1201/9781003281764-13

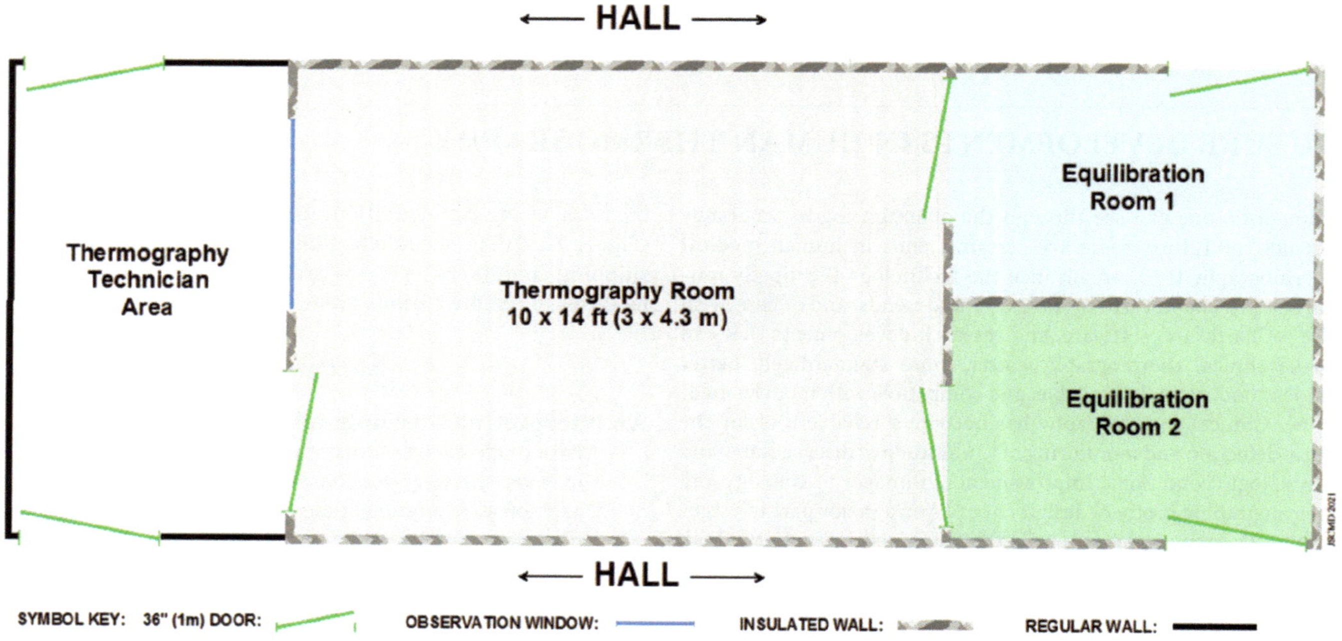

FIGURE 12.1 Possible design of a professional thermography suite. Two equilibration rooms allow a thermal imaging examination to proceed while the next patient is being cooled. The door between an equilibration room and the thermography area can only be opened from the thermography room side.

history of mammography regulation. In the 1990s, there was a lack of confidence in the overall quality of mammography, along with concerns that it was causing an increase in breast cancer mortality in screened women compared to controls under age 50.[4] Federal law addressed these concerns in 1992, granting oversight of mammography practice to the US Food and Drug Administration (FDA). Analogous regulations may be needed to ensure quality in the practice of breast thermography; standardization needs to be delineated and agreed upon by the regulatory agencies.

Recommended for thermography education and regulation are the following:

- A universal radiometric file format needs to be developed and supported by thermal imager manufacturers.
- A universal, graded spectral color display palette is needed along with a graded greyscale clinical display standard. Other non-spectral and stepped palettes should be relegated to the historical archives except for special research or display purposes.

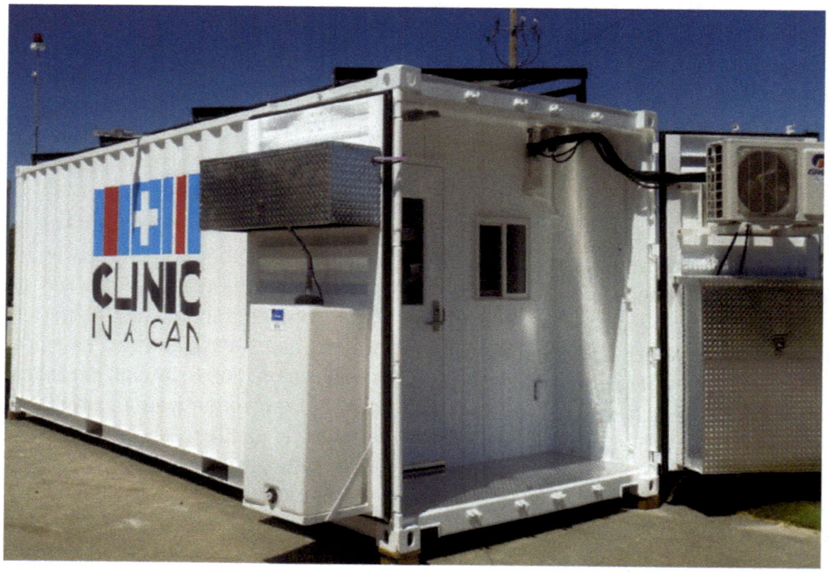

FIGURE 12.2 A standard 20-ft (6.1-m) steel shipping container can be outfitted as a medical clinic complete with R-19 insulation, solar power, air conditioning, heating, and plumbing. An internal windowless and temperature-controlled exam area is ideal for thermal imaging.[2]

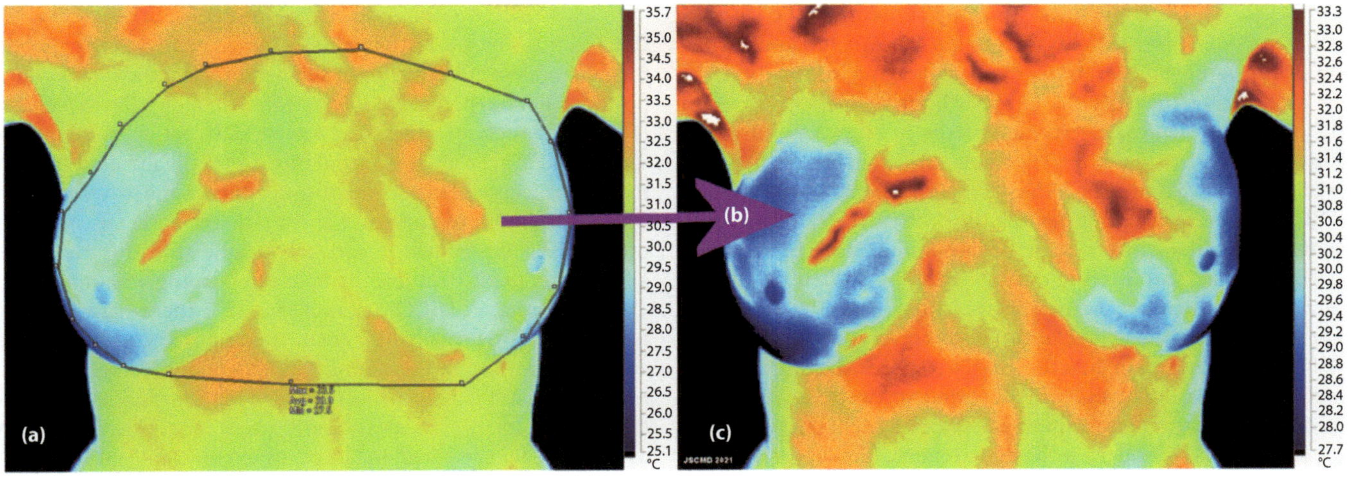

FIGURE 12.3 Automatic full-span formatting. (a) The region of interest is outlined, providing the maximum, mean, and minimum temperatures enclosed. (b) On operator command (arrow), the image is spanned so that the area within the outline displays the full blue-red visual spectrum. (c) The resulting image is ready for qualitative interpretation.

- Standard equilibration and imaging protocols should be adopted for thermography of the body and breasts.
- Protocols for thermal imaging of complex regional pain syndrome (CRPS), Raynaud's disease, and other conditions requiring dynamic thermographic procedures should be made standard.
- A patient's right to scientific, private, timely, and pain-free thermal imaging should be protected. Unnecessarily long cooling times, ice-water immersion, and non-validated protocols should be eliminated from screening exams, especially breast exams.
- Clinical thermography training courses should be offered by medical, nursing, paramedical, and technical schools. Official certification of thermography training and continuing education will be needed for acceptance by the medical community.
- As human thermal imaging grows, at some point, it will likely be subsumed into the specialty of Radiology, which would assure quality control through accreditation.

Adapting DICOM image standards for clinical thermography

Hypothesis: Adapting DICOM medical imaging standards will provide a base for thermal image handling and will advance thermography's standing in professional medical practice.

The integration of thermographic data into clinical information systems is of utmost importance if thermography is to be accepted into clinical medicine; the Digital Imaging and Communications in Medicine (DICOM) image file standard must expand to include thermographic radiometric files, formatted images, and metadata.[5] DICOM is the international standard for the dissemination of medical images and is commonly used

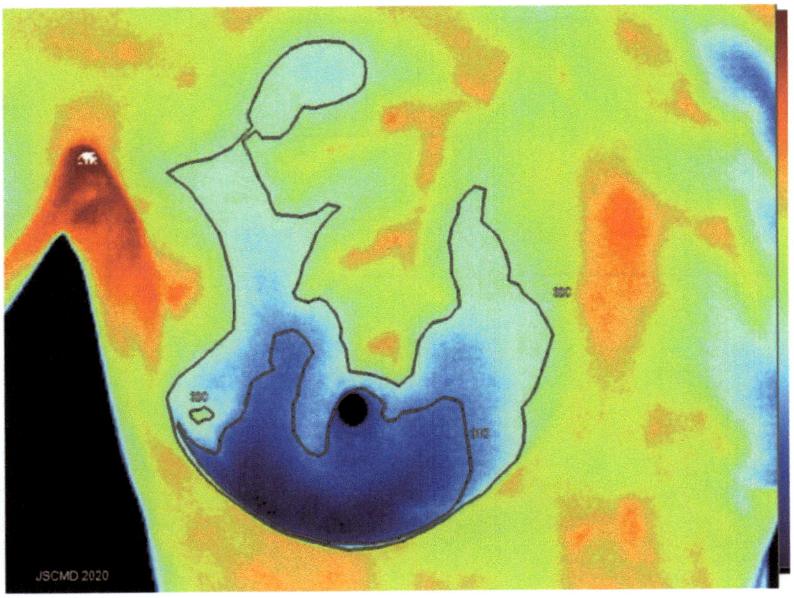

FIGURE 12.4 Selectable and adjustable thermal contour lines on a full-span color image, shown here at 31°C and 32°C. This type of display improves differential temperature measurements with little loss of qualitative information.

for MRIs, CT scans, and other imaging modalities. The DICOM standard encompasses the transmission, storage, retrieval, printing, processing, and display of medical imaging information.[6]

By utilizing the DICOM format, thermal imaging data can be stored in medical electronic records in such a way that all imaging information is interoperable and transferable between various medical entities.[7] The term *interoperable* means that DICOM ensures that all devices (in particular, those made by different manufacturers) can be accommodated. Specifically, DICOM integrates imaging devices with PACS (Picture Archive and Communication System) workstations. PACS is the infrastructure needed to (a) perform the storage of medical images in DICOM format and (b) link the imaging devices, diagnostic workstations, image archives, image routing software, and medical record information into a single integrated system (Figure 12.5).

The DICOM standard is being extended to support applications in infrared thermography.[8] Upon scheduling a thermography session, the patient demographics, scheduled procedure type, and protocol information will be made available to the PACS. Images are captured in DICOM format. The completed DICOM images are then stored in the PACS after being checked for accuracy and completeness by the PACS gateway computer. By implementing PACS in DICOM format, clinical thermographers can manage and display images and keep track of patient files in a timely manner.[9]

In addition to the standard HIPAA-protected private information (patient's name, birthdate, ID number, etc.), there are public metadata relevant to the image acquisition device and procedure protocol. Public thermographic metadata includes the model and make of the thermal imager, the palette used, patient cooling protocols, and other data (e.g., serial number of the infrared imager, the device's thermal offset and gain, distance to the patient, region of interest (ROI), temperature span, and any thermal challenge procedures). Subsequent images can be guided by this metadata, allowing for greater uniformity between imaging sessions.

The adoption of DICOM standard within thermographic systems is certainly feasible, since all the required capabilities are contained within the standard.[10] With enough demand, infrared imager software can be upgraded to generate a DICOM-compatible image. In the meantime, a thermographer can manually enter the image and its pertinent metadata into DICOM format, as a CSV (comma-separated value) radiometric matrix, or a scaled and annotated image in PNG or other format. This is done using a DICOM-writing application program. Basic DICOM software can be downloaded for free via this website: www.pacsone.net. Mathworks' MATLAB also provides a DICOM Writer (dicomwrite). A method for converting raw thermographic data using DICOM and XML configuration files has been developed, setting the stage for thermal imager manufacturers to integrate infrared imaging into the DICOM standard.[11]

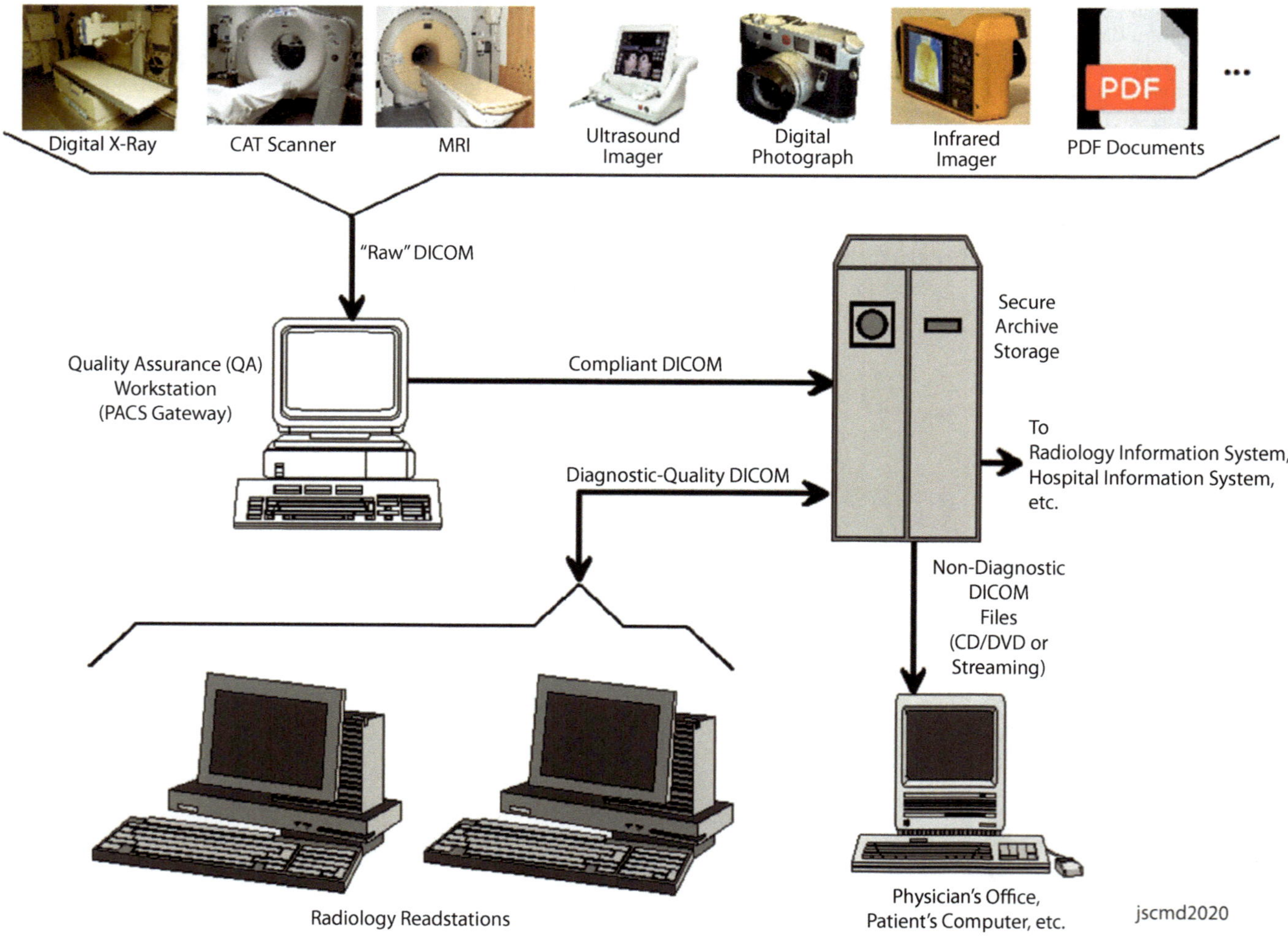

FIGURE 12.5 Schematic showing the flow of DICOM-formatted image files through a typical PACS (picture archiving and communication system). Individual systems and features may vary depending on institutional requirements.

Presently, the DICOM standard is actively maintained by the committee to meet the evolving needs of medical imaging. This committee must approve any proposed DICOM metadata standards; the DICOM specifications document presently encompasses 13 volumes. Since the implementation of DICOM is complicated, an urgent need for thermography organizations is to arrive at a consensus regarding the appropriate metadata fields for DICOM's adoption of clinical thermography.

SIDEBAR 12.1 SUGGESTIONS FOR TOMORROW'S RESEARCHERS

- Document imager type(s) and temperature offset and gain calibration for each in all papers
- Document imaging environment: temperature, significant infrared sources present, airflow, etc.
- Use calibrated contact thermometers to accurately record a subject's core temperature
- Document the time of day that imaging was performed
- Menstrual cycle timing may be important for women's studies
- Document the patient temperature equilibration protocol
- Document the test procedure fully, especially any dynamic thermal protocols
- Using a greyscale or spectral color palette, scale all images to maximize the thermal visual contrast

Future research

First: A fair breast cancer trial

Hypotheses: 21st Century thermography is a more effective primary screening tool than mammography. Thermography can detect tumors missed by mammography in women with dense breasts. Breast thermography is an effective screening tool in younger women (under age 40).

In the 1970s, Breast Cancer Detection and Demonstration Project (BCDDP), thermography "lost" to X-ray mammography. The low-resolution thermal scanners and displays of that time, the lack of proper thermographic protocols, and inadequate training of the scan interpreters all played major roles in that decision. While rejecting breast thermography, however, the BCDDP strongly advised further development and study of thermal imaging under controlled conditions.[12] These developments and studies have now been accomplished. With the vastly-improved thermal and spatial resolution of modern imagers and well-developed protocols for breast thermography, the time has come for a rematch of X-ray mammography and thermal breast imaging in the early detection and screening of breast malignancy.

To allow sufficient time for follow-up, this rematch would continue 10 to 12 years, with imaging provided annually. As with the X-ray mammographers, only well-trained thermographers would be included, all using calibrated, top-of-the-line thermal imagers and applying the same practice guidelines for optimal infrared image interpretation.

A similar randomized study could examine thermographic prognostic significance in early-stage breast cancer patients, with risk stratification based on age, breast density, tumor size, tumor grade, tumor margins, lymph node involvement, body fat distribution, and other factors.[13]

Another study could undertake a retrospective analysis of data from multiple well-established thermography clinics using modern thermographic equipment and established practice guidelines. Study size would need to be large in order to maximize statistical power. The women would be matched with a group of women who had chosen screening mammography during the same period of time. The study would determine whether thermographic screening examinations could effectively detect breast tumors in women aged 40 to 74 years.

Pre-invasive or noninvasive melanomas

Hypothesis: Thermography can be used to monitor melanomas in lower-risk groups to avoid excessive surgeries and other treatments.

Early diagnosis may improve survival rates for many types of cancer, but not all cancers detected early will go on to become aggressive or potentially life-threatening. Cancer screening may pick up substantial numbers of indolent or benign lesions. Neoplasms that follow a more indolent course may never advance, and many will spontaneously regress.[14] The increasing incidence of some tumor types has not been matched by an increase in mortality.[15] Early diagnosis of indolent neoplasms may translate into unnecessary and harmful treatments that could worsen overall morbidity and mortality.[16]

Cutaneous malignant melanoma can follow a very slow and non-threatening course.[17] There has been a marked increase in the incidence of melanoma in the past few decades. This increase has occurred despite a huge increase in the excision of *benign* skin lesions.[18] Detection of early stage and lower-grade melanoma has increased, with little change seen in melanoma mortality rates.[19] Taken together, these findings suggest an over-diagnosis of malignant melanoma.[20]

Many thin cutaneous melanomas will never progress if left untreated, or will only progress at such a slow rate that the individual does not develop metastatic disease in his or her lifetime.[21] If indeed many melanomas tend to be biologically benign, a more conservative approach to treatment and management may be warranted.

Investigations are needed to determine whether thermography can be used to monitor melanomas in lower-risk groups (e.g., younger women) to avoid excessive surgeries and other treatments. Progression of melanoma with increased inflammation and angiogenesis may be detected using the QUAINT procedure described in Chapter 10.[22] This method is in need of clinical testing.

Breast cancer – Avoidance of overtreatment

Hypothesis: thermography can identify which of the lower-risk DCIS cases (grades 1 and 2) are likely to progress or recur as invasive breast cancer, and which cases will remain indolent.

Breast thermography can detect breast lesions that are often missed by screening mammography. The question then becomes: If such small lesions can be found by thermography, will this increase the chances of overdiagnosis and overtreatment? The question has relevance because of the remarkable phenotypic heterogeneity within many cancers.[23] Indolent lesions with low malignant potential are extremely common, and screening has greatly increased the detection rate for indolent lesions and their precursors (e.g., DCIS). It has been estimated that one-third to one-half of all mammography-detected breast cancers are being over-diagnosed.[24] This high detection of indolent lesions often results in overtreatment.[25] Patients with low-grade DCIS who do not undergo surgery show no difference in breast cancer survival rates.[26] There is considerable evidence that low-to-intermediate grade DCIS is being over-treated.[27] Much of this is due to mammography (which picks up most DCIS due to calcifications) being unable to identify tumors that have a lethal potential.

The transition from DCIS to an invasive breast cancer can be detected by thermography better than mammography. The activity of nitric oxide synthase (NOS) isoforms is significantly higher in DCIS than in normal surrounding tissues, and increased NOS activity may be associated with angiogenesis and the early development of invasive breast cancer and other cancers.[28]

Factors linked with rapid tumor growth rate are strongly associated with abnormal thermograms.[29] Cancer prognosis is significantly correlated with the thermal patterns of the tumor and surrounding tissues.[30] Thus the more indolent and less aggressive tumors are likely to have a smaller thermal signature compared to more rapidly growing tumors.

Serial thermography can be used to help guide decision-making around the monitoring of DCIS cases and appropriate treatment strategies. Smaller indolent lesions can be treated more conservatively.[31] Minimally toxic approaches could be used to induce tumor regression without the need for more substantial surgery and treatment.[32]

Monitoring response to cancer treatment

Hypothesis: During and after cytotoxic treatments, serial monitoring of skin temperatures in the tumor region provides clinical information concerning treatment efficacy, making it possible to adjust the treatment regimen and individualize treatment schedules.

Patients undergoing radiotherapy demonstrate vascular changes during treatment to the tumor area, which can be thermographically monitored and evaluated.[33] Damage to the tumor's vasculature is a critical determinant of radiotherapy's effectiveness.[34] Quantifiable changes in vasculature during radiotherapy show a reduction in the number of vessels during the treatments (Figure 12.6). Thermal monitoring of treatment response could be extended to chemotherapy and immunotherapy. Multiple images can reveal changes in the tumor state, which can be correlated with other indicators of treatment efficacy. More research into these algorithmic methods is needed.

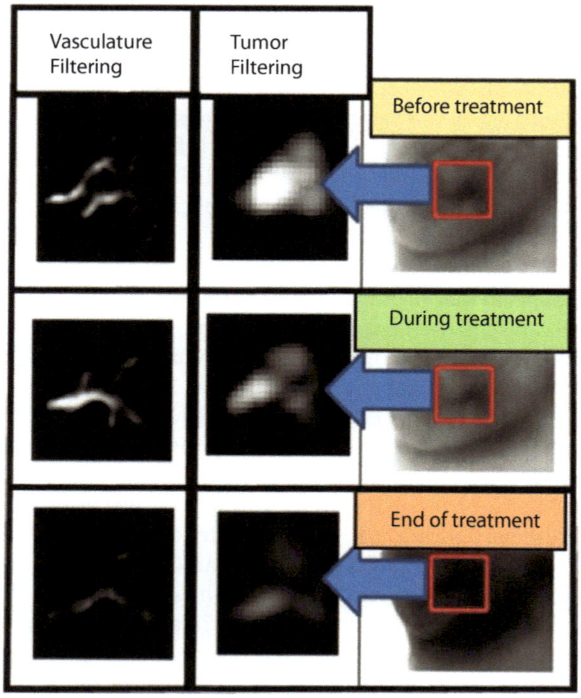

FIGURE 12.6 Thermal monitoring of BrCA radiation treatment showing a reduction in vascularity and size.[35]

Monitoring breast cancer relapses

Hypotheses: Thermography is prognostic of BrCA metastasis. Thermography can detect local recurrence. Thermography can help assess BrCA treatments.

A very abnormal breast thermograph portends a more "active" disease with a less favorable prognosis; angiogenic and inflammatory processes generate a stronger thermal signal, indicating more aggressive disease behavior.[36] With the increased spatial resolution of modern imagers, it is now possible to detect inflamed lymphatics coursing over the breast, tracks that are distinct from venous patterns. Because this inflammation suggests carcinomatous lymphatic spread, it may correlate qualitatively with both the size and overall direction of metastatic invasion. A combined thermography-histopathology study of this phenomenon is needed to determine if the lymphatic pattern is due to invading cells, a reaction to their upstream presence, or other factors.

Studies have focused on breast thermography as a prognostic tool for predicting tumor growth and survival in breast cancer patients. In node-negative breast cancer patients who undergo thermal imaging prior to surgery, those with an abnormal thermal pattern have a much greater risk of mortality.[37] Breast cancer patients with severe thermographic abnormalities have more aggressive tumors that are more likely to recur or metastasize.[38] It is now time to conduct trials to see how thermography can be used to assess the short- and long-term efficacy of cancer treatment in breast cancer patients.[39]

Intraoperative support for lumpectomy

Hypothesis: Thermography can help localize breast tumor margins.

Lumpectomy is commonly used to treat early-stage breast cancer. During the procedure, the tumor is removed and the surgical margins are routinely sampled for the presence of cancer cells via frozen section histology. When malignant cells are found at the margins, additional tissue may be removed, often leading to prolonged procedures and an increased the risk of surgical complications. New methods such as fluorescent imaging and photoacoustic imaging are being investigated but are either time-consuming or tend to have a limited field of view. Thermography has the potential to provide real-time imaging to guide tissue excision during a lumpectomy by delineating tumor margins.

An approach known as Enhanced Thermal Imaging (ETI) is designed to detect the vascular networks associated with malignant growth. The technique selectively heats the blood by approximately 0.5°C by using strong 530 nm (green) LED light. The warmer blood gives better thermal contrast between the vessels and surrounding tissue. Thermal images then reveal a clear delineation of the vascular structures. The enhanced images display a corona of bright emission along the edges of cancer associated with the surgical margin.[40] More research is needed to bring ETI into clinical use.

Support for breast reconstruction

Hypothesis: Thermography can help plan plastic surgery pedicle and free flaps.

During autologous flap procedures, the plastics surgeon is confronted with multiple challenges, notably the selection of a suitable vascular perforator bundle with sufficient blood supply for the flap, surgical excision of that perforator, determination of perfusion area of the perforator, microsurgical anastomosis, and shaping the completed flap. Dynamic Infrared Thermography (DIRT) has been proposed to help identify perforators. DIRT can map the influence of each perforator on the flap perfusion, monitor the perforator's integrity after dissection, and monitor vascular patency of the free flap after anastomosis. DIRT appears to be a useful, non-invasive tool for all the phases of flap transplantation with minimal interference to the operative procedure.[41] More research to simplify and integrate DIRT into plastic surgery procedures is needed.

Monitoring oral mucositis in cancer patients

Hypothesis: Thermography can detect early mucositis caused by cancer therapies.

Oral mucositis, a painful inflammation linked to cancer treatment, is seen in up to 80% of patients receiving high-dose chemotherapy and in up to 100% of patients receiving radiation for head and neck cancer. Mucositis occurs in approximately 40% of patients receiving conventional chemotherapy.[42] Mucositis usually becomes symptomatic 4–5 days after beginning treatment, reaching a peak at around day 10 and then slowly improving over the course of a few weeks. Mucositis associated with radiotherapy usually appears at the end of the second week of treatment and may last for six to eight weeks.[43]

Thermography can detect small and early changes in skin surface temperature associated with the development of mucositis in patients undergoing chemoradiotherapy.[44] Areas of mucositis average 2°C (3.6°F) warmer than the oral mucosa of normal controls. Necrotic plaque over the mucositis ulcers can be detected as a cool area equal to normal mucosal temperatures.[45]

Future studies should investigate thermographic findings in cancer patients undergoing chemotherapy or radiotherapy.

Pediatrics and neonatal care

Hypothesis: Thermographic monitoring can improve outcomes in neonatal care.

In neonatal care, monitoring the temperature of the newborn is essential for ensuring the infant's ongoing health and for detecting early signs of disease or dysfunction. Thermography has the advantage of not disturbing the infant or disrupting their sleep. Thermal imaging can monitor a neonate's temperature, respiration, and limb warmth (Figure 12.7). "Thermal imaging is a reliable and non-invasive method for continuous monitoring of the emitted temperature of the neonates, with potential for contributing to the assurance of wellbeing, and to the diagnosis of pathologies, including internal abnormalities."[46]

Large prospective studies are needed to get a clearer understanding of the benefits and the barriers to the use of thermal imaging in neonatology. Recent improvements in miniaturization now allow the placement of wide-angle imagers *inside* the incubator, where they can provide an unobstructed thermal view of the infant that can be monitored at the nursing station.

For older children, thermal imaging has been shown to be an effective tool in other pediatric specialties, namely in fracture screening, detection of bacterial throat infections, osteogenic pattern recognition, and burn wound assessments.[48] The use of thermal imaging in young children holds special appeal because its non-contact, non-invasive nature reduces anxiety in the child. Pediatric thermography holds great possibilities; research in this field is encouraged.

Monitoring for diabetic foot problems

Hypothesis: Thermal monitoring can improve outcomes of diabetic foot conditions.

Thermography is useful for early detection of abnormalities of the foot by analyzing asymmetries and local temperature changes over time. Foot ulcers are an extremely common diabetic complication and a leading cause of amputation. An increase of 2°C (3.6°F) in the skin temperature on the plantar surface of the

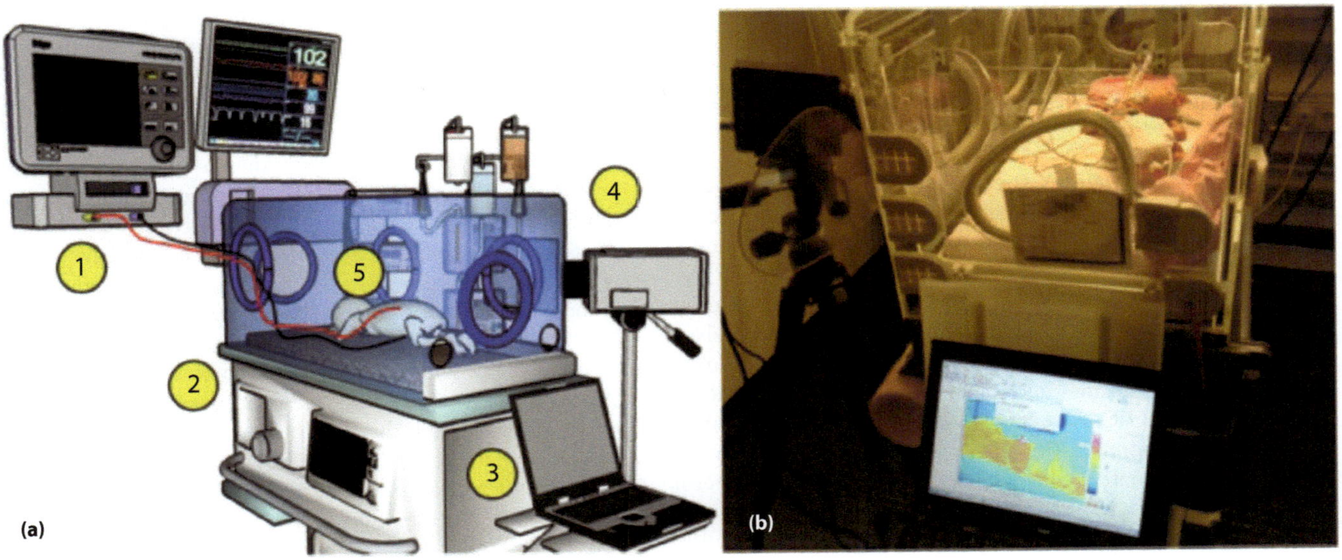

FIGURE 12.7 Experimental setup for neonatal IR thermography. This setup employs thermography in association with clinical temperature measurement (a) three-dimensional schematic showing components and elements of the setup: (1) patient monitoring system, (2) convective infant incubator unit, (3) analysis workstation, (4) IR imager, and (5) the infant with two skin electrodes connected. (b) Photograph of typical clinical setting.[47]

foot can serve as an early indication of injury or inflammation. Early detection of a hotspot region can lead to interventions that reduce the risk of developing a foot ulcer.[49] Handheld infrared thermography is a useful home-monitoring tool for reducing the risk of a foot ulcer recurrence.[50] Thermal images of plantar footprints are another way to detect incipient problems, and may be easier to obtain.

The rapid development of handheld smartphone-based thermal infrared imagers presents a creative solution for better managing this chronic condition. Such devices can generate clinically useful thermal foot images for assessing skin temperatures in the diabetic foot.[51] Small thermographic devices can help screen high-risk patients for timely intervention, as well as improve adherence to protective footwear.[52] Further studies are needed to optimize smartphone technologies and grade the thermal findings of diabetic foot conditions.

Atherosclerosis detection

Hypothesis: Thermology can detect arterial endothelial inflammation.

Atherosclerosis entails the buildup of fatty plaque in the artery walls, ultimately restricting blood flow or flaking off as emboli. Atherosclerosis is a chronic inflammatory process.[53] The inflammation is both local and systemic, with both the innate and adaptive immune systems playing key roles in its initiation and progression.[54] Arteries are generally located too deep anatomically to be detected by thermal imaging (except during surgery), but they can be studied by other thermological methods.

The endothelial inflammatory component provides heat to the intraluminal blood flow. Thermology can detect this local temperature variation, aiding the detection of atherosclerotic plaques in the coronary vessels. Several cardiac catheter designs utilizing micro-thermistor technology have been employed to study this inflammation. Coronary thermology research has generated some important pathophysiological information.

Coronary inflammation and cardiac muscle contractions both increase the blood temperature as it flows through the coronary arteries and into the venous coronary sinus. Blood temperature differences have been measured in patients with symptomatic coronary artery disease. Compared to subjects without coronary artery disease, patients with angiographically significant lesions show a greater coronary blood temperature rise.

Thermal heterogeneity is the difference in blood temperature adjacent to an inflamed arterial endothelium compared to blood temperature adjacent to normal endothelium. Acute coronary syndromes are characterized by diffuse thermal heterogeneity of up to 1.5°C (2.7°F) as measured by intra-arterial thermistors.[55] How well this temperature profile can be visualized thermographically during open-chest heart procedures is under study.[56] Thermal heterogeneity is reduced in patients treated with HMG-CoA reductase inhibitors, independent of the clinical syndrome.[57] These "statin" medications appear to have anti-inflammatory effects beyond lowering cholesterol levels.

Dietary changes that lower cholesterol levels significantly decrease thermal heterogeneity of atherosclerotic plaque.[58] Plant-based "heart friendly" diets could improve cardiovascular outcomes.[59] Furthermore, supplementation with omega-3 fatty acids may inhibit vascular inflammation.[60] Thermography may aid in assessments of these nutritional regimens.

Computer-aided thermography and artificial intelligence

Hypothesis: Development and validation of artificial intelligence (AI), fractal, and other computer-aided (C-A) methods for thermal pattern analysis will improve the speed and accuracy of thermographic image interpretation.

Today's third-generation thermal imagers utilize large focal plane array (FPA) detectors and on-board image processing to increase thermal sensitivity, spatial resolution, and reliability.[61] These uncooled microbolometer-based infrared imagers have immensely improved medical thermal imaging.[62] Professional thermal imagers currently have a minimum resolution of 320 × 240 pixels, allowing detection of tiny thermal features.[63] Thermal imagers that have a resolution of 640 × 480 pixels are becoming available.

Eventually, automated methods will overcome the limitations of manual thermographic analysis. There are limits regarding how many thermograms even the most skilled human thermographer can view, process, and successfully interpret. Computers, however, can quickly process an image and extract the relevant information without tiring. C-A thermography can objectify the findings and minimize the inter-observer variability that occurs with human interpretation.

To improve the accuracy of thermal image processing, future research will focus on three technical aspects: (1) feature extraction and classification; (2) smart image enhancement; and (3) asymmetry analysis. Ongoing progress in software image analysis will integrate signal processing algorithms as well as manage a huge knowledge base. Nevertheless, C-A thermography will require high-level training and experience to ensure quality outcomes.

The four steps of C-A thermography are (1) preprocessing of the thermogram, (2) segmentation or extraction of the ROI, (3) extraction of features within the ROI, and (4) classification of a particular ROI as normal versus abnormal, or healthy versus diseased.

Various techniques are involved in preprocessing, such as resizing the images using template and interpolation techniques, mapping the input to the output image pixel intensity values, and using algorithms such as the adaptive histogram equalization method.[64] The further refinement of these and other preprocessing methods will be essential to improving the accuracy of thermographic analysis.

Automated segmentation can be used to better analyze hotspots and asymmetries within the thermogram. Accurate segmentation is a challenging task, however, because it must establish an accurate contour and then derive the ROI accordingly. Shape, color, and texture are features commonly incorporated into segmentation algorithms. A blood vessel segmentation method has been proposed to map out regions based on the vessels' shape and intensity.[65] Automated segmentation is expected to undergo major improvements in the coming years.

Asymmetry analysis can be improved using Artificial Intelligence (AI) and thermal radiomics.[66] Much of the AI research in thermography has focused on image mining – the uncovering of hidden information within images. Image mining, in turn, is dependent on deep learning without input from humans. A complex set of algorithms models high-level abstractions in data to find information within the thermogram. Multiple processing layers (analogous to layers of neurons) exist between the input and output. Deep-learning algorithms employ multiple linear and non-linear transformations that comprise the processing layers.[67]

In breast thermography, multiple images are used to inform the input layer and then the hidden layers. The output of the last hidden layer provides input to the output layer, where a clinical decision is made.[68] Drawing from a dataset of thermograms of known disease, algorithms for segmentation using deep learning can achieve a 99% accuracy rate for breast cancer detection.[69] A similar approach can detect breast tumors independent of the image capture and view angle, enabling automated image analysis.[70]

The use of fractals can further improve the process of AI-based thermography. Fractal analyses show that the boundaries of benign tumors are well defined, while boundaries of malignant tumors are irregular, i.e., have more fractal dimensions.[71] Fractal analyses of thermograms reveal more fractal dimensions within increasingly malignant tumors.[72] In fractal AI, the thermal edge and core of a cancerous area in a thermogram can be detected by a "fuzzy active contour" which may actually be detecting the wispy lymphatic patterns accompanying a tumor. This particular contour has been found to circumscribe an area of malignant tissue.[73]

Future generation C-A thermography will make thermographic analysis more cost-effective; the operational costs for computer-based systems are low when compared with those based on manual analysis.[74] This integration and reduced dependency on human labor results in rapid throughput and centralized processing, factors that can create a higher level of thermographic accuracy and reliability.[75]

Conclusion

Major improvements in thermal sensitivity and resolution, a better understanding of proper calibration practices, and availability of low-cost professional imagers now allow clinicians to take full advantage of thermography within their disciplines. Published peer-reviewed medical research is constantly expanding the range of applications for medical thermography. Unfortunately, many older studies did not provide information on imager calibration, putting much of the reported temperature data in doubt; these studies will need repeating. In this chapter, some of the more promising future directions for the practice of clinical thermography have been described. With the advent of novel applications as well as improved imaging devices and testing protocols, an expanding use of thermal imaging will continue to improve the medical and surgical practices of the future.

Notes

1. Source: Photonics Spectra Reference Chart © 2021 Laurin Publishing, Pittsfield, MA.
2. Image Credit: Michael Joseph Wawrzewski III, PA-C; Clinic in a Can, Wichita, KS, USA; Used by permission.
3. https://aathermology.org/organization-2/guidelines/
4. Baines CJ, Breast J. 2005; Doi.org/10.1111/j.1075-122X.2005.217162.x
5. Graham RNJ et al., Clin Radiol. 2005; PMID: 16223609. Doi: 10.1016/j.crad.2005.07.003. See also: DICOM reference guide. Health Devices. 2001; PMID: 11258234.
6. Gibaud B., NATO Security through Science Series B: Physics and Biophysics, Springer, Dordrecht, 2008. Doi: 10.1007/978-1-4020-8752-3_13
7. Noumeir R, J Digit Imaging 2005; PMCID: PMC3046723.
8. Bidgood WD Jr et al., J Am Med Inform Assoc. 1997; Doi: 10.1136/jamia.1997.0040199
9. Vardasca T et al., EAT 2012 Book of Proceedings (2012). ISSN-1560-604X, p79. See also: Robertson I, Clin Tech Small Anim Pract. 2007; Doi: 10.1053/j.ctsap.2007.05.008
10. Schaefer, G et al., IEEE Engineering in Medicine and Biology Society. Conference 2006. Doi: 10.1109/IEMBS.2006.259523
11. Rumiński J, 29th Annual International Conference of the IEEE Engineering in Medicine and Biology Society, Doi: 10.1109/IEMBS.2007.4352273 Corpus ID: 21341714
12. Bronzino JD (ed.), The Biomedical Engineering Handbook, 3rd Ed, CRC Press, 2006, Section 26.1.2 ISBN 0-8493-2122-0.
13. Syed YY, Mol Diagn Ther. 2020; PMID: 32613290. Doi: 10.1007/s40291-020-00482-7
14. Zahl PH, et al., Arch Intern Med. 2008; PMID: 19029493. Doi: 10.1001/archinte.168.21.2311. See also: Esserman L et al., JAMA 2009, PMID: 19843904. Doi: 10.1001/jama.2009.1498
15. Esserman L et al., J Natl Cancer Inst. 2010. Doi:10.1093/jnci/djq119
16. Welch HG et al., J Natl Cancer Inst. 2010; PMID: 20413742. Doi: 10.1093/jnci/djq099
17. Glasziou PP et al., Med J Aust. 2020; PMID: 31858624, PMCID: PMC7065073. Doi: 10.5694/mja2.50455
18. Esserman LJ et al., JAMA 2013; PMID: 23896967. Doi: 10.1001/jama.2013.108415. See also: Geller AC et al., J Clin Oncol. 2013; PMID: 24043747, PMCID: PMC3906570, Doi: 10.1200/JCO.2012.47.3728
19. Welch HG et al., BMJ 2005; PMID: 16081427, PMCID: PMC1199022. Doi: 10.1136/bmj.38516.649537.E0
20. Nørgaard C et al., Acta Derm Venereol. 2011; PMID: 21874217, Doi: 10.2340/00015555-1177
21. Erickson C et al., Clin Dermatol. 2010; PMID: 20541680. Doi: 10.1016/j.clindermatol.2009.06.021. See also: Shuster S, Br J Dermatol. 2009; PMID: 19785614. Doi: 10.1111/j.1365-2133.2009.09399.x
22. Melnikova VO et al., Pigment Cell Melanoma Res. 2009; PMID: 19368690. Doi: 10.1111/j.1755-148X.2009.00570.x. See also: Lee JT et al., J Cell Biochem. 2007; PMID: 17171636. Doi: 10.1002/jcb.21204. See also: Emmett MS et al., Am J Cancer Res. 2011; PMCID: PMC3196284.
23. Shieh Y et al., Nat Rev Clin Oncol. 2016, PMCID: PMC6585415. Doi: 10.1038/nrclinonc.2016.50
24. Autier P et al., Eur J Cancer. 2018; PMID: 29272783. Doi: 10.1016/j.ejca.2017.11.002
25. Welch HG et al., J Natl Cancer Inst. 2010; PMID: 20413742. Doi: 10.1093/jnci/djq099
26. Sagara Y et al., Front Oncol. 2017; Doi: 10.3389/fonc.2017.00192
27. Van Seijen M et al., Br J Cancer. 2019; PMCID: PMC6697179. Doi: 10.1038/s41416-019-0478-6. See also: Groen EJ et al., Breast 2017; PMID: 27671693. Doi: 10.1016/j.breast.2016.09.001. See also: Van der Borden CL et al., Trends Cancer. 2019; PMID: 31311652. Doi: 10.1016/j.trecan.2019.05.005
28. Ehrenfeld P et al., Nitric Oxide 2019; PMID: 30862477. Doi: 10.1016/j.niox.2019.03.002. See also: Monteiro HP et al., Nitric Oxide 2019; PMID: 31009708. Doi: 10.1016/j.niox.2019.04.009
29. Head JF et al., Ann N Y Acad Sci. 1993; PMID: 8279754. Doi: 10.1111/j.1749-6632.1993.tb17203.x
30. Amalu WC et al., Infrared Imaging of the Breast – An Overview. In JD Bronzino (ed.), Biomedical Engineering Handbook, 3rd Ed, Medical Devices and Systems, CRC Press, 2006, p. 20.
31. Shehata M et al., J Breast Imaging 2019; PMCID: PMC6735611. Doi: 10.1093/jbi/wbz039. See also: Li Y et al., Nutrients 2017; Doi: 10.3390/nu9070728. PMID: 28698459; PMCID: PMC5537842. See also: Bodai BI et al., Perm J. 2018; https://doi.org/10.7812/TPP/17-025
32. Fritz H et al., Integr Cancer Ther. 2014. Doi: 10.1177/1534735414534463, PMID: 24867961.
33. Hoffer OA et al., J Biomed Opt. 2018; PMCID: PMC5933077. Doi: 10.1117/1.JBO.23.5.058001
34. Garcia-Barros M et al., Science 2003; PMID: 12750523. Doi: 10.1126/science.1082504
35. Image from Hoffer OA et al., J Biomed Opt. 2018. Doi: 10.1117/1.JBO.23.5.058001, CC-BY-4.0

36. Ham M et al., Arch Pharm Res. 2013; PMID: 24222504. Doi: 10.1007/s12272-013-0271-7
37. Wu LA et al., BMC Cancer 2016. Doi: 10.1186/s12885-016-2602-9
38. Head JF et al., Ann N Y Acad Sci. 1993; PMID: 8279754. Doi: 10.1111/j.1749-6632.1993.tb17203.x
39. Mustacchi G et al., Tumori 1984; PMID: 6506231. See also: Ikeda T et al., Gan To Kagaku Ryoho. 1989; PMID: 2658842.
40. Case JR et al., J Biomed Opt. 2015. Doi: 10.1117/1.JBO.20.11.116003
41. Thiessen FEF et al., Eur J Obstet Gynecol Reprod Biol. 2020; PMID: 32623250. Doi: 10.1016/j.ejogrb.2020.05.038
42. Pico JL et al., Oncologist 1998; PMID: 10388137. See also: Lalla RV et al., Dent Clin North Am. 2014; PMID: 24655526. Doi: 10.1016/j.cden.2013.12.005
43. Rubenstein, EB et al., Cancer 2004. Doi:10.1002/cncr.20163. PMID 15108223.
44. Cohen EE et al., Oral Oncol. 2013; PMCID: PMC3797568. Doi: 10.1016/j.oraloncology.2013.07.009
45. White BA et al., Int J Tissue React. 1987; PMID: 3610508.
46. Topalidou A et al., BMC Pregnancy Childbirth. 2019. Doi: 10.1186/s12884-019-2533-y
47. Figure and caption from: Abbas AK, Leonhardt S, BMC Med Imaging 2014. Doi: 10.1186/1471-2342-14-9. PMID: 24580961. PMCID: PMC4015601. CC-BY-2.0.
48. Owen R et al., BMJ Paediatr Open 2017. Doi: 10.1136/bmjpo-2017-000080
49. Ilo A et al., J Diabetes Sci Technol. 2020; PMCID: PMC7189167. Doi: 10.1177/1932296819871270
50. Hazenberg CEVB et al., Diabetes Metab Res Rev. 2020; doi: 10.1002/dmrr.3247.
51. van Doremalen RFM, et al., J Diabetes Sci Technol. 2020; PMCID: PMC7189170. Doi: 10.1177/1932296819854062
52. Najafi B et al., Diabetes Metab Res Rev. 2020; PMID: 31909547. Doi:10.1002/dmrr.3239
53. Talepoor AG et al., Endocr Metab Immune Disord Drug Targets 2020; PMID: 31622224. Doi: 10.2174/1871530319666191016095725
54. Herrero-Fernandez B et al., Int J Mol Sci. 2019; PMCID: PMC6862594. Doi: 10.3390/ijms20215293
55. Toutouzas K et al., J Interv Cardiol. 2005; PMID: 16336430. Doi: 10.1111/j.1540-8183.2005.00090.x
56. Suma H et al., Ann Thorac Surg. 2000; PMID: 11093537. Doi: 10.1016/s0003-4975(00)01886-5
57. Toutouzas K et al., Am Heart J. 2004; PMID: 15523307. Doi: 10.1016/j.ahj.2004.05.013. See also: Stefanadis C et al., Eur Heart J. 2002. Doi: 10.1053/euhj.2002.3174
58. Verheye S et al., Eur Heart J. 2004. Doi 10.1016/j.ehj.2003.10.023
59. Ventegodt S et al., Sci World J. 2006. Doi: 10.1100/tsw.2006.330. See also: Tuso P et al., Perm J. 2015; PMCID: PMC4315380. Doi: 10.7812/TPP/14-036. See also: Kerley CP, Card Fail Rev. 2018; PMCID: PMC5971679. Doi: 10.15420/cfr.2018:1:1
60. Carracedo M et al., Semin Immunopathol. 2019; PMCID: PMC6881483.
61. Lahiri BB et al., Medical Applications of Infrared Thermography: A Review. Infrared Phys Technol. 2012. Doi 10.1016/j.infrared.2012.03.007
62. Ring EFJ, High Resolution Infrared Imaging. Eur J Thermol. 1998;8:121.
63. Poerbaningtyas E et al., J Biomed Phys Eng. 2020; PMCID: PMC7321399.
64. Faust O et al., Infrared Phys Technol. 2014; PMCID: PMC7108233. See also: Blu T et al., Linear Interpolation Revitalized. IEEE Trans. Image Process 2004. Doi: 10.1109/TIP.2004.826093. See also: Gonzalez RC et al., Digital Image Processing Using MATLAB, vol. 2. Gatesmark Publishing, Knoxville, 2009. ISBN-13: 978-0982085400.
65. Kakileti ST et al., JCO Glob Oncol. 2020; PMCID: PMC7605380.
66. Francis SV et al., J Med Eng Technol. 2013; PMID: 23194447. Doi: 10.3109/03091902.2012.728674. See also: Kakileti ST et al., Artif Intell Med. 2020. Doi:10.1016/j.artmed.2020.101854
67. Ramesh V, International Journal of Engineering and Management Research (IJEMR). 2017; https://www.ijemr.net/DOC/AReviewOnApplicationOfDeepLearningInThermography.PDF
68. Mambou SJ et al., Sensors (Basel). 2018. Doi: 10.3390/s18092799
69. Ekici S et al., Med Hypotheses. 2019. Doi: 10.1016/j.mehy.2019.109542
70. Kakileti ST et al., Conf Proc IEEE Eng Med Biol Soc. 2019. Doi: 10.1109/EMBC.2019.8856628
71. Silva TAED et al., Sensors (Basel). 2020. Doi: 10.3390/s20143866
72. Zade MA et al., IET Syst Biol. 2019; PMID: 30774110 DOI: 10.1049/iet-syb.2018.5020
73. Ghayoumi Zadeh H et al., Segmenting Breast Cancerous Regions in Thermal Images Using Fuzzy Active Contours. EXCLI J. 2016; PMCID: PMC5225687.
74. Ng EY et al., BMC Cancer 2004. Doi: 10.1186/1471-2407-4-17
75. Faust O et al., Infrared Phys Technol. 2014; PMCID: PMC7108233.

AN ATLAS OF NORMAL HUMAN THERMOGRAPHY

Unless you know what is thermographically normal, you cannot know what is abnormal. Especially with a new field such as high-resolution human thermography, an atlas of normal images is essential. One problem arises, however, when assembling an atlas of normals: What is normal? A thermogram read as "normal" by a qualified thermologist does not mean that the subject is "healthy," only that the thermogram in question appears within normal limits. A normal thermogram of a 20-year-old woman will be very different from a normal 70-year-old man. As a person ages, they develop small thermographic blemishes such as moles, skin creases, or small venous markings that can be considered normal. Also, a "normal" thermographic appearance will depend on the subject's position and activity during the temperature equilibration period. The superficial muscles of balance in the legs will appear warm in a standing position because they must remain active to maintain an upright posture. These muscles may appear cooler if equilibration is done sitting or supine. The trapezius and posterior neck muscles may appear warm if equilibration is done in a sitting or standing position. These thermal appearances can be considered normal once body position is taken into account. Despite postural differences, there are certain thermographic normals that pertain to all ages, sexes, and body types. This atlas is a collection of qualitative normal static images; no images taken with dynamic cooling or heating are included. To aid the user of this atlas, each subject's sex and age are provided, and small anomalies in the image may be explained. The images are presented anatomically from head to foot. Where possible, both male and female examples are shown. All subjects have been thermally equilibrated at 68°F (20°C) for at least 15 minutes in a standing/walking position. The images (Figures 13.1-13.24) were taken under standard thermographic environmental conditions and are presented in a standard Blue–Red spectral color palette using the full-span scaling technique.

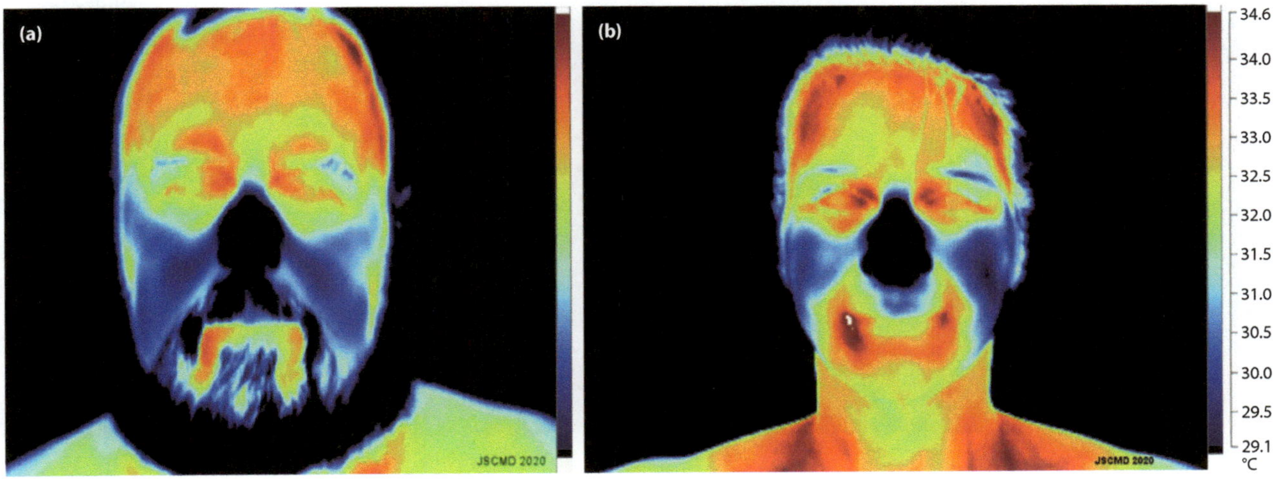

FIGURE 13.1 (a) Face frontal view, normal – bearded 66 yoM. (b) Face frontal view, normal – 27 yoF. The right side of the face is often slightly warmer than the left.

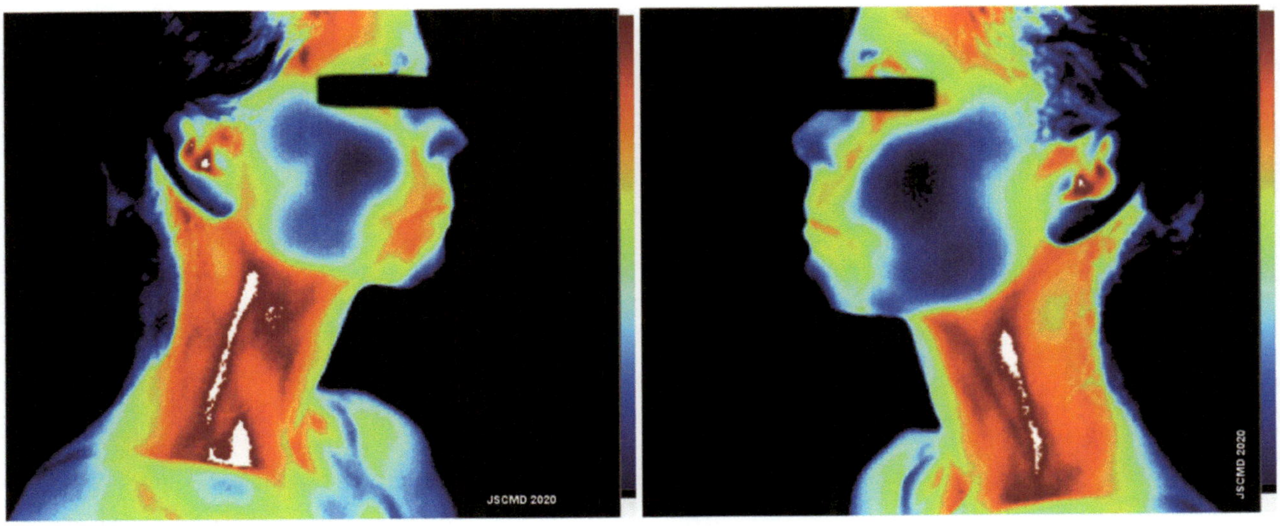

FIGURE 13.2 Face and neck lateral oblique views, isothermal, normal – 65 yoF.

DOI: 10.1201/9781003281764-14

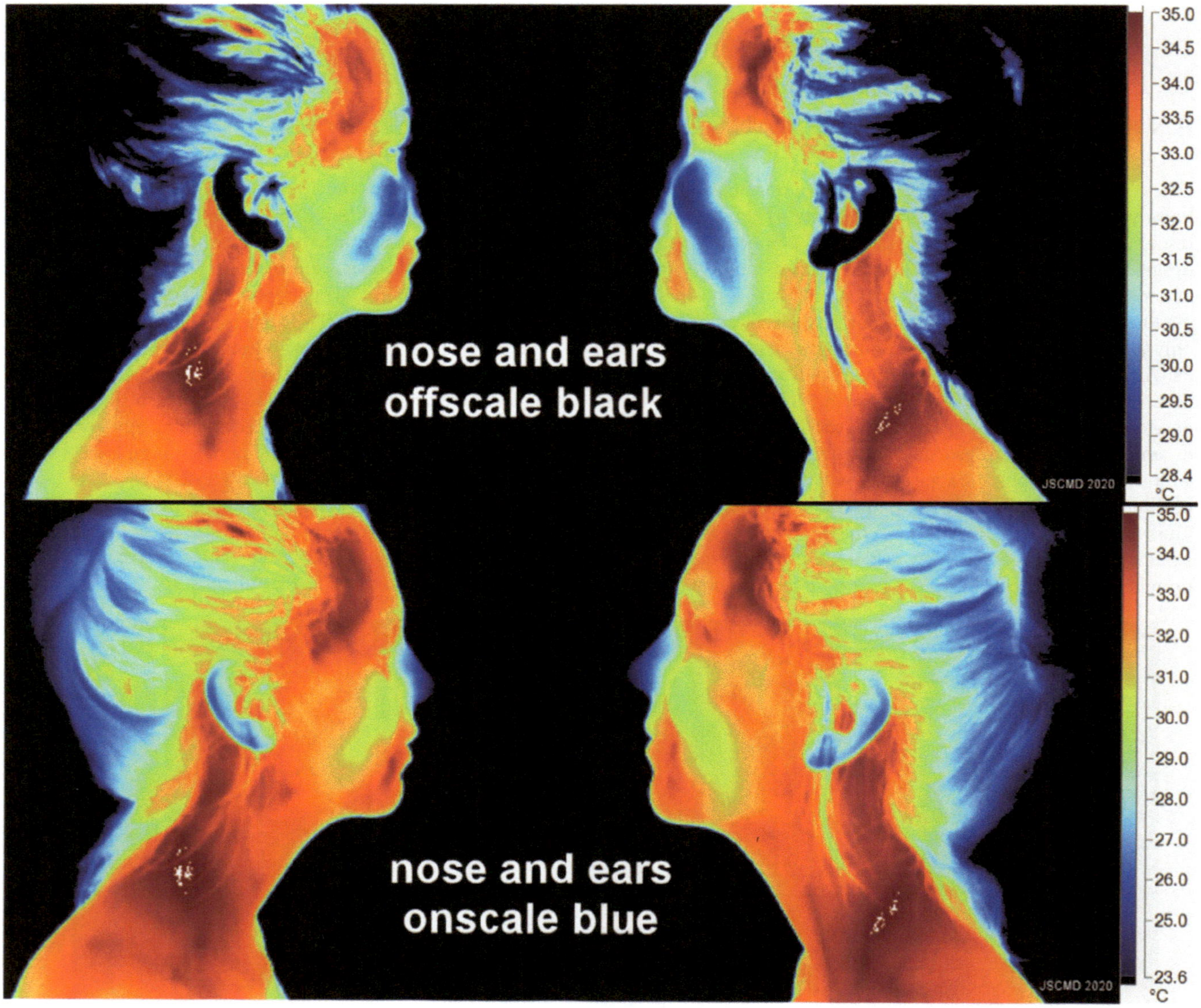

FIGURE 13.3 Face and neck lateral views, normal – 27 yoF. The upper and lower images are identical, but scaled differently to bring out the features of the face (*upper*) or show the cold nose and ears at the expense of face thermal detail (*lower*).

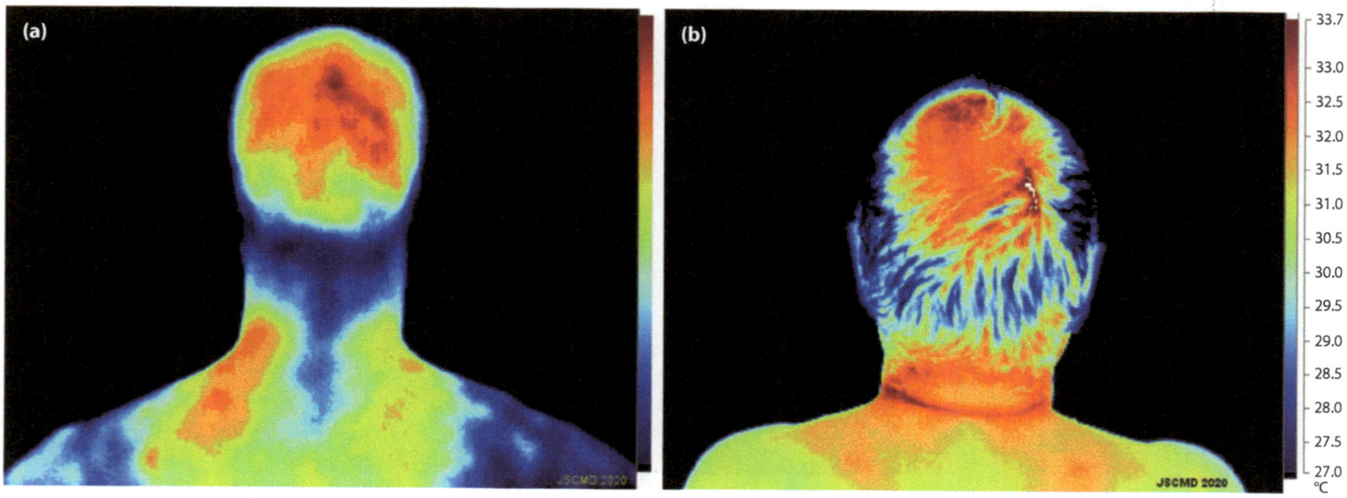

FIGURE 13.4 (a) Cranium and neck, posterior view, normal, head shaved – 28 yoM. (b) Cranium and neck, posterior view, normal – 70 yoM.

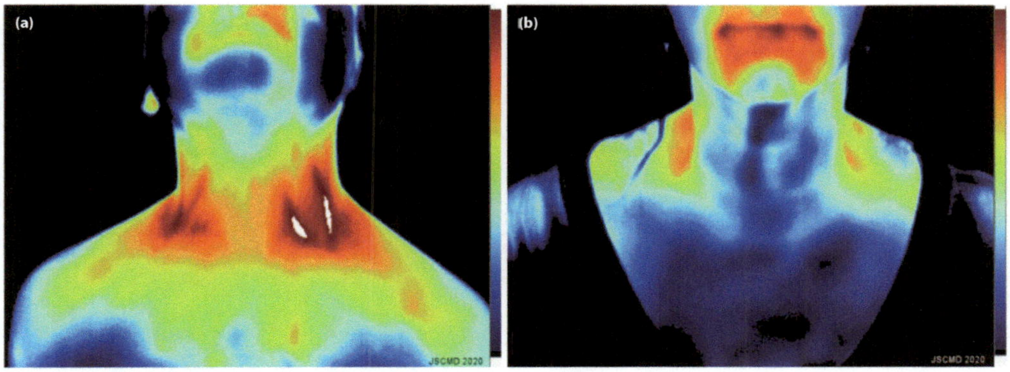

FIGURE 13.5 (a) Neck anterior view, normal – 8 yoM. Both the anterior and exterior jugular veins are seen, greater on the left. (b) Neck anterior view, normal – 33 yoF.

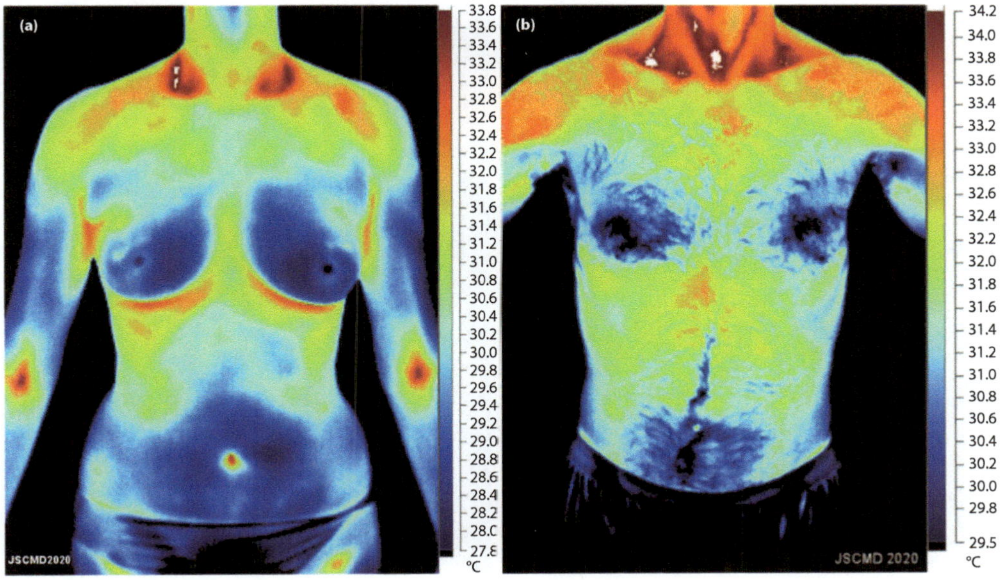

FIGURE 13.6 (a) Thorax frontal view, normal – 49 yoF. (b) Thorax frontal view, normal – 45 yoM.

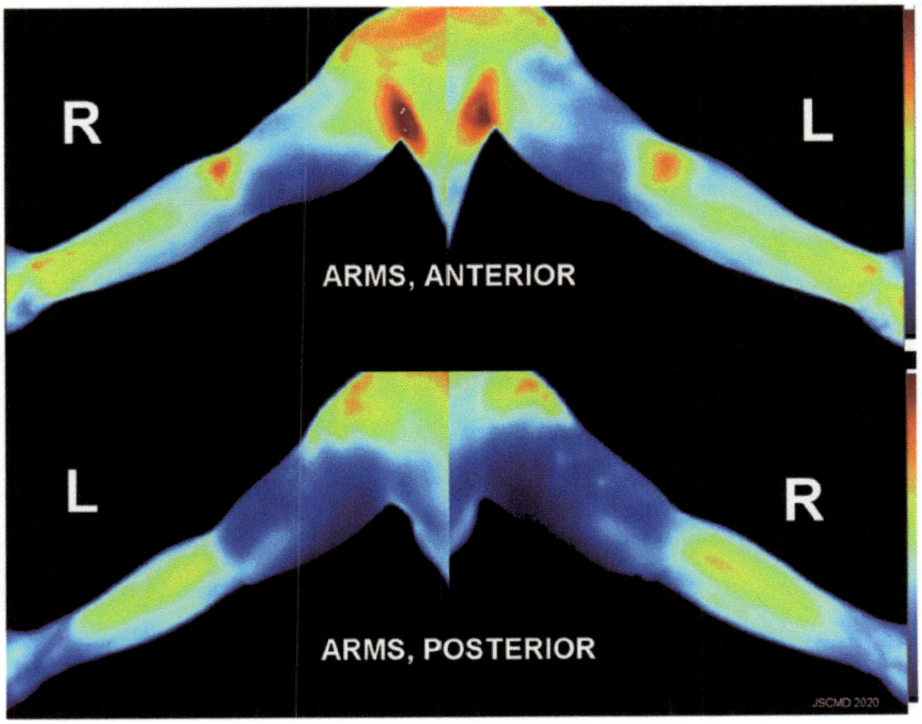

FIGURE 13.7 Arms normal, isothermal anterior and posterior bilateral views – 48 yoF.

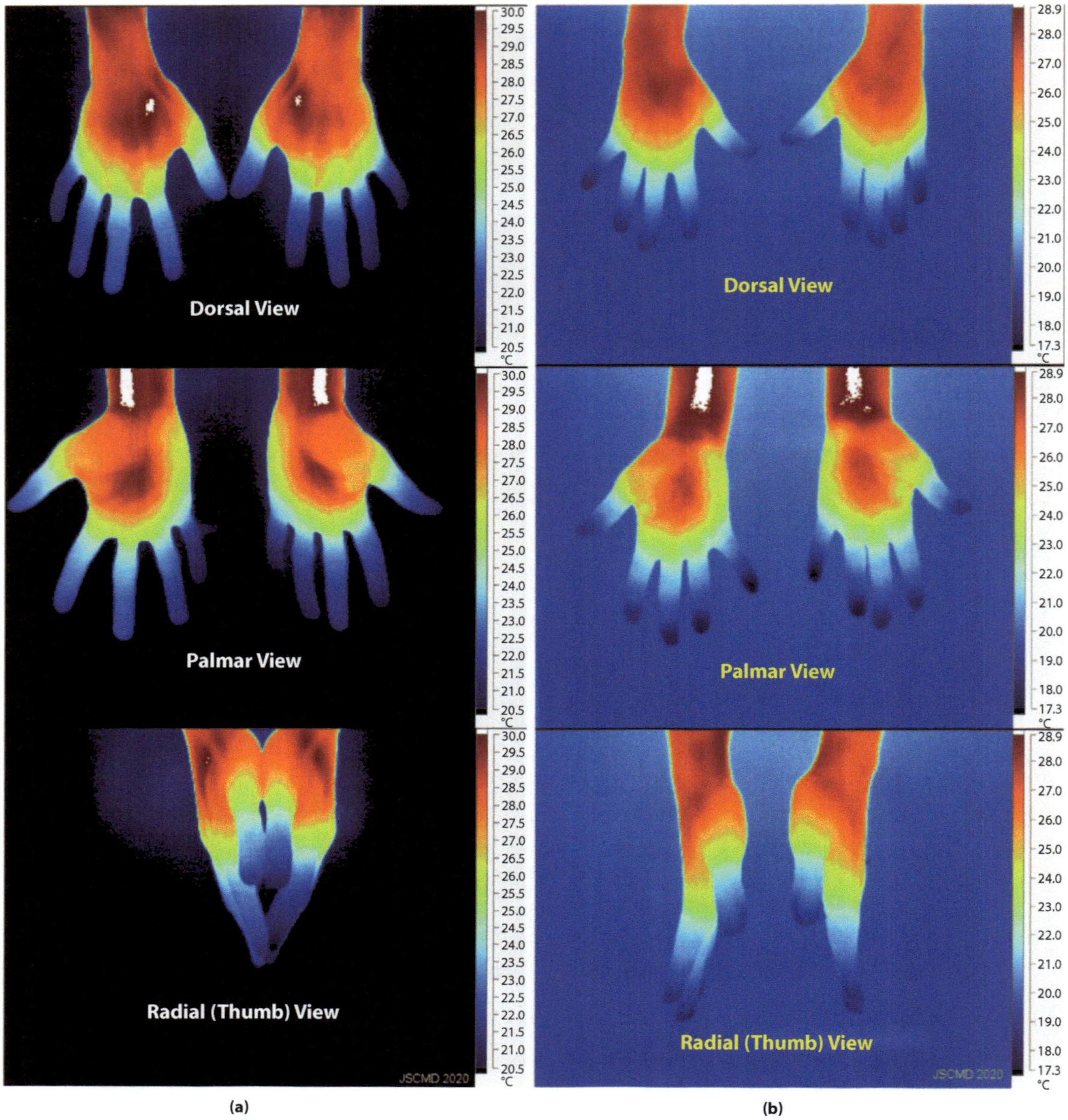

FIGURE 13.8 (a) Hands normal, isothermal views – 53 yoM. (b) Hands normal, isothermal views – 46 yoF.

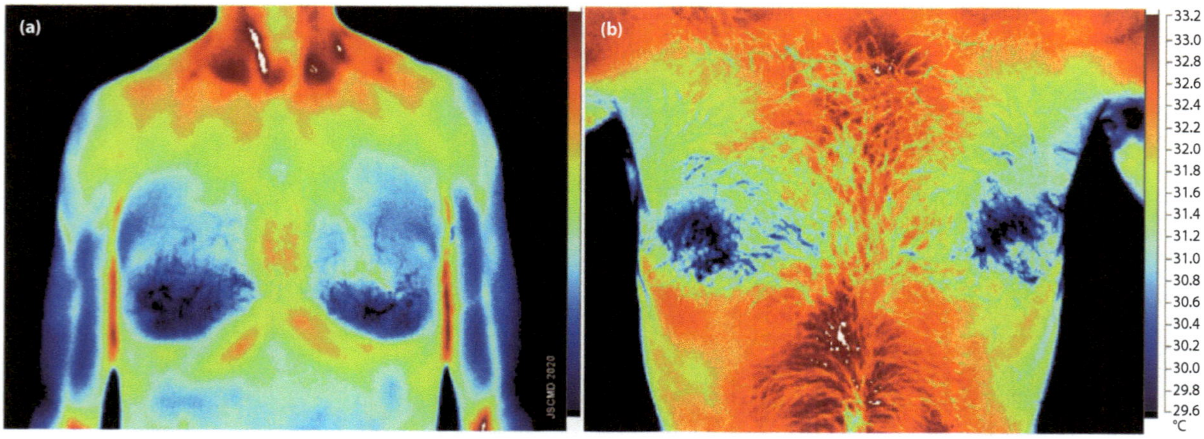

FIGURE 13.9 (a) Chest anterior view, normal. A single vascular trace appears over the left pectoral area. The right anterior jugular vein appears warm, as do the cephalic veins bilaterally – 54 yoM. (b) chest anterior view, normal – 45 yoM.

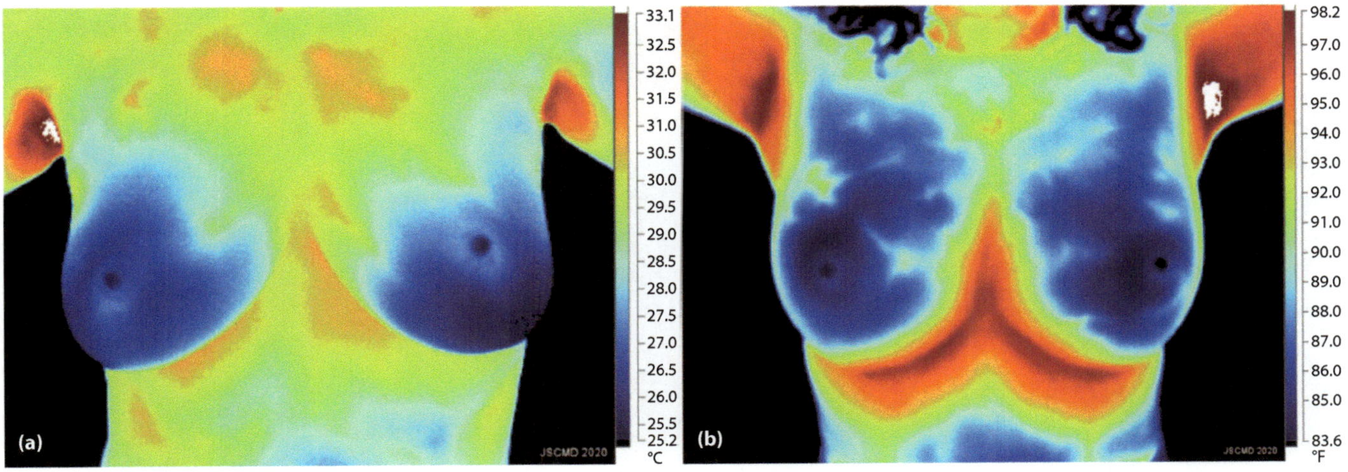

FIGURE 13.10 (a) Chest anterior view, normal, breasts TH-1 bilaterally – 65 yoF. (b) Chest anterior view, normal, breasts TH-2 bilaterally – 60 yoF.

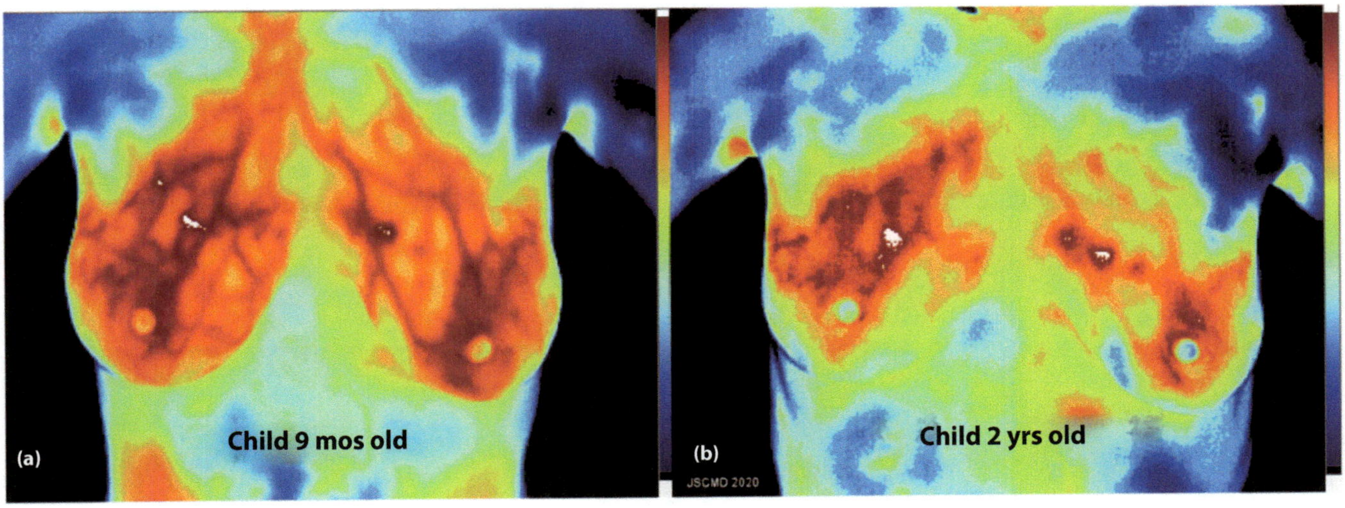

FIGURE 13.11 Chest anterior views of a breastfeeding woman showing active lactation appearance over time, normal. (a) Child 9 months old. (b) Child 24 months old – 32–33 yoF.

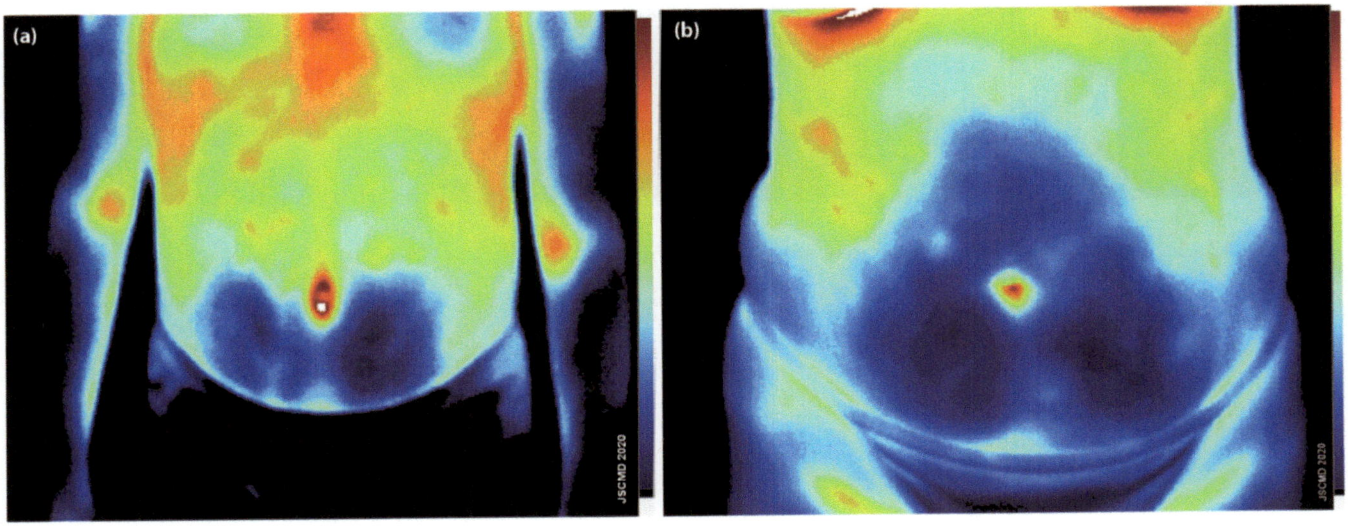

FIGURE 13.12 (a) Abdomen view, normal – 8 yoM. Note split umbilicus. (b) Abdomen view, normal – 48 yoF.

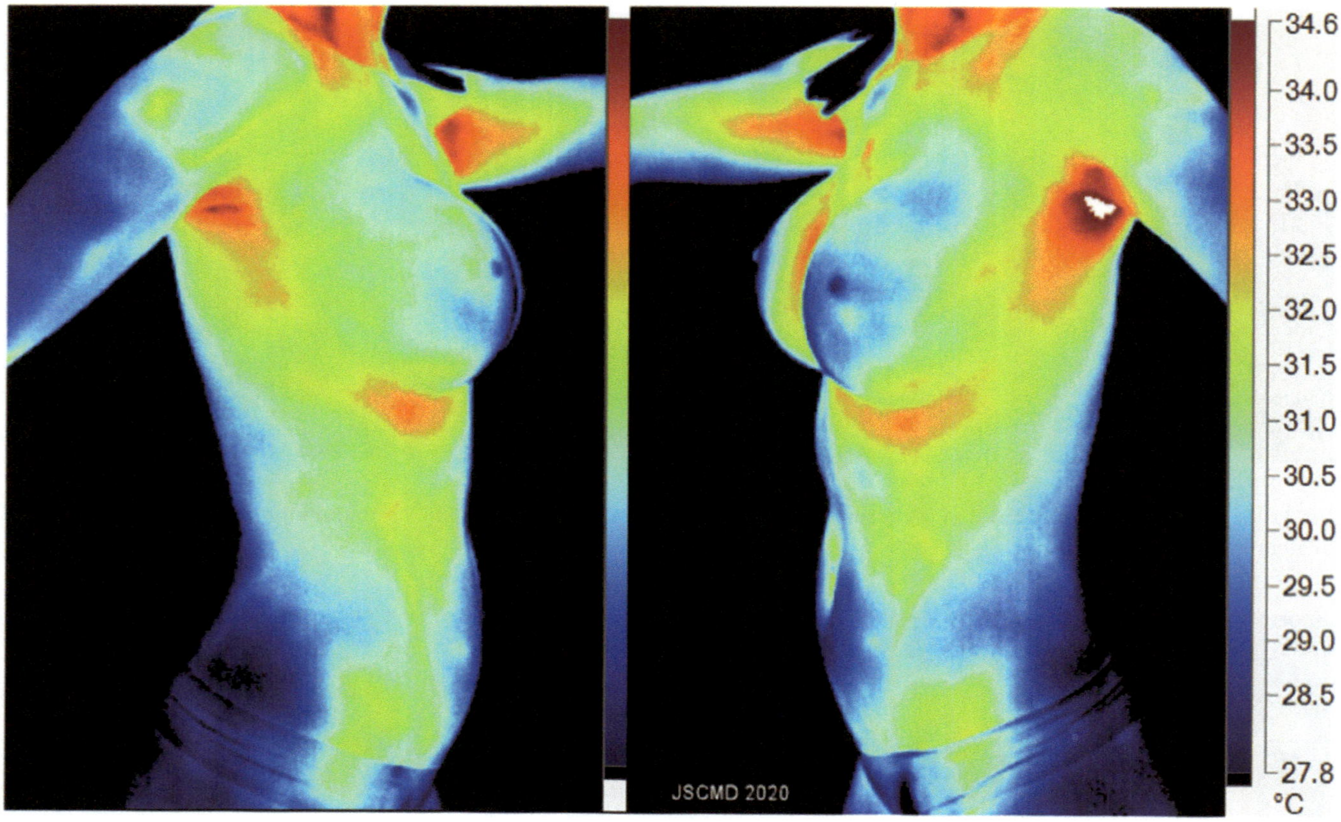

FIGURE 13.13 Thorax lateral views, isothermal, normal – 40 yoF.

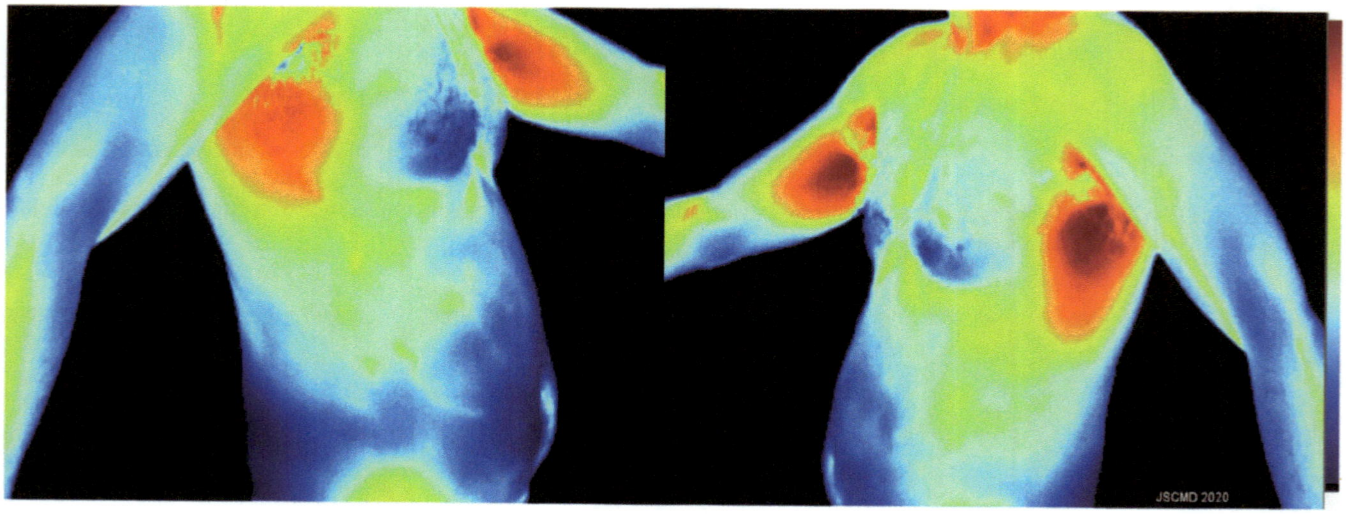

FIGURE 13.14 Thorax lateral views, isothermal, normal – 54 yoM.

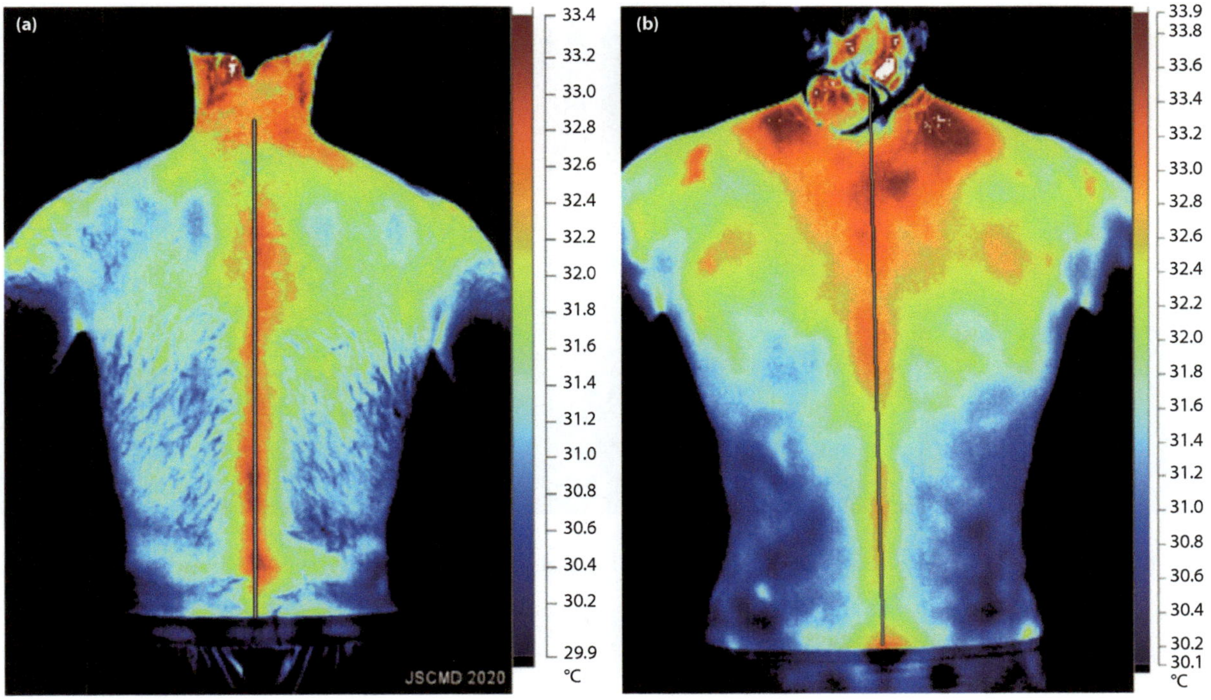

FIGURE 13.15 (a) Spinal view, normal. Slight right trapezius and lumbar warmth are present – 45 yoM. (b) Spinal view, normal. Warmth over the trapezii can be normal in upright subjects – 27 yoF. The added line is useful for detecting scoliosis.

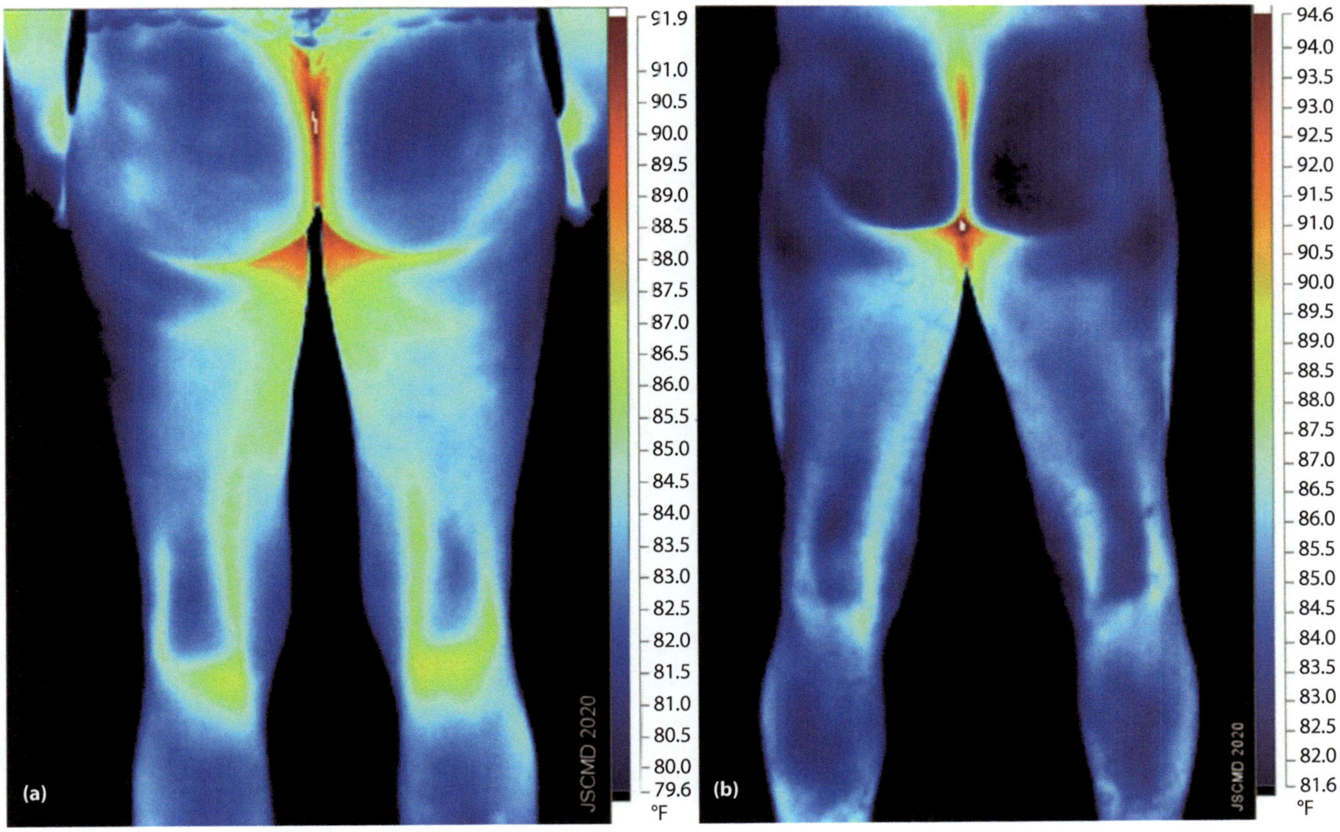

FIGURE 13.16 (a) Buttocks and posterior upper legs, normal – 39 yoF. (b) Buttocks and posterior upper legs, normal – 33 yoM.

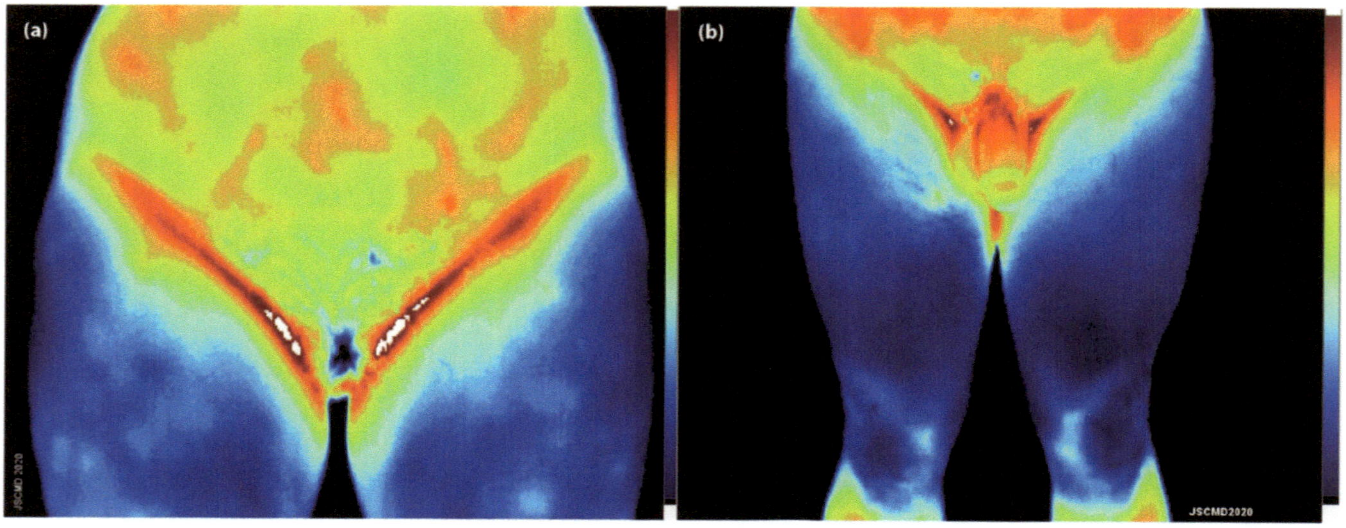

FIGURE 13.17 (a) Pelvis anterior view, normal – 64 yoF. (b) Pelvis anterior view, normal; penis circumcised; small pubic mole – 28 yoM.

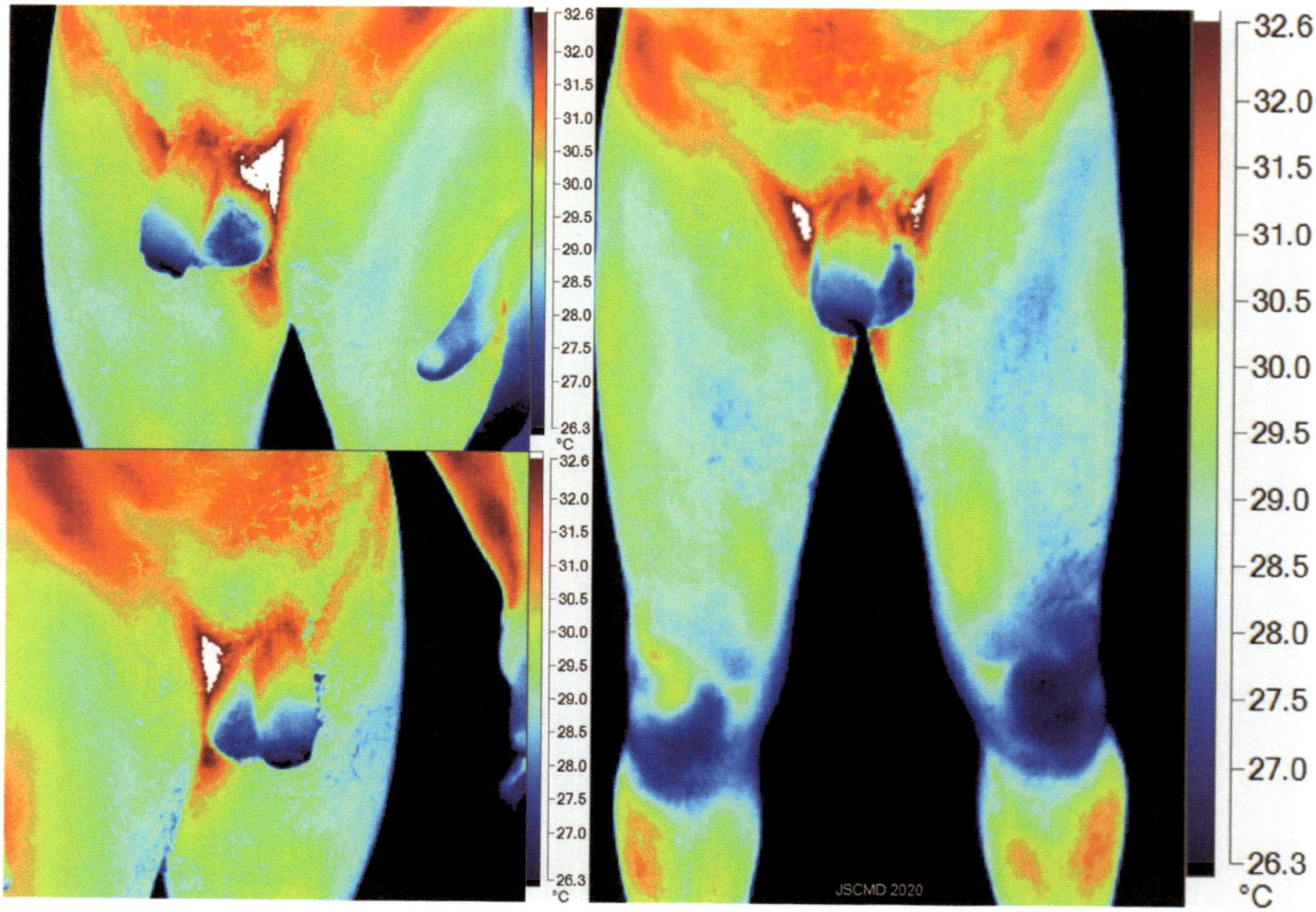

FIGURE 13.18 Pelvis and genitals, isothermal anterior and oblique views, normal. Penis uncircumcised, pubic hair shaved – 33 yoM. Note: The right knee shows slight inflammation superiorly.

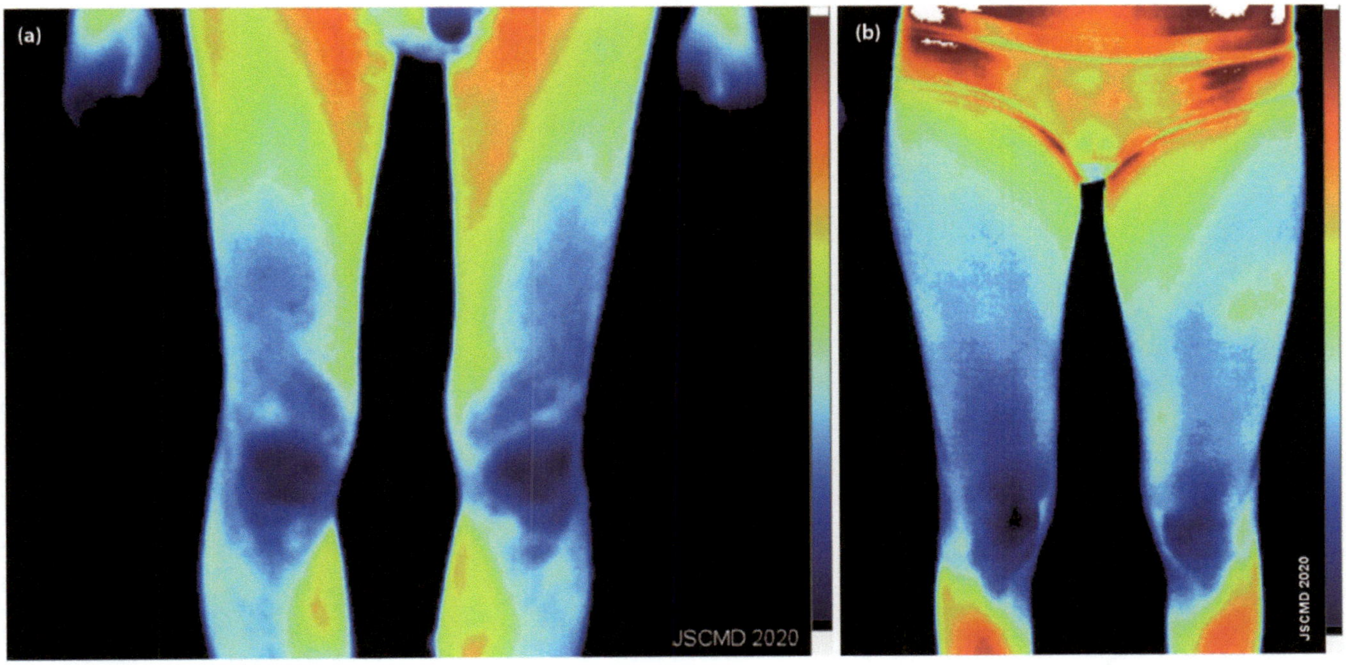

FIGURE 13.19 (a) Legs upper anterior view with knees, normal – 68 yoM. (b) Legs upper anterior view with knees, normal – 32 yoF.

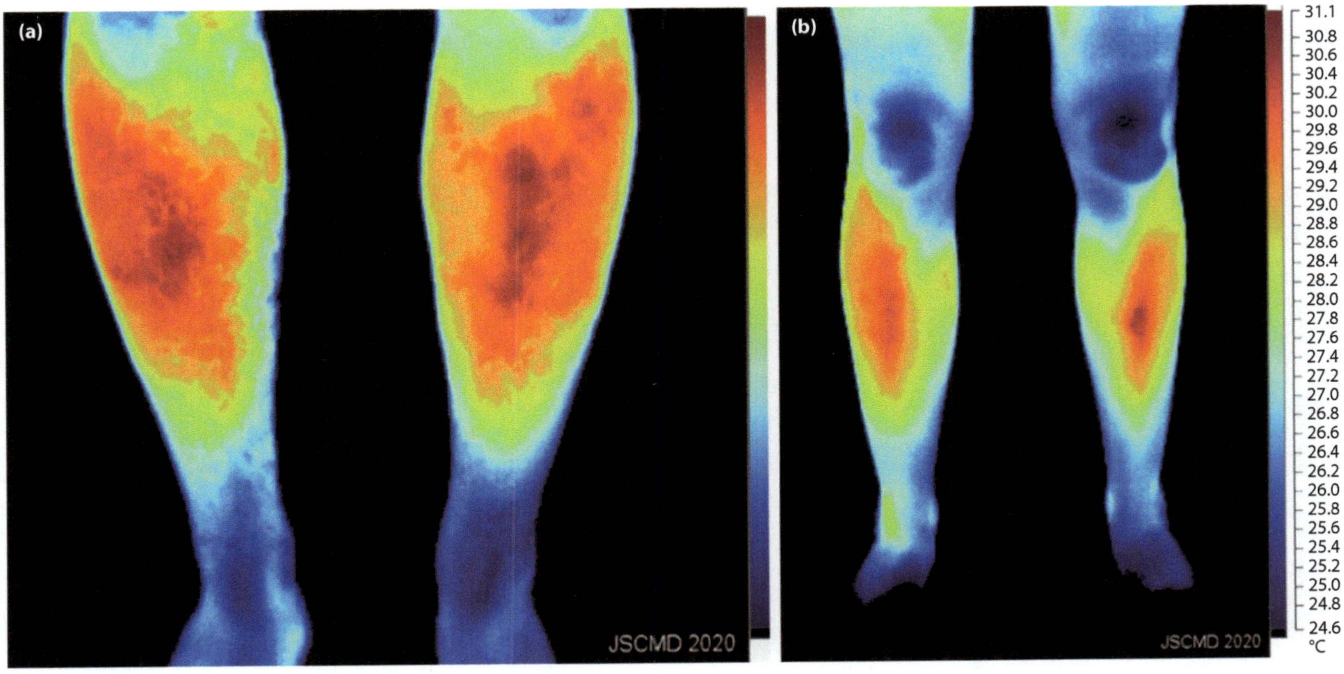

FIGURE 13.20 (a) Legs lower anterior view, normal – 47 yoM. (b) Knees and lower legs, anterior, normal – 45 yoF. The muscles maintaining balance are warm in these standing subjects.

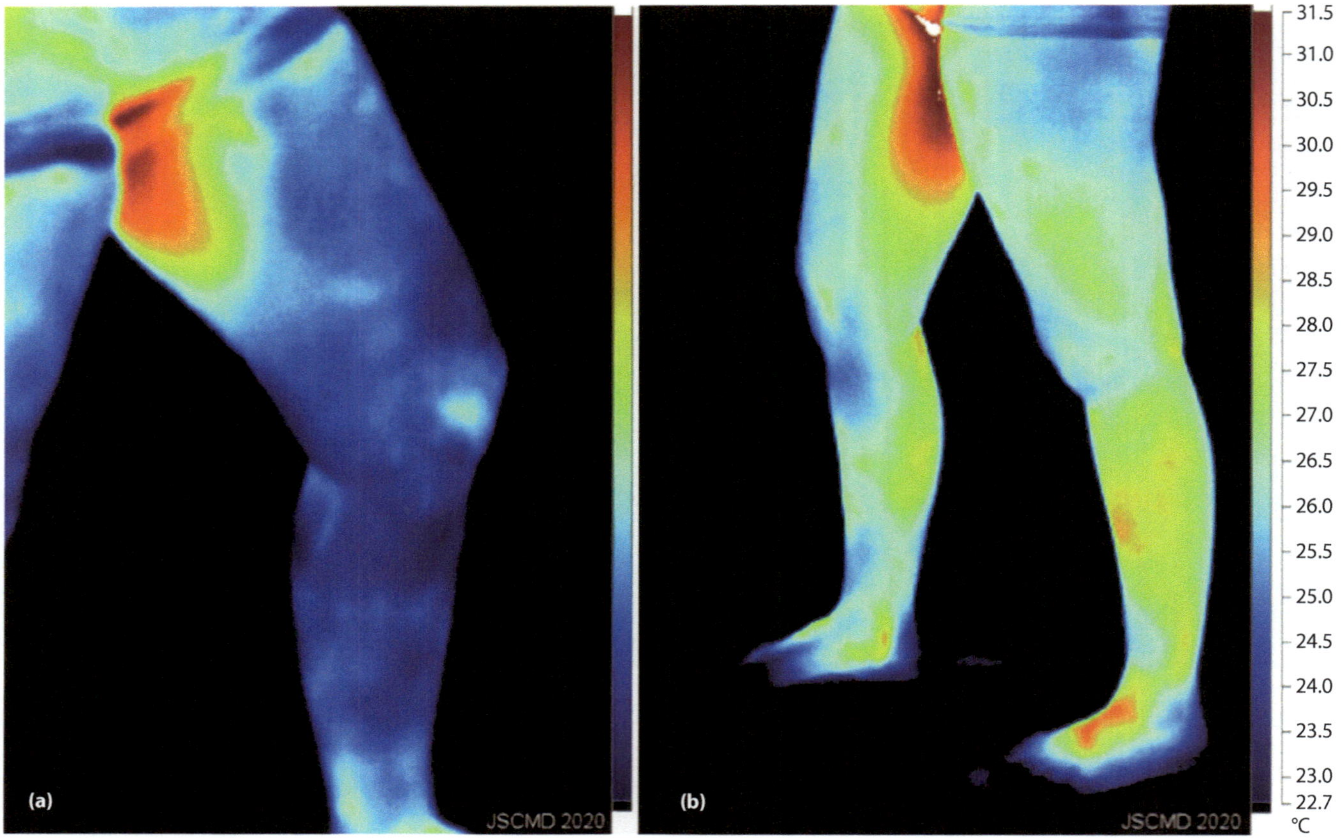

FIGURE 13.21 (a) Left leg, medial view, normal – 65 yoF. (b) Legs, left lateral view, normal –32 yoF.

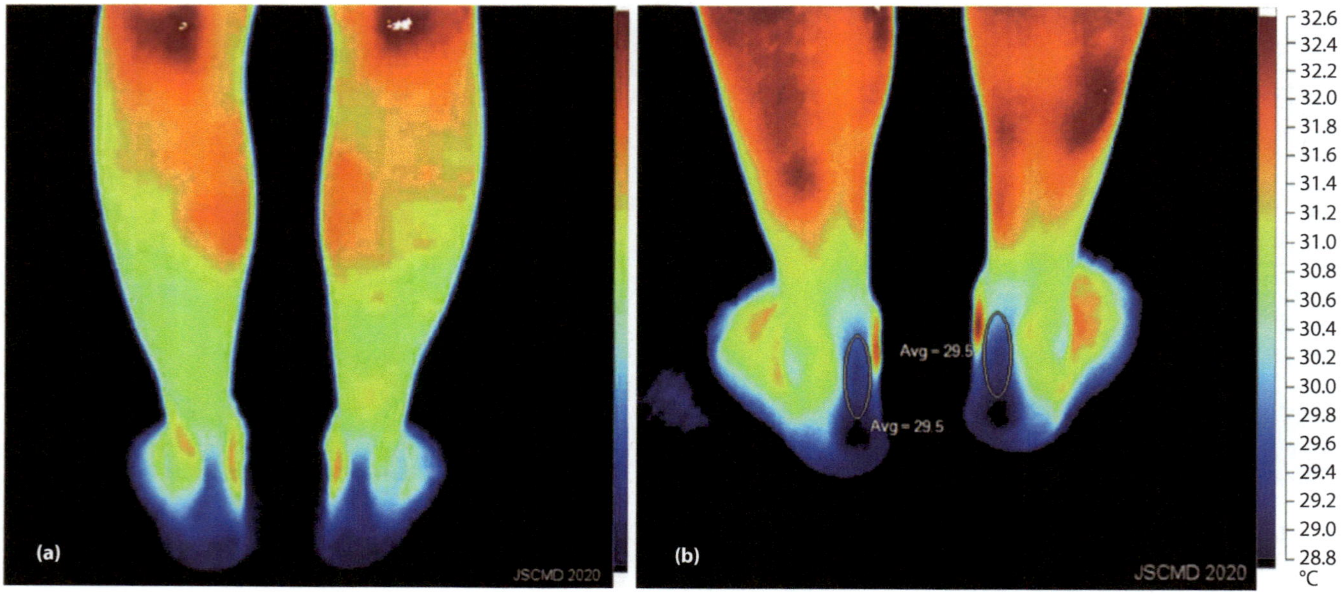

FIGURE 13.22 (a) Lower legs, posterior view, normal – 47 yoF. (b) Achilles tendon view, normal – 67 yoM.

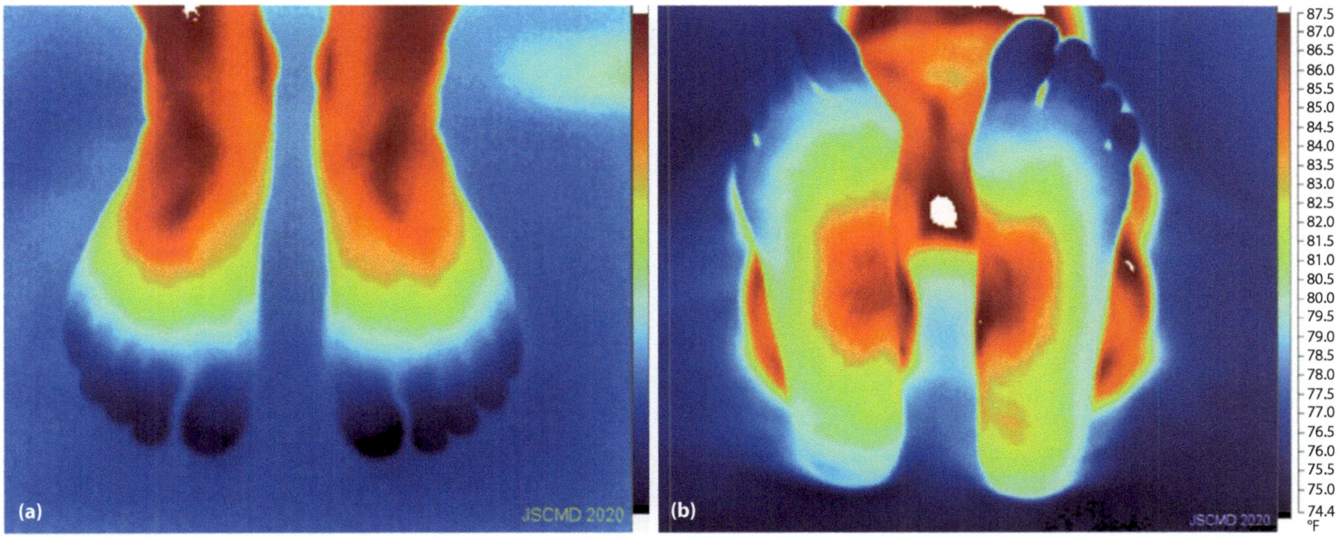

FIGURE 13.23 (a) Feet dorsal view, normal – 38 yoF. (b) Feet plantar view, normal. Moderate hallux valgus is present on the right – 70 yoF.

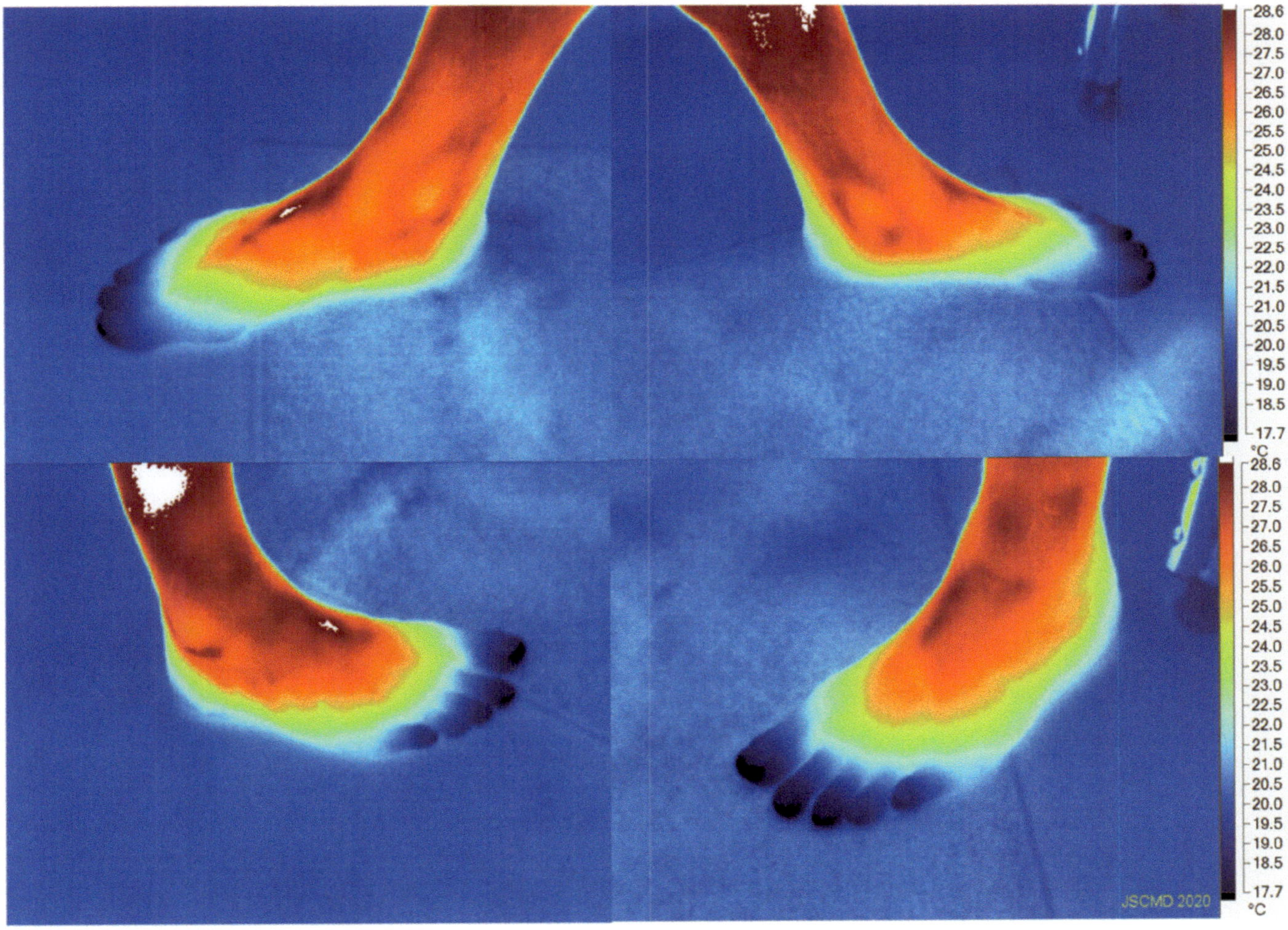

FIGURE 13.24 Feet – Lateral and medial views, isothermal, normal. The dorsalis pedis artery is seen over the metatarsal area bilaterally – 46 yoM.

APPENDIX I – LIST OF ABBREVIATIONS

ABI	ankle-brachial index
ACE (ACEI)	angiotensin-converting enzyme inhibitor
ACH	air-conditioner/heater
AD	Alzheimer's dementia
ADT	Active dynamic thermography
AGE	Advanced Glycation End Product
AI	Artificial Intelligence
AmNO	Amyl Nitrate
ARB	Angiotensin II Receptor Blocker
AS	Ankylosing Spondylitis
AVA	Arterio-Venous Anastomosis; Glomus Body
AVM	arterio-venous malformation
BAT	Brown Adipose Tissue
BCDDP	Breast Cancer Detection and Demonstration Project
BL	Baseline
BMI	Body Mass Index
BrCA	Breast Cancer
BRCA1	Gene affecting breast cancer occurrence
BRCA2	Gene affecting breast cancer occurrence
C-A	Computer-Aided
CABG	coronary artery bypass graft
CE	cauda equina
CHPP	cold-heat pathologic patterns
CNO	chronic nonbacterial osteomyelitis
CNS	central nervous system
CP	cerebral palsy
CPT	current procedural terminology
CPU	central processing unit
CRIB	chronic radial inflammation of the breast
CRPS	chronic regional pain syndrome
CS	compartment syndrome
CSF	cerebrospinal fluid
CSV	comma-separated value
CT	computerized tomography
CTS	Carpal tunnel syndrome
CV	cervicogenic vertigo
DCIS	ductal carcinoma in situ
DICOM	Digital Imaging and Communications in Medicine
ΔT	temperature difference
DIRT	dynamic infrared thermography
DPN	diabetic peripheral neuropathy
DSP	digital signal processor
DVT	deep venous thrombosis
ε	emissivity (infrared)
ED	emergency department
EDRF	endothelium-derived relaxing factor (nitric oxide)
eNOS	endothelial nitric oxide synthase
ETI	enhanced thermal imaging
FAX	facsimile
FDA	(US) Food and Drug Administration
fIRI	functional infrared imaging
FNA	fine needle aspiration
FPA	focal plane array
fps	frames per second
GCA	giant cell arteritis
GLD	Gynoid lipodystrophy
HER-2	Human epidermal growth factor receptor-2
HIPAA	Health Insurance Portability and Accountability Act (US)
HVAC	heating, ventilating, air conditioning
ICD	International Classification of Diseases
ID	identification
IIBC	invasive inflammatory breast cancer
ILSITS	Integrative Life Solutions Thermography Service
IMGR	imager
iNOS	Inducible nitric oxide synthase
IR	infrared
IUT	Instrument (or Imager) Under Test
Ki-67	a proliferative index of cancer activity
LED	light-emitting diode
LFCN	lateral femoral cutaneous nerve
LSCI	Laser Speckle Contrast Imaging
LSS	lumbar spinal stenosis
MCL	medial collateral ligament
MGD	meibomian gland dysfunction
mK	milliKelvin (degrees)
MRI	magnetic resonance imaging
ms	millisecond
MWL	modality worklist
NADPH	nicotinamide adenine dinucleotide phosphate
NCIT	non-contact infrared thermometry
NCT	non-contact thermometer
NETD	noise equivalent temperature difference
NIBP	non-invasive blood pressure
NIST	National Institute of Science and Technology, Gaithersburg, MD, USA
NO	nitric oxide
NOS	nitric oxide synthetase
NUC	nonuniformity correction
OA	osteoarthritis
PACS	picture archiving and communication system
PAD	peripheral artery disease
PD	Parkinson's disease
PDE5	phosphodiesterase type 5
PDF	Portable Document Format
PET	positron emission tomography
PGD	paradoxical glomus dilation
PMD	percent mammographic density
PORH	post-occlusion reactive hyperemia
ppm	parts per million
PsA	psoriatic arthritis
PsD	psoriatic dermatitis
QUAINT	quantification analysis of induced thermography
RA	rheumatoid arthritis
RH	relative humidity
ROI	region of interest
RP	Raynaud's phenomenon
SAA	spot-averaging analysis
SAP	sub-areolar lymphatic plexus

SC	spinal cord
SEM	scanning electron microscope
SLE	systemic lupus erythematosus
SSA	spot-slope analysis
SSI	surgical site infection
SVM	support vector machine
Tbody	body temperature
Tcor	temperature offset correction
Tcore	core temperature
TDD	temperature detection difference
TED	thyroid eye disease
TENS	transcutaneous electrical nerve stimulation
TFI	thigh-foot index
Timgr	temperature sensed by imager
TMJ	temporomandibular joint
TMJD	temporomandibular joint disorder
TOS	thoracic outlet syndrome
Troom	room temperature
Tstd	temperature standard
UV	ultraviolet
V-M	Ville-Marie (Infrared Grading Scale)
VNA	vendor neutral archives
Vox	vanadium oxide
VWF	vibration white finger
WATD	wound – abdominal temperature difference
yoF	year old Female
yoM	year old Male

APPENDIX II – INFRARED IMAGER SPECIFICATIONS FOR MEDICAL THERMOGRAPHY

A. **Imager Hardware**:
1. Imager system spectral bandwidth: 8–12 μm, Typical
2. Lens: Coated Germanium crystal; f/0.8, Typical
3. Detector Type: Uncooled Microbolometer
4. Detector resolution of 76,800 thermal pixels (320 × 240 array), Minimum.
5. [640 × 480 pixel detectors available, but must meet thermal noise specification (NETD)].
6. Noise Equivalent Temperature Difference (NETD) <0.050°C (50 mK), Maximum @ 30°C (86°F). (single, non-averaged image)
7. Field of View: 23° by 17°, Typical.
8. Spatial Resolution: 1.3 milliradian (mrad) Instantaneous Field of View (IFOV), Maximum
9. Focal Distance: 0.15 meters to infinity, Typical
10. Focus Mechanism: Manual method, Minimum. Autofocus preferred.
11. Thermal drift correction by an automatic or manually-initiated calibration routine; shutter-based calibration preferred.
12. Radiometric digital image output calibrated for the physiologic temperature range of 20–45°C:
    a. 1:1 Thermal Gain Error 5% over 20–45°C (68–113°F), Maximum
    b. Temperature Detection Difference (TDD) over 20–45°C of 0.56°C (1°F), Maximum.
    c. Absolute Temperature Accuracy within ±2°C (±3.6°F), Maximum.
    d. Radiometric Output Temperature Resolution: ±0.1°C (0.18°F), Maximum.
    e. Image Flatness: ±0.1°C radiometric 9-pixel average over entire image, Maximum (conditions: isothermal target at temperature of 20–45°C)
    f. Radiometric temperature correction set to Emissivity of 0.98 (human skin).
13. Non-Radiometric output for Qualitative Image analysis calibrated for the physiologic temperature range of 20–45°C:
    a. Output in standard imaging formats such as. jpg, png, or. bmp.
    b. Temperature Color Scale embedded in the infrared image recommended.
14. Video Outputs
    a. Radiometric video output file format preferred for thermal analysis.
    b. Video Frame Rate: 9 Hz, Minimum.
    c. Non-Radiometric files formats: MPEG or AVI, Typical
15. Visual images taken automatically with the thermal images. Recommended.
16. Digital Image Transfer to Interpreting Computer
    a. Standard Universal Serial Bus (USB) or Ethernet, Typical
    b. Secure Digital Memory Card (SD) transfer recommended for emergency backup if wired connection fails.
    c. Wireless (WiFi, Bluetooth) transfer may be used; wired USB or SD transfer capabilities advised should the wireless connection fail.

B. **Imager Software:**
1. Note: Interpretation software is generally supplied with the infrared imager. Software from one manufacturer may not open radiometric images taken with imagers from other manufacturers. DICOM software compatibility recommended.
2. The interpretation software must meet these minimum specifications as well as the requirements of the imaging clinic:
    a. Emissivity correction adjustable to or fixed at 0.98 (human skin).
    b. Included Palettes: Blue-Red ("Spectrum") and Graded Greyscale palettes, Minimum.
    c. Thermal Palette Resolution: 12 bits, Minimum; 14 to 16 bits Preferred. [8 to 10-Step (4-bit) Palettes no longer recommended for clinical thermography.]
    d. Temperature range adjustable to cover range of human emissions (20–45°C).
    e. Out-of-Range indicators: White for off-range High, Black for off-range Low recommended. Sharp Out-of-Range color transitions recommended.
    f. Infrared-to-Visual color scale controls to allow both Full-Scale and Fixed-Scale interpretation preferences.
    g. Software parallax correction for alignment of visual and infrared images.
    h. User-Selected Image Area, Line, and Point temperature measurement display capabilities, Minimum. Automatic temperature comparisons recommended.
    i. An embedded calibrated Temperature Color Scale accompanying each non-radiometric thermal image recommended.
    j. The date and time of image acquisition to accompany each image as metadata; this data should be visible with each image on any report or exported image.
    k. Report Generation: The software should export annotated non-radiometric images and temperature measurement data in a professional report format.
    l. Software to allow saving all original images, annotated images, and written reports in one folder unique to each patient. This facilitates comparison of images across several imaging sessions for improved interpretation over time.

INDEX

Page numbers in *italics* refer to figures and those in **bold** refer to tables.

D

E

F

G

M

N

O

P

Q